FLUID AND ELECTROLYTE BALANCE

NURSING CONSIDERATIONS

FLUID AND ELECTROLYTE BALANCE

Nursing Considerations

Second Edition

Norma Milligan Metheny, PhD, RN, FAAN

Professor of Medical–Surgical Nursing
Coordinator of Graduate Medical–Surgical Nursing Major
St. Louis University School of Nursing
St. Louis, Missouri

With 15 contributors

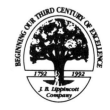

J. B. LIPPINCOTT COMPANY
Philadelphia
New York • London • Hagerstown

Sponsoring Editor: **David P. Carroll**
Editorial Assistant: **Amy Stonehouse**
Project Editor: **Anne-Adele Wight**
Indexer: **Victoria Boyle**
Art Director: **Susan Hermansen**
Designer: **Doug Smock**
Production Manager: **Helen Ewan**
Production Coordinator: **Nannette Winski**
Compositor: **G & S Typesetters, Inc.**
Printer/Binder: **Courier Book Company**

Second Edition

Portions of this book have been reproduced from Metheny N: Quick Reference to Fluid Balance, Philadelphia, JB Lippincott, 1984; and Metheny N, Snively WD: Nurses' Handbook of Fluid Balance, 4th ed, Philadelphia, JB Lippincott, 1983.

6 5 4

Library of Congress Cataloging-in-Publication Data

Fluid and electrolyte balance: nursing considerations / [edited by]
  Norma Milligan Metheney; with 15 contributors. — 2nd ed.
      p.   cm.
  Rev. ed. of: Fluid and electrolyte balance / Norma Milligan
Metheney. ©1987.
  Includes bibliographical references and index.
  ISBN 0-397-54891-5
    1. Body fluid disorders.   2. Body fluid disorders—Nursing.
  I. Metheny, Norma Milligan. Fluid and electrolyte balance.
    [DNLM: 1. Water–Electrolyte Balance—nurses' instruction.
  2. Water–Electrolyte Imbalance—nursing.   WD 220 F646]
RC630.F556   1992
616.3'9—dc20
DNLM/DLC
for Library of Congress   92-33727
                                            CIP

This book is dedicated to the memory of Roberta Scofield, RN, MSN, OCN, an exceptional teacher and clinician, a compassionate nurse, and a steadfast friend of the profession.

CONTRIBUTORS

Charold L. Baer, RN, PhD, FCCM, CCRN
Professor, Department of Adult Health and Illness,
Oregon Health Sciences University, Portland, Oregon
Chapter 18: Renal Failure

Linda K. Book, RN, BSN
Burn Nurse Specialist, Burn Center, St. John's Mercy
Medical Center, St. Louis, Missouri
Chapter 22: Major Thermal Injuries

Evelyn M. Burns, RN, MSN, CNM
Perinatal Clinical Specialist, St. Mary's Health Center,
St. Louis, Missouri
Chapter 23: Pregnancy

Susan Cole, RN, MSN, CCRN
St. Louis University Hospital, St. Louis, Missouri
Chapter 15: Cirrhosis with Ascites

Loretta Forlaw, RN, MSN
Army Nurse Corps, Olney, Maryland
Chapter 12: Total Parenteral Nutrition

Mary Ellen Grohar-Murray, RN, PhD
School of Nursing, St. Louis University, St. Louis,
Missouri
Chapter 20: Fluid Balance in the Head-Injured Patient

Marilyn Hackethal, RN, MSN
Professor of Nursing, Lewis and Clark Community
College, Alton, Illinois
Chapter 17: Acute Pancreatitis

Mary Kay Knight Macheca, RN, MSN(R), CDE
Diabetes Clinical Nurse Specialist, Barnes Hospital at
Washington University, St. Louis, Missouri
Chapter 21: Diabetic Ketoacidosis and Hyperosmolar Coma

Jeannie Mollohan, RN, MSN
Head Nurse, Pediatric Intensive Care Unit, Cardinal
Glennon Children's Hospital, St. Louis, Missouri
Chapter 25: Fluid Balance in Infants and Children

Irene I. Riddle, PhD, RN
Professor and Director, PhD Program in Nursing,
St. Louis University, St. Louis, Missouri
Chapter 25: Fluid Balance in Infants and Children

Sherry Robinson, RN, MSN
Assistant Professor of Nursing, Millikin University,
Decatur, Illinois
Chapter 26: Fluid Balance in the Elderly Patient

Darnell Roth, RN, CRNI, AA
CEO and President, D/R Intravenous Therapy
Consulting Inc, St. Louis, Missouri
Chapter 10: Intravenous Therapy

Marilyn Schallom, RN, MSN, CCRN
Surgical Nurse Specialist, Barnes Hospital at
Washington University, St. Louis, Missouri
Chapter 14: Fluid Balance in the Surgical Patient

Sandra Siehl, RN, MSN
Director of Oncology Services, Barnes Hospital at
Washington University Medical Center, St. Louis,
Missouri
Chapter 24: Oncologic Conditions

Martha Spies, RN, MSN
Deaconess College of Nursing, St. Louis, Missouri
Chapter 19: Heart Failure

PREFACE

Like its predecessor, the second edition of *Fluid and Electrolyte Balance: Nursing Considerations* is intended to provide the nurse with a current, integrated approach to the care of patients with fluid, electrolyte, and acid–base imbalances. This pragmatic book has relevance to both students and practitioners of nursing. Because the concept of fluid and electrolyte balance cuts across nursing boundaries, the scope of the book is wide. It is written simply for easy assimilation of information, yet it contains enough material to stimulate the interest of advanced practitioners. Available research findings related to conditions affecting fluid and electrolyte balance are integrated throughout the text. The first three units present, respectively, fundamental concepts and systematic assessment for fluid and electrolyte disturbances, an overview of major fluid and electrolyte disturbances, and principles of parenteral fluid therapy. The first two units are necessary for understanding the clinical chapters and offer numerous tables for quick reference. Case studies are included in the chapters dealing with specific imbalances to enhance understanding of these conditions. The unit on parenteral fluid therapy provides comprehensive information on the care of patients with peripheral and central intravenous devices. Types and applications of parenteral fluids, along with nursing considerations in their administration, are also described. The unit on clinical situations has sufficient chapters to allow for quick reference to specific information. A final unit offers a concise explanation of special fluid and electrolyte problems in the very young and the very old.

While the overall structure of the second edition remains the same as the first, numerous revisions have been made. For example, an enlarged discussion of the pathophysiology of common causes of third-space fluid shifts is included. Also helpful to the nurse is the expanded explanation of therapies to alleviate fluid volume excess (caused by, eg, sodium restriction, bedrest, and diuretics). The iatrogenic influence of drugs on electrolyte balance is explained in greater depth throughout the text. Because disruptions in antidiuretic hormone levels (eg, syndrome of antidiuretic hormone and diabetes insipidus) and heat disorders are closely related to sodium imbalance, these entities have been incorporated into the basic sodium chapter in Unit One. The chapter on parenteral fluids has been substantially enlarged to include discussion of nursing responsibilities in the administration of colloids and blood, as well as the pros and cons of crystalloids versus colloids. The issue of how much water to give tube-fed patients is addressed in greater depth in the tube-feeding chapter, as is assessment for fluid and electrolyte disturbances in the same population. Imbalances likely to occur in the perioperative period are covered in greater depth. Research-based guidelines are included in the chapter on cirrhosis for the rate and volume of ascitic fluid removal. The effect on fluid balance of laxatives, enemas, and various types of bowel preparations for diagnostic studies are covered more thoroughly in the gastrointestinal chapter. The renal chapter has been completely rewritten, with a greater emphasis on assessment. A number of skilled master clinicians have thoroughly revised the chapters related to their clinical specialties to reflect current practice regarding fluid balance. In all chapters, pathophysiology is discussed to promote understanding of rationales for nursing intervention. Extensive reference lists, including nursing and medical research studies when available, are provided to allow the reader to pursue particular areas of interest.

To facilitate integration of the information into nursing practice, the book has a strong nursing focus with frequent discussion of application of the nursing process. Of course, assessment is a primary concern in the care of patients with potential or actual fluid and electrolyte problems. In fact, much of what nurses do in caring for these patients revolves around monitoring for the occurrence or worsening of imbalances. The monitoring role entails the identification of patients at risk for specific imbalances, as well as frequent observations and analyses of the physiologic indices of fluid balance, so that derangements can be detected early and corrective measures instituted. Throughout the text, patients at risk for specific imbalances are identified, as are the common indicators of these problems. Examples of nursing diagnoses related to fluid and electrolyte problems are presented when appropriate. While some of these diagnoses are as yet untested, they are offered to assist the reader in integrating the vital area of fluid and electrolyte balance into nursing practice. In an attempt to contribute to the standardization of terminology for nursing diagnoses, labels recommended by the North American Nursing Diagnosis Association are used in the text whenever possible. Following identification of nursing diagnoses in the clinical chapters, nursing interventions are described. By their nature, these interventions often involve manipulation of fluid and nutrient intake. Therefore, the electrolyte content of common beverages and foods has been included. Nursing responsibilities related to the parenteral administration of fluids, electrolytes, and nutrients are also discussed. To facilitate quick access to vital information about these interventions, tables summarize important facts. When appropriate, health teaching and health promotion interventions are described because a major emphasis of nursing care of patients with potential fluid and electrolyte disturbances is prevention. When prevention is not possible, interventions are described to prevent worsening of the imbalances.

Historically, nurses have recognized responsibilities related to care of patients with fluid and electrolyte problems. For example, in the mid-1800s Florence Nightingale wisely wrote of the beneficial qualities of "beef tea."[1] In modern practice we are aware that one of the major features of bouillon is its high sodium content, which contributes to the buildup of extracellular fluid volume. Several decades ago Virginia Henderson identified the patient's need to "eat and drink adequately."[2] Currently, the nursing care of patients with fluid and electrolyte problems is complicated by the almost daily advances in health care technology. Clearly a comprehensive, yet pragmatic, nursing text on fluid and electrolyte balance is needed to facilitate the incorporation of this important area into nursing practice.

In short, this text was written with the intent of fostering critical thinking in those providing care for patients with potential or actual fluid and electrolyte disturbances. Designed for nurses in all areas of practice (such as hospitals, home-health agencies, nursing homes, and clinics), it provides the nurse with information necessary to deliver safe, effective, scientifically based nursing care.

Norma Milligan Metheny, PhD, RN, FAAN

REFERENCES

1. Nightingale F: Notes on Nursing. New York, Dover, 1969
2. Henderson V: The Nature of Nursing. New York, Macmillan, 1966

PREFACE TO
THE FIRST EDITION

This pragmatic book on fluid and electrolyte balance is intended for both students and practitioners of nursing. Since the concept of fluid and electrolyte balance cuts across nursing boundaries, the scope of the book is wide. It is simply written for easy assimilation of information, yet it contains enough material to stimulate the interest of advanced practitioners. The first three units present, respectively, fundamental concepts and systematic assessments for fluid and electrolyte disturbances, an overview of major fluid and electrolyte disturbances, and principles of parenteral fluid therapy. Requisite for an understanding of the clinical chapters, the first two offer numerous tables for quick reference. Case studies are included in the chapters dealing with specific imbalances to enhance understanding of these conditions. The unit on parenteral fluid therapy provides comprehensive information on the care of patients with peripheral and central intravenous devices. Types and applications of parenteral fluids, along with nursing considerations in their administration, are also described. The unit on clinical situations has sufficient chapters to allow for quick access to specific information.

To facilitate integration of the information into nursing practice, the book has a strong nursing focus with frequent discussion of application of the nursing process. Of course, assessment is a primary concern in the care of patients with potential or actual fluid and electrolyte problems. In fact, much of what nurses do in caring for these patients revolves around monitoring for the occurrence or worsening of imbalances. The monitoring role entails the identification of patients at risk for specific imbalances as well as frequent observations and analyses of the physiologic indices of fluid balance so that derangements can be detected early and

corrective measures instituted. Throughout the text, patients at risk for specific imbalances are identified, as are the common indicators of these problems. Examples of nursing diagnoses related to fluid and electrolyte problems are presented as appropriate. While some of these diagnoses are as yet untested, they are offered to assist the reader in integrating the vital area of fluid and electrolyte balance into nursing practice. In an attempt to contribute to the standardization of terminology for nursing diagnoses, labels recommended by the North American Nursing Diagnosis Association are used in the text whenever possible. Following the identification of nursing diagnoses in the clinical chapters, nursing interventions are described. By their nature, these interventions often involve manipulation of fluid and nutrient intake. Therefore, the electrolyte content of common beverages and foods has been included. Nursing responsibilities related to the parenteral administration of fluids, electrolytes, and nutrients are also discussed. In order to facilitate quick access to vital information about these interventions, tables summarize important facts. When appropriate, nursing interventions related to health teaching and health promotion are described since a major emphasis of nursing care of patients with potential fluid and electrolyte disturbances is prevention. When prevention is not possible, interventions are described to prevent worsening of the imbalances.

Historically, nurses have recognized responsibilities related to the care of patients with fluid and electrolyte problems. For example, in the mid-1800s Florence Nightingale wisely wrote of the beneficial qualities of "beef tea."[1] In modern practice we are aware that one of the major features of bouillon is its high sodium content, which contributes to the buildup of extracellular fluid volume. Several decades ago Virginia Henderson identified the patient's need to "eat and drink adequately."[2] Similarly, Faye Abdellah verified through research that "maintenance of fluid and electrolyte balance" is an important nursing problem in the care of all patients.[3] Currently the nursing care of patients with fluid and electrolyte problems is complicated by the almost daily advances in health care technology. Clearly a comprehensive, yet pragmatic nursing text on fluid and electrolyte balance is needed to facilitate the incorporation of this important area into nursing practice. Working toward this goal, a number of expert nurses with clinical expertise in various areas of practice have made significant contributions to the text. When appropriate, pathophysiology is discussed to promote understanding of rationales for nursing intervention. Reference lists, including nursing and medical research studies when available, are provided to allow the reader to pursue particular areas of interest.

In short, this text was written with the intent of fostering critical thinking in those providing care for patients with potential or actual fluid and electrolyte disturbances. Designed for nurses in all areas of practice (such as hospitals, home-health agencies, nursing homes, and clinics), it provides the nurse with information necessary to deliver safe, effective, scientifically based nursing care.

Norma Milligan Metheny, RN, PhD

REFERENCES

1. Nightingale F: *Notes on Nursing.* New York, Dover Publishers, 1969
2. Henderson V: *The Nature of Nursing.* New York, Macmillan, 1966
3. Abdellah F: Patient-Centered Approaches to Nursing. New York, Macmillan, 1960

CONTENTS

unit one

BASIC CONCEPTS

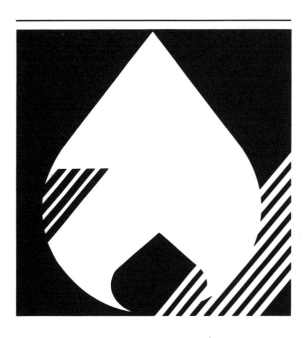

1

Fundamental Concepts and Definitions

BODY FLUIDS

In the typical adult, approximately 60% of weight consists of *fluid* (water and electrolytes). This fluid is either *intracellular* (within the cells) or *extracellular* (outside the cells). Extracellular fluid (ECF) is further subdivided into *intravascular fluid* (plasma) and *interstitial fluid* (fluid lying between the cells, or tissue fluid). See Figure 1-1. Also part of the ECF are transcellular fluids, primarily representing secretions from epithelial cells and having ionic compositions different from the plasma and interstitial fluids. Examples of transcellular fluid include cerebrospinal, pleural, peritoneal, and synovial fluids.[1] Approximately two thirds of the body fluid in adults exists in the intracellular

space (primarily in the skeletal muscle mass). The remaining one third is primarily found between the cells and in the plasma space. Microscopically, one might visualize the body fluids as in Figure 1-2.

Total body water content varies with body fat content, sex, and age. Fat cells contain little water, while lean tissue is rich in water. Thus, women have less body fluid than men because they have proportionately more body fat. The elderly have less body fluid than their younger counterparts for the same reason. Obese individuals in general have considerably less fluid than those of lean build (see Fig. 1-3).

Infants have a high body fluid content (approximately 70% to 80% of their body weight). In addition to having proportionately more body fluid than the

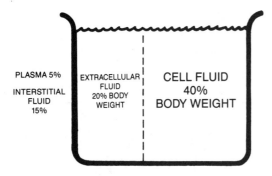

FIGURE 1–1.
Total body fluid, 60% body weight.

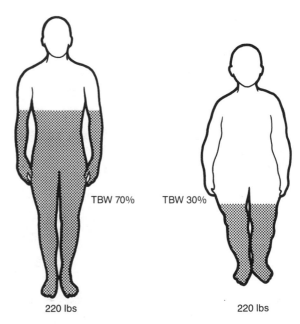

FIGURE 1–3.
Body composition of a lean and an obese individual. Although these individuals weigh the same, the body fluid content (total body water or TBW) of the lean individual is more than twice that of the obese one. Therefore, it follows that, if an adequate fluid and electrolyte ration is given to the lean individual, this same ration given to the obese person may actually represent double the amount required. (Adapted from Statland H: Fluid & Electrolytes in Practice, 3rd ed. Philadelphia, JB Lippincott, 1963)

adult, the infant has relatively more ECF. Indeed, more than half of the newborn's body fluid is extracellular, while in the adult only a third or less is extracellular. Because ECF is more readily lost from the body than is cellular fluid, the infant is more vulnerable to fluid volume deficit. As the infant becomes older, his or her total body fluid percentage decreases; the change is most rapid during the first 6 months. By the end of the second year, the total body fluid approaches the adult percentage of approximately 60% (36% cellular and 24% extracellular). At puberty, the adult body composition is attained (40% cellular and 20% extracellular). For the first time there is a sex differentiation in fluid content.

After 40 years of age, mean values for total body fluid in percentage of body weight decrease for both men and women; however, the sex differentiation remains. After 60 years of age the percentage may decrease to approximately 52% in men and 46% in women (even less in obese persons). Again, the reduction in body fluid is explained by the fact that with aging there is a decrease in lean body mass in favor of fat. Variations in total body fluid with age are listed in Table 1-1.

ELECTROLYTES

Body fluid is composed primarily of water and electrolytes. An *electrolyte* is defined as a substance that develops an electrical charge when dissolved in water. Examples of electrolytes are sodium, potassium, cal-

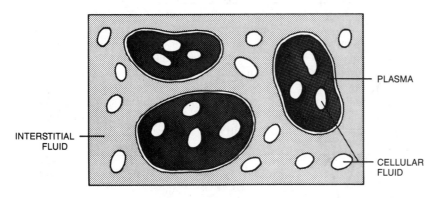

FIGURE 1–2.
Microscopic visualization of body fluid distribution.

TABLE 1–1.
Approximate Values of Total Body Fluid as a Percentage of Body Weight in Relation to Age and Sex

AGE	TOTAL BODY FLUID (% BODY WEIGHT)
Full-term newborn	70%–80%
1 year	64%
Puberty to 39 years	Men: 60% Women: 52%
40 to 60 years	Men: 55% Women: 47%
More than 60 years	Men: 52% Women: 46%

cium, chloride, and bicarbonate. Those that develop a positive charge in water are called *cations;* examples are sodium (Na^+), potassium (K^+), calcium (Ca^{2+}), and magnesium (Mg^{2+}). Electrolytes that develop negative charges when dissolved in water are called *anions;* examples are chloride (Cl^-) and bicarbonate (HCO_3^-).

The electrolyte content of intracellular fluid (ICF) differs significantly from that of ECF. Table 1-2 lists the electrolytes in plasma (ECF) and Table 1-3 lists those in ICF. Because special techniques are required to measure the concentration of electrolytes in the ICF, it is

TABLE 1–2.
Plasma Electrolytes

ELECTROLYTES	mEq/L
Cations:	
Sodium (Na^+)	142
Potassium (K^+)	5
Calcium (Ca^{2+})	5
Magnesium (Mg^{2+})	2
Total cations	154
Anions:	
Chloride (Cl^-)	103
Bicarbonate (HCO_3^-)	26
Phosphate (HPO_4^{2-})	2
Sulfate (SO_4^{2-})	1
Organic acids	5
Proteinate	17
Total anions	154

TABLE 1–3.
Approximation of Major Electrolyte Content in Intracellular Fluid

ELECTROLYTES	mEq/L
Cations:	
Potassium (K^+)	150
Magnesium (Mg^{2+})	40
Sodium (Na^+)	10
Total cations	200
Anions:	
Phosphates Sulfates	150
Bicarbonate (HCO_3^-)	10
Proteinate	40
Total anions	200

customary to measure the electrolytes in the ECF, namely plasma. Plasma electrolyte concentrations are used in assessing and managing patients with electrolyte imbalances. Some tests are performed on *serum* (the portion of plasma left after clotting); for practical purposes, the terms *serum electrolytes* and *plasma electrolytes* are used interchangeably.

The major electrolytes in the ECF are sodium (Na^+) and chloride (Cl^-) with a great preponderance of sodium ions (142 mEq/L) compared with other cations. About 90% of the ECF osmolality (concentration) is determined by the sodium concentration. Sodium is of primary importance in regulating body fluid volume; it has long been recognized that retention of sodium is associated with fluid retention. Whenever excessive quantities of sodium are lost, body fluid volume tends to decrease.

The electrolyte content of interstitial fluid is not measured in clinical situations; however, it is essentially the same as that of plasma except that it contains less proteinate. (Recall that plasma protein is necessary to maintain oncotic pressure and keep the intravascular fluid inside the blood vessels.)

The major electrolytes in the ICF are potassium and phosphate. Because the ECF can tolerate only small potassium concentrations (approximately 5 mEq/L), release of large stores of intracellular potassium by cellular trauma can be extremely dangerous.

The body expends a great deal of energy maintaining the extracellular preponderance of sodium and the intracellular preponderance of potassium. It does so by means of cell membrane pumps, which exchange sodium and potassium ions.

UNITS OF MEASURE

Concentrations of solutes can be expressed in several ways: for example, milligrams per deciliter (mg/dL), milliequivalents per liter (mEq/L), or millimoles per liter (mmol/L). Because all of these units may be used in clinical settings, a brief review of their meanings is appropriate. *Milligrams per 100 mL (deciliter)* expresses the weight of the solute per unit volume. In contrast, a milliequivalent is a measure of chemical activity. By definition, a *milliequivalent of an ion* is its atomic weight expressed in milligrams divided by the valence. This measure is most favored in the United States for expressing the small concentrations of electrolytes in body fluids because it emphasizes the principle that ions combine milliequivalent for milliequivalent, not millimole for millimole or milligram for milligram.[2] Also, the important concept of *electroneutrality* is clarified when using milliequivalents, because milliequivalents of cations and anions exist in equal numbers in the body fluids (see Fig. 1-4). This obligatory relationship is not evident if the ionic concentrations are measured in millimoles per liter or in milligrams per deciliter. In other words, because electrolytes in body fluids are active chemicals (anions and cations) that unite in varying combinations, many consider it more logical to express their concentration as a measure of chemical activity, rather than as a measure of weight. An analogy offered by Statland[3] states the point clearly. When a hostess creates a guest list for a dance, she does not invite 1000 pounds of boys per 1000 pounds of girls; she invites the same number of boys and girls.

Countries using the Système Internationale (S.I.) units express electrolyte content in body fluids in millimoles. To understand millimoles, it is necessary to review the definition of a mole. One *mole* (mol) of a substance is defined as the molecular (or atomic) weight of that substance in grams. For example, a mole of

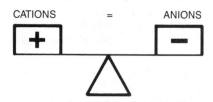

FIGURE 1–4.
The number of cations always equals the number of anions.

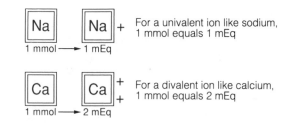

FIGURE 1–5.
Millimoles versus milliequivalents for univalent and divalent ions.

sodium is equivalent to 23 g (the atomic weight of sodium is 23). A *millimole* is one thousandth of a mole, or the molecular or atomic weight expressed in milligrams. Thus, a millimole of sodium is equivalent to 23 mg. Univalent elements, such as sodium (Na^+), chloride (Cl^-), and potassium (K^+), have identical numbers for milliequivalents and millimoles; that is, 140 mEq of Na^+ = 140 mmol of Na^+ and 5 mEq of K^+ = 5 mmol of K^+. However, different numbers are required for electrolytes that are not univalent. To convert from units of millimoles per liter to milliequivalents per liter, use the following formula: mEq/L = mmol/L × valence. For example, because the valence of calcium is 2, 1 mmol of calcium = 2 mEq of calcium[4] (see Fig. 1-5). Although the milliequivalent is not an S.I. unit, it is so widely employed and conceptually useful that it is likely to be used for some time.

FUNCTIONS OF BODY FLUIDS

Body fluids are in constant motion, maintaining healthy living conditions for body cells. The ECF interfaces with the outside world and is modified by it, but the ICF remains stable. Nutrients are transported by the ECF to the cells, and wastes are carried away from them by means of the capillary bed.

The capillary bed in the adult provides approximately 6300 square meters of filtering surface.[5] Normal movement of fluids through the capillary wall into the tissues depends on the force of the hydrostatic pressure at both the arterial and the venous ends of the vessel. Conversely, the osmotic pressure exerted by the protein of the plasma draws fluid back into the capillary. Direction of fluid movement depends on the differences in these two opposing forces. Because the hydrostatic pressure is greater than the colloid osmotic pressure at the arterial end of the capillary, the fluids move out of the vessel. However, the osmotic force is greater than the hydrostatic pressure at the venous end of the capillary, so fluid reenters the capillary here (see Fig. 1-6).[6]

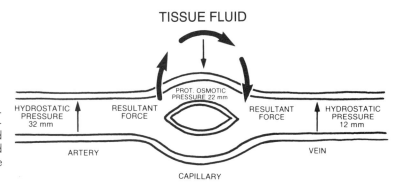

FIGURE 1–6.
Fluid movement at capillary bed. Plasma protein osmotic pressure is approximately 22 mmHg, whereas blood pressure is 32 mmHg at the arterial end of the capillary and 12 mmHg at the venous end.

REGULATION OF BODY FLUID COMPARTMENTS

OSMOSIS

When two different solutions are separated by a membrane impermeable to the dissolved substances, a shift of water occurs through the membrane from the region of low solute concentration to the region of high solute concentration until the solutions are of equal concentration (see Fig. 1-7). The magnitude of this force depends on the number of particles dissolved in the solutions and not on their weights.

The number of dissolved particles in a unit of water determines the solution's concentration, and can be expressed as either osmolality or osmolarity. *Osmolality* refers to the number of osmoles per kilogram of water; thus, the total volume will be 1 L of water plus the relatively small volume occupied by the solute.[6] On the other hand, *osmolarity* refers to the number of osmoles per liter of solution. In this instance, the volume of water is less than 1 L by an amount equal to the solute volume. Because of the very low solute concentration in body fluids, the difference between osmolality and

osmolarity is negligible. Nonetheless, osmolality is the correct term to use when referring to body fluids because osmotic activity in the body depends on the concentration of active particles per kilogram of water.[7] The term *tonicity* is sometimes used instead of osmolality.

DIFFUSION

Diffusion is defined as the natural tendency of a substance to move from an area of higher concentration to one of lower concentration. It occurs through the random movement of ions and molecules. Exchange of oxygen and carbon dioxide between the alveoli and capillaries occurs by diffusion.

FILTRATION

Filtration is the transfer of water and dissolved substances from a region of high pressure to a region of low pressure; the force behind it is hydrostatic pressure. An example of filtration is the passage of water and electrolytes from the arterial capillary bed to the interstitial fluid; in this instance, the hydrostatic pressure is furnished by the pumping action of the heart.

SODIUM–POTASSIUM PUMP

Sodium concentration is greater in ECF than in ICF; therefore, there is a tendency for sodium to enter by diffusion. This tendency is offset by the *sodium–potassium pump*, which is located in the cell membrane and, in the presence of adenosine triphosphate (ATP), actively moves sodium from the cell into the ECF. Conversely, the high intracellular potassium concentration is maintained by pumping potassium into the cell. Active transport occurs to move other ions (such as calcium and hydrogen) from areas of lesser concentration to areas of greater concentration. By definition, active transport implies that energy expenditure must take place for the movement to occur against a concentration gradient.

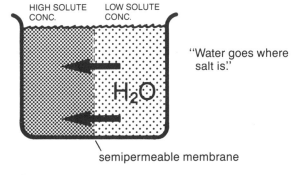

FIGURE 1–7.
Osmosis.

ROUTES OF GAINS AND LOSSES

Water and electrolytes are gained in various ways. In health, one gains fluids by drinking and eating (much of solid food is actually fluid). In illness, fluids may be gained by the parenteral route (intravenously or subcutaneously) or by means of an enteral feeding tube in the stomach or intestine. For critically ill patients, even small gains of fluid (such as that provided by humidifiers) must be considered. When fluid balance is critical, *all routes of gain* and *all routes of loss* must be recorded and the volumes compared. Organs of fluid loss include the kidneys, skin, lungs, and the gastrointestinal tract.

KIDNEYS

The usual urine volume in the adult is between 1 and 2 L a day. A general rule of thumb is approximately 1 mL of urine per kilogram of body weight per hour (1 mL/kg/hr), with boundaries of 0.5 mL to 2 mL per kilogram of body weight per hour.[8]

SKIN

Visible water and electrolyte loss through the skin occurs by sweating (*sensible perspiration*). Sweat is a hypotonic fluid containing several solutes; the chief ones are sodium chloride and potassium. Actual sweat losses vary according to environmental temperature (from 0 mL to 1000 mL or more an hour). Significant sweat losses occur if the patient's body temperature exceeds 101° F (38.3° C) or if room temperature exceeds 90° F (32.2° C).

Continuous water loss by evaporation (approximately 600 mL/day) occurs through the skin as *insensible perspiration,* a nonvisible form of water loss. The presence of fever greatly increases insensible water loss through the lungs and the skin. Loss of the natural skin barrier in major burns also increases water loss by this route.

LUNGS

The lungs normally eliminate water vapor (insensible loss) at a rate of approximately 300 to 400 mL a day. The loss is much greater with increased respiratory rate, depth, or both.

GASTROINTESTINAL TRACT

The usual loss through the gastrointestinal (GI) tract is only about 100 to 200 mL a day, although approximately 8 L of fluid circulate through the GI system every 24 hours (the "GI circulation"). The bulk of fluid is reabsorbed in the small intestine; obviously, large losses can be incurred from the GI tract if abnormal conditions such as diarrhea or fistulas occur.

Of note, Table 2-1 shows that in health the 24-hour average intake and output of water in the healthy adult are approximately equal.

HOMEOSTATIC MECHANISMS

The body is equipped with homeostatic mechanisms to keep the composition and volume of body fluid within narrow limits of normal. Organs involved in this mechanism include the kidneys, lungs, heart, blood vessels, adrenal glands, parathyroid glands, and pituitary gland (see Fig. 1-8).

KIDNEYS

The kidneys are vital to the regulation of fluid and electrolyte balance. They normally filter 170 L of plasma a day in the adult, while excreting only 1.5 L of urine. They act both autonomously and in response to blood-borne messengers, such as aldosterone and antidiuretic hormone (ADH).

Major functions of the kidneys in fluid balance homeostasis include

- Regulation of ECF volume and osmolality by selective retention and excretion of water and electrolytes
- Regulation of electrolyte levels in the ECF by selective retention and excretion
- Regulation of pH of ECF by excretion or retention of hydrogen ions
- Excretion of metabolic wastes (primarily acids) and toxic substances

Renal failure results in multiple fluid and electrolyte problems (see Chapter 18).

HEART AND BLOOD VESSELS

Plasma must reach the kidneys in sufficient volume to permit regulation of water and electrolytes. The pumping action of the heart provides circulation of blood through the kidneys under sufficient pressure for urine to form; renal perfusion makes renal function possible. Stretch receptors in the atria and blood vessels react to hypovolemia by stimulating fluid retention.

LUNGS

The lungs are also vital in maintaining homeostasis. Alveolar ventilation is responsible for the daily elimination of approximately 13,000 mEq of hydrogen ions

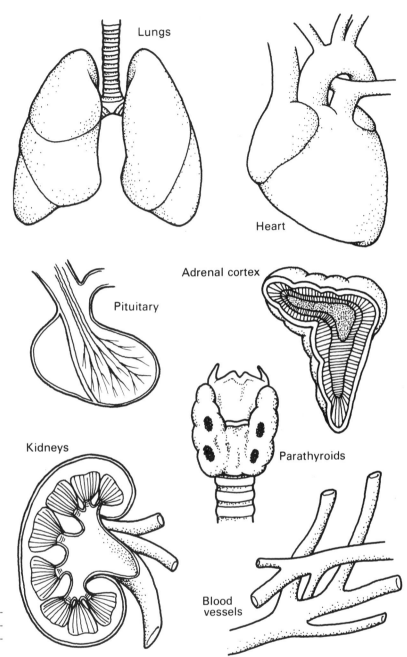

FIGURE 1–8.
Homeostatic mechanisms. (Metheny N: Quick Reference to Fluid Balance, p 9. Philadelphia, JB Lippincott, 1984; with permission.)

(H^+), as opposed to only 40 to 80 mEq excreted daily by the kidneys.

Under control of the medulla, the lungs act promptly to correct metabolic acid–base disturbances by regulating the level of carbon dioxide (a potential acid) in the ECF. For example, to compensate for metabolic alkalosis, the lungs hypoventilate to retain CO_2; the increased acidity helps correct excess alkalinity of the body fluids. Just the opposite occurs with metabolic acidosis; the lungs hyperventilate to remove CO_2, which helps decrease the excess acidity of body fluids.

Pulmonary dysfunction can produce a rapid change (matter of seconds) in the plasma H^+ concentration (acid–base balance). Hypoventilation causes respiratory acidosis; hyperventilation causes respiratory alkalosis. When the lungs are at fault, the kidneys must compensate for the pH disturbances. Acid–base regulation is discussed in depth in Chapter 9.

The lungs also remove approximately 300 mL of water daily through exhalation (insensible water loss) in the normal adult. Abnormal conditions such as hyperpnea or continuous coughing increase this loss; mechanical ventilation with excessive moisture decreases it.

PITUITARY GLAND

The hypothalamus manufactures a substance known as *antidiuretic hormone* (ADH), which is stored in the posterior pituitary gland and released as needed. Because ADH makes the body retain water, it is sometimes referred to as the "water-conserving" hormone.

The amount of water retained or excreted by the kidneys is regulated by ADH. As ADH secretion increases, water retention increases. Conversely, water loss is greater in the face of diminished ADH production. Minor changes in body fluid osmolality constantly occur during normal living and lead to minor physiological changes in ADH production. A rising osmolality, such as that which occurs with salt intake, increases ADH production and thus water retention; a falling osmolality, such as that which occurs with water intake, decreases ADH production and enhances water excretion. It is evident, therefore, that osmolality and ADH are normally in constant interaction. In the presence of a falling blood volume, ADH secretion and subsequent water retention are stimulated by volume stimuli (probably arising from sensors in the heart and great vessels).

Syndrome of inappropriate antidiuretic hormone (SIADH) and *diabetes insipidus* (DI) are disorders of water balance due to ADH disturbances at opposite ends of a continuum. In SIADH, excessive ADH secretion causes water retention. Just the opposite happens in DI, which is characterized by large urine volumes due to inadequate amounts of ADH. These pathological states are discussed in depth in Chapter 4.

ADRENAL GLANDS

The primary adrenocortical hormone in the influence of fluid balance is *aldosterone,* a mineralocorticoid secreted by the outer zone of the adrenal cortex. This hormone acts chiefly on the distal tubules of the kidney to promote Na^+ reabsorption in exchange for K^+ and H^+ ions (which are excreted). Thus, aldosterone production causes sodium retention and expansion of the ECF, along with renal excretion of potassium. Occurrences that can stimulate aldosterone secretion include a fall in the plasma sodium concentration or an increase in the potassium concentration. However, the primary regulator of aldosterone secretion appears to be angiotensin II, which is produced by the renin–angiotensin system. A decreased blood volume or flow activates this system and increases aldosterone secretion. The aldosterone, in turn, increases renal retention of sodium (along with water) to correct the volume deficit. The opposite happens when a state of volume overexpansion exists.

Cortisol, another adrenocortical hormone, has only a fraction of the mineralocorticoid potency of aldosterone. However, secretion of cortisol in large quantities can produce sodium and fluid retention, and potassium deficit.

PARATHYROID GLANDS

Most persons have four parathyroid glands. These pea-sized glands, embedded in the corners of the thyroid gland, regulate calcium and phosphate balance by means of parathyroid hormone (PTH). Control of calcium ion concentration by PTH is largely due to this hormone's effect on bone reabsorption. Fall in calcium ion concentration stimulates PTH secretion. This, in turn, acts directly on the bones to increase reabsorption of bone salts, releasing large amounts of calcium into the ECF. Conversely, when the extracellular calcium level is too high, PTH secretion is depressed so that almost no bone reabsorption occurs. Long-term control of calcium ion concentration results from the effect of PTH on calcium reabsorption from the kidney tubules and calcium absorption from the gut through the GI mucosa. Both of these effects are significantly increased by PTH.

A reciprocal relationship exists between extracellular calcium and phosphate levels in that an elevation of one usually causes depression of the other. Thus, a high extracellular phosphate concentration causes a secondary depression of extracellular calcium; as a result, PTH release is stimulated (a condition often seen in renal failure).

Another hormone that bears consideration in the regulation of calcium is calcitonin, a substance secreted by the thyroid gland. Calcitonin's action on calcium is opposite to that of PTH; in other words, calcitonin reduces plasma calcium concentration. The calcium-lowering effect of calcitonin occurs primarily through inhibition of osteoclast bone resorption.[9] Its effect on plasma calcium concentration is relatively stronger in children than in adults because the action of calcitonin involves bone remodeling, which is more rapid in children.[10] Pharmacological use of calcitonin in the treatment of hypercalcemia is discussed in Chapters 6 and 24.

REFERENCES

1. Kokko J, Tannen, R: Fluids and Electrolytes, 2nd ed, p 4. Philadelphia, WB Saunders, 1990
2. Rose B: Clinical Physiology of Acid–Base and Electrolyte Disorders, 3rd ed, p 4. New York, McGraw-Hill, 1989
3. Statland H: Fluid and Electrolytes in Practice, 3rd ed, p 4. Philadelphia, JB Lippincott, 1963
4. Smith K, Brain E: Fluids and Electrolytes: A Conceptual Approach, p 14. New York, Churchill Livingstone, 1980
5. Willatts S: Lecture Notes of Fluid and Electrolyte Balance, p 13. Oxford, Blackwell Scientific Publications, 1982
6. Rose, p 17
7. Smith, Brain, p 19
8. Pestana C: Fluids and Electrolytes in the Surgical Patient, 4th ed, p 223. Baltimore, Williams & Wilkins, 1989
9. Maxwell M, Kleeman C, Narins R: Clinical Disorders of Fluid & Electrolyte Metabolism, 4th ed, p 771. New York, McGraw-Hill, 1987
10. Guyton A: Textbook of Medical Physiology, 7th ed, p. 436. Philadelphia, WB Saunders, 1986

2

Nursing Assessment

Much of what the nurse does to care for patients with actual or potential fluid and electrolyte problems revolves around monitoring for the occurrence or worsening of the imbalances. It is logical for nursing to assume this vital role since the nurse is directly respon- sible for hospitalized patients 24 hours a day and is often the primary contact for patients both in extended-care facilities and in the home setting. Monitoring for fluid balance disturbances involves more than simple observations, and is based on an understanding of normal physiological mechanisms as well as of the indicators of disrupted fluid balance.

The monitoring role entails identifying patients at risk for specific imbalances as well as continuously observing and analyzing the physiological indices of fluid balance so that disturbances can be detected early and corrective measures can be initiated. As with many conditions, a high level of suspicion is necessary to detect fluid and electrolyte problems. The suspicion that electrolyte abnormalities exist is strengthened by the presence of clinical features known to occur with them, and often by the results of laboratory tests and electrocardiographical findings.

Nursing assessment of fluid balance requires a review of the patient's history and laboratory data, as well as careful clinical observation. In summary, one must know "what to look for," "where and how often to look," and when to expect certain changes as a result of interventions (outcome criteria).

HISTORY

The following questions should be considered in the nursing history:

1. Is there a disease process or injury state present that can disrupt fluid and electrolyte balance? (Examples might include diabetes mellitus, pancreatitis, and bowel obstruction.) In what type of imbalance(s) does this condition usually result?
2. Is the patient receiving any medication or treatment that can disrupt fluid and electrolyte balance? (Examples include steroids, diuretics, and total parenteral nutrition [TPN].) If so, how might this therapy upset fluid balance?
3. Is there an abnormal loss of body fluids and, if so, from what source? What types of imbalances are usually associated with the loss of these fluids?
4. Have any dietary restrictions (for example, low-sodium diet) been imposed? If so, how might fluid balance be affected?
5. Has the patient taken adequate amounts of water and other nutrients orally or by some other route? If not, how long has the inadequate intake been present?
6. How does the total intake of fluids compare with the total fluid output?

After evaluating information gained from the above questions in the nursing history, it becomes easier to identify patients at risk for specific fluid and electrolyte disturbances. Because the anticipation of an imbalance makes its appearance easier to detect, it is important to focus on "expected" imbalances. It is extremely difficult to recognize significant changes in the patient when one does not know "what to look for." It is also important to consider that the symptoms of an imbalance, and their severity, depend on (1) how long the imbalance has been present, (2) its magnitude and rapidity of onset, and (3) how efficiently the homeostatic mechanisms compensate for it. Also, one must remember that imbalances rarely occur alone; usually more than one is present, making identification more difficult.

As stated above, certain disease or injury states put the patient at risk for specific fluid and electrolyte imbalances. These are discussed in Chapters 3 through 9 and in chapters dealing with specific clinical entities.

Unfortunately, there are a number of imbalances that can be *created* by medical therapy. It is important to be aware of these disturbances and alert for their appearance since many times they can be prevented by early nursing and medical interventions. Some medical therapies that can produce fluid and electrolyte disturbances are discussed in Chapters 3 through 9 and in the relevant later chapters. See these chapters for specific imbalances or clinical situations.

CLINICAL ASSESSMENT

After the history described above has been reviewed, one should be able to identify potential problems related to fluid and electrolyte balance.

At this point, a thorough nursing assessment is indicated. Remember that nursing assessment is not a "one-time" procedure but must be done at regular intervals to detect changes and reformulate nursing diagnoses. The following parameters should be considered in clinical assessment for fluid and electrolyte status:

- Comparison of total intake and output of fluids
- Urine volume and concentration
- Skin and tongue turgor
- Degree of moisture in oral cavity
- Body weight
- Thirst
- Tearing and salivation
- Appearance and temperature of skin
- Facial appearance
- Edema
- Temperature, pulse, and respirations
- Blood pressure
- Neck vein filling
- Hand vein filling
- Central venous pressure
- Neuromuscular irritability
- Other signs

Nursing observations must be *interpreted*, using one's knowledge of the patient's history and pathophysiological condition, to determine whether the information gained from the assessment suggests normal or abnormal signs or measurements, and to what degree. Then, the appropriate nursing action(s) must be determined. One must know when medical intervention is required, and a close working relationship with the physician is necessary for optimal care.

COMPARISON OF INTAKE AND OUTPUT

Many serious fluid balance problems can be averted by maintaining a careful vigil on patient intake and output (I & O) and keeping accurate records. (Totals for several consecutive days should be compared.) If the total intake is substantially less than the total output, it is obvious that the patient is in danger of fluid volume deficit (FVD). On the other hand, if the total intake is substantially more than the output, the patient is in danger of fluid volume excess (FVE) (or, in the case of inappropriate secretion of antidiuretic hormone [ADH], water excess). To understand abnormal states better, it is helpful to review the 24-hour average I & O in a normal adult (Table 2-1).

Balance of I & O is desirable only in steady-state conditions. In pathophysiological conditions, therapy is directed at promoting recovery. For example, in shock and trauma states, more fluid than has been lost will be needed to restore plasma volume to optimal levels.[1]

It is important to initiate I & O records for any patient with a real or potential water and electrolyte problem: do not wait for an order from the physician.

1. Intake should include all fluids taken into the body (oral fluids, foods that are liquid at room temperature, intravenous fluids, subcutaneous fluids, fluids instilled into drainage tubes as irrigants, tube feeding solutions, water given through feeding tubes, and even enema solutions in patients requiring strict fluid intake recording, such as those suffering renal failure).

2. Output should include urine, vomitus, diarrhea, drainage from fistulas, and drainage from suction apparatus. Perspiration should be noted and its amount estimated. The presence of prolonged hyperventilation should also be noted since it is an important route of water-vapor loss. Drainage from lesions (such as from large decubitus ulcers) should be noted and estimated.

3. The I & O record should include the time of day and the type of fluid gained and lost. This information is necessary in planning therapy.

4. The type of I & O record used often depends on the patient's condition. A patient with a severe fluid balance problem may require an hourly summary of his or her fluid gains and losses so that the fluctuating needs can be dealt with quickly. Many patients require only 8-hour summaries of their fluid gains and losses. Figure 2-1 depicts a bedside record suitable for this purpose. Note that the record lists the volumes of containers used.

Although it is not technically difficult to measure fluid I & O or to record the measurements, persistent effort is required if one is to achieve an accurate account. There are innumerable possibilities for error in the measurement and recording of fluid gains and losses; however, some errors occur much more frequently than others. Common errors and suggestions for overcoming them are shown in Table 2-2.

Pflaum[2] examined the accuracy of a routine I & O technique in a general hospital and found it lacking; when compared with measurement of body weight, the mean daily error was 800 mL. From her results Pflaum concluded that measurement of I & O is of little value and that a more accurate indicator, body weight, should be adopted. While it is generally recognized that I & O records are often sorely lacking, one should use *both*

(text continues on page 18)

TABLE 2–1.
Average Intake and Output in an Adult for a 24-Hour Period

INTAKE		OUTPUT	
Oral liquids	1300 mL	Urine	1500 mL
Water in food	1000 mL	Stool	200 mL
Water produced by metabolism	300 mL	**Insensible:**	
Total	2600 mL	Lungs	300 mL
		Skin	600 mL
		Total	2600 mL

BARNES

17-4 Rev. 6/89

FROM 2300 / / TO 2300 / /

Addressograph Plate

INTAKE				OUTPUT	
Coffee mug - 180cc Ice tea container to clear line (without ice) - 250cc Ice cream container (melted) - 30cc Sherbet container (melted) - 50cc Juice container - 120cc Milk carton - 240cc Paper cup (1/4 from brim) - 240cc Soup bowl (broth) - 180cc Gelatin container (melted) - 100cc		ORDERS: (CIRCLE) NPO WATER CLEAR FLUIDS FULL FLUIDS AMT. DESIRED CC	SOURCE KEY: V = VOIDED C = CATHETER INC = INCONTINENT	SOURCE KEY: VOM. = VOMITUS LIQ. S. = LIQUID STOOL HV. = HEMOVAC L.T. = LEVIN TUBE T.T. = T. TUBE OTHER	
RATE GTTS/MIN. CC/HR.					

TIME	PARENTERAL			ORAL		URINE		OTHER	
	SOLUTION IN BOTTLE KIND AMT. (CC)		AMT. (CC) ABSORBED	KIND	AMT. (CC)	SOURCE	AMT. (CC)	SOURCE	AMT. (CC)
2300 2400									
2400 0100									
0100 0200									
0200 0300									
0300 0400									
0400 0500									
0500 0600									
0600 0700									
8 HR. TOT.				8 HR. TOT.		8 HR. TOT.		8 HR. TOT.	
0700 0800									
0800 0900									
0900 1000									
1000 1100									
1100 1200									
1200 1300									
1300 1400									
1400 1500									
8 HR. TOT.				8 HR. TOT.		8 HR. TOT.		8 HR. TOT.	
1500 1600									
1600 1700									
1700 1800									
1800 1900									
1900 2000									
2000 2100									
2100 2200									
2200 2300									
8 HR. TOT.				8 HR. TOT.		8 HR. TOT.		8 HR. TOT.	
24 HR. TOT.				24 HR. TOT.		24 HR. TOT.		24 HR. TOT.	

FIGURE 2–1.
Eight-hour fluid intake and output record. (Courtesy Barnes Hospital, St Louis, MO)

TABLE 2–2.
Overcoming Common Errors in Measuring Intake and Output

COMMON ERRORS	SUGGESTIONS
Errors Involving Both Intake and Output:	
Failure to communicate to the entire staff which patients require intake–output measurement (Body fluids are often discarded without being measured, and oral fluids are not recorded, merely because staff members are not aware of the patients on intake–output.)	1. A "measure intake–output" sign should be attached to the patient's bed to serve as a reminder. 2. A list of all patients requiring intake–output measurement should be posted in a convenient work area for quick reference. 3. Also, for quick reference, the card file should contain a list of all patients requiring intake–output measurement. 4. An adequate patient report should be given to all personnel.
Failure to explain intake–output to the patient and family (Most patients will cooperate *if* they know what is expected of them.)	1. Both the patient and the family should receive a simple explanation of why intake–output measurement is necessary. 2. Careful instructions are necessary to acquaint the patient and family with their role in helping to achieve an accurate intake–output record.
Well-meaning intentions to record a drink of water or an emptied urinal at a later, more convenient time are often forgotten.	Measurements should be recorded at the time they are obtained.
Failure to measure fluids that can be directly measured because it takes less time to guess at their amounts	Measure *all* fluids amenable to direct measurement—guesses should be reserved for fluids that cannot be measured directly.
Errors Related to Intake:	
Failure to designate the specific volume of glasses, cups, bowls, and other fluid containers used in the hospital (Each person may ascribe a different volume to the same glass of water.)	The bedside record should list the volumes of glasses, cups, bowls, and other fluid containers used in the hospital (see Fig. 2–1).
Failure to obtain an adequate measuring device for small amounts of oral fluids (Patients frequently drink small quantities of fluids; the amounts must be estimated unless a calibrated cup is available—frequent estimates increase the margin of error.)	Small calibrated paper cups should be kept at the bedside for such a purpose.
Failure to consider the volume of fluid displaced by ice in iced drinks frequently causes an overstatement of ingested oral fluids	Only small amounts of ice should be used for iced drinks so that the accurate amount of fluid ingested can be recorded.
Overstatement of fluid volume given as ice chips; note that the liquid volume of a glass of ice chips is only about half a glass	Record fluid intake from ice chips as approximately half of the ice chips volume (for example: an ounce of ice chips is approximately 15 mL of water).
Failure to consider that parenteral fluid bottles are over-filled; a 1000-mL bottle may actually contain 1100 mL; a 500-mL bottle may contain 550 mL	Run excess fluid through tubing during set-up, or record actual volume infused.
Assuming that the contents of empty containers were drunk by the patient (Patients sometimes give their coffee or juice to a visiting relative or other patients in the room; they may forget to tell the person checking the tray.)	The patient should be asked what fluids were drunk.

(continued)

TABLE 2–2.
(continued)

COMMON ERRORS	SUGGESTIONS
Errors Related to Output:	
Failure to estimate fluid lost as perspiration	1. An attempt should be made to describe the amount of clothing and bed linen saturated with perspiration—it has been estimated that one necessary bed change represents at least 1 L of lost fluid. 2. Some intake–output records require the nurse to estimate perspiration as +, + +, + + +, or + + + + (+ represents sweating that is just visible, and + + + + represents profuse sweating).
Failure to estimate "uncaught" vomitus (Frequently, "uncaught" emesis is recorded merely as a lost specimen.)	The amount of fluid lost as vomitus should be estimated and recorded as an estimate—it is better to guess than to give no indication at all as to the amount.
Failure to estimate the amount of incontinent urine (Intake–output records often indicate the number of incontinent voidings but give no indication of the amounts; obviously, such records are of little value.)	The amount of incontinent urine should be estimated—it is helpful to note the amount of clothing and bed linen saturated with urine.
Failure to estimate fluid lost as liquid feces	1. The patient should be encouraged to use the bedpan or a measuring device over the toilet so that the fluid loss can be directly measured. 2. The amount of fluid lost in incontinent liquid stools should be estimated.
Failure to estimate fluid lost as wound exudate	1. The amount of drainage on a dressing should be measured and charted—this can be done by measuring the width of the stained area and determining the thickness of the dressing. 2. If extreme measures are necessary, the dressing can be weighed before application and again when removed. 3. If a fistula is present, a stoma bag should be applied to catch the drainage.
Failure to check a urinary catheter for patency when there is decreased drainage of urine (It is sometimes too quickly assumed that decreased drainage from a catheter is due to decreased urine formation.)	Decreased drainage from a urinary catheter is an indication to check for patency before charting the absence of, or decrease in, urinary output.
Failure to obtain an adequate measuring device for hourly or more frequent checks on urinary output (An error of even 10 mL could be significant when dealing with small amounts of urine.)	A collecting device calibrated to measure *small amounts* of urine should be used (see Fig. 2–2).
Failure to record the amount of solution used to irrigate tubes and the amount of fluid withdrawn during the irrigation	1. One method for dealing with this problem is to add the amount of irrigating solution to the intake column, and the amount of fluid withdrawn to the output column. 2. Another method is to compare the amount of irrigating solution used with the amount of fluid withdrawn during the irrigation—if more fluid was put in than was taken out, the excess is added to the intake column; if more fluid was taken out than was put in, the excess is added to the output column.

I & O measurements and body weights to best evaluate a patient's fluid balance status. Unfortunately, body weight measurements are also often inaccurate.

URINE VOLUME

As a general rule of thumb, the normal urinary output is about 1 mL per kilogram of body weight per hour, with boundaries of 0.5 to 2 mL/kg/hr.[3] Table 2-1 shows that the usual urine volume in adults is approximately 1500 mL/day (ranges from 1000 to 2000 mL/day). This is equivalent to approximately 40 to 80 mL/hr in the typical adult. Urine volume in children is less, and is dependent on age and weight.

During periods of stress, the 24-hour urine volume in the adult may diminish to 750 to 1200 mL/day (or 30 to 50 mL/hr). Urine volume is somewhat less during periods of stress because of increased aldosterone and ADH secretion.

A low urine volume suggests FVD, and a high urine volume suggests FVE. Several factors can alter urinary volume, including

▶ Amount of fluid intake
▶ Losses from skin, lungs, and gastrointestinal tract
▶ Amount of waste products for excretion (Urine volume is increased in conditions with high solute loads, such as diabetes mellitus, high-protein tube feedings, thyrotoxicosis, and fever.)
▶ Renal concentrating ability (When concentrating ability is diminished, urine volume is increased to allow adequate solute excretion.)
▶ Blood volume (Hypovolemia causes decreased renal perfusion and, thus, oliguria; hypervolemia causes increased urinary volume if the kidneys are functioning normally.)
▶ Hormonal influences (primarily aldosterone and ADH)

Nursing Considerations

1. Maintain I & O records on all patients with real or potential fluid balance problems. Measure all fluid gains and losses according to routes.
2. Be alert for fluid intake greatly exceeding fluid output, or fluid output greatly exceeding fluid intake. Totals of I & O records for several consecutive days should be obtained for a clearer understanding of fluid balance status.
3. Be aware that the usual urine output in adults is 1 to 2 L/day (or approximately 750 to 1200 mL/day during periods of stress).
4. Use a device calibrated for small volumes of urine when hourly urine volumes must be measured (see Fig. 2-2).

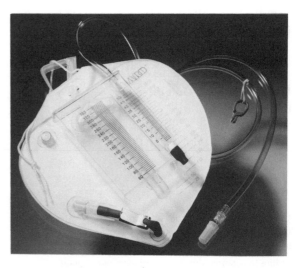

FIGURE 2–2.
Device suitable for measuring small urine volume. (350-mL urine meter bag). (Courtesy of Bard Urological Division, Covington, GA)

5. Be aware that the usual urine output in adults is 40 to 80 mL/hr (or 30 to 50 mL/hr during periods of stress).
6. Be aware that patients taking in high-solute loads (as in high-protein tube feedings) need extra water to aid in solute elimination.
7. Be aware that individuals with diminished renal concentrating ability (such as the aged) need more fluid to excrete solutes than do those with normal renal function.
8. Be aware that a low urine volume with a high specific gravity (SG) indicates fluid volume deficit.
9. Be aware that a low urine volume with a low SG is indicative of renal disease.
10. Evaluate I & O levels and urinary SG in relation to other clinical signs.
11. Be aware of common sources of errors in I & O measurements (see Table 2-2).

URINE CONCENTRATION

Urinary SG measures the kidneys' ability to concentrate urine. In this test, the concentration of urine is compared with the 1.000 SG of distilled water. Because urine contains electrolytes and other substances, its SG is greater than 1.000. The range of SG in urine is from 1.003 to 1.035; most random specimens are between 1.012 and 1.025. Typical urine osmolality (another measure of urine concentration) ranges from 500 to 800 mOsm/kg; extreme ranges are from 50 to 1400 mOsm/kg.

Urinary SG is elevated when there is a FVD as the

normal kidney seeks to retain needed fluid, thus excreting solutes in a small concentrated urine volume. However, one should be aware that heavy molecules not normally present in large quantities in urine can falsely affect SG readings. For example, glucose, albumin, or radiocontrast dyes will elevate urinary SG out of proportion to the actual concentration. Thus, it is more accurate to measure urine osmolality in patients with glycosuria, proteinuria, or recent use of radiopaque dyes.

Specific gravity can be measured with a refractometer, a dipstick that has a reagent area for SG, or with a urinometer. Freshly voided urine specimens at room temperature are desirable for testing SG. Refrigerated samples may have falsely elevated readings, as may specimens exposed to excessive heat and dryness (a result of evaporation). Ideally, urinary SG should be measured immediately after the specimen is collected. However, in some situations this is not possible.

To determine the variability in specimens tested immediately after voiding and at intervals up to 4 hours after voiding, a study of 20 ill infants with disposable diapers was conducted.[4] Urine was aspirated from each diaper immediately after voiding and tested with a refractometer. Subsequently the diaper was folded, rolled, and taped so that the urine was not exposed to air, heat, or light. Specific gravity measurements of urine aspirated from each diaper at up to 4-hour intervals after voiding were not significantly different from those obtained at the time of urination.

SKIN TURGOR

In a normal person, pinched skin will immediately fall back to its normal position when released. This elastic property, referred to as turgor, partially depends on interstitial fluid volume. In an individual with a FVD, the skin flattens more slowly after the pinch is released, and may remain elevated for several seconds.

Tissue turgor is best measured by pinching the skin over the sternum, inner aspects of the thighs, or forehead (see Fig. 2-3), although some prefer to test skin turgor in children over the abdominal area and on the medial aspects of the thighs.

Although the purpose of the skin turgor test is to measure only interstitial fluid volume, it also measures skin elasticity. Because they have less skin elasticity relative to younger patients, reduced skin turgor is common in patients older than 55 to 60 years of age. Skin turgor may be difficult to assess in the elderly or in those with recent weight loss and is not diagnostic in the absence of other signs of FVD.

In children, skin turgor begins to diminish after 3% to 5% of the body weight is lost. However, severe malnutrition, particularly in infants, can cause depressed

skin turgor even in the absence of fluid depletion. Obese infants with FVD may have skin turgor that is deceptively normal. Infants with hypernatremia may have firm skin that feels thick.

In summary, tissue turgor can vary with age, nutritional state, and even race and complexion. Observations are most meaningful if done sequentially before the development of a fluid balance abnormality.

A group of researchers recently reported the use of an experimental device to measure interstitial fluid pressure (IFP) as a means to assess interstitial fluid volume.[5] Included in the study were seven healthy volunteers and 25 patients in varying fluid volume states (hypervolemia, normovolemia, or hypovolemia). The device consisted of a catheter inserted into the subcutaneous space and connected to an electronic monitoring device. The authors reported that the results suggest IFP is a sensitive measure for reflecting the hydration status of the interstitial compartment.

TONGUE TURGOR

In a normal person, the tongue has one longitudinal furrow. In the person with FVD, there are additional longitudinal furrows, and the tongue is smaller (due to fluid loss). Unlike skin turgor, tongue turgor is not appreciably affected by age and therefore is a useful assessment for all age groups. Note that sodium excess causes the tongue to appear red and swollen.

MOISTURE IN ORAL CAVITY

A dry mouth may be the result of FVD or of mouth breathing. If it is due to FVD, all of the oral tissues will be dry. In contrast, if the dryness is due to mouth breathing, the areas where the gums and cheek membranes meet will remain moist. Dry, sticky mucous membranes are noted in sodium excess (hypernatremia).

BODY WEIGHT

Weighing patients with potential or actual fluid balance problems daily is of great clinical importance for the following reasons. (1) Accurate body weight measurements are usually easier to obtain than accurate fluid I & O measurements. (2) Rapid variations in weight, when measured correctly, reflect changes in body fluid volume.

When analyzing changes in a patient's weight, it is important to consider factors that may hinder the accuracy of weight measurement. For example, there may be errors in the weighing technique or in the recording of results, or the scales themselves may be faulty. A recent study indicated that a small but signifi-

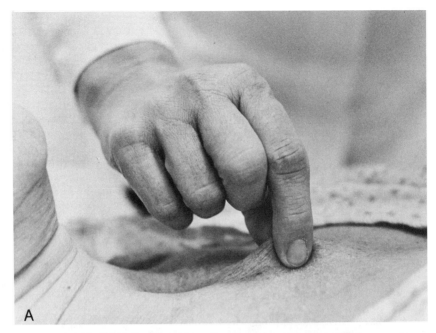

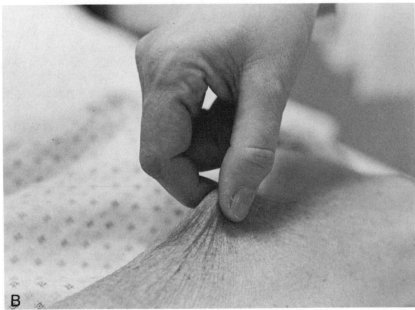

FIGURE 2–3.
(**A**) Testing skin turgor on sternum. (**B**) Testing turgor of same older person on forearm is less valid due to decreased skin elasticity in this area.

cant percentage of scales in clinical use are inaccurate and imprecise to a clinically important degree.[6] The investigators perceived the problem to be related to breakage and wear rather than manufacturing defects. To minimize inaccuracies in weight measurements, medical institutions should test the accuracy of their clinical scales periodically. Before obtaining the patient's weight, it is helpful to test one's own weight on the scale to note any obvious discrepancy. Indicators of an inaccurate scale may include the following: one's own weight seems to be in error, a change greater than 1 lb occurs when one's weight is shifted on the scale's platform, the platform is wobbly, or other defects in the scale's structure are apparent.

The following practices should be followed in weighing patients:

1. Use the same scale each time since there may be significant variation among scales. Because this may present a problem when the patient is transferred from unit to unit, the need for accurate scales throughout an institution is obvious. This point emphasizes the need to test the accuracy of clinical scales routinely.
2. Measure weight in the morning before breakfast and after voiding.
3. Be sure the patient is wearing the same or similar clothing each time and that the clothing is dry.
4. If the patient is unable to stand for weighing on a small portable scale or a stand-on scale (see Fig. 2-4), use a sling-type scale (see Fig. 2-5). Wheelchair and under-bed scales are also commercially available.

Body weight as an index of fluid balance is based on the assumption that the patient's dry weight remains relatively stable. Over a short period (hour-to-hour), this assumption is valid, and changes in body weight reflect changes in body fluid volume rather than tissue mass changes. To assess these small hourly changes, it is necessary to use extremely accurate metabolic scales, which are not available on most patient care units.

Most patients are weighed only once a day on scales calibrated in units of ¼ lb, ½ lb, or 1 lb. Long-term (day-to-day) body weight variations reflect changes in tissue mass as well as body fluid volume. Thus, factors affecting tissue mass (caloric intake and metabolic status) must also be evaluated. Tissue loss occurs in catabolic states (such as severe stress) and tissue mass gain occurs in anabolic states. Therefore, long-term measurements of body weight should be corrected for tissue loss in catabolic states (up to 500 g/day) or for lean tissue gain in anabolic states (80 to 150 g/day).[7] (A pound is roughly equivalent to 454 g.) It is generally assumed that a relative deficit of 3400 calories is needed to lose 1 lb of tissue mass; this deficit can be the result of inadequate caloric intake, increased metabolic rate, or both.

Body weight loss will occur when the total fluid intake is less than the total fluid output. A rapid 2% loss of total body weight indicates mild FVD, while a 5% loss represents moderate FVD and a rapid loss of 8% or more represents severe FVD. Conversely, body weight gain will occur when the total fluid intake is greater than the total fluid output. A rapid 2% gain of total body weight indicates mild fluid volume excess (FVE), while a 5% gain represents a moderate FVE and an 8% or greater gain a severe FVE.

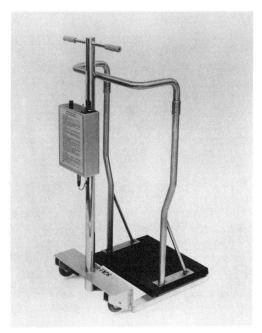

FIGURE 2–4.
Stand-on scale. (Model 5005, Scale-Tronix, White Plains, NY)

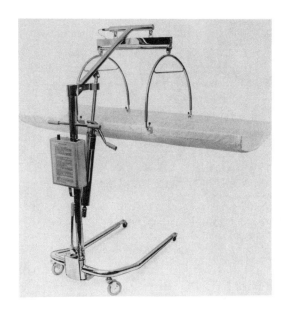

FIGURE 2–5.
Sling scale. (Model 2001, Scale-Tronix, White Plains, NY)

A rapid body weight gain or loss of 1 kg (2.2 lb) is approximately equivalent to the gain or loss of 1 L of fluid (or expressed another way, a gain or loss of 500 mL of fluid is equivalent to a gain or loss of 1 lb). A patient may have a severe FVD, although body weight is essentially unchanged or even increased, when there is a "third-space" shift of body fluid (see Chapter 3).

THIRST

Thirst is a subjective sensory symptom that has been defined as an awareness of the desire to drink. Increased concentration of the extracellular fluid will osmotically pull fluid from the cells in the thirst control center and stimulate thirst. Any factor that causes intracellular dehydration will in general cause the sensation of thirst.

The sense of thirst is so protective of the normal serum sodium level that hypernatremia virtually never occurs unless thirst is impaired or rendered ineffective because of unconsciousness or inaccessibility of water. In adults, hypernatremia is most often seen in persons older than 60 years of age,[8] partially because age is associated with diminished osmotic stimulation of thirst.[9]

Thirst is prominent in patients who have increased water losses as occur in, for example, hyperglycemia, high fever, or diarrhea. An infant can be tested for thirst by offering water, although the presence of nausea may mask the symptom. Unfortunately, patients with altered states of consciousness do not experience normal thirst. Also, many patients are debilitated and unable to respond to thirst. It is no wonder that hypernatremia is a relatively common imbalance on neurologic units.

TEARING AND SALIVATION

Tearing and salivation are decreased in patients with FVD.[10] These signs are particularly helpful in pediatric situations to detect FVD.

APPEARANCE OF SKIN AND SKIN TEMPERATURE

Metabolic acidosis can cause warm, flushed skin due to peripheral vasodilatation. Severe FVD causes the skin to be pale and cool due to peripheral vasoconstriction, which occurs to compensate for hypovolemia.

FACIAL APPEARANCE

An individual with a severe FVD has a pinched facial expression. A significant FVD causes decreased intraocular pressure; thus, the eyes appear sunken and feel soft to the touch.

EDEMA

Edema is defined as an excessive accumulation of interstitial fluid (the body fluid that bathes the cells). Edema usually does not become clinically apparent until the interstitial volume has increased by at least 2.5 to 3 L.[11]

Causes of edema include (1) increased capillary permeability, which allows fluid to leak into the interstitium (as in burns or localized trauma); (2) increased capillary hydraulic pressure, which forces fluid into the interstitium (as in heart failure or venous obstruction); (3) decreased plasma oncotic pressure of hypoalbuminemia, which fosters the transfer of fluid into the interstitium (particularly when the plasma albumin level is less than 2 g/dL); and (4) lymphatic obstruction, which permits local edema (as in node enlargement of malignancy).[12]

Edema formation may be either localized (as in thrombophlebitis) or generalized (as in heart failure and the nephrotic syndrome). An excess of interstitial fluid accumulating predominantly in the lower extremities of ambulatory patients and in the presacral region of bedridden patients is referred to as *dependent edema*. *Generalized edema* is spread throughout the body, and may accumulate in periorbital and scrotal regions because of the relatively lower tissue hydrostatic pressure in these regions.[13] Edema related to salt retention is generally pitting and can be manifested by pressing one's finger into the soft tissues (see Fig. 2-6). After the pressure is removed, the "pit" gradually disappears. Barely perceptible pitting edema indicates that total body sodium content has increased by approximately 400 mEq (2.7 L of saline).[14]

Describing peripheral edema by appearance is somewhat subjective. For example, it is sometimes indicated by using plus signs to represent the amount, ranging from +1 to +4, with +1 indicating barely perceptible, +2 and +3 moderate, and +4 severe edema. Measuring an extremity or body part with a millimeter tape in the same area each day is the most exact method (see Fig. 2-7).

There is no peripheral edema with only water retention (as occurs in excessive secretion of ADH). Instead, there is cellular swelling that can be detected by pressing one's finger over the sternum (or other bony prominence) and producing a visible fingerprint.

Pulmonary Edema

Pulmonary edema results from excessive shifting of fluid from the vascular space into the pulmonary interstitium and air spaces. Such accumulation of extravascular water (EVW) affects pulmonary functioning and gas exchange to varying degrees depending on both the site of accumulation (interstitial versus alveolar) and the quantity of fluid involved. Cardiogenic causes of increased EVW usually result in alveolar fluid, and noncardiogenic causes in interstitial edema.[15]

Clinical symptoms of EVW result primarily from either one or both of two phenomena: (1) fluid entering the air spaces and (2) increased interstitial pressure impinging on bronchioles and blood vessels, which results in increased airway and vascular resistances, leading to abnormal distribution of perfusion and ventilation.[16]

BODY TEMPERATURE

Changes in body temperature as *symptoms* of fluid and electrolyte imbalances may include

1. Elevation in body temperature in hypernatremia may occur due to excessive water loss. The temperature may reach 105° F or greater when water loss is marked.[17] The elevated body temperature is probably related to lack of available fluid for sweating. Also, dehydration probably has a direct effect on the hypothalamus.
2. In a cool room, a patient with an isotonic FVD may be slightly hypothermic (probably related to the decreased basal metabolic rate). After partial correction of the FVD, the temperature generally increases to an appropriate level. With moderate FVD, tem-

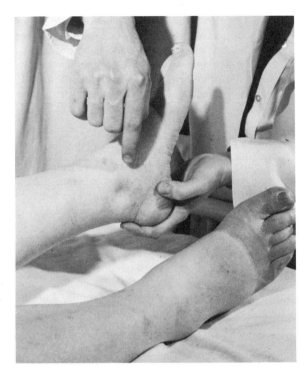

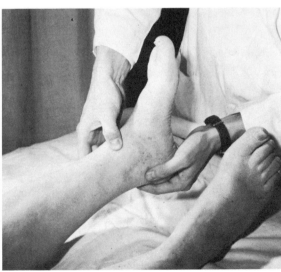

FIGURE 2–6.
Pitting edema of feet and lower legs (*Top*). Same patient has been relieved by treatment (*Bottom*). (Courtesy of CIBA Pharmaceutical Co, Summit, NJ)

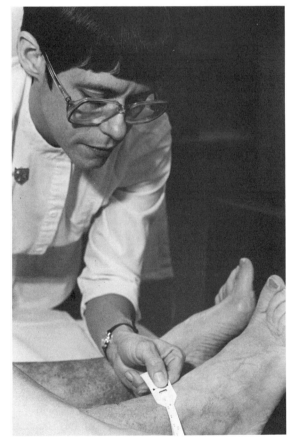

FIGURE 2–7.
Measuring degree of edema with millimeter tape.

perature taken rectally may be 97° F (36.1° C) to 99° F (37.2° C); with severe FVD, it may be 95° F (35° C) to 98° F (36.7° C).[18]

Body temperature changes do not reflect only fluid balance problems. Fever can *cause* fluid balance problems if not promptly recognized and treated. Fever causes an increase in metabolism rate and, thus, in formed metabolic wastes, which require fluid to make a solution for renal excretion; fluid loss, therefore, is increased. Fever also causes hyperpnea, an increase in breathing rate resulting in extra water vapor loss through the lungs. Because fever increases loss of body fluids, temperature elevations must be detected early and appropriate interventions taken.

A temperature elevation between 101° F (38.3° C) and 103° F (39.4° C) increases the 24-hour fluid requirements by at least 500 mL, and a temperature higher than 103° F (39.4° C) increases it by at least 1000 mL.[19]

PULSE

Tachycardia is usually the earliest sign of the decreased vascular volume associated with FVD. It may also be associated with deficits of magnesium or potassium. Conversely, excesses of magnesium or potassium can cause decreased pulse rate. Irregular pulse rates also occur with potassium imbalances and magnesium deficit.

Pulse volume is decreased in FVD and increased in FVE.

RESPIRATIONS

Deep, rapid respirations may be a compensatory mechanism for metabolic acidosis or a primary disorder causing respiratory alkalosis. Slow, shallow respirations may be a compensatory mechanism for metabolic alkalosis or a primary disorder causing respiratory acidosis.

Weakness or paralysis of respiratory muscles is likely in severe hypokalemia or hyperkalemia and in severe magnesium excess (the respiratory center may be paralyzed at a serum magnesium level of 10 to 15 mEq/L).

Moist rales, in the absence of cardiopulmonary disease, indicate FVE.

BLOOD PRESSURE

A sensitive method for detecting volume depletion is measurement of the blood pressure and pulse with the patient in a lying and then standing position. Standing from a supine position causes an abrupt drop in venous return, for which sympathetically mediated cardiovascular adjustments normally compensate. In the healthy individual, cardiac return is maintained by increased peripheral resistance and a slight increase in heart rate; systolic pressure falls only slightly and diastolic pressure may actually rise a few millimeters of mercury. In contrast, a fall in systolic pressure greater than 15 mmHg or an increase in the pulse rate greater than 15 beats/min is suggestive of intravascular volume deficit.[20] Of course, conditions, such as diabetes, associated with autonomic neuropathy can also produce these orthostatic blood pressure and pulse changes.

Hypotension may occur with magnesium excess, perhaps first occurring at a level of 3 to 5 mEq/L. Hypertension can occur with magnesium deficit and with FVE.

NECK VEINS

The jugular veins provide a built-in manometer for the following changes in central venous pressure (CVP): no invasive maneuvers are required, and the procedure can be reliable when done correctly (see Fig. 2-8).

Changes in fluid volume are reflected by changes in neck vein filling, provided the patient is not in heart failure. Normally, with the patient supine, the external jugular veins fill to the anterior border of the sternocleidomastoid muscle. Flat neck veins in the supine position indicate a decreased plasma volume. With the patient positioned sitting at a 45-degree angle, the venous distentions normally should not extend higher than 2 cm above the sternal angle. Elevated venous pressure is indicated by neck veins distended from the

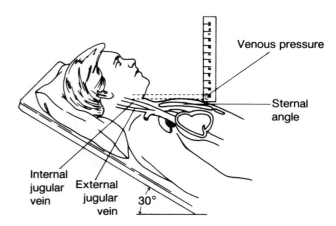

FIGURE 2–8.
An assessment of jugular venous pressure. The highest point at which jugular vein pulsations can be seen is noted. The vertical distance between this point and the sternal angle is measured and recorded as centimeters "above or below" the sternal angle. (Adapted from Brunner L, Suddarth D: Textbook of Medical-Surgical Nursing, 6th ed. p 523. Philadelphia, JB Lippincott, 1988)

top portion of the sternum to the angle of the jaw; this is often seen in severe heart failure.

To estimate jugular venous pressure, the nurse should do the following:

1. Position the patient in a semi-Fowler's position (head of bed elevated to a 30- to 60-degree angle), keeping the neck straight.
2. Remove any of the patient's clothing that could constrict the neck or upper chest.
3. Provide adequate lighting to visualize effectively the external jugular veins on each side of the neck.
4. Measure the level to which the veins are distended on the neck about the sternal angle. The vertical distance between this point and the sternal angle is measured and reported as centimeters above or below the sternal angle.

HAND VEINS

Observation of hand veins can be helpful in evaluating the patient's plasma volume. Usually, elevation of the hands causes the hand veins to empty in 3 to 5 seconds; placing the hands in a dependent position causes the veins to fill in 3 to 5 seconds (see Figs. 2-9 and 2-10).

A decreased plasma volume causes the hand veins to take longer than 3 to 5 seconds to fill when the hands are in a dependent position. An increased plasma volume causes the hand veins to take longer than 3 to 5 seconds to empty when the hands are elevated. When this is the case, the peripheral veins are engorged and clearly visible.

CENTRAL VENOUS PRESSURE

Central venous pressure (CVP) refers to pressure in the right atrium or vena cava and provides information about the following parameters:

▶ Blood volume
▶ Effectiveness of the heart's pumping action
▶ Vascular tone

Pressure in the right atrium is usually 0 to 4 cm of water; pressure in the vena cava is approximately 4 to 11 cm of water. A low CVP may indicate

▶ Decreased blood volume or
▶ Drug-induced vasodilation (causing pooling of blood in peripheral veins)

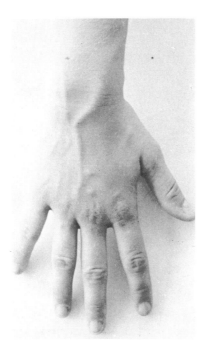

FIGURE 2–9.
Appearance of hand veins when the hand is held in a dependent position. (Metheny N: *Quick Reference to Fluid Balance*, p 40. Philadelphia, JB Lippincott, 1984; with permission.)

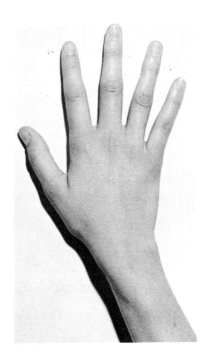

FIGURE 2–10.
Appearance of hand veins when the hand is held in an elevated position. (Metheny N: *Quick Reference to Fluid Balance*, p 41. Philadelphia, JB Lippincott, 1984; with permission.)

A high CVP may indicate

▸ Increased blood volume or
▸ Heart failure or
▸ Vasoconstriction (causing the vascular bed to become smaller)

More important than absolute values are the upward or downward trends; these trends are determined by taking frequent readings (often every 30 to 60 minutes).

It is always important to evaluate CVP in reference to other available clinical data such as

▸ Blood pressure
▸ Pulse
▸ Respirations
▸ Breath and heart sounds
▸ Fluid intake
▸ Urinary output

Example: A rise in CVP paralleling that of systolic blood pressure (BP) is an indication of adequate fluid volume replacement. A low CVP persisting after fluid volume replacement may be a sign of continued occult bleeding.

In those patients with normal cardiac function and relatively normal pulmonary function, the CVP remains an acceptable guide to blood volume. Patients with acute cardiopulmonary decompensation require more extensive hemodynamic monitoring with a device that reflects pressures in both sides of the heart.

Sometimes the rate of an infusion is titrated according to the patient's CVP; when this is necessary, the physician should designate the desired limits so that the nurse can adjust the flow rate accordingly. For example, in acute hypercalcemia, the physician may order isotonic saline at a rate of 250 mL/hr, provided that the CVP does not exceed 10 cm.

Nursing Considerations

1. Measure CVP with the patient flat in bed if possible. If not, have the patient in the same position each time CVP is measured. Indicate the patient's position on the chart when recording the pressure. Place the zero point of the manometer at the level of the patient's right atrium (see Fig. 2-11). The point selected may be marked on the patient's side so that the zero mark may be used consistently.
2. Be aware that a falsely high reading will result if the patient is being ventilated on a respirator.[21] When recording the measurement, be sure to note that it was made during artificial ventilation.
3. Be aware that the fluid should fluctuate 3 to 5 cm in the manometer with respirations when the catheter is patent and properly positioned in the vena cava.

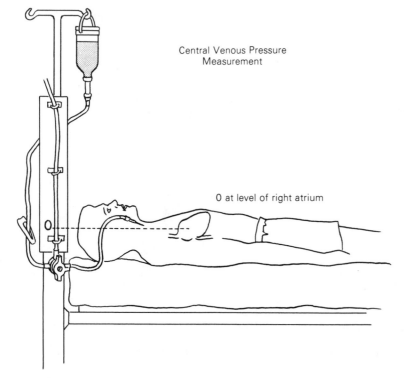

Central Venous Pressure Measurement

0 at level of right atrium

FIGURE 2–11.
Central venous pressure measurement with zero point of manometer at level of right atrium. (Metheny N: *Quick Reference to Fluid Balance,* p 43. Philadelphia, JB Lippincott, 1984; with permission.)

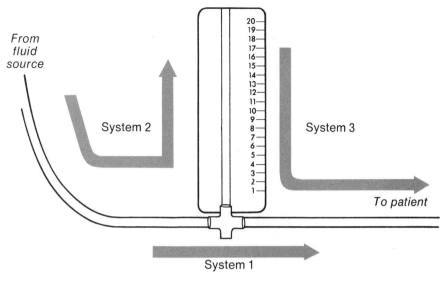

FIGURE 2–12.
Fluid flow systems in central venous pressure measurement. *System 1* allows flow from the container to the patient (routine infusion). *System 2* allows flow from the container to the manometer (allows manometer to fill). *System 3* allows flow from the manometer to the patient (allows reading of CVP). (Hudak et al: Critical Care Nursing, 5th ed, p 122. Philadelphia, JB Lippincott, 1990; with permission.)

4. Take the following steps to read CVP:
   A. First, turn the stopcock so that the solution will flow from the container to the manometer (see Fig. 2-12, System 2).
   B. Second, turn the stopcock to direct manometer flow to the patient (see Fig. 2-12, System 3). The fluid level should drop, reaching a reading level in about 15 seconds.
   C. Third, record the reading at the upper level of the respiratory fluctuation of fluid in the manometer (fluid falls slightly on inspiration and rises slightly on expiration).
5. Use meticulous aseptic technique for dressing changes, catheter care, and tube changes.
6. Check frequently for signs of redness, swelling, and purulent drainage at the injection site.
7. Secure connections to prevent the occurrence of air embolism. Remember that air emboli are more likely to occur when a catheter is placed in the central veins where pressure is low. (Air embolism is discussed in Chapter 10.)

NEUROMUSCULAR IRRITABILITY

It is sometimes necessary to assess patients for increased or decreased neuromuscular irritability, particularly when imbalances in calcium, magnesium, and sodium are suspected.

The nurse may, as necessary, check for Chvostek's sign and Trousseau's sign; also, deep tendon reflexes can be tested to monitor neuromuscular irritability.

To test Chvostek's sign (Fig. 2-13), the facial nerve should be percussed about 2 cm anterior to the earlobe. A positive response shows a unilateral twitching

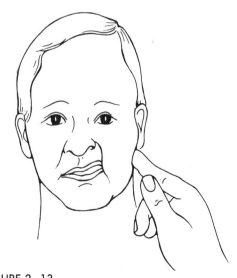

FIGURE 2–13.
Tapping the facial nerve approximately 2 cm anterior to the earlobe will elicit Chvostek's sign (unilateral twitching of the facial muscles) in some patients with hypocalcemia or hypomagnesemia.

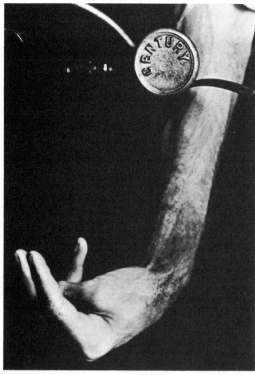

FIGURE 2–14.
Carpopedal attitude of hand (Trousseau's sign). (Ezrin C, Godden JO, Volpe R, Wilson R: Systematic Endocrinology, 2nd ed, p. 510. Hagerstown, MD, Harper & Row, 1979)

of the facial muscles, including the eyelid and lips. Chvostek's sign is indicative of hypocalcemia or hypomagnesemia.

To test for Trousseau's sign, place a blood pressure cuff on the arm and inflate above systolic pressure for 3 minutes. A positive reaction is the development of carpal spasm (Fig. 2-14).[22]

The common deep tendon reflexes include the biceps, triceps, brachioradialis, patellar, and Achilles reflexes.

A deep tendon reflex is elicited by briskly tapping a partially stretched tendon with a rubber percussion hammer, preferably over the tendon insertion of the muscle. The broad head of the hammer is used to stroke easily accessible tendons (eg, the Achilles) and the pointed end for less accessible tendons (eg, the biceps). The response in the prospective muscle is a sudden contraction. The muscle being tested should be slightly stretched (by the position of the limb), and the patient should be relaxed. With too little or too much muscle stretch the reflex cannot be elicited.

The reflexes are usually graded on a 0 to 4+ scale

- ▶ 0 = no response
- ▶ 1+ = somewhat diminished, but present
- ▶ 2+ = normal
- ▶ 3+ = brisker than average and possibly but not necessarily indicative of disease
- ▶ 4+ = hyperactive

Deep tendon reflexes may be hyperactive in the presence of hypocalcemia, hypomagnesemia, hypernatremia, and alkalosis. They may be hypoactive in the presence of hypercalcemia, hypermagnesemia, hyponatremia, hypokalemia, and acidosis.

Of course, many factors other than electrolyte disturbances can produce abnormalities in deep tendon reflexes. As with most other signs, deep tendon reflexes should be evaluated in light of other clinical signs, patient history, and laboratory data.

OTHER SIGNS

Other areas to consider in clinical assessment include changes in

- ▶ Behavior
- ▶ Sensation
- ▶ Fatigue level

Since these changes are often vague, they are best evaluated in context with specific imbalances (see Chapters 3 through 9).

EVALUATION OF LABORATORY DATA

Data from laboratory tests provide the nurse with valuable information about the patient's fluid and electrolyte status. However, it is important that specimens be collected properly to obtain valid results and that the findings be evaluated in light of the patient's history and clinical status. Treatment for an abnormality reported on an improperly performed laboratory test can be quite serious. For example, assume that the laboratory erroneously reports a serum potassium of 8.0 mEq/L (due to an accidentally hemolyzed blood sample) in a patient with an actual serum potassium of 4.0 mEq/L. Initiation of aggressive treatment for nonexistent hyperkalemia could reduce the serum level to dangerously low levels. When in doubt, it is wise to confirm a grossly abnormal test result.

OBTAINING SPECIMENS

Venous Blood Samples

Several general principles should be kept in mind when obtaining venous blood samples:

1. *Avoid drawing blood samples from a site above an infusing IV line.* Data from a recent study indicate that specimens for serum biochemical and hematologic profiles should be drawn from the opposite arm or *below* the IV while it is infusing or out of the IV needle after the IV fluids have been stopped for two minutes.[23]

   The study was conducted to address the question of where blood samples should be drawn in patients receiving IV fluids. Intravenous fluids were infused into the forearms of 18 healthy volunteers after baseline hematologic and serum biochemical profiles were obtained. Fluids (either 5% dextrose in water or 5% dextrose in half-normal saline) were administered at a rate of 125 mL/hr. Thirty minutes after beginning the infusions, blood was drawn from the opposite arm, and from above and below the IV in the same arm. The IV fluids were then stopped. After two minutes, another blood sample was drawn from the IV needle. In blood drawn from above the infusing IV a dilutional effect was apparent in most of the analytes, with results falling greater than two standard deviations below baseline levels; only serum glucose showed values above baseline. (Of note, serum glucose and phosphorus levels differed from preinfusion baseline levels regardless of sites from which they were drawn.)

2. Avoid conditions that can predispose to hemolysis of blood samples:[24]
   ▶ Skin too wet with antiseptics
   ▶ Prolonged use of tourniquet
   ▶ Use of small-gauge needle to withdraw a large volume of blood
   ▶ Vigorous shaking of the blood specimen
   Hemolysis of the sample is particularly disruptive when the test is for serum potassium, magnesium, or phosphate levels. (Recall that these electrolytes are primarily found *intra*cellularly; rupture of the blood cells causes a falsely high reading of serum levels.)

3. Avoid prolonged use of tight tourniquets and opening and closing of the patient's hand when drawing blood for potassium levels. A tight tourniquet around an exercising extremity (eg, an opening and closing hand) can elevate the plasma potassium as much as 2.7 mEq/L.[25]

4. It is recommended that a needle used to obtain blood samples for electrolyte determinations be at least 20 gauge in diameter.[26]

5. Be aware that the blood-drawing procedure should be performed as skillfully and atraumatically as possible. Watson et al[27] suggest that, when there is difficulty with phlebotomy, test results may show great variation and should be reviewed with care.

Arterial Blood Samples

See Chapter 9 for guidelines on obtaining arterial blood samples.

Urine Specimens

Twenty-Four-Hour Specimens

Since 24-hour urine specimens are often indicated in the measurement of urinary excretion of electrolytes, it is helpful to review the steps in the procedure:

1. Obtain a collection bottle from the laboratory; if a preservative is needed, it should be obtained with the bottle.
2. Follow directions from the laboratory with regard to any special preparation of the patient (for example, some tests may require dietary modifications or the withholding of certain drugs).
3. To begin collection, ask the patient to void and discard the specimen; note the exact time on the lab slip.
4. Save *all* urine for the next 24 hours and pour it into the collection bottle (omission of even one specimen invalidates the test).
5. Include a final voiding as close to 24 hours after the initiation of the test as possible (record exact finish time on lab slip).
6. For infants, obtain specimens in pasted-on collection devices.
7. Be sure to explain the test to the patient and gain his or her cooperation. This is imperative to any successful 24-hour test (for example, patients who are using bedpans should be instructed to void before having a bowel movement, and not to place toilet paper in the collection container).
8. Remind the staff and patient (with signs) of the importance of saving all urine.

Single Urine Specimens

For a single urine specimen, the first voided morning specimen is ideal because of its greater concentration. However, a fresh specimen collected at any time is reliable for most purposes. To avoid false readings, the specimen must be collected in a clean container. If a specimen is kept more than 1 hour before analysis, it should be refrigerated to avoid changes in the urine.

UNDERSTANDING TESTS USED TO MEASURE FLUID BALANCE

Blood and urine tests that can be used to assess fluid and electrolyte status are listed in Tables 2-3 and 2-4. Usual reference ranges for the tests and significance of

(text continues on page 34)

TABLE 2–3.
Blood Tests Used to Evaluate Fluid and Electrolyte Status

TEST	USUAL REFERENCE RANGE	COMMENTS
Serum potassium	3.5–5.0 mEq/L (3.5–5.0 mmol/L)	Alterations in acid–base balance significantly affect potassium distribution: ▶ Acidosis results in a shift of potassium out of the cells, causing the serum potassium concentration to increase. ▶ Alkalosis results in a shift of potassium into the cells, causing a decrease in serum potassium concentration. ▶ On the average, every 0.1 unit change in arterial pH causes a reciprocal change of 0.5 mEq/L in plasma potassium concentration.[28] ▶ Insulin promotes entry of extracellular potassium into cells and thus temporarily lowers the serum potassium concentration. There are a number of causes of factitious hyperkalemia.[29] ▶ Tight tourniquet around an exercising extremity (as in opening and closing the hand) can elevate potassium as much as 2.7 mEq/L ▶ Hemolysis of sample releases potassium from blood cells into the serum, thus elevating the serum potassium level ▶ Leukocytosis in range of 70,000 per cubic millimeter, as in leukemia, or platelet counts greater than one million per cubic millimeter (Leukocytes and platelets, which are rich in potassium, may release their large intracellular potassium stores during the clotting process.)
Serum sodium	135–145 mEq/L (135–145 mmol/L)	Serum sodium level is closely related to body water status: ▶ For the adult, it can be roughly estimated that each 3 mEq elevation of serum sodium above normal range represents a deficit of approximately 1 L of body water.[30] ▶ An elevated plasma glucose level pulls water out of the cells into the extracellular fluid; by dilution, this lowers the plasma sodium concentration. In theory, every 62 mg/dL increment increase in plasma glucose will draw enough water out of the cells to dilute the plasma sodium concentration 1 mEq/L.[31] For example, if the plasma glucose is 1000 mg/dL (930 mg/dL above normal), the plasma sodium should fall 15 mEq/L. This expected change does not always occur, however, because of the effect of osmotic diuresis associated with hyperglycemia. ▶ The measured plasma sodium concentration may be artifactually reduced when marked hyperlipidemia is present.[32]
Serum calcium	Total Calcium: 8.9–10.3 mg/dL (2.23–2.57 mmol/L) Total calcium in serum is the sum of the ionized (47%) and nonionized (53%) calcium components. The nonionized portion consists of calcium bound to albumin (40%) and the portion (13%) chelated to anions (such as citrate and phosphate).	▶ Total calcium is the test performed in most clinical settings. To evaluate the actual calcium level, the clinician must first know the serum albumin level to apply the following rule: In the noncritically ill, the total serum calcium may be corrected for variations in the serum albumin by estimating that a change in the serum albumin of 1.0 g/dL (10 g/L) will change the total serum calcium by 0.8 mg/dL (0.2 mmol/L).[33] ▶ The above estimation is not valid when situations are present that affect pH (which changes the percentage of ionized calcium) or the quantity of substances available to bind with calcium is altered. Alkalosis increases the binding of calcium to albumin, as does an increased free fatty acid level (common in stressed patients). Other factors that can acutely lower ionized calcium are increased levels of lactate, bicarbonate, citrate, phosphate, and some substances in radiographic contrast media.[34]

(continued)

TABLE 2–3.
(continued)

TEST	USUAL REFERENCE RANGE	COMMENTS
	Ionized Calcium: 4.6–5.1 mg/dL (1.15–1.27 mmol/L)	Many laboratories now have the capability to directly measure the ionized calcium level. This is desirable, especially in critically ill patients, since it is the ionized calcium that is physiologically active and thus clinically important. One should be aware that variations in the sample collection technique can affect the results. For example, acid–base changes from prolonged tourniquet application and variations in the amount of heparin in the collecting syringe can both artifactually alter the measured Ca^{++}.[35]
Serum magnesium	1.3–2.1 mEq/L (0.65–1.05 mmol/L)	Hemolysis of the sample will invalidate the results by releasing magnesium from the red blood cells into the serum (recall that magnesium is primarily an intracellular ion).
Serum chloride	97–110 mEq/L (97–110 mmol/L)	▶ Less than normal concentration indicates hypochloremia (commonly associated with hypokalemia and metabolic alkalosis). ▶ Greater than normal concentration indicates hyperchloremia, which may be associated with excessive administration of isotonic saline.
Carbon dioxide content	22–31 mEq/L (22–31 mmol/L)	▶ This test measures total bicarbonate and carbonic acid in venous blood and is a general measure of the degree of alkalinity or acidity. (It should not be confused with the partial pressure of carbon dioxide, pCO_2, obtained from arterial blood gas analysis.) ▶ A level below normal indicates metabolic acidosis. ▶ In the absence of chronic obstructive pulmonary disease, an elevated level indicates metabolic alkalosis.
Serum phosphate	2.5–4.5 mg/dL (0.81–1.45 mmol/L)	▶ Hemolysis of the sample will invalidate the results by releasing phosphate from the red blood cells into the serum (recall that phosphate is primarily an intracellular ion). ▶ Phosphate levels are evaluated in relation to calcium levels since there is an inverse relationship between the two (eg, an increased phosphorus level causes the calcium level to decrease). ▶ Phosphate levels normally higher in children than adults. ▶ Drugs containing high phosphate levels may temporarily increase the serum phosphate level for several hours after the dose. ▶ Insulin promotes entry of extracellular phosphorus into cells. ▶ Intravenous glucose running before or at the time of the test causes a lowered serum phosphorus level (due to carbohydrate metabolism).
Plasma ammonia	11–35 μmol/L (Reported values vary according to laboratory.)	▶ The body is less able to handle high ammonia levels when the serum potassium is low or when alkalosis is present. ▶ Ammonia level varies with protein intake and is affected by some antibiotics.
Serum osmolality	280–295 mOsm/kg Can be measured by lab or can be calculated by the following formula: $$pOsm = 2(Na) + \frac{G}{18} + \frac{BUN}{2.4}$$	▶ Serum osmolality is determined mainly by serum sodium concentration (recall that serum sodium makes up 90% of the osmotic pressure generated by plasma). ▶ Finding is increased in dehydration (hypernatremia). ▶ Finding is decreased in overhydration (hyponatremia). ▶ Finding is increased in hyperglycemia and in presence of elevated BUN

(continued)

TABLE 2–3.
(continued)

TEST	USUAL REFERENCE RANGE	COMMENTS
Anion gap	12–15 mEq/L $AG = Na - (Cl + HCO_3)$	▸ Anion gap is useful in ascertaining cause of metabolic acidosis. ▸ A level greater than 15 mEq/L indicates presence of excessive organic acids (as in diabetic ketoacidosis, lactic acidosis, uremic renal failure, and salicylate intoxication). ▸ Normal anion gap acidosis may be due to diarrhea, ureterostomies, excessive chloride administration, and distal tubular acidosis.
BUN	8–25 mg/dL (2.9–8.9 mmol/L)	▸ Elevated BUN can be due to reduced renal blood flow secondary to fluid volume deficit (causing reduced urea clearance). ▸ Excessive protein intake can elevate BUN by increasing urea production. ▸ Increased catabolism due to trauma, starvation, bleeding into the intestines, or catabolic drugs can also increase the BUN by increasing urea production. ▸ A low BUN is often associated with overhydration and may also be associated with low protein intake.
Creatinine	0.6–1.5 mg/dL (53–133 μmol/L)	▸ As an indicator of renal disease is more specific and sensitive than BUN since nonrenal causes of elevation are few. ▸ Test is useful in evaluating renal dysfunction when a large number of nephrons have been destroyed (not increased above normal until at least half of nephrons are nonfunctioning)[36] ▸ In patients with large muscle mass or acromegaly, it may be slightly above normal. ▸ A slightly elevated creatinine level may occur in severe fluid volume depletion, which results in a reduction in glomerular filtration rate.
BUN:creatinine ratio	10:1 (approximate)	▸ This ratio is useful in evaluating hydration status. ▸ When the ratio increases in favor of the BUN (ratio > 10:1), conditions such as hypovolemia, low perfusion pressures to the kidney, or increased protein metabolism may be present. ▸ When the ratio is < 10:1, conditions such as low protein intake, hepatic insufficiency, or repeated dialysis may be present. ▸ When both the BUN and creatinine levels rise, maintaining the 10:1 ratio, the problem is likely intrinsic renal disease (although it may also be seen when fluid volume depletion results in reduction in the glomerular filtration rate).
Hematocrit (%)	Male: 44–52 Female: 39–47	▸ Hematocrit determines the percentage of red blood cells in plasma. ▸ Changes are interpretable in terms of fluid balance only when no changes in the red blood cell mass (such as bleeding or hemolysis) are occurring. ▸ Hematocrit is elevated in fluid volume deficit (because red blood cells are contained in a relatively smaller plasma fluid volume). ▸ Hematocrit is decreased in fluid volume excess (because the red blood cells are contained in a relatively larger plasma fluid volume).
Fasting plasma glucose	65–110 mg/dL (3.58–6.05 mmol/L)	A markedly elevated glucose level in bloodstream causes osmotic diuresis and resultant fluid volume deficit. ▸ Results will be elevated above baseline if patient is receiving parenteral glucose (regardless of site from which the specimen is drawn.)[37]

(continued)

TABLE 2–3.
(continued)

TEST	USUAL REFERENCE RANGE	COMMENTS
Plasma lactate	0.3–1.3 mEq/L (0.3–1.3 mmol/L)	▶ Lactic acidosis is considered to be present if the plasma lactate level is greater than 4 to 5 mEq/L.[38] ▶ Most cases of lactic acidosis are due to marked tissue hypoperfusion. ▶ False low values occur with high lactic dehydrogenase levels; elevations may occur with exercise, alcohol, glucose, and sodium bicarbonate infusions.[39]
Albumin	3.5–4.8 g/dL (35–48 g/L)	▶ Decreased serum albumin level causes reduced colloidal osmotic pull in intravascular space, allowing fluid to shift to the interstitial space and produce edema. ▶ It is important to know the albumin level when evaluating total calcium values.

TABLE 2–4.
Urine Tests Used to Evaluate Fluid and Electrolyte Status

TEST	USUAL REFERENCE RANGE	COMMENTS
Urinary sodium	40–220 mEq/24 hr[40] (40–220 mmol/24 hr) Random specimen usually > 40 mEq/L[41] Varies with diet	▶ Less than 10–15 mEq/L in hypovolemic states, reflecting renal sodium conservation to maintain blood volume[42] ▶ Greater than 20 mEq/L in hypovolemic states associated with the following:[43] Underlying renal disease Diuretics (while drug is acting) Osmotic diuresis Hypoaldosteronism ▶ Greater than 20 mEq/L in SIADH and psychogenic polydipsia[44] ▶ Important to record dietary intake during 24-hour period because measurement of urinary sodium without knowledge of dietary intake is of limited value ▶ Urinary sodium levels must be evaluated in view of total clinical picture. ▶ To evaluate ECF volume contraction in patients with recent vomiting, it is preferable to use urinary Cl as an index rather than Na because the urine Na concentration is often not low in this instance.[45]
Urinary potassium	25–125 mEq/24 hr (25–125 mmol/24 hr) Random specimen usually > 40 mEq/L[46] Varies with diet	▶ Primary use of a 24-hour urine measurement for potassium is to assess hormonal functioning and to determine if hypokalemia is of renal or nonrenal origin[47] ▶ Amount of potassium in urine varies with amount of serum aldosterone or cortisol (increased amounts of which cause increased potassium excretion) ▶ Renal failure causes decreased potassium excretion in urine. ▶ In the presence of hypokalemia, excretion of less than 20 mEq/d is evidence that the hypokalemia is not from renal loss.[48]

(continued)

TABLE 2–4.
(continued)

TEST	USUAL REFERENCE RANGE	COMMENTS
Urinary chloride	110–250 mEq/24 hr (110–250 mmol/24 hr) Varies with salt intake	▸ Usually similar to that of sodium in hypovolemic states because sodium and chloride are generally reabsorbed together[49] ▸ Helpful in differentiating between types of metabolic alkalosis[50] Less than 10–15 mEq/L when metabolic alkalosis is due to vomiting, gastric suction, or diuretic use (late) Usually greater than 20 mEq/L when metabolic alkalosis is due to mineralocorticoid excess or profound potassium depletion[51]
Urinary calcium (quantitative) (qualitative, Sulkowitch's test)	50–300 g/24 hr in adults (depending on dietary intake)[52] Fine white cloud	▸ May be as high as 800–900 mg/24 hr in hypercalcemia associated with metastatic tumors[53] ▸ May be quite low when hypocalcemia is present ▸ Heavy white precipitate indicates more than normal calcium in urine ▸ Clear specimen indicates less than normal calcium in the urine ▸ Measured on single specimen by observing urine for precipitate after adding a few drops of calcium oxalate
Urinary specific gravity (SG)	1.003–1.035[54] Most random samples have SG of 1.012–1.025. Aged may have a lower range due to decreased renal concentrating ability.	▸ SG depends on the state of hydration and varies with the urine volume and the load of solutes to be excreted. ▸ SG is elevated in fluid volume deficit as the normal kidney seeks to retain needed fluid and thus excretes solutes in a small concentrated urine volume. ▸ SG fixed at 1.010 signals significant renal disease (isothenuria). ▸ Heavy molecules such as glucose, albumin, or dyes will elevate SG of urine out of proportion to the actual concentration. Thus, it is more accurate to measure urine osmolality in patients with glycosuria, proteinuria, or recent use of radiopaque dyes.
Urine osmolality	Typical urine is 500–800 mOsm/kg (extreme range is 50–1400 mOsm/kg)[55] After an overnight fast of 14 hours, the urine osmolality should be at least three times the serum osmolality.[56]	▸ Elevated in fluid volume deficit (healthy kidneys conserve needed fluid, causing urine to be more concentrated). ▸ Decreased in fluid volume excess (healthy kidneys excrete unneeded fluid, causing urine to be diluted). ▸ Simultaneous measurement of serum and urine osmolality is a more accurate way to measure renal concentrating ability than is urinary SG.
Urinary pH	4.5–8.0 Pooled daily output averages around 5.0; most random samples are less than 6.6.	▸ Urine pH reflects serum pH and helps confirm the presence of acidosis or alkalosis (with the exception of paradoxical aciduria in hypokalemic alkalosis, alkaline urine due to urea-splitting infections, and alkaline urine in renal tubular acidosis).[57] ▸ Finding is increased with use of alkalinizing agents such as sodium bicarbonate and potassium citrate. ▸ Urinary pH is decreased with use of acidifying agents such as ascorbic acid, sodium acid phosphate, and methenamine mandelate. ▸ Urine should be examined soon after collection because urine that is left standing too long becomes alkaline due to bacterial-induced splitting of urea into ammonia. ▸ Urinary pH normally fluctuates throughout the day.

ECF, extracellular fluid; SG, specific gravity; SIADH, syndrome of inappropriate antidiuretic hormone secretion.

variations are also included. Commonly used units of measures are reported with Système Internationale (S.I.) units in parentheses.

EVALUATING TEST RESULTS

Laboratory reports in the chart should be reviewed at regular intervals to note the patient's current status and to detect trends in the data. Because normal ranges for laboratory tests vary slightly from institution to institution, it is necessary to evaluate results according to those listed by the laboratory performing the tests. Also, one must consider variables that can affect the results of specific tests (Tables 2-3 and 2-4).

INITIATING NURSING INTERVENTIONS

After evaluating the significance of test results, initiate interventions as indicated. In some instances, the nurse can act independently (as in increasing oral intake in the patient with FVD). In other situations, the problem may require input from both nursing and medicine. In the latter situation, it is often the nurse who first detects the problem and initiates efforts to deal with it. For example, the nurse may note FVD in a patient unable to take oral fluids; in this situation, the nurse needs to seek medical directives for intravenous fluids, initiate the fluids, and monitor the patient's response to the therapy. Deciding whether or not the response is adequate requires good nursing judgment; when desired outcomes are not achieved, further collaboration between the nurse and physician is indicated to deal with the problem.

Nursing interventions required in specific fluid and electrolyte imbalances are more appropriately discussed in later chapters. See Chapters 3 through 9 for specific imbalances and later chapters for interventions indicated in commonly occurring clinical situations.

REFERENCES

1. Shoemaker et al: Textbook of Critical Care, 2nd ed, p 137. Philadelphia: WB Saunders, 1989
2. Pflaum S: Investigation of intake-output as a means of assessing body fluid balance. Heart Lung 8:495, 1979
3. Pestana C: Fluids and Electrolytes in the Surgical Patient, 4th ed, p 223. Baltimore, Williams & Wilkins, 1989
4. Stebor A: Posturination time and specific gravity in infants' diapers. Nurs Res 38(4): 244, 1989
5. Fisher R, Papoff P, Fisher A: The interstitial fluid monitor: A device to aid in the determination of patient fluid requirements. J Am Board Fam Pract 3:7–17, 1990
6. Schlegal-Pratt K, Heizer W: The accuracy of scales used to weigh patients. Nutr Clin Pract 5(6): 254, 1990
7. Condon R, Nyhus L: Manual of Surgical Therapeutics, 7th ed, p 170. Boston, Little, Brown, 1988
8. Snyder N, Feigal D, Arieff, A: Hypernatremia in elderly patients: A heterogenous, morbid, and iatrogenic entity. Ann Intern Med 107:309, 1987
9. Phillips et al: Reduced thirst after water deprivation in healthy elderly men. N Engl J Med 311:753, 1984.
10. Goldberger E: A Primer of Water, Electrolyte and Acid–Base Syndromes, 7th ed, p 34. Philadelphia, Lea & Febiger, 1986
11. Rose B: Clinical Physiology of Acid–Base and Electrolyte Disorders, 3rd ed, p 417. New York, McGraw-Hill, 1989
12. Ibid, p 420
13. Schrier R: Renal and Electrolyte Disorders, 3rd ed, p 96. Boston, Little, Brown, 1986
14. Condon, Nyhus, p 171
15. Askanazi J, Starker P, Weissman C: Fluid and Electrolyte Management in Critical Care, p 235. Boston, Butterworths, 1986
16. Ibid
17. Goldberger, p 34
18. Schwartz S, Shires T, Spencer F: Principles of Surgery, 4th ed, p 74. Baltimore, Williams & Wilkins, 1989
19. Condon, Nyhus, p 177
20. Kokko J, Tannen R: Fluids and Electrolytes, 2nd ed, p 72. Philadelphia, WB Saunders, 1990
21. Hudak C, Gallo B, Benz J: Critical Care Nursing, 5th ed, p 123. Philadelphia, JB Lippincott, 1990
22. Maxwell M, Kleeman C, Narins R: Clinical Disorders of Fluid and Electrolyte Metabolism, 4th ed, p 777. New York, McGraw-Hill, 1987
23. Watson K, O'Kell R, Joyce J: Data regarding blood drawing sites in patients receiving intravenous fluids. Am J Clin Pathol 79:119, 1983
24. Corbett J: Laboratory Tests in Nursing Practice, 2nd ed, p 9. East Norwalk, CT, Appleton-Century-Crofts, 1987
25. Schrier, p 235
26. Jaffe M, Skidmore L: Diagnostic and Laboratory Cards for Clinical Use. Bowie, MD, Robert J Brady, 1984
27. Watson et al, p 119
28. Condon, Nyhus, p 159
29. Schrier, p 235
30. Condon, Nyhus, p 164
31. Rose, p 685
32. Ibid, p 686
33. Olinger M: Disorders of calcium and magnesium metabolism. Emerg Med Clin North Am 7(4): 798, 1989
34. Ibid
35. Ibid
36. Corbett, p 88
37. Watson et al, p 119

38. Rose, p 514
39. Corbett, p 148
40. Ibid, p 111
41. Condon, Nyhus, p 173
42. Rose, p 371
43. Ibid
44. Ibid, p 354
45. Kamel et al: Urine electrolytes in the assessment of extracellular fluid volume contraction. Am J Nephrol 9:344, 1989
46. Condon, Nyhus, p 173
47. Corbett, p 117
48. Ibid
49. Rose, p 371
50. Ibid, p 490
51. Ibid
52. Corbett, p 163
53. Ibid
54. Fischbach F: A Manual of Laboratory Diagnostic Tests, 3rd ed, p 125. Philadelphia, JB Lippincott, 1988
55. Corbett, p 90
56. Ibid
57. Condon, Nyhus, p 173

unit two

OVERVIEW OF FLUID AND ELECTROLYTE PROBLEMS: NURSING CONSIDERATIONS

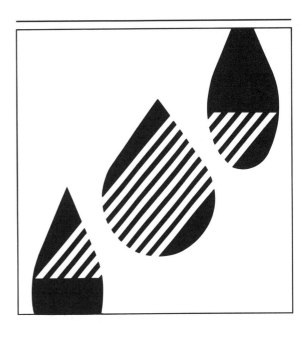

3

Fluid Volume Imbalances

Fluid volume imbalances are commonly seen in nursing practice. Although they may occur alone, they most frequently occur in combination with other imbalances. Thus, events leading to fluid volume disturbances also frequently lead to electrolyte problems. For the purposes of this chapter, however, fluid volume imbalances will be discussed in their "pure" form, that is, without the presence of other disturbances. There is much the nurse can do to prevent the occurrence of fluid volume imbalances, or at least decrease their severity. This chapter will describe assessment for fluid volume disturbances and explain rationales for nursing interventions.

ISOTONIC FLUID VOLUME DEFICIT

Fluid volume deficit (FVD) results when water and electrolytes are lost in an isotonic fashion (see Fig. 3-1). It should not be confused with the term "dehydration," which refers to a loss of water alone (leaving the patient with sodium excess). Fluid volume deficit may occur alone or in combination with other imbalances. Unless other imbalances are present concurrently, serum electrolyte levels remain essentially unchanged.

ETIOLOGICAL FACTORS

Fluid volume deficit is almost always due to loss of body fluids and occurs more rapidly when coupled with decreased intake for any reason. It *is* possible to develop FVD solely on the basis of inadequate intake, provided the decreased intake is prolonged.

Losses of Gastrointestinal Fluids

In review, many liters of gastrointestinal (GI) secretions are produced each day; most of these secretions are reabsorbed in the ileum and proximal colon, leaving only approximately 150 mL of relatively electrolyte-free fluid to be excreted daily in the feces. When any abnormal route of loss is present, such as vomiting, diarrhea, GI suction, fistulas, or drainage tubes, it becomes evident how large losses can occur (resulting in FVD).

Fluids trapped in the GI tract, as is the case with intestinal obstruction, are physiologically outside the body (third-space effect). Indeed, any condition that interferes with the absorption of fluids from the GI tract can cause serious FVD.

Polyuria

Any condition that causes excessive urine formation can produce FVD. This situation is commonly seen in patients with profound hyperglycemia, as either diabetic ketoacidosis or nonketotic hyperosmolar coma. To excrete a large solute load, the kidneys must also excrete a large urine volume. One also sees polyuria associated with a large solute load in individuals receiving hyperosmolar tube feedings. No matter what the cause of the high solute load, absence of sufficient exogenous fluid to allow for excretion of the solute will cause fluid to be "pulled in" from the plasma, tissue space, and even from the cells.

Fever

An elevated body temperature can cause FVD if extra fluids are not supplied as indicated. Fever causes an increase in metabolism and thus in formed metabolic wastes, which require fluid to make a solution for renal excretion; in this way, fluid loss is increased. Fever also causes hyperpnea, an increase in breathing resulting in extra water vapor loss through the lungs.

A temperature elevation between 101° F (38.3° C) and 103° F (39.4° C) generally increases the 24-hour fluid requirement in adults by at least 500 mL, and a temperature higher than 103° F (39.4° C) increases it by at least 1000 mL.[1] A respiratory rate greater than 35 per minute further increases fluid needs.[2] Individual patients must be assessed clinically to determine precise fluid requirements.

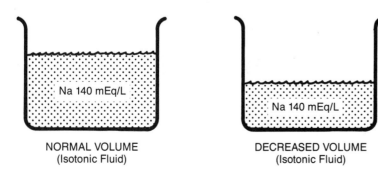

NORMAL VOLUME
(Isotonic Fluid)

DECREASED VOLUME
(Isotonic Fluid)

FIGURE 3–1.
Fluid volume deficit (sometimes called "isotonic dehydration").

Sweating

Recall that sweat is a hypotonic fluid containing primarily water, sodium, chloride, and potassium. Sweat can vary in volume from 0 to 1000 mL/hr, or more. Thus, it is conceivable that a person can become volume depleted from severe perspiration in the absence of adequate fluid replacement. Frequently, a sodium imbalance is superimposed on the volume depletion (either hyponatremia if excessive water is ingested, or hypernatremia if no liquids are consumed).

Third-Space Fluid Losses

Because third-space fluid losses are unique in character, a separate section has been devoted to this subject immediately after the discussion of FVD.

Decreased Intake

Unfortunately, several circumstances can interfere with normal fluid intake. Among these are anorexia, nausea, and fatigue. Patients unable to swallow because of neurological impairment are frequently noted to have at least some degree of FVD. Others prone to this condition are those who are reluctant to swallow because of oral or pharyngeal pain or those unable to gain access to fluids because of decreased mobility. Depression can be so severe as to interfere with normal fluid intake.

DEFINING CHARACTERISTICS

A fluid volume deficit can develop slowly or with great rapidity, and can be mild, moderate, or severe, depending on the degree of fluid loss. Important characteristics of FVD are discussed below and listed in the Summary of Fluid Volume Deficit.

Weight Loss

Rapid weight loss reflects loss of body fluid because fluctuations in lean body mass do not occur quickly. For example, it has generally been assumed that it takes a caloric deficit of approximately 3400 kcal to lose 1 lb (0.45 kg) of weight.[3] Theoretically, then, a typical adult on bedrest with a normal metabolism would have to take in zero calories to achieve a "real" weight loss of 1 lb in two days. On the other hand, a liter of fluid weighs approximately 2 lbs; this amount of fluid can easily be lost in a short period. Indeed, some patients lose much more than this quickly.

Decreased Skin and Tongue Turgor

Recall that in a normal person pinched skin will immediately fall back to its normal position when released. This elastic property, or turgor, is partially dependent on interstitial fluid volume. In a person with FVD, the skin may remain slightly elevated for many seconds after being pinched, indicating a deficit of fluid in the interstitial compartment (one segment of extracellular fluid). It is important to remember that, because tissue turgor also reflects the degree of skin elasticity, it is less valid as a sign of FVD in elderly persons. Chapter 2 provides helpful hints for testing skin turgor.

In a person with FVD, the tongue is smaller and has additional longitudinal furrows, again reflecting loss of interstitial fluid. Fortunately, tongue turgor is not affected appreciably by age and thus is a useful assessment for all age groups.

Decreased Moisture in Oral Cavity

A dry mouth may be due to FVD or to mouth breathing. If due to FVD, all of the oral tissues will be dry. In contrast, if the dryness is due to mouth breathing, the areas where the gums and cheek membranes meet will remain moist. If the serum sodium is elevated in conjunction with FVD, the mucous membranes will be dry and sticky.

Decreased Urinary Output

Decreased urinary output reflects inadequate perfusion of the kidney because there is not enough extracellular fluid (ECF) to bring the requisite amount of plasma to the glomeruli. A urine volume less than 30 mL/hr in an adult is cause for concern if it persists. One must be constantly aware that persistent oliguria in the severely volume depleted patient can result in renal tubular damage (discussed later in this chapter).

Increased Urinary Specific Gravity

Elevation of urinary specific gravity (SG) is a reflection of compensatory fluid conservation by the kidneys. Recall that urinary SG can range from 1.003 to 1.035 in normal situations. Thus, a healthy renal response would be one toward the upper limits of normal.

Disrupted Blood Urea Nitrogen/Creatinine Ratio

The blood urea nitrogen (BUN) level rises slowly out of proportion to the serum creatinine with a longstanding FVD of sufficient magnitude to reduce glomerular filtration rate, thus interfering with clearance of nitrogenous wastes.

Changes in Vital Signs

Body temperature is subnormal, due to decreased metabolism, unless infection is present. In contrast, note that body temperature is often elevated in patients with water deficit (hypernatremia), also referred to as "dehydration." Rectal temperatures as low as 95° F (35° C) to 97° F (36.1° C) have been ascribed to FVD in patients free of infection.[4]

Postural hypotension and increased pulse rate are signs of hypovolemia. On changing from a lying to an upright position, a drop in systolic pressure greater than 15 mmHg or an increase in the pulse rate greater than 15 beats/min suggests intravascular volume deficit.[5] As fluid volume depletion worsens, blood pressure (BP) becomes low in all positions due to loss of compensatory mechanisms. Tachycardia occurs as the heart pumps faster to compensate for the decreased plasma volume.

Changes in Central Venous Pressure and Peripheral Veins

The jugular veins provide a built-in manometer for following changes in central venous pressure, and thus fluid volume status, and do not involve an invasive maneuver. Direct measurement of central venous pressure is frequently performed in acutely ill patients and will reveal a reading less than normal in those with FVD (provided cardiopulmonary function is not impaired). Slow-filling hand veins are also indicative of FVD. Chapter 2 provides a description of the assessment of these parameters.

Other Changes

Altered sensorium is the result of decreased cerebral perfusion, secondary to decreased blood volume. Cold extremities reflect peripheral vasoconstriction, which occurs to build up central blood volume. The hematocrit is elevated above baseline due to loss of intravascular fluid and subsequent concentration of the formed elements of blood.

TREATMENT

In planning fluid replacement for the patient with FVD, it is necessary to consider usual maintenance fluid volume requirements and other factors (such as fever) that can influence fluid needs. When the deficit is not severe, the oral route is preferred for replacement, provided the patient is able to drink. However, when fluid losses are acute, the intravenous (IV) route is required. Chapter 11 discusses formulas used in determining maintenance as well as replacement fluid requirements.

Isotonic electrolyte solutions (such as lactated Ringer's or 0.9% NaCl) are frequently used to treat the hypotensive patient with FVD because such fluids expand plasma volume. As soon as the patient becomes normotensive, a hypotonic electrolyte solution (such as 0.45% NaCl) is often used to provide both electrolytes and free-water for renal excretion of metabolic wastes. These and additional fluids are discussed in Chapter 11.

If the patient with severe FVD is oliguric, it is necessary to determine whether the depressed renal function is the result of reduced renal blood flow secondary to FVD (prerenal azotemia) or, more seriously, to acute tubular necrosis due to prolonged FVD. The therapeutic test used in this situation is the *fluid challenge test.* One version of the test, as described by Goldberger,[6] is presented below.

1. An initial fluid test volume (200–300 mL in an adult) can be given over a 5- to 10-minute period provided the central venous pressure (CVP) is below 15 cm water; the patient should be observed for changes in the CVP, BP, and lung sounds.
   ▸ Constant CVP or pulmonary artery wedge monitoring is required to adequately assess the patient's response to the fluid load. A Foley catheter facilitates accurate measurement of urinary output.
   ▸ The type of fluid used for the fluid challenge depends on the clinical situation.
2. If the CVP remains unchanged or does not elevate more than 2 or 3 cm above the initial reading, the BP remains stable (or becomes elevated, if hypotension was initially present), and lung sounds remain normal or become no worse, an additional fluid load is given (200 mL over a 10-minute period).
3. If the CVP continues below 15 cm, and if vital signs remain unchanged, the infusion is continued at a rate of 500 mL/hr until the urinary output improves and other parameters (such as CVP and BP) return to normal. It is necessary to monitor the CVP, BP, and lung sounds every 15 minutes.
4. If the problem is prerenal azotemia, the urinary output will increase to more than 20 mL/hr within a few hours. Failure to induce an increased urinary output may indicate the presence of acute renal failure or urinary obstruction.
5. If the patient remains oliguric after the fluid load, and if the CVP and BP have returned to normal, it is necessary to determine whether the oliguria is still prerenal and will respond to further expansion of the blood volume, or whether the volume depletion has led to acute renal failure. If renal failure has occurred, the administration of additional fluids can be dangerous. The physician may elect to use the mannitol infusion test or IV injection of furosemide to evaluate the situation further.

Be aware that prompt treatment of FVD is imperative to prevent the occurrence of renal damage. If

FVD is allowed to progress to acute tubular necrosis, the patient will require strict renal management (see Chap. 18).

NURSING INTERVENTIONS

1. Assess for presence, or worsening, of FVD:
   - Measure and evaluate intake and output (I & O) at 8-hour intervals at least; sometimes hourly measurements are critical. For a valid picture of the patient's fluid balance status, total I & O measurements for 2 or 3 consecutive days and compare (see section on I & O in Chap. 2).
   - Monitor daily body weights. Consider factors necessary to obtain accurate readings (see Chap. 2). Remember that an acute weight loss of 1 lb represents a fluid loss of approximately 500 mL.
   - Monitor for postural hypotension (that is, a drop in the systolic reading >15 mmHg when the patient is moved from a lying to sitting position).
   - Monitor for tachycardia (pulse increase >15 beats/min) particularly when patient is moved from a lying to sitting position.
   - Monitor skin and tongue turgor (see Chap. 2).
   - Monitor condition of mucous membranes. Remember that oral membranes will be dry in a mouth breather regardless of fluid status. When in doubt, run a finger over the gum folds to determine if dryness is present; if it is, FVD is likely present.
   - Monitor concentration of urine; use a urinometer if one is available (see Chap. 2). Be aware that a low urinary SG in the presence of oliguria is a sign of renal disease. In a volume depleted patient the urinary SG should be above 1.020 (indicating healthy renal conservation of fluid).
   - Monitor BUN/creatinine ratio. In FVD, BUN will elevate out of proportion to serum creatinine level (see Table 2-3).
   - Monitor CVP and pulmonary artery wedge pressures if devices are in use. Central venous pressure monitoring is discussed in Chapter 2, wedge pressures in Chapter 19.
   - Monitor body temperature; be aware that it will drop below normal when isotonic FVD is moderate or severe, unless infection is present. (Rectal temperatures of 95° F [35° C] have been observed in severe FVD.)
   - Monitor level of sensorium; expect that it will decrease as FVD progresses in severity.
2. Give oral fluids if indicated.
   - Consider the patient's "likes" and "dislikes" when offering fluids.
   - Consider the type of fluid the patient has lost. For example, one would select fluids containing sodium and potassium for a patient who has a FVD due to vomiting. See Tables 3-1 and 25-4 for the electrolyte content of commonly available beverages. See Table 16-1 for a summary of the electrolyte content of selected body fluids.
   - If the patient is reluctant to drink because of oral discomfort, select fluids that are nonirritating to the mucosa, and provide frequent mouth care (offer saline gargles and apply lubricant to lips).
   - Offer fluids at frequent intervals.
   - Explain the need for fluid replacement to the patient and attempt to gain his or her cooperation.
   - Administer medications as needed if nausea is present to provide relief before fluids are offered.
3. Consider the following interventions for patients with impaired swallowing:
   - Assess gag reflex and ability to swallow water before offering solid foods; have a suction apparatus on hand.
   - Position the patient upright with head and neck flexed slightly forward during feeding (tilting the head backward during swallowing predisposes to aspiration because this position opens the airway).
   - Provide thick fluids or semi-solid foods (such as puddings or gelatin). These are more easily swallowed because of their consistency and weight than are thin liquids.[7]
4. If the patient is unable to eat and drink, discuss the possibility of tube feedings with the physician.
5. Consult with the physician for parenteral fluid directives if the patient is unable to consume fluids by the enteral route. This intervention is important to prevent renal damage related to prolonged FVD.
   - Be aware that the IV route is favored in acute situations and when large volumes of fluid are needed.
6. Be aware that a carefully kept I & O record is necessary to determine the amount and type of fluids to be administered. Usually, abnormally lost fluids are replaced in the volume that has been lost.
7. Be familiar with the usual types of fluids used to treat FVD (review Treatment above and see Chapter 11).
8. Understand principles of fluid challenge test and parameters for nursing assessment (see Treatment above).
9. Monitor response to fluid intake, either orally or parenterally. If therapy is adequate, one should observe the following:
   - Increased urinary volume, toward 40 to 60 mL/hr in adult

TABLE 3–1.
Electrolyte Content of Selected Beverages

BEVERAGE	SODIUM (mg)	POTASSIUM (mg)	CALCIUM (mg)	MAGNESIUM (mg)	PHOSPHORUS (mg)
Orange juice, canned, 8 fl oz	6	436	21	27	36
Tomato juice, 6 fl oz	658	400	16	20	34
Peach nectar, canned, 8 fl oz	17	101	13	11	16
Dole pineapple juice, canned, 6 fl oz	2	280	28		17
Prune juice, canned, 8 fl oz	11	706	30	36	64
Black tea, instant, 1 tsp	1	46	0	3	3
Coffee, powdered instant, 1 round tsp	1	64	3	6	5
Pepsi Cola, 12 fl oz	2		0		55
Diet Pepsi Cola, 12 fl oz	2	30	0		29
Diet Coca-Cola, 12 fl oz	8	18			24
Sprite, 12 fl oz	46	0			
Thirst Quencher, bottled, 8 fl oz	96	26	0	1	22
Kool-aid, powdered, all flavors, 8 fl oz	8	1	15		8
Tang, orange, powdered, 6 fl oz	2	45	20		12
Milk, 2% fat, 8 fl oz	122	377	297	33	232
Beef broth, 1 cube	864	15		2	8
Chicken broth, 1 cube	1152	18		3	9

Pennington J, Church H: Bowes and Church's Food Values of Portions Commonly Used, 15th ed, Philadelphia, JB Lippincott, 1989; with permission

---

▶ If previously hypotensive, increased BP toward normal
▶ Return of pulse rate to baseline
▶ Improved sensorium and sense of vitality
▶ Improved skin and tongue turgor
▶ Decreased dryness of oral mucosa
▶ Increased CVP, toward normal
▶ Normal, or no worse, breath sounds
▶ Decreased urinary SG as urinary volume increases
▶ Increased body weight, toward preillness level

10. Report inadequate response to fluid therapy to physicians and seek appropriate fluid directives before renal damage occurs.
11. Monitor patients with tendency for abnormal fluid retention (such as renal or cardiac problems) for signs of overload during aggressive fluid replacement.
   ▶ A cardiac patient requiring fluid replacement for FVD should be monitored with pulmonary wedge pressures or CVP determinations during fluid replacement.[8]

12. When administering fluids, either orally or parenterally, consider other illnesses that are occurring concurrently.
   ▶ For example, patients with syndrome of inappropriate antidiuretic hormone secretion (SIADH), potential or actual increased intracranial pressure, renal failure, or preeclampsia require complex management. (These conditions are discussed in later chapters.)
13. Take safety precautions if altered sensorium is present.
14. Turn patient frequently; apply moisturizing agents to skin and massage bony prominences to avoid skin breakdown.
15. Give frequent oral care.

Case Studies

1. An 80-year-old man developed FVD as a result of overzealous diuretic use. After a 13-lb weight loss over 4 days, the CVP dropped to 1 cm of water. Skin turgor over the sternum and medial aspect of the thigh was poor (when skin was pinched, it remained

---

Summary of Fluid Volume Deficit

ETIOLOGICAL FACTORS	DEFINING CHARACTERISTICS
Loss of water and electrolytes, as in: ▸ Vomiting ▸ Diarrhea ▸ Excessive laxative use ▸ Fistulas ▸ GI suction ▸ Polyuria ▸ Fever ▸ Excessive sweating ▸ Third-space fluid shifts Decreased intake, as in: ▸ Anorexia ▸ Nausea ▸ Inability to gain access to fluids ▸ Depression	Weight loss over short period (except in third-space losses) ▸ 2% (mild deficit, such as 2.4-lb loss in 120-lb person) ▸ 5% (moderate deficit, such as 6-lb loss in 120-lb person) ▸ 8% or > (severe deficit, such as 10-lb loss or > in 120-lb person) Decreased skin and tongue turgor Dry mucous membranes Urine output < 30 mL/hr in adult Postural hypotension (systolic pressure drops by more than 15 mmHg when patient moves from lying to standing or sitting position) Weak, rapid pulse Slow-filling peripheral veins Decreased body temperature, such as 95°–98° F (35°–36.7° C) unless infection is present Central venous pressure less than 4 cm of water in vena cava BUN elevated out of proportion to serum creatinine Urinary specific gravity high Hematocrit elevated Flat neck veins in supine position Marked oliguria, late Altered sensorium Cold extremities, late

---

elevated for 6 seconds). Urine output was low at 20 mL/hr and the BUN was greatly elevated at 80 mg/dL (normal is 10–20 mg/dL). Body temperature was 97.4° F (36.3° C), pulse was 96 and weak in volume, and BP was 140/90 supine and 122/84 in a sitting position.

Commentary: This patient had lost 6 L of fluid in a relatively short period; his CVP was far below the normal level of 4 to 11 cm of water. His BUN was elevated; the urine volume was low, particularly for an elderly person. These factors, plus positional hypotension and increased pulse rate, were indicative of FVD. Note that the body temperature was not elevated, probably reflecting the slowed metabolic rate associated with FVD not complicated by infection.

2. A 35-year-old woman developed FVD after 4 days of severe diarrhea and poor intake. She weighed 119 lb on admission (preillness weight 128 lb). Her BUN was 40 mg/dL and serum creatinine was 1.3 mg/dL. Skin turgor was poor and urine output was 15 mL/hr (SG 1.030). Blood pressure was 120/80 recumbent and fell to 98/60 when erect. Pulse was 110, weak, and regular.

Commentary: This patient lost 7% of her body weight in 4 days; her BUN was twice normal whereas her serum creatinine was normal. Postural hypotension, poor turgor, and oliguria, all point to FVD.

THIRD-SPACING OF BODY FLUIDS

Third-spacing of body fluids is a unique situation leading to decreased intravascular volume and largely presenting with the same characteristics as those of FVD. However, because it is more difficult to diagnose than direct loss of body fluids, it is given a separate section in this chapter. In addition, third-space fluid losses are discussed in the clinical chapters dealing with specific conditions associated with this phenomenon.

DEFINITION

Third-spacing refers to a shift of fluid from the vascular space into a portion of the body from which it is not easily exchanged with the rest of the ECF. These third-space losses stem from the vascular portion of the ECF and thus produce a deficit in the ECF volume. The trapped fluid, although still technically within the body, is essentially unavailable for functional use. Termed *nonfunctional* because it is not able to participate in the normal functions of the ECF compartment, the third-spaced fluid might just as well have been lost externally. Fluid can be sequestered from the intravascular space into potential body spaces (such as the pleural, peritoneal, pericardial, or joint cavities) or it can become trapped in the bowel by obstruction or in the interstitial space as edema after burns or other trauma. Further, it can be trapped in inflamed tissue, as in peritonitis, pancreatitis, or fasciitis.

Major considerations in differentiating the FVD associated with third-spacing from that associated with fluid lost through vomiting or diarrhea are that (1) the latter fluid losses can be observed and measured whereas the former cannot; and (2) decreased body weight does not occur in third-spacing as it does in actual fluid loss. Indeed, patients with third-spacing may *gain* weight as IV fluids are administered to replace the diminished intravascular volume.

PHASES OF THIRD-SPACE FLUID SHIFTS AND ASSOCIATED CLINICAL MANIFESTATIONS

Third-space fluid shifts occur in two phases. The first is described above and involves a shift of fluid from the intravascular space into a nonfunctional fluid space. Clinical manifestations expected with a significant shift of fluid are essentially those of FVD because, although the fluid is in the body, it is functionally unavailable for use. During this period, expect the following:

- Tachycardia and hypotension (effective blood volume is reduced as the fluid shifts out of the vascular space)
- Urine volume less than 30 mL/hr in the adult (decreased plasma volume causes a fall in renal perfusion and thus less urine formation)
- High urinary SG and osmolality (renal attempt to conserve needed water)
- Elevated hematocrit (red blood cells become suspended in a smaller plasma volume as the fluid shifts out of the intravascular space)
- Postural hypotension
- Low CVP
- Poor skin and tongue turgor
- Insignificant body weight changes

During this phase, the body attempts to compensate for the third-space losses of ECF by renal conservation of sodium and water. Transfer of intracellular fluid (ICF) to the extracellular compartment for replenishment of the third-space fluid loss is insignificant.[9] As with any cause of FVD, it is important to correct the reduced plasma volume before renal perfusion is compromised to the extent that acute tubular necrosis occurs.

After a variable number of days, the fluid shifts back to the vascular space and may impose a temporary hypervolemia. Resolution of the third-space is slower than its accumulation. In some instances the shift of fluid back to the intravascular space occurs within 48 to 72 hours. In others, it may not occur for 10 days or longer.[10] As the extra fluid in the tissues or body spaces shifts back into the intravascular compartment, it is excreted through the kidneys. During this phase, fluid administration is carefully regulated to prevent circulatory overload. Assessment is primarily directed at detecting hypervolemia before serious effects occur. For example, observe for polyuria (hourly urine volume may be as high as 200 mL as the excess fluid is excreted), distended neck veins (a sign of fluid overload), moist lung sounds, shortness of breath, elevated CVP, and elevated systolic BP. In some situations, diuretics may be necessary to aid in the removal of excess fluid volume in the vascular space.[11]

PATHOPHYSIOLOGY OF CLINICAL SITUATIONS ASSOCIATED WITH THIRD-SPACE FLUID SHIFTS

Sequestration of fluids (third-spacing) is at least partially the result of altered capillary permeability due to injury, ischemia, or inflammation.[12] Because the third-space fluid stems from the ECF, it understandably has the same composition as the ECF. The magnitude of these losses is often greater than losses due to I & O imbalance but is more difficult to recognize. Redistribution of fluid within the body does not appear as a change in the patient's weight or on the fluid I & O records; instead, these losses can be detected only by physiological changes in organ function.

If there is no oral or IV intake of fluid, the effective circulating volume will decline to a point at which hypotension develops. If fluids are replaced to maintain the vascular volume, the ECF volume will expand and be reflected in weight gain. Because the exact mechanism of third-spacing varies somewhat with the specific cause, it is helpful to consider each separately.

Nonthermal Trauma and Surgery

Traumatic injury results in redistribution of intravascular fluid into the area of injury, thereby reducing the functional ECF volume. The volume of third-spacing varies with the severity of injury. For example, a patient with a fractured hip may lose 1500 to 2000 mL of blood into the tissues surrounding the injury site.[13] Although this fluid will eventually reabsorb (over a period of days or weeks), the deficit can cause an acute reduction in the vascular volume if it is not replaced.

Varying degrees of third-spacing occur in surgical procedures and are related to tissue manipulation and injury. The amount of fluid lost from the extracellular space varies with the extent and nature of the surgical undertaking. Minor operative procedures (such as appendectomy) are associated with considerably less fluid sequestration than are major operative procedures (such as extensive retroperitoneal dissection).[14] For example, a simple laparotomy with a total small bowel exploration can result in 700 mL of ECF distributional loss, whereas an extensive colon resection can cause as much as 2 to 3 L of ECF to sequester into the peritoneal cavity in 2 to 4 hours.[15] After abdominal surgery, particularly pelvic surgery, fluid accumulates in the peritoneum, bowel wall, and other traumatized tissues. Formation of a third-space after nonthermal traumatic injury occurs immediately and is maximal by 5 to 6 hours.[16] Unrecognized deficits of ECF during the early postoperative period are manifested primarily as circulatory instability; signs of volume deficiency in other organ systems may be delayed for several hours with this type of fluid loss.[17]

Burns

Altered capillary permeability of burned tissue results in an exudation of plasma at the burn site. There is also an increase in fluid flux across capillaries in nonburned tissue that apparently results from hypoproteinemia rather than an alteration in capillary permeability. Formation of edema occurs primarily in the first 24 hours, with the greatest losses being incurred during the first 8 hours. For this reason, thermally injured patients should receive 50% of their estimated fluid losses in the first 8 hours; colloids should be given on the second day to minimize edema formation in the nonburned tissue.[18]

Intestinal Obstruction

Patients suffering from mechanical intestinal obstruction or from adynamic ileus may sequester large quantities of ECF equal to many liters.[19] In acute intestinal obstruction, as much as 6 L or more can accumulate within the lumen and wall of the gut.[20] Although it is difficult to calculate the actual volume of sequestered fluid in bowel obstruction, the presence of air fluid levels on an upright abdominal radiograph generally indicates a minimum of 1500 mL of fluid within the lumen of the gut.[21]

Inflammation of Intraabdominal Organs

Important third-space fluid losses can occur into the peritoneum, the bowel wall, and other tissues in the resence of inflammatory lesions of the intraabdominal orans. The extent of these losses may not be fully appreciated unless one considers that the peritoneum alone has approximately 1 m² of surface area.[22] A slight increase in thickness from sequestration of fluid may result in a functional loss of several liters of fluid.[23] Swelling of the bowel wall and mesentery and secretion of fluid into the lumen of the bowel will cause even larger losses.

Sepsis

Sepsis produces a generalized capillary leak that produces a decrease in the functional ECF volume (while producing interstitial edema).[24] As sepsis persists, protein malnutrition produces hypoproteinemia, which in turn may increase the formation of edema. Therefore, the administration of colloid solutions during early sepsis when a capillary leak is present (in the absence of hypoproteinemia) may be unadvisable as it may serve to increase tissue edema further; once hypoproteinemia ensues, colloid administration may be helpful.[25]

Pancreatitis

In pancreatitis, inflammation and autodigestion by pancreatic enzymes lead to peripancreatic edema as well as fluid loss into the retroperitoneal tissue. A dramatic decrease in plasma volume (as much as 30% to 40% over a 6-hour period) causes systemic hypovolemia.[26] Associated clinical signs of fluid loss include hypotension, tachycardia, oliguria, and increased hematocrit due to hemoconcentration. (In the presence of hemorrhagic pancreatitis, the hematocrit may drop rather than elevate.) A balanced electrolyte solution, such as lactated Ringer's solution, is usually sufficient to replace fluid lost into the retroperitoneum.[27] However, in severe cases of hemorrhagic pancreatitis, blood products and colloid solutions are also indicated.

Ascites

Ascites in hepatic cirrhosis accumulates slowly enough for renal sodium and water retention to replenish the circulating blood volume while at the same time causing symptoms of edema. However, patients with marked ascites may suffer significant third-space fluid problems after rapid removal of ascites by paracentesis because the fluid quickly reaccumulates and may significantly decrease the circulating intravascular volume, producing hypotension and other signs of circulatory instability.[28] For this reason, ascites is usually managed with sodium restriction and diuretics rather than rapid direct removal. See Chapter 15 for a discussion of the pathophysiology of ascites formation in patients with liver disease.

FLUID REPLACEMENT

Treatment is directed at correcting the cause of the third-space shift of body fluids. As is the case with any cause of FVD, the reduced plasma volume must be corrected before renal damage occurs.

Most third-space losses are properly replaced with a balanced salt solution such as lactated Ringer's solution. Attempts to correct the fluid deficit with hypotonic solutions (such as 5% dextrose in water or half-strength saline) are not recommended because clinically significant hyponatremia may result.[29] Any deficits in red blood cell mass should be corrected by the administration of packed cells or whole blood to maintain optimal oxygen-carrying capacity of the blood. Large quantities of replacement fluids are often needed to maintain an effective circulating volume.

A distinction is made between those processes that lead to significant protein depletion (such as burns and peritonitis) and those that do not (such as intestinal obstruction and pleural effusion).[30] In the former conditions, plasma or plasma substitutes are given as well as replacement electrolyte solutions.[31]

Fluid replacement therapy must be tailored to the patient's response. For example, during the first phase, when fluid has shifted from the intravascular space, the aim of fluid therapy is to stabilize BP and pulse and maintain an adequate urine volume (usually 30–50 mL/hr). Although an adequate hourly urine output is usually a reliable index of volume replacement, it may be misleading when excessive administration of glucose (more than 50 g in a 2- to 3-hr period) has occurred, possibly producing osmotic diuresis, or when an osmotic agent such as mannitol has produced urine formation at the expense of the vascular volume.[32] Also, recall that patients with chronic renal disease or incipient acute renal damage from shock and injury may have inappropriately high urinary volumes.

FLUID VOLUME EXCESS

Fluid volume excess (FVE) is the result of the abnormal retention of water and sodium in approximately the same proportions in which they normally exist in the ECF (see Fig. 3-2). It is always secondary to an increase in the total body sodium content, which, in turn, leads to an increase in total body water. Because there is isotonic retention of both substances, the serum sodium concentration remains essentially normal.

ETIOLOGICAL FACTORS

This imbalance may be caused by simple overloading with fluids or by diminished function of the homeo-

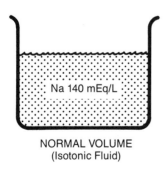

NORMAL VOLUME
(Isotonic Fluid)

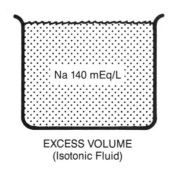

EXCESS VOLUME
(Isotonic Fluid)

FIGURE 3–2.
Fluid volume excess.

static mechanisms responsible for regulating fluid balance. Etiological factors can include the following:

1. Compromised regulatory mechanisms, as in congestive heart failure, renal failure, cirrhosis of the liver, and steroid excess.
2. Overzealous administration of sodium-containing fluids, particularly to patients with impaired regulatory mechanisms. The commonly used isotonic fluids, 0.9% NaCl and lactated Ringer's solution, contain sizable amounts of sodium and, if used to excess, can easily exceed the tolerance of patients with impaired regulatory mechanisms. Note that 0.9% NaCl contains 154 mEq/L of sodium and that lactated Ringer's has 130 mEq/L.
3. Excessive ingestion of sodium chloride or other sodium salts in the diet. See Table 3-3 for sodium content of compounds used to improve texture or flavor of food, or to extend freshness. Other "hidden" gains of sodium may result from the use of proprietary drugs such as Alka-Seltzer or the frequent use of hypertonic enemas (such as Fleet enema).

DEFINING CHARACTERISTICS

The defining characteristics of FVE are linked with an excess of fluid in the extracellular compartment and are listed in the Summary of Fluid Volume Excess.

TREATMENT

Therapy is directed at the causative factors when possible, such as reversal of cardiac failure due to hypothyroidism by thyroid hormone replacement. When reversal of the primary problem is impossible, symptomatic treatment often consists of restriction of sodium and fluids and the administration of diuretics. In some conditions, only one of these therapies is necessary. Sodium-restricted diets and diuretic administration are discussed below, along with the effect of bedrest on mobilization of edematous fluid.

Sodium-Restricted Diets

Sodium content in foods may be expressed as grams of salt, milligrams of sodium, or milliequivalents of sodium. To understand conversions of grams of salt to grams of sodium, recall that sodium represents about 40% of the weight of salt (sodium chloride). Therefore, a gram of sodium chloride is equivalent to 0.4 g of sodium. Dietary prescriptions are more sensibly stated in terms of sodium rather than salt content. According to usual definitions, a mildly restricted diet contains 4 to 5 g of sodium, a moderately restricted one contains 2 g, and a severely restricted diet contains 0.5 g of sodium.[33] To convert milligrams of sodium to milliequivalents, divide the number of milligrams by 23 (the atomic weight of sodium); for example, 1000 mg of sodium is equivalent to 43 mEq of sodium.

The typical diet in Western societies greatly exceeds daily sodium needs.[34] Of the total dietary sodium, approximately one third comes from the salt shaker, one third from processed foods, and one third from the food itself.[35] Recall that processed foods often have hidden sources of sodium in the form of preservatives, such as monosodium glutamate, baking powder, baking soda, brine, and disodium phosphate. Tables 3-1 and 3-2 list the sodium and potassium contents of some common beverages and foods. Table 3-3 summarizes the sodium content of common food additives. These figures clearly indicate how plentiful sodium is in the average diet.

Sodium-restricted diets are commonly prescribed for patients with fluid excess problems, such as occur with congestive heart failure, hepatic failure with ascites, renal failure, and hypertension. Some patients do well with only mildly restricted diets while others require severe restrictions. A mild sodium-restricted diet requires only light salting of food (about half the usual amount) in cooking and at the table, no addition of salt to foods that are already seasoned (such as canned foods and foods ready to cook or eat), and avoidance of foods that are high in sodium. Examples of such foods include the following:

► Sauerkraut and other vegetables prepared in brine
► Bacon, luncheon meats, frankfurters, ham, kosher meats, and sausages
► Relish, horseradish, catsup, mustard, and Worcestershire sauce
► Processed cheese
► Olives and pickles
► Potato chips, pretzels, and other salty snack foods
► Bouillon cubes

Patients should be made aware that most canned and ready-to-eat foods already have added salt and thus should be used only as their specific diets allow. Foods that may be used freely include most fresh vegetables and fruits and unprocessed cereals. Cooking from scratch is usually the best way to prepare low-sodium food, and several excellent cookbooks are available for this purpose. Low-sodium baking powder can be found in the dietetic section of many grocery stores, and low-sodium milk, milk products, and bakery goods are available in most large cities.

Because a substantial portion of sodium is ingested in the form of seasoning, use of substitute seasonings plays a major role in cutting sodium intake. Lemon juice, onion, and garlic are excellent substitute flavor-

TABLE 3–2.
Sodium, Potassium, and Caloric Content of Various Foods

FOOD	SODIUM (mg)	POTASSIUM (mg)	CALORIES
Fruits:			
Apple, raw with skin, 1 medium	1	159	81
Apricots, raw, 3 medium	1	313	51
Banana, raw, 1 medium	1	451	105
Raisins, golden seedless, ⅔ cup	12	746	302
Orange, navel, raw, 1 medium	1	250	65
Vegetables:			
Carrot, raw, 1 medium	25	233	31
Potato, baked, without skin, 1	8	610	145
Tomato, raw, 1	10	254	24
Spinach, canned, ½ cup	29	370	25
Meats:			
Bologna, beef, 1 slice	226	36	72
Frankfurter, beef, 1 frank (8/1-lb pkg)	585	94	180
Turkey, roasted, light meat, without skin, 3.5 oz	64	305	157
Cereals:			
Cheerios, General Mills, 1¼ cups	290	105	111
Corn flakes, Kellogg's, 1¼ cups	351	26	110
Grape-Nuts, Post, ¼ cup	188	85	104
Raisin-Bran, Kellogg's, ¾ cup	269	192	115

Pennington J, Church H: Bowes and Church's Food Values of Portions Commonly Used, 15th ed. Philadelphia, JB Lippincott, 1989; with permission

TABLE 3–3.
Sodium Content of Common Food Additives

ADDITIVE	SODIUM CONTENT
Salt	2300 mg/tsp
Baking powder (Calumet)	426 mg/tsp
Baking powder (sodium aluminum silicate)	1205 mg/tbl
Mustard, brown	65 mg/tsp
Catsup	156 mg/tbl
Horseradish, prepared	14 mg/tbl
Soy sauce	3300 mg/¼ cup
Worcestershire sauce (Heinz)	234 mg/tbl

Adapted from Pennington J, Church H: Bowes and Church's Food Values of Portions Commonly Used, 15th ed. Philadelphia, JB Lippincott, 1989

ing agents, although some patients prefer salt substitutes. Most salt substitutes contain potassium and should be used cautiously by those taking potassium-conserving diuretics (listed in Table 3-4) and by those who have renal impairment. Salt substitutes containing ammonium chloride can be harmful to patients with liver damage. (Salt substitutes are discussed further in Chapter 5 and are listed in Table 5-4).

In certain communities, the drinking water may contain too much sodium for a sodium-restricted diet. Depending on its source, water may have as little as 1 mg or more than 1500 mg/L. When the local water supply has a high sodium content, it may be necessary for patients to use distilled water. Also, patients on sodium-restricted diets should be cautioned to avoid water softeners that add sodium to water in exchange for other ions, such as calcium. Finally, patients on sodium-restricted diets should consider the sodium content in "over-the-counter" drugs. For example, one Alka-Seltzer tablet contains 311 mg of sodium.[36]

Diuretics

Diuretics are commonly used drugs that promote increased urine flow. More specifically, they act by inhibiting salt and water reabsorption by the kidney tubules. By inducing a negative fluid balance, these medications are useful in the treatment of conditions associated with FVE.

For the most part, diuretics can be grouped into three major classes:

▶ Loop diuretics (such as furosemide, bumetanide, and ethacrynic acid), which act in the thick ascending loop of Henle
▶ Thiazide-type diuretics (such as chlorothiazide and hydrochlorothiazide), which act in the distal tubule and connecting segment
▶ Potassium-sparing diuretics (such as amiloride, spironolactone, and triamterene), which act in the cortical collecting tubule

Examples of other diuretics are acetazolamide, a carbonic anhydrase inhibitor, and mannitol, a nonreabsorbable polysaccharide that acts as an osmotic diuretic.

To achieve excretion of excess fluid, either a single diuretic (such as a thiazide) or a combination of agents may be selected (such as thiazide and spironolactone). The latter combination is particularly helpful in that the two drugs have different sites of action and thus allow more effective control of FVE.

Diuretics can have undesirable effects. Following are some that affect fluid and electrolyte balance:

▶ Extracellular fluid volume depletion
▶ Hyponatremia
▶ Alterations in potassium excretion

TABLE 3–4.
Commonly Used Diuretic Agents

DRUG	COMMENTS
Thiazides Examples: chlorothiazide (Diuril), hydrochlorothiazide (Esidrix)	Act by inhibiting sodium reabsorption in the distal tubule and, to a lesser extent, the inner medullary collecting duct Cause loss of sodium, chloride, and potassium Decrease urinary calcium excretion and sometimes result in slightly elevated serum calcium level Potassium supplements or extra dietary potassium may be necessary when these agents are used routinely
Loop diuretics Examples: furosemide (Lasix), ethacrynic acid (Edecrin), bumetanide (Bumex)	Powerful diuretics that act primarily in the thick segment of the medullary and cortical ascending limbs of Henle's loop Cause loss of sodium, chloride, and potassium Potassium supplements or extra dietary K may be necessary when these agents are used routinely
Potassium-conserving diuretics Examples: spironolactone (Aldactone), triamterene (Dyrenium), amiloride	Cause loss of sodium and chloride Conserve potassium Spironolactone inhibits action of aldosterone (Recall that the hormone aldosterone causes sodium retention and potassium excretion.) Triamterene acts on the distal renal tubule to depress the exchange of sodium Effect of Amiloride apparently due to inhibition of sodium entry into the cell from luminal fluid These drugs reduce potassium excretion and may lead to hyperkalemia; thus, potassium supplements are contraindicated, as are salt substitutes containing potassium Often combined with thiazides for effective diuresis; in this case, the hypokalemic tendency of the thiazides may offset the hyperkalemic tendency of triamterene and spironolactone (examples of such combinations are Dyazide and Aldactazide.)

▶ Magnesium wasting
▶ Alterations in calcium excretion
▶ Metabolic acid–base disturbances

Extracellular Fluid Volume Depletion

Depletion of the ECF volume is a common complication of diuretic use, especially when the potent loop-acting diuretics are used.[37] Although the duration of sodium loss with diuretic use is limited, some patients have a relatively large initial response and develop true volume depletion.[38] This complication is most likely to occur in patients who are concurrently losing fluids from other routes (as in vomiting or diarrhea) or who are unable to take in sufficient amounts of salt and water. It is also more likely in patients with mild edema who begin daily diuretic therapy that is continued after the edema has subsided.[39] Clinical signs of fluid volume depletion include weakness, malaise, muscle cramps, and postural dizziness.[40] Reduction of the effective circulatory volume decreases renal perfusion and can lead to prerenal azotemia, manifested by an increase in the BUN and plasma creatinine concentrations. In general, volume depletion causes a greater rise in the BUN than in the plasma creatinine level. If the patient has an underlying renal insufficiency, the ECF deficit can lead to overt uremia.

Note that when diuretics are administered, the fluid that is lost initially comes from the vascular space. The resultant drop in venous pressure, and consequently, in the capillary hydraulic pressure, promotes movement of the edematous fluid into the vascular space to restore the reduced volume. How quickly this chain of events can safely occur depends on the degree and distribution of excess fluid. Fluid from patients with marked generalized edema due to heart failure can have edematous fluid mobilized rapidly because most of the capillary beds are involved. (Removal of as much as 2 to 3 L of edematous fluid in 24 hours can occur without much reduction in the plasma volume.[41]) However, use of diuretics to remove ascitic fluid from cirrhotic patients without peripheral edema must be accomplished more slowly because fluid can only be mobilized by the peritoneal capillaries. Therefore, approximately 500 to 750 mL/day is the maximum amount that can be safely achieved in most of these patients.[42]

Hyponatremia

Mild-to-moderate hyponatremia (120–134 mEq/L) often occurs shortly after the institution of diuretic therapy.[43] This imbalance is most associated with thiazide-type diuretics.[44] Hyponatremia is relatively common in edematous patients with heart failure or hepatic cirrhosis who are treated with diuretics. The development of hyponatremia is related both to an effective volume depletion, leading to enhanced secretion of antidiuretic hormone, and to an unexplained increased water intake.[45] The result is retention of ingested water, leading to a dilution of the serum sodium level.

Hypokalemia

Urinary potassium losses are increased by the thiazide and loop diuretics, often leading to the development of hypokalemia. Reports of the actual occurrence of hypokalemia due to diuretics are varied. One study found that the administration of 50 to 100 mg of hydrochlorothiazide per day to treat hypertension was associated with a mean reduction in the plasma potassium level of approximately 0.6 mEq/L, with about half of the patients having plasma potassium concentrations at or below 3.5 mEq/L.[46] Another study found that only 15% of 83 subjects taking either furosemide or a thiazide-type diuretic over a prolonged period developed mild hypokalemia (serum K < 3.5) and that none developed a serum of K 3.0 or less.[47] Although potassium supplements are indicated in some patients, it is believed that restriction of dietary sodium to approximately 87 mEq/day is the most appropriate way to abolish excessive urinary potassium wasting.[48] Obviously, the smallest dosage of a diuretic necessary to achieve the desired degree of fluid excretion should be used.

Potassium depletion can lead to defects in renal concentration and perhaps eventually to the development of interstitial fibrosis. Severe potassium depletion can cause cardiac muscle irritability, especially in the presence of digitalis therapy. It can also slow the release of insulin from the pancreas, leading to carbohydrate intolerance.

Hyperkalemia

The potassium-conserving diuretics (spironolactone, amiloride, and triamterene) act on the distal nephron to block potassium secretion, and are capable of contributing to hyperkalemia in patients with renal insufficiency. These drugs should be used with extreme caution, if at all, in patients with renal failure or those receiving potassium supplements.[49]

Magnesium Wasting

Magnesium depletion can be induced by diuretic therapy, with loop diuretics causing more profound depletion than thiazides.[50] (In contrast, potassium-sparing diuretics tend to diminish urinary magnesium losses.) In a study of 33 patients treated with loop diuretics, hypomagnesemia was found to be present in all and was associated with a marked reduction in muscle magnesium content.[51] Other authors found that the plasma magnesium level often remains within normal limits because most of the magnesium loss comes from cellular stores.[52] Clinical significance of magnesium depletion is not clear, although it has been suggested that it predisposes to cardiac arrhythmias, particularly if there is a concurrent hypokalemia.

Alterations in Calcium Excretion

Thiazide diuretics can cause hypercalcemia, especially when there is an underlying condition that may perpetuate the increase in serum calcium.[53] Because thiazides decrease calcium excretion in the urine, they are sometimes used to minimize new stone formation in patients with idiopathic hypercalciuria. The net retention of calcium in this setting may also increase bone mineralization.[54]

In contrast, the loop diuretics (furosemide, bumetanide, and ethacrynic acid) increase renal calcium excretion. Therefore, a loop diuretic is often used in conjunction with saline infusions to treat patients with severe hypercalcemia. There have been reports of kidney stone formation in patients receiving loop diuretics, particularly in infants in whom there can be a more than 10-fold increase in calcium excretion.[55]

Metabolic Acid—Base Disturbances

Hypokalemia occurring with use of thiazide and loop diuretics is often accompanied by metabolic alkalosis. In contrast, the potassium-sparing diuretics can result in both hyperkalemia and metabolic acidosis.

Bedrest

Bedrest alone can induce a diuresis, particularly in cases of heart failure.[56] Mobilization of edematous fluid by the supine position is probably related to diminished peripheral venous pooling and a resultant increase in the effective circulating blood volume, and, thus, in renal perfusion.

Metabolic requirements of peripheral tissues are usually decreased by bedrest so that, in patients with congestive heart failure, there is less demand placed on the compromised myocardium. This action can transfer as much as 400 to 500 mL of interstitial fluid into the central circulation over a few days.[57] Additional beneficial effects of bedrest include the facilitation of diuresis by decreased circulating levels of aldosterone, antidiuretic hormone, and catecholamines.[58]

A recent study of 14 patients with hypoalbuminemic fluid-retaining states (seven with cirrhosis, five with nephrotic syndrome, one with nutritional hypoproteinemia, and one with protein-losing enteropathy) compared the effects of various body positions (sitting, supine, 10-degree head-down tilt) on renal fluid and electrolyte handling. The authors reported that the head-down tilt position acted as a physiological diuretic.[59] Excluded from the study were patients with cardiac or respiratory problems. The authors recommended further study.

NURSING INTERVENTIONS

1. Assess for the presence, or worsening, of FVE:
   - ▶ Monitor I & O and evaluate at regular intervals for excessive fluid retention.
   - ▶ Monitor changes in body weight; be alert for acute weight gain.
   - ▶ Assess breath sounds at regular intervals for presence, or worsening, of rales.
   - ▶ Monitor degree of peripheral edema; look for edema in most dependent parts of body (feet and ankles in ambulatory patients, sacral region in bedridden patients). Check for pitting edema (see Fig. 2-6) and measure extent of edema with millimeter tape (see Fig. 2-7).
   - ▶ Monitor degree of distention of peripheral veins.
   - ▶ Monitor laboratory values (look for low BUN and hematocrit; however, realize that there may well be other causes for abnormalities in these values, such as low protein intake and anemia).
2. Encourage adherence to sodium-restricted diet, if prescribed. Assist dietitian in diet instruction. Review section of sodium-restricted diets under treatment.
3. Instruct patients requiring sodium restriction to avoid "over-the-counter" drugs without first checking with the health-care adviser.
4. When fluid retention persists despite adherence to dietary sodium intake, consider hidden sources of sodium, such as water supply or use of water softeners.
5. When indicated, encourage rest periods. Lying down favors diuresis of edematous fluid.[60]
6. Monitor the patient's response to diuretics. Discuss significant findings with physician.
7. Monitor rate of parenteral fluids and the patient's response. Discuss significant findings with physician.
8. Teach self-monitoring of weight and I & O measurements to patients with chronic fluid retention (such as those with congestive heart failure, renal disease, or cirrhosis of liver).
9. Monitor for worsening of underlying cause of FVE. See Chapters 15, 18, and 19 for specific interventions for patients with cirrhosis and renal and heart failure.
10. If dyspnea and orthopnea are present, position the patient in semi-Fowler's position to favor lung expansion.

Summary of Fluid Volume Excess

ETIOLOGICAL FACTORS	DEFINING CHARACTERISTICS
Compromised regulatory mechanisms: ▶ Renal failure ▶ Congestive heart failure ▶ Cirrhosis of liver ▶ Cushing's syndrome Overzealous administration of sodium-containing IV fluids Excessive ingestion of sodium-containing substances in diet or sodium-containing medications	Weight loss over short period: ▶ 2% (mild excess, such as 2.4-lb in 120-lb person) ▶ 5% (moderate excess, such as 6-lb in 120-lb person) ▶ 8% or > (severe excess, such as 10-lb gain or > in 120-lb person) Peripheral edema (excess of fluid in interstitial space) Distended neck veins Distended peripheral veins Slow-emptying peripheral veins Central venous pressure > 11 cm of water in vena cava Moist rales in lungs Polyuria (if renal function is normal) Ascites, pleural effusion (when fluid volume excess is severe, fluid transudates into body cavities) Decreased BUN (due to plasma dilution) Decreased hematocrit (also due to plasma dilution) Bounding, full pulse Pulmonary edema, if severe

11. Turn and position the patient frequently; be aware that edematous tissue is more prone to skin breakdown than is normal tissue.

Case Studies

1. A 70-year-old woman with congestive heart failure was admitted to an acute care facility. In addition to distended neck veins and pedal edema, pulmonary edema was present. The CVP was 20 cm of water and the BUN was 8 mg/dL.

Commentary: See Figures 2-6 and 2-7 for examples of pitting edema and distended neck veins. Note in this case study the relatively low BUN, especially for an elderly person (indicating plasma dilution). The CVP was greatly elevated because normal is 4 to 11 cm of water.

2. A 10-year-old girl was inadvertently given 3.5 L of isotonic saline (0.9% NaCl) for 3 days postoperatively. A gain of approximately 6 lb over the admission weight was noted. According to laboratory data, the BUN was 6 mg/dL on the third postoperative day.

Commentary: This case is an example of fluid overloading during a period in which the kidneys were less able to excrete the excess. Recall that in the early postoperative period there is a tendency to retain fluids because of increased secretion of adrenal hormones (stress reaction). Fluid overload was reflected by the weight gain and low BUN. A review of the I & O record would also have reflected the problem. Had the staff paid attention to the far greater intake than output, the problem could have been alleviated early.

REFERENCES

1. Condon R, Nyhus L: Manual of Surgical Therapeutics, 7th ed, p 177. Boston, Little, Brown, 1988
2. Ibid
3. Alpers D, Clouse R, Stenson W: Manual of Nutritional Therapeutics, 2nd ed, p 143. Boston, Little, Brown, 1988
4. Schwartz S, Shires T, Spencer F: Principles of Surgery, 5th ed, p 74. New York, McGraw-Hill, 1989

5. Kokko, J, Tannen, R: Fluids and Electrolytes, 2nd ed, p 72. Philadelphia, WB Saunders, 1990
6. Goldberger E: A Primer of Water, Electrolytes and Acid–Base Syndromes, 7th ed, p 220. Philadelphia, Lea & Febiger, 1986
7. Gettrust K, Ryan S, Engleman D: Applied Nursing Diagnoses: Guides for Comprehensive Care Planning, p 17. New York, John Wiley & Sons, 1985
8. Vannata J, Fogelman M: Moyer's Fluid Balance, 4th ed, p 152. Chicago, Year Book Medical Publishers, 1988
9. Schwartz et al, p 84
10. Ibid, p 51
11. Young M, Flynn K: Third-spacing: When the body conceals fluid loss. RN August: 46, 1988
12. Schwartz et al, p 51
13. Rose B: Clinical Physiology of Acid–Base and Electrolyte Disorders, 3rd ed, p 365. New York, McGraw-Hill, 1989
14. Schwartz et al, p 51
15. Vanatta & Fogelman, p 164
16. Ibid
17. Maxwell et al, p 920
18. Schwartz et al, p 51
19. Berk J, Sampliner J (eds): Handbook of Critical Care, 2nd ed, p 324. Boston, Little, Brown, 1982
20. Maxwell et al, p 907
21. Berk & Sampliner, p 324
22. Shires T: Fluids, Electrolytes, and Acid Bases, p 18. New York, Churchill Livingstone, 1988
23. Berk & Sampliner, p 324
24. Schwartz et al, p 84
25. Ibid, p 51
26. Askanazi J, Starker P, Weissman C (eds.): Fluid and Electrolyte Management in Critical Care, p 257. Boston, Butterworths, 1986
27. Ibid
28. Goldberger, p 359
29. Berk & Sampliner, p 324
30. Maxwell et al, p 907
31. Ibid
32. Schwartz et al, p 84
33. Alpers et al, p 325
34. Ibid, p 64
35. Ibid
36. Physician's Desk Reference for Nonprescription Drugs, p 610. Oradell, NJ, Medical Economics, 1990
37. Maxwell et al, p 442
38. Rose B: Clinical Physiology of Acid–Base and Electrolyte Disorders, 3rd ed, p 397. New York, McGraw-Hill, 1989
39. Ibid
40. Ibid, p 398
41. Ibid, p 432
42. Ibid
43. Maxwell et al, p 884
44. Rose, p 401
45. Ibid
46. Morgan D, Davidson C: Hypokalemia and diuretics: An analysis of publications. Br Med J 280:905, 1980
47. Davidson C et al: Effect of long-term diuretic treatment on body-potassium in heart disease. Lancet 2:1044, 1976
48. Maxwell et al, p 443
49. Rose, p 401
50. Maxwell et al, p 834
51. Dyckner T, Wester P: Intracellular magnesium loss after diuretic administration. Drugs 28:161, 1984
52. Rose, p 402
53. Maxwell et al, p 768
54. Coe F, Parks J, Bushinsky D et al: Chlorthalidone promotes mineral retention in patients with idiopathic hypercalciuria. Kidney Int 33:1140, 1988
55. Hufnagel et al: Renal calcifications: A complication of long-term furosemide therapy in pre-term infants. Pediatrics 70:360, 1982
56. Schrier R: Renal and Electrolyte Disorders, 3rd ed, p 117. Boston, Little, Brown, 1986
57. Gauer O et al: The regulation of extracellular fluid volume. Physiol Rev 50:547, 1970
58. Maxwell et al, p 432
59. Karnad et al: Head-down tilt as a physiological diuretic in normal controls and in patients with fluid-retaining states. Lancet Sept 5:525, 1987
60. Schrier, p 117

4

Sodium Imbalances

SODIUM BALANCE

Disturbances in sodium balance frequently occur in clinical practice and develop under circumstances varying from the simple to the complex. These imbalances and the nurse's role in their management are discussed in this chapter. First, however, some basic facts about the role of sodium in physiological activities are reviewed.

Sodium is the most plentiful electrolyte in the extracellular fluid (ECF), with a concentration ranging from 135 to 145 mEq/L. More than 95% of the body's physiologically active sodium is in the ECF. In contrast, the intracellular concentration of sodium is small.

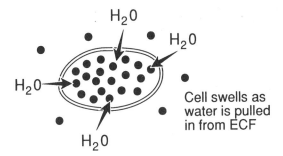

Hyponatremia:
Na less than 130 mEq/L

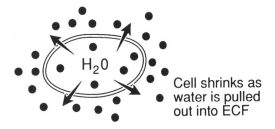

Hypernatremia:
Na greater than 150 mEq/L

FIGURE 4–1.
Effect of extracellular sodium level on cell size.

Maintenance of this asymmetric distribution across cell membranes requires transporting sodium out of the cell against an electrochemical gradient by the ATPase pump.

The fact that sodium does not easily cross the cell-wall membrane, in addition to being the dominant electrolyte in quantity, accounts for its primary role in controlling water distribution as well as ECF volume. In general, a loss or gain of sodium is accompanied by a loss or gain of water.

Extracellular sodium concentration has a profound effect on body cells. That is, a low serum sodium level (*hyponatremia*) results in a relatively diluted ECF and allows water to be drawn into the cells. Conversely, a high serum sodium level (*hypernatremia*) results in a relatively concentrated ECF and allows water to be pulled out of cells (Figure 4-1).

Provided there are no abnormal losses, the usual daily sodium requirement in adults is approximately 100 mEq.[1] More than this amount is readily plentiful in the diet, in a liter of lactated Ringer's solution or isotonic saline (0.9% NaCl), or in 2 L of half-strength saline (0.45% NaCl) (see Table 4-1).

HYPONATREMIA

DEFINITION

Hyponatremia refers to a serum sodium level that is below normal (<135 mEq/L). A low serum concentration does not necessarily mean that the total body sodium is less than normal. In fact, many patients have hyponatremia when there is an excess of total body sodium (as occurs with congestive heart failure or cirrhosis of the liver). When marked hyperlipidemia or hypoproteinemia are present, the serum sodium may appear to be lower than it actually is (pseudohyponatremia).[2]

Syndrome of inappropriate antidiuretic hormone secretion (SIADH) produces a special kind of hyponatremia that is associated with excessive water retention. In conditions producing SIADH, there is either too much antidiuretic hormone released or the renal response to the hormone is intensified. Release of ADH is termed *inappropriate* because in normal situations a low serum sodium level would depress ADH activity.

PATHOPHYSIOLOGY

Hyponatremia may result from a loss of sodium or a gain of water; in either event, it is due to a relatively greater concentration of water than of sodium. A common imbalance, hyponatremia can range from mild to severe. When severe, it is often a marker of serious underlying disease. In addition, severe hyponatremia can itself cause major neurological damage and death. As

TABLE 4–1.
Approximate Sodium Content of Selected Parenteral Fluids

PARENTERAL FLUID	SODIUM (mEq/L)
0.9% NaCl ("Isotonic saline")	154
0.45% NaCl (half-strength saline)	77
0.33% NaCl	56
0.22% NaCl	38
.011% NaCl	19
3% NaCl*	513
5% NaCl*	855
Lactated Ringer's solution	130

* *Extremely hypertonic fluids*

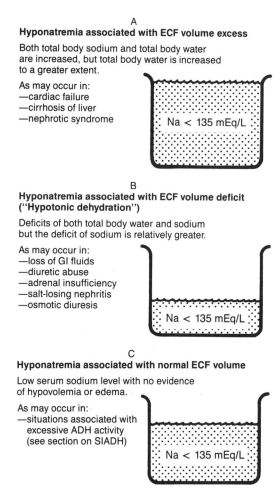

A

Hyponatremia associated with ECF volume excess

Both total body sodium and total body water are increased, but total body water is increased to a greater extent.

As may occur in:
—cardiac failure
—cirrhosis of liver
—nephrotic syndrome

Na < 135 mEq/L

B

Hyponatremia associated with ECF volume deficit ("Hypotonic dehydration")

Deficits of both total body water and sodium but the deficit of sodium is relatively greater.

As may occur in:
—loss of GI fluids
—diuretic abuse
—adrenal insufficiency
—salt-losing nephritis
—osmotic diuresis

Na < 135 mEq/L

C

Hyponatremia associated with normal ECF volume

Low serum sodium level with no evidence of hypovolemia or edema.

As may occur in:
—situations associated with excessive ADH activity (see section on SIADH)

Na < 135 mEq/L

FIGURE 4–2.
Hyponatremic states.

noted in Figure 4-1, a decrease in the serum sodium concentration is expected to cause a shift of water from the ECF to the intracellular space, resulting in generalized cellular edema. Unlike other tissues, the brain's capacity to expand is limited by the bony cranium. Herniation of the brain stem has been found on autopsy in patients who died from severe acute hyponatremia.

Regardless of the primary underlying pathology, free water intake (orally, by tube, or intravenously [IV]) must exceed free water output for hyponatremia to occur. As illustrated in Figure 4-2, hyponatremia can be superimposed on a normal fluid volume, on fluid volume deficit (FVD), or on fluid volume excess (FVE).

Mechanisms accounting for hyponatremia coupled with ECF volume excess in patients with cirrhosis of the liver and cardiac failure are described in Chapters 15 and 19, respectively. The effect of hyperglycemia on the serum sodium level is discussed in Chapter 21. In general, note that hyperglycemia promotes an osmotic gradient that causes water to move out of the cells into the ECF, thereby diluting the serum sodium level. For every 100 mg/100 mL rise in plasma glucose, the osmotic water shift dilutes the plasma sodium concentration by 1.6 mEq/L.[3]

ETIOLOGICAL FACTORS

Etiological factors associated with hyponatremia are listed in Table 4-2 and are briefly described below.

Diuretics

Hyponatremia is a fairly common and usually mild complication of diuretic therapy. However, severe hyponatremia may develop at times. Diuretic-induced severe hyponatremia is primarily a complication of thiazide-type drugs, and most often affects elderly women.[4] A recent study found that thiazides were either the sole cause or a major contributing factor to more than half the hospital admissions for hyponatremia.[5]

Adrenal Insufficiency

Hyponatremia is a common complication of adrenal insufficiency and is due to the effects of aldosterone and cortisol deficiencies. Lack of aldosterone increases renal sodium loss, and cortisol deficiency is associated with increased release of ADH (causing water retention).

Gastrointestinal Fluid Losses

Gastric fluid loss by vomiting or gastric suction can predispose to hyponatremia by the direct loss of sodium. The act of vomiting also predisposes to water retention, and thus hyponatremia, because it is a potent stimulus for the release of ADH. Even then, however, hyponatremia is not likely to be severe without the intake of free water. When vomiting occurs at home, oral intake is usually greatly curtailed. However, in hospital settings, the erroneous administration of excessive electrolyte-free solutions (such as 5% dextrose in water) can seriously dilute the serum sodium concentration. In many situations, the loss of gastric fluid results in simple FVD uncomplicated by hyponatremia.

Loss of intestinal fluid by diarrhea can also result in an isotonic FVD, leaving the serum sodium within a normal range. The volume depletion induced by diarrhea can also serve as a stimulus for ADH release, leading to renal water retention and hyponatremia. The amount of free-water intake orally or IV frequently determines the severity of hyponatremia. Water loss through diarrhea can at times exceed sodium loss, leading to hypernatremia.

TABLE 4–2.
Etiological Factors Associated With Hyponatremia

Loss of Sodium:
▶ Use of thiazide diuretics, particularly in combination with low-salt diet, vomiting, diarrhea, or sweating
▶ Adrenal insufficiency
▶ Gastrointestinal fluid losses, coupled with excessive water replacement
▶ Heavy sweating, coupled with excessive water intake
▶ Salt-losing nephritis

Water gains:
▶ Use of drugs predisposing to SIADH
  ▶ Intravenous cyclophosphamide (Cytoxan)
  ▶ Vincristine (Oncovin)
  ▶ Chlorpropamide (Diabenese)
  ▶ Tolbutamide (Orinase)
  ▶ Carbamazepine (Tegretol)
  ▶ Amitriptyline (Elavil)
  ▶ Haloperidol (Haldol)
  ▶ Thioridazine (Mellaril)
  ▶ Thiothixene (Navanel)
  ▶ Nonsteroidal antiinflammatory drugs
▶ Presence of tumors predisposing to SIADH
  ▶ Oat-cell carcinoma of lung
  ▶ Tumors of pancreas and duodenum
  ▶ Leukemia
  ▶ Hodgkin's disease
▶ Presence of central nervous system disorders predisposing to SIADH
  ▶ Subarachnoid hemorrhage
  ▶ Head injury
  ▶ Encephalitis
  ▶ Brain tumor
▶ Pulmonary disorders
  ▶ Tuberculosis
  ▶ Pneumonia
  ▶ Asthma
  ▶ Acute respiratory failure
▶ Release of vasopressin after anesthesia and surgery
▶ Labor induction with oxytocin
▶ Irrigation of prostatic bed during transurethral prostatectomy
▶ Psychotic polydipsia
▶ Acquired immunodeficiency syndrome (related to multisystem morbidity)
▶ Excessive administration of dextrose and water solutions (such as 5% dextrose in water), particularly during periods of stress when patient is likely to retain fluids excessively

Sweating

Sweat is a hypotonic fluid with a sodium concentration of approximately 40 to 50 mEq/L; however, there is considerable variation from one person to another.[6]

With exercise in a hot environment, sweat losses can exceed 200 mEq/day.[7] Hyponatremia develops in situations in which large volumes of sweat are produced and replaced with water alone.

Salt-Losing Nephritis

A variety of kidney conditions can result in renal salt wasting. Among these are chronic interstitial nephropathy, medullary cystic disease, and polycystic kidney disease.[8] The degree of renal sodium wasting can range from mild to severe.

Drugs Predisposing to SIADH

Several drugs (Table 4-2) can impair renal water excretion, thus causing a special form of hyponatremia sometimes referred to as SIADH. A few of the major ones are discussed below.

Chlorpropamide, an oral hypoglycemic agent, is the most common cause of drug-induced SIADH.[9] This drug enhances ADH release and potentiates its action on the kidney. One study reported that 4% of patients in a clinical population receiving chlorpropamide were hyponatremic (suggesting excessive ADH effect).[10]

Cyclophosphamide is an antineoplastic alkylating agent that can increase renal sensitivity to ADH and perhaps its release when given IV in high doses. Because a high fluid intake is generally prescribed to lessen the possibility of hemorrhagic cystitis, severe hyponatremia can result. Use of isotonic saline rather than water to maintain a high urine output can minimize this complication.[11] Another antineoplastic drug that can cause hyponatremia is vincristine, apparently by a neurotoxic effect on the hypothalamus.[12]

Carbamazepine, used as an anticonvulsant, can cause hyponatremia by inducing the release of ADH. Apparently, the hyponatremia caused by this drug is dose related.

Nonsteroidal antiinflammatory drugs (NSAID) decrease renal water excretion because decreased synthesis of prostaglandins potentiates the action of ADH on the kidney. Despite this effect, hyponatremia due solely to these agents is uncommon.[13] Instead, NSAID tend to exacerbate the tendency toward hyponatremia in patients with other causes of SIADH.

Tumors Predisposing to SIADH

Probably the most frequent cause of SIADH is oat-cell carcinoma of the lung. Other malignancies associated with this syndrome include carcinomas of the duodenum and pancreas, Hodgkin's disease, leukemia, and lymphoma. Malignant cells from patients with SIADH have been shown, in some instances, to synthesize and release a substance similar to native ADH ("ectopic

ADH production"). In Chapter 24 SIADH in oncology patients is discussed further.

Central Nervous System Disorders Associated with SIADH

Conditions associated with damage to or inflammation of the central nervous system (CNS) can promote vasopressin (ADH) release and lead to SIADH. For example, SIADH can occur in over 20% of patients having subarachnoid hemorrhage.[14] In Chapter 20 SIADH in central nervous system disorders is discussed further.

Psychogenic Polydipsia

Excessive water intake is relatively common in psychiatric patients and can occasionally cause severe symptomatic hyponatremia. This syndrome is also referred to as "compulsive water drinking" and "self-induced water intoxication." Epidemiological studies indicate that the incidence of polydipsia ranges from 6% to 17% in chronically ill psychiatric patients.[15] Among patients with polydipsia, schizophrenia is by far the most frequent diagnosis, although patients with other types of disorders may also have this problem. This dilutional hyponatremia is thought to occur when the rapid ingestion of voluminous quantities of water exceeds the excretory capacity of normally functioning kidneys. As soon as water intake is interrupted by sleep or a convulsion, the kidneys manage to excrete the excess water load and the serum sodium level returns to normal.[16]

Hyponatremia in psychiatric patients has been attributed to selected medications used to treat psychoses. For example, carbamazepine is a well-established cause of vasopressin release. (Vasopressin, of course, favors water retention.) It has been suggested that patients who smoke may be more likely to be symptomatic because nicotine contributes to transient release of vasopressin, as may the psychosis itself.[17]

Labor Induction with Oxytocin

Oxytocin, like vasopressin (ADH), is synthesized in the hypothalamus and released by the pituitary gland. Although its primary effects are on uterine function and milk production, it also possesses significant antidiuretic activity. Administration of oxytocin to induce labor, therefore, can cause hyponatremia if improperly performed.

In the past, little attention was paid to the water-retentive capacity of oxytocin, and excessive fluid (usually in the form of 5% dextrose in water) was administered. Numerous reports exist of women who became comatose from hyponatremia within 48 hours of receiving improperly administered oxytocin infusions.[18] Safe guidelines for oxytocin administration are discussed in Chapter 23.

Postoperative Hyponatremia

In a recent study of 1088 postoperative patients, Chung et al[19] reported a 4.4% incidence of hyponatremia (serum $Na^+ < 130$ mEq/L) within 1 week of surgery. Predisposing factors included a temporary increase in vasopressin release after anesthesia and the stress of surgery. Pain enhances the release of vasopressin by direct stimulation of the hypothalamus. Because of the tendency for hyponatremia in new postoperative patients, the excessive administration of electrolyte-free solutions during the first 3 to 5 postoperative days should be avoided. Postoperative hyponatremia is evidently more common in women than in men.[20] Also at increased risk are patients who have undergone mitral commissurotomy to relieve mitral stenosis, probably due to ADH release from activation of the atrial volume receptors.[21]

Pulmonary Disorders

Several pulmonary conditions may be associated with SIADH, including tuberculosis, pneumonia, acute asthma, atelectasis, empyema, pneumothorax, and acute respiratory failure.[22] Bioassay of tuberculosis lung tissue has demonstrated ADH activity.[23] The mechanisms for hyponatremia in other pulmonary infections and conditions are not clear.

Postprostatectomy Via Transurethral Resection

During transurethral resection of the prostate, the urologist must irrigate the prostatic bed with an electrolyte-free solution. If the procedure is prolonged or if the irrigating solution is introduced under pressure, large volumes of the fluid may be absorbed into the circulation. In the past, distilled water was used but has been replaced by solutions containing isotonic or slightly hypotonic glycine, mannitol, or sorbitol.[24] Nonetheless, serum sodium concentration can still be lowered by the irrigating solution. Exact effects vary with the type of irrigant.

Acquired Immunodeficiency Syndrome

Recent studies have indicated that hyponatremia is very common in patients with acquired immunodeficiency syndrome (AIDS). For example, Vitting et al[25] reported that 56% of the AIDS patients followed prospectively in their study were hyponatremic (mean serum sodium level was 126 ± 4 mEq/L). The authors reported that the hyponatremic states did not result from any new or pathophysiologically distinct mechanism, but were the result of accumulated multiorgan morbidity unique to patients with AIDS. In addition, the below normal serum sodium levels often followed the administration of hypotonic fluids.

In another study, Agarwal et al[26] found that approximately 35% of 103 patients with AIDS admitted for opportunistic infections had serum sodium levels lower than or equal to 130 mEq/L. The authors reported that contributing factors to the hyponatremic states in this population included SIADH and volume depletion.

DEFINING CHARACTERISTICS

The defining characteristics of hyponatremia depend on its magnitude, rapidity of onset, and cause. In general, the lower the serum sodium level, the more likely symptoms are to be severe (see Table 4-3). Another major factor is the rapidity of onset. For example, two patients having similarly low serum sodium values may have greatly different symptoms if hyponatremia developed slowly in one and quickly in the other. In acute hyponatremia, symptoms develop at a higher level than they do when hyponatremia is chronic; in the latter case, symptoms may not become evident until the serum sodium is quite low (eg, 110 mEq/L). Severity of symptoms may also vary with the cause. For example, acute water overloading is more likely to cause severe symptoms than is the chronic loss of sodium.

Early manifestations of hyponatremia include those involving the gastrointestinal (GI) system, such as nausea and abdominal cramps. However, most of the major manifestations of hyponatremia are of a neuropsychiatric nature and are related to cellular swelling. Recall that cellular swelling occurs in hyponatremia as the relatively diluted ECF is pulled into the cells. Because the swollen brain has limited room for expansion within the skull, cerebral edema becomes a potentially

TABLE 4–3.
Clinical Manifestations of Hyponatremia

Chronic Versus Acute Hyponatremia:

Chronic (slow developing, usually due to a combination of sodium loss and water gain)
- Anorexia
- Nausea
- Emesis
- Muscular weakness
- Irritability
- Personality changes (uncooperative, confused, hostile)
- If very severe, gait disturbances, stupor, and seizures may occur

Acute (fast developing, due primarily to water overload):
- All of the above, but neurological manifestations tend to be more severe as the serum sodium usually falls rapidly to low levels in acutely water-overloaded patients

Severity of Drop in Serum Concentration:

Patients are often asymptomatic when the serum sodium level is >125 mEq/L.
<125 mEq/L[30]
- Nausea
- Malaise
<110 to 115 mEq/L
- Seizures
- Coma

Volume Status[31]:
- Hyponatremia coupled with ECF volume depletion may produce added symptoms of weakness, fatigue, muscle cramps, and postural dizziness.
- Hyponatremia due to SIADH does not produce peripheral edema (although water retention has occurred) because about two thirds of the retained water is stored in the cells.

Laboratory Data
- By definition, serum sodium level is <135 mEq/L
- Urinary sodium <15mEq/L indicates renal conservation of sodium and that loss of sodium is from a nonrenal route
- Urinary sodium >20 mEq/L in SIADH

ECF, extracellular fluid; SIADH, syndrome of inappropriate antidiuretic hormone secretion.

TABLE 4–4.
Clinical Manifestations of SIADH

Water retention
- ▶ Intake of fluid greatly exceeds urinary output (as evidenced by I & O records)
- ▶ Weight gain (reflecting water retention)
- ▶ No peripheral edema (water is primarily retained inside the cells, not the interstitium)
- ▶ Fingerprint edema over sternum (reflecting cellular edema)
- ▶ Signs of cerebral edema (see neurological symptoms below)

Gastrointestinal symptoms
- ▶ Anorexia
- ▶ Nausea
- ▶ Vomiting
- ▶ Abdominal cramps

Neurologic symptoms
- ▶ Lethargy
- ▶ Headaches
- ▶ Personality changes
- ▶ Absence of diminished deep tendon reflexes
- ▶ Seizures
- ▶ Pupillary changes
- ▶ Coma

Laboratory findings
- ▶ Hyponatremia
  - ▶ Symptoms usually do not appear unless serum sodium level is <125 mEq/L
  - ▶ Plasma osmolality below normal (reflecting low serum sodium level)
- ▶ Low BUN and creatinine
  - ▶ Reflecting state of overhydration
- ▶ Urinary signs
  - ▶ Urinary sodium >20 mEq/L (As opposed to hyponatremia due primarily to sodium loss, where much lower sodium levels are expected due to renal conservation of the needed cation.)
  - ▶ Urinary SG >1.012
  - ▶ Urine osmolality is usually higher than plasma osmolality (urine contains important amounts of sodium and plasma is diluted with water)

SG, specific gravity; SIADH, syndrome of inappropriate antidiuretic hormone secretion.

lethal problem. In general, patients having acute declines in serum sodium levels have higher mortality rates than do those with more slowly developing hyponatremia. In laboratory animals, it has been found that cerebral swelling is less marked when hyponatremia is chronic rather than acute, even when there are comparable decrements in serum sodium.[27]

A test sometimes done to demonstrate intracellular water excess is placement of firm finger pressure over the sternum or other bony surface for a period of 15 to 30 seconds.[28] On removal of the finger, a positive sign consists of a visible fingerprint, similar to that seen when a fingerprint is made on paper with ink.

Because SIADH presents a unique set of circumstances, the clinical manifestations of this disorder are spelled out in Table 4-4.

TREATMENT

The obvious treatment for hyponatremia due to sodium loss is sodium replacement. This may be accomplished orally, by nasogastric tube, or by the parenteral route. For patients able to eat and drink, replacement is easily accomplished because sodium is plentiful in a normal diet. For those unable to take sodium orally or by gastric tube, the parenteral route is necessary. If the plasma volume is below normal, lactated Ringer's solution or isotonic saline (0.9% NaCl) may be prescribed. If the plasma volume is normal or excessive, however, it may be necessary to administer cautiously a small volume of 3% or 5% NaCl (an extremely dangerous fluid when used incorrectly). The sodium content of some parenteral fluids is listed in Table 4-1. When the primary problem is water retention, it is safer to restrict water than to administer sodium.

Syndrome of Inappropriate Antidiuretic Hormone Secretion

If the problem is SIADH, treatment is directed at eliminating the underlying cause if possible (eg, radiation therapy for a tumor secreting ectopic ADH-like substances, or discontinuing a drug that increases ADH secretion). If this is not possible, alleviation of water overload by fluid restriction is indicated. Fluid is restricted to the extent that urinary and insensible losses induce a negative water balance (ie, fluid loss exceeds intake). Laboratory values and clinical status are used as guides for fluid restriction. The most important parameters are serum and urine electrolytes and osmolality, fluid intake and output, and body weight records.

For patients with mild hyponatremia, fluid restriction may be all that is needed. More severe cases may require the IV administration of a small amount of hypertonic saline (3% or 5% NaCl), in addition to fluid restriction, to provide sodium in a minimal fluid volume. Furosemide is often used concomitantly to promote water excretion and decrease the risk of FVE and its dangerous sequelae (such as pulmonary edema). Use of hypertonic saline alone only transiently elevates the serum sodium level because most of the administered sodium is rapidly lost in the urine.

If the underlying cause of SIADH is chronic, other therapeutic measures must be used. Fluid restriction is not tolerated well by most patients over a prolonged period. For such patients, the administration of demeclocycline (Declomycin) is most common. Demeclocycline apparently interferes with the effects of ADH on the kidney, causing increased water excretion and, thus, an elevated sodium level. Because its effects take several days to begin, it is not solely relied on in acute phases.

NURSING INTERVENTIONS

1. Identify patients at risk for hyponatremia. As noted in Table 4-2, many common conditions can lower the serum sodium concentration.
   ▶ Being aware of patients at risk for hyponatremia is crucial to monitoring for the occurrence of subtle early changes associated with this imbalance. As explained earlier in the chapter, a profound hyponatremia can be fatal if not detected early and treated appropriately.
2. Review medications the patient is receiving, noting those that predispose to hyponatremia (such as thiazides or the drugs listed in Table 4-2 associated with SIADH).
3. Monitor fluid losses and gains for all patients at risk for hyponatremia. Look for loss of sodium-containing fluids (such as GI secretions or sweat), particularly in conjunction with a low-sodium diet or excessive water intake either orally or IV.
4. Monitor laboratory data for serum sodium levels lower than normal.
5. Monitor for presence of GI symptoms, such as anorexia, nausea, vomiting, and abdominal cramping, as these may be early signs of hyponatremia. Of course, these symptoms must be evaluated in relation to other findings, such as fluid gains and losses, amount of sodium intake, and laboratory data.
6. Monitor for CNS changes, such as lethargy, confusion, muscular twitching, convulsions, and coma. Be aware that more severe neurological signs are associated with very low sodium levels that have fallen rapidly due to water overloading.
7. For patients able to consume a general diet, encourage foods and fluids with a high sodium content. For example, broth made with one beef cube contains approximately 900 mg (39 mEq) of sodium; 8 oz of canned tomato juice contains approximately 700 mg (30 mEq) of sodium.[32] Sodium content of additional fluids can be found in Table 3-1.
8. When administering sodium-containing IV fluids to patients with cardiovascular disease, monitor for signs of circulatory overload especially closely. These include moist rales in the lungs (the greater the sodium concentration, the greater the risk). Sodium content of some of the major IV fluids is listed in Table 4-1.
8. Avoid giving large water supplements to patients receiving isotonic tube feedings, particularly if routes of abnormal sodium loss are present or water is being retained abnormally (as in SIADH) (see Chapter 13).
9. Use extreme caution when administering hypertonic saline solutions (3% or 5% NaCl). Be aware that these fluids can be lethal if infused carelessly (see Table 4-5).
10. Be aware of the effect a low serum sodium level can have on patients receiving lithium. A low serum sodium level causes a relative increase in lithium retention and predisposes to toxicity. Because of this, decreased tolerance to lithium occurs in patients with protracted sweating and diarrhea. In such instances, supplemental salt and fluid should be administered. Because diuretics promote sodium loss, patients taking lithium should not use

TABLE 4–5.
Summary of Important Nursing Considerations in Administration of Hypertonic Saline Solutions (3% and 5% NaCl)

1. Check the serum sodium level before administering these solutions and frequently thereafter.
2. Be aware that these solutions are dangerous and should be used only in critical situations in which the serum sodium is very low (such as less than 110 mEq/L) and neurological symptoms are present.
3. Administer these solutions only in intensive care settings where the patient can be closely monitored. Watch for signs of pulmonary edema and worsening of neurological signs. Use with great caution in patients with congestive heart failure or renal failure.
4. Be aware that only small volumes are needed (such as 5 mL or 6 mL/kg body weight of 5% NaCl) to elevate the serum sodium level by 10 mEq/L.[33] For example, elevating the serum sodium level of a 70-kg patient from 110 to 120 mEq/L would require approximately 350 to 420 mL.
5. The serum sodium should not be raised more rapidly than 2 mEq/L/hr unless the clinical state of the patient indicates the need for more rapid treatment.[34]
6. Use a volume-controlled apparatus to administer the fluid; maintain close vigilance on the device as none are foolproof.
7. Be aware that the aim of therapy is not to elevate the serum sodium level to normal quickly; rather, it is to elevate it only enough to alleviate neurological signs. It has been recommended that the serum concentration be raised no higher than 125 mEq/L with hypertonic saline.[35]
8. Be aware that the physician may prescribe furosemide to promote water loss and prevent pulmonary edema. Urine should be saved as renal sodium and potassium losses may need to be measured to allow for replacement.

---

diuretics unless they are under close medical supervision. For all patients on lithium therapy, an adequate salt intake should be assured. The patient's food intake should be checked and the physician informed of anorexia. (Seek a dietary consultation if indicated.)

11. To avoid serious sodium deficiency, instruct patients with adrenal insufficiency to do the following:
   ► Take steroid-replacement medications as prescribed
   ► Keep several days' dosage on their person when traveling
   ► Wear an identification bracelet stating need for steroids in case of emergency
   ► Seek medical consultation in times of excessive stress (Some physicians instruct patients how to take added dosages in times of need.)
   ► Monitor their weight and fluid intake and output (I & O) changes and report significant findings to the health care provider
   ► Increase dietary salt intake as indicated during presence of excessive sweating or diarrhea (or other causes of sodium loss)
12. Monitor patients with decreased adrenal function for signs of acute adrenocortical insufficiency (adrenal crisis) when they are exposed to severe stress (such as surgery, trauma, emotional upset, excessive heat, or prolonged medical illness). Look for extreme weakness, acute onset of nausea and vomiting, hypotension, confusion, and even shock.

Because SIADH requires special nursing management, an assessment for this condition is provided in Table 4-6 and nursing interventions during therapy for SIADH are described in Table 4-7. Recovery from this dilutional state is usually rapid if the condition is recognized early and appropriate measures are initiated. The nurse plays a vital role in preventing serious consequences of this disorder. Nursing interventions related to SIADH in part involve monitoring to detect the disturbance before it becomes severe, and to determine if the response to therapeutic interventions is adequate. Change interventions involve restricting fluids (step 1 in Table 4-7) and initiating safety precautions when indicated (step 5 in Table 4-7).

Case Studies
1. A 50-year-old man was started on hydrochlorothiazide and a low-sodium diet for the treatment of hypertension. After 2 weeks, he began to complain of weakness, abdominal cramping, leg cramps, and postural dizziness. On examination he was found to have decreased skin turgor and flat neck veins in the supine position. Laboratory data included the following:

TABLE 4–6.
Nursing Assessment for SIADH

1. Identify patients at risk (see Table 4-2).
2. Maintain accurate I & O.
   ▶ Look for fluid intake greatly exceeding output; I & O should be totaled and the overall picture observed for several consecutive days.
3. Maintain daily body weight records.
   ▶ Look for sudden weight gain (recall that 1 L of fluid weighs approximately 2.2 lb).
   ▶ Although there will be an acute weight gain, do not expect to detect peripheral edema because most (approximately two thirds) of the excess fluid will be retained inside the cells, not in the interstitial space.
4. Monitor serum sodium concentrations.
5. Observe for gastrointestinal symptoms, which usually occur early.
   ▶ Be alert for anorexia, nausea, vomiting, and abdominal cramping.
6. Observe the neurologic status carefully.
   ▶ Be particularly alert for lethargy because this is usually the first symptom. Also, look for personality changes, decreased or absent deep tendon reflexes, headache, convulsions, and coma.

TABLE 4–7.
Nursing Interventions Related to Therapy for SIADH

1. Restrict fluids to the prescribed level.
   ▶ Consider all routes of intake (eg, oral fluids, "keep-open" IV, piggyback medications).
   ▶ Gain the patient's cooperation, if he or she is rational, by explaining the need for fluid restriction.
   ▶ Place "fluid restriction" signs at the bedside.
   ▶ Remove the water pitcher.
   ▶ Explain the need for fluid restriction to visitors.
   ▶ Space the allotted fluid allowance over the 24-hour period.
   ▶ Minimize the risk of accidental overadministration of IV fluids by using a volume-controlled device.
2. Maintain an accurate I & O record and study its pattern.
   ▶ A greater urinary output than fluid intake is desired because it indicates a negative water balance. (Remember, the excessive water load must be excreted before significant improvement occurs.)
3. Maintain an accurate body-weight record.
   ▶ With proper therapy, expect to see an acute decline in body weight due to excretion of excess water. Recall that a liter of fluid is equivalent to 2.2 lb; for example, a weight loss of 6.6 lb over a period of 1 to 2 days indicates a loss of approximately 3 L.
4. Assess neurologic signs.
   ▶ With appropriate therapy, an increased level of consciousness and increased muscle strength is hoped for. Unfortunately, neurological damage induced by SIADH is not always reversible, particularly if treatment is delayed.
5. Initiate safety precautions.
   ▶ Elevate siderails for the patient with a decreased level of consciousness; be prepared for seizure activity; modify other aspects of the patient's environment as indicated.
6. Monitor serum sodium levels.
   ▶ With appropriate therapy, the sodium concentration should elevate slowly toward normal. It is important that the correction not take place too rapidly.
7. Administer hypertonic saline, when prescribed, with great caution.
   ▶ Review the facts regarding administration of hypertonic saline (Table 4-5).

SIADH, syndrome of inappropriate antidiuretic hormone secretion.

Summary of Hyponatremia

ETIOLOGICAL FACTORS	DEFINING CHARACTERISTICS
Loss of sodium	Anorexia
▸ Use of diuretics	Nausea
▸ Loss of GI fluids	Vomiting
▸ Adrenal insufficiency	Lethargy
▸ Osmotic diuresis	Confusion
▸ Salt-losing nephritis	Muscular twitching
Gains of water	Seizures
▸ Excessive administration of D_5W	Coma
▸ Psychogenic polydipsia	Papilledema
▸ Excessive water administration with isotonic or hypotonic tube feedings	Hemiparesis
Disease states associated with SIADH	Serum Na <135 mEq/L
▸ Oat-cell carcinoma of lung	Serum osmolality <285 mOsm/kg
▸ Carcinoma of duodenum or pancreas	Urinary Na level varies with cause of hyponatremia
▸ Head trauma	
▸ Stroke	
▸ Pulmonary disorders (tuberculosis, pneumonia, asthma, respiratory failure)	
Pharmacologic agents that may impair renal water excretion	
▸ Chlorpropamide (Diabenese)	
▸ Cyclophosphamide (Cytoxan)	
▸ Vincristine (Oncovin)	
▸ Thioridazine (Mellaril)	
▸ Fluphenazine (Prolixin)	
▸ Carbamazepine (Tegretol)	
▸ Oxytocin (Pitocin)	

Na = 118 mEq/L   K = 22 mEq/L
Cl = 66 mEq/L   pOsm = 240 mOsm/kg

Commentary: This patient was obviously hyponatremic, as indicated by the low plasma sodium level and osmolality. In this instance, the hyponatremia was accompanied by decreased fluid volume (as evidenced by the decreased skin turgor and flat neck veins). In addition, the plasma potassium and chloride levels were quite low. Thiazide diuretics promote both sodium and potassium excretion and predispose to hypochloremic alkalosis (metabolic alkalosis). Sodium loss, coupled with a low sodium intake, caused hyponatremia.

2. A 40-year-old man with polycystic kidney disease developed nausea, vomiting, and diarrhea. He stopped eating but drank large quantities of water. Over a period of 4 days, he developed progressive lethargy and had a grand mal seizure. Laboratory data included:

Na = 108 mEq/L   Cl = 72 mEq/L
BUN = 142 mg/dL   Creatinine = 12 mg/dL

Commentary: This patient lost sodium through vomiting and diarrhea and replaced only water. He continued to lose sodium through the kidneys because of his renal disease. The neurological symptoms were due to dilution of the already low serum sodium level by excessive water intake, resulting in brain swelling.

3. A 58-year-old man with a history of inoperable oat-cell carcinoma of the lung was admitted to the hospital; according to his family, he had a 2-week history of progressive lethargy. Laboratory data included the following:

Plasma Na = 105 mEq/L   Urinary Na = 76 mEq/L
Cl = 72 mEq/L   Urinary osmolality = 800 mOsm/kg

Commentary: The history of an oat-cell lung tumor strongly suggests the presence of ectopic ADH production. Lethargy is a prominent symptom of hyponatremia due to water excess. Lab data revealed an extremely low plasma sodium level. In contrast, note the relatively high urinary sodium level, indicative of the "salt-wasting" of SIADH.

4. After an automobile accident, a 30-year-old woman was admitted to the emergency department of a small suburban hospital. She had sustained facial fractures and a possible head injury (evidenced by temporary loss of consciousness at the accident scene). During the first 3 days of her hospitalization, she received an average of 4 L of fluid daily (despite persistent low urinary output). She became increasingly lethargic and complained of headache and nausea. On the 4th day she had a grand mal seizure and was noted to have papilledema and Babinski's sign. At that time, her serum sodium level was 110 mEq/L. Despite intensive treatment, she died within a week. On autopsy, her brain was found to be swollen, and she weighed 10 pounds more than when admitted (despite almost no caloric intake during her hospitalization).

Commentary: Patients with head injuries (especially when facial injuries are also present) are at risk for SIADH and should be monitored closely for it. Care should be taken to avoid fluid overloading head-injured individuals (see Chapter 23). Note that this patient did not have any concomitant injuries that necessitated large fluid volume replacement. Weight on autopsy was greater than on admission because water was abnormally retained in cells throughout her body. No peripheral edema was present because the excess water was retained *intracellularly,* not in the interstitial space. (Recall that peripheral edema is due to retention of both sodium and water in the interstitial space.) This patient's death could have been prevented had those providing care looked at the I & O record and paid attention to the obvious warning signs of SIADH. For example, despite the 4000 mL/day intake, she excreted less than 600 mL on most days. Nurses' notes made frequent mention of the presence of lethargy, nausea, abdominal cramping, and headache.

HYPERNATREMIA

DEFINITION

Hypernatremia refers to a greater-than-normal serum sodium level, that is, a serum level greater than 145 mEq per liter.

PATHOPHYSIOLOGY

Normally, the body defends itself against the development of hypernatremia by both increased release of ADH and stimulation of thirst by osmoreceptors in the hypothalamus.[36] Thus, when the serum sodium begins to elevate, the resultant retention of water and increased water intake lower the sodium concentration. Failure of these responses naturally can lead to hypernatremia. Hypernatremia is virtually never seen in an alert patient with a normal thirst mechanism and access to water.

Causes of hypernatremia include a gain of sodium in excess of water, or a loss of water in excess of sodium. Disease states capable of causing a significant acute alteration in the serum sodium frequently produce a concomitant change in the ECF volume. Thus, hypernatremia often occurs with either FVD or FVE. See Figure 4-3 for further explanation.

As noted in Figure 4-1, hypernatremia initially favors shrinkage of cells as fluid is pulled from them into the hypertonic ECF. It is this cellular dehydration in the brain that produces its contraction and is largely

Hypernatremia associated with a near normal ECF volume

Loss of water causes elevation of serum sodium level; does not lead to volume contraction unless water losses are massive.

As may occur in:
—increased insensible
  water loss
  (as in hyperventilation)

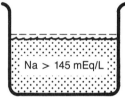

Hypernatremia associated with ECF volume deficit ("Hypertomic dehydration")
Losses of both sodium and water but relatively greater loss of water.

As may occur in:
—profuse sweating
—diarrhea, particularly
  in children
—aged individuals with poor
  water intake (recall that
  the aged kidney loses part
  of its ability to concentrate
  urine and thus cannot conserve water as it should)

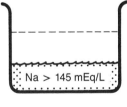

Hypernatremia associated with fluid volume excess

Gains of both sodium and water, but relatively greater gain of sodium.

As may occur:
—administration of hyper-
  tonic sodium solutions
  or substances (such as
  sodium bicarbonate in
  cardiac arrest)

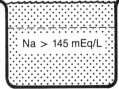

FIGURE 4–3.
Hypernatremic states.

responsible for the neurologic symptoms of hypernatremia. Contraction of the brain may put mechanical traction on delicate cerebral vessels and produce vascular trauma. Autopsies on patients who died from hypernatremia have shown widespread cerebral vascular bleeding.

The cerebral shrinking caused by hypernatremia is transient. Usually within 24 hours, by means of complex mechanisms, the brain begins to adapt to the extracellular hyperosmolality by raising the amount of intracellular solutes and, thereby, minimizing its water loss. With increased intracellular solute, water movement back into the brain is initiated and the brain volume moves toward normal. This adaptation accounts for the relative absence of symptoms in patients with slow developing high serum sodium levels (sometimes up to levels of 170–180 mEq/L).[37] Conversely, severe hypernatremia that develops over a period of less than 24 hours is often fatal. As will be noted in the section describing treatment of hypernatremia, overly rapid correction of the hypernatremia with free water can lead to dangerous cellular swelling. Recall that water administered into the bloodstream can quickly dilute the serum sodium level; however, because of the blood–brain barrier, the cellular fluid does not dilute at a similar rate. As a result, the cellular fluid becomes relatively more concentrated and creates a reversed osmotic gradient, pulling water into the cells.

ETIOLOGICAL FACTORS

Etiological factors associated with hypernatremia are listed in Table 4-8 and are briefly described below. In general, it should be noted that the etiology of hypernatremia is quite different in children and adults. For example, the most common cause in infants is diarrhea, whereas in the elderly, it is infirmity with inability to obtain sufficient free-water intake.

Water Deprivation

Hypernatremia may occur in any patient with a diminished mental status because the ability to perceive and respond to thirst are impaired. In adults, hypernatremia is most often seen in patients older than 60 years.[38] Not only are older persons at increased risk for illness and diminished mental status, increasing age is associated with lowered osmotic stimulation of thirst and decreased ability of the kidneys to conserve water in times of need. Infants, because they are unable to ask for water, are also at increased risk.

Insensible Water Loss

A typical adult patient with normal body temperature will lose approximately 1000 mL of water per day through respiration and evaporation from the skin (insensible water loss). When any condition is present that increases this insensible water loss (such as hyper-

---

TABLE 4–8.
Etiological Factors Associated With Hypernatremia

Deprivation of water, most common in unconscious or debilitated patients unable to perceive or respond to thirst (such as the elderly stroke patient)

Deprivation of water in infants, very young children, or retarded individuals unable to communicate thirst

Hypertonic tube feedings without adequate water supplements (see Chapter 13)

Greatly increased insensible water loss (as in hyperventilation or in extensive denuding effects of uncovered second- or third-degree burns)

Watery diarrhea

Ingestion of salt in unusual amounts (as in faulty preparation of oral electrolyte-replacement solutions)

Excessive parenteral administration of sodium-containing fluids
▶ Hypertonic saline (3% or 5% NaCl)
▶ Sodium bicarbonate ($NaHCO_3$) in cardiac arrest or treatment of lactic acidosis
▶ 0.9% NaCl (when primary fluid loss is water)

Diabetes insipidus if the patient does not experience, or cannot respond to, thirst; or, if fluids are excessively restricted

Less common are heatstroke, near drowning in sea water (which contains a sodium concentration of approximately 500 mEq/L), accidental introduction of hypertonic saline into maternal circulation during therapeutic abortion, and malfunction of either hemodialysis or peritoneal dialysis systems

ventilation or massive burns), hypernatremia may result. For example, patients with tracheostomies in dry environments can, with excessive minute volume air exchange, lose as much as 1 to 1.5 L of water by this route each day.[39]

Watery Diarrhea

Gastrointestinal fluid losses are a major cause of hypernatremia in children, and apparently result from a combination of hypotonic fluid loss in diarrheal stools, increased insensible water loss associated with concomitant fever, and excessive sodium administration in formulas or IV fluids. Fortunately, the incidence of this imbalance has decreased in recent years because more appropriate lower-solute replacement fluids are used (providing adequate amounts of free water). Loss of hypotonic fluid in the stool of cirrhotic patients treated with lactulose may also result in severe hypernatremia.[40]

Excessive Sodium Intake

Ingestion or IV infusion of too much salt can induce hypernatremia. Acute fatal hypernatremia due to excessive sodium intake has been reported after the accidental substitution of sodium chloride for sugar in infant formulas. It can also result from improperly prepared oral electrolyte solutions (addition of too much NaCl or $NaHCO_3$). Due to failure to check parenteral fluid containers carefully, fatalities have resulted from the administration of 5% sodium chloride solution instead of the intended 5% dextrose solution. Other causes of hypernatremia include excessive administration of $NaHCO_3$ during cardiac arrest or in the treatment of lactic acidosis. Elevated serum sodium levels can even occur from the administration of an isotonic sodium chloride solution (0.9% NaCl) if the patient's fluid deficit is primarily water.

Ingestion of sea water (which has a sodium concentration of 450 to 500 mEq/L can lead to severe hypernatremia. Accidental or purposeful excessive salt ingestion by children or incompetent adults has resulted in fatalities. (Drinking of a saturated salt solution has been reported as a method of suicide in China.[41]) Also, cases have been reported in which fatalities followed the accidental administration of hypertonic salt solutions into the maternal circulation during therapeutic abortion attempts.

Diabetes Insipidus

Diabetes insipidus (DI) is a water balance disorder with which is associated either a lack of ADH or an end-organ (kidney) resistance to its effects, leading to water diuresis. Hypernatremia will result if insufficient water is replaced either orally or IV. As a rule, however, the serum sodium remains normal because the individual with DI experiences thirst and drinks sufficient fluid to replace the lost urine volume. There are two types of DI, central and nephrogenic. Central DI (CDI) is sometimes referred to as neurogenic. Nephrogenic DI (NDI) is sometimes referred to as renal.

Central DI is due to a relative lack of ADH and is sometimes called vasopressin-sensitive DI because it responds favorably to vasopressin (ADH) administration. This form of DI may occur after head trauma (particularly caused by fractures at the base of the skull or surgical procedures near the pituitary) or as a result of infection, primary tumor, or metastatic tumor. It may also be idiopathic; approximately half of the patients with CDI have no known underlying pathology.

Nephrogenic DI is due to failure of the kidney to respond to ADH, not to a deficit of the hormone. This condition is sometimes referred to as vasopressin-resistant DI because the administration of vasopressin does not relieve the disorder. It may occur as a rare genetic disorder or may be acquired. Acquired NDI is much more common and may be the result of electrolyte disorders (such as hypokalemia or hypercalcemia), chronic renal failure, or drugs such as lithium, alcohol, demeclocycline, amphotericin, and vinblastine.[42] Fortunately, the NDI caused by hypercalcemia and hypokalemia is usually reversible within 1 to 12 weeks after correction of the imbalance.[43] Although usually reversible, the dose-related concentrating defect associated with lithium may become permanent after prolonged use of the drug.[44]

Other Causes

Although far less common than in the past, high protein intake in enteral feedings may produce an increased osmotic load of urea, which necessitates the excretion of large volumes of water. Hypernatremia, azotemia, and ECF volume deficit may follow. Osmotic diuretics (such as mannitol or urea) may also produce an obligatory water loss, resulting in hypernatremia.

Hypernatremia may occur in patients receiving peritoneal dialysis or hemodialysis. This imbalance was more prevalent when a 7% dextrose dialysate was available for peritoneal dialysis. Although the 7% dextrose dialysate is no longer used, mild hypernatremia can still occur with currently used preparations. The dextrose concentration in the dialysate and the length of the dwell period appear to be major factors governing this complication. Because of the high diffusibility of sodium across the dialyzer membrane, the serum sodium after a hemodialysis treatment reflects the dialysate sodium. Thus, use of a dialysate with a sodium concentration in excess of 140 mEq/L can result in postdialysate hypernatremia.[45] Other causes of hypernatremia in dialysis patients include accidents in the dialysate delivery system.

DEFINING CHARACTERISTICS

Defining characteristics of hypernatremia are given in Table 4-9. When the patient is awake, thirst is the usual early sign of developing hypernatremia. It should be noted that thirst, by stimulating water intake, normally protects against hypernatremia. Thus, hypernatremia generally occurs in individuals either unable to perceive or respond to thirst (eg, adults with an altered mental status or infants). An awake, alert patient with hypernatremia can be assumed to have a hypothalamic lesion affecting the thirst center.

Like hyponatremia, the primary manifestations of hypernatremia are neurological in nature. The earliest signs are lethargy, weakness, and irritability. These symptoms can progress to twitching, seizures, coma, and death if the hypernatremia is severe. They are presumably the consequence of cellular dehydration (resulting from pulling of fluid from the cells into the hyperosmotic ECF). If hypernatremia is severe, permanent brain damage can occur, especially in children. Brain damage is apparently due to subarachnoid hemorrhages that result from tearing of vessels during brain contraction. Because of rupture of cerebral vessels, a lumbar puncture may reveal blood in the cerebrospinal fluid. Symptoms in infants often include marked irritability and a high-pitched cry, with a depressed sensorium ranging from lethargy to frank coma. In adults, the symptoms of hypernatremia are often difficult to separate from those of the underlying pathology, which is often of a catastrophic nature.

As is the case with hyponatremia, the rapidity of onset is an important determinant of the severity of symptoms as well as the eventual outcome of hypernatremia. Chronic hypernatremia that evolves over more than 2 days is associated with a much lower incidence of mortality than acute hypernatremia. Recall that the body initiates a series of events to protect the brain within 24 hours of the development of hypernatremia.

If the hypernatremia is accompanied by FVD (sometimes referred to as hypertonic fluid volume depletion), other symptoms such as postural hypotension may occur. Conversely, if associated with FVE, pulmonary edema and increased venous pressure may be evident.

Hypernatremia is the only imbalance with which dry, sticky mucous membranes are associated.[52] The tongue may appear red and swollen and the skin flushed. Body temperature is generally elevated and may approach a lethal level, as in the patient suffering from heatstroke.[53] Fever will generally occur if the room temperature exceeds 65°F (18.3°C).[54]

Diabetes Insipidus

The most prevalent signs of DI are polyuria and polydipsia. Depending on the severity of the disease, the degree of polyuria in central DI can range from 3 to 15 L in 24 hours. It is usually much less in acquired NDI

TABLE 4–9.
Defining Characteristics of Hypernatremia

Thirst (Note that thirst is so strong a defender of serum sodium in normal individuals that hypernatremia never occurs unless the person is rendered unconscious or is denied access to water; ill persons may have an impaired thirst mechanism.)

Elevated body temperature may occur if room temperature is higher than 65°F (18.3°C)[46]

Tongue dry and swollen; dry and sticky mucous membranes[47]

Restlessness and weakness in moderate hypernatremia

Disorientation, delusions, and hallucinations in severe hypernatremia[48]; or, patient may be lethargic when undisturbed and irritable and hyperreactive when stimulated[49]

Lethargy, stupor, or coma. (The level of consciousness depends not only on actual sodium levels, but on the rate of development of hypernatremia. For example, a patient may have a serum sodium level of 170 mEq/L and remain conscious if the imbalance developed slowly.)

Muscle irritability and convulsions[50]

Signs of irritability and high-pitched cry in infants[51]

Laboratory data
▸ Serum sodium >145 mEq/L
▸ Serum osmolality >295 mOsm/kg
▸ Urinary specific gravity >1.015 as the kidneys attempt to conserve water (provided water loss is from a route other than the kidneys)

TABLE 4–10.
Clinical Manifestations of Diabetes Insipidus

Excessive urinary output regardless of fluid intake

Urinary output often exceeds 200 mL/hr

Urinary specific gravity <1.005; urine osmolality <200 mOsm/L

Serum osmolality and sodium levels greater than normal if water intake does not match urinary losses

Intense thirst in the alert patient (volume of intake corresponds to urine volume)

Inability of kidneys to concentrate urine by fluid restriction (a common test for this disorder)

Polyuria in central diabetes insipidus ranges from 3 to 15 L per 24 hours (depending on the severity of the disease) and usually from 3 to 4 L per 24 hours for acquired nephrogenic diabetes insipidus

(such as 3–4 L/day).[55] Patients with CDI often crave ice water to quench their thirst. Clinical manifestations of DI are summarized in Table 4-10.

As a rule, the patient with an intact thirst mechanism will drink sufficient fluids to maintain balance (ie, an essentially normal serum sodium and serum osmolality). Unfortunately, the frequency of urination and drinking often interferes with other activities when the condition is severe.

If the patient is not able to perceive or respond to thirst or if parenteral fluid replacement is inadequate, polyuria will lead to severe dehydration (hypernatremia and hyperosmolality of plasma) with weight loss, tachycardia, and even shock.

TREATMENT

Too rapid correction of hypernatremia can result in cerebral edema, seizures, permanent neurological damage, and death. As discussed in the section on pathophysiology, hypernatremia initially pulls water from brain cells and produces brain contraction. After a period of approximately 24 hours, however, the brain begins to adapt by increasing the intracellular solute level. Rapid lowering of the plasma sodium can render the plasma relatively hypoosmotic to the brain cells and allow water to be pulled into the cells, producing cerebral edema. (Note that the blood–brain barrier prevents the intracellular solutes from being diluted at the same rate as the solute in the plasma.) To minimize the risk of complications, it is generally recommended that the plasma sodium concentration be gradually lowered to normal over a minimum of 48 hours and at a maximum rate of 2 mEq/L/hr.[56]

Standard formulas exist for calculating the degree

of free-water deficit in hypernatremic patients. Generally, sufficient free water is given in the form of hypotonic fluids (ranging from 5% dextrose in water to 0.45% sodium chloride solution) to lower the plasma sodium level gradually over a period of approximately 48 hours.[57] Patients who have sustained both water and sodium losses and who show evidence of circulatory insufficiency may need to receive isotonic saline (0.9% NaCl) until they become hemodynamically stable. After stabilization, 0.45% NaCl may be infused.[58]

Diabetes Insipidus

The standard treatment of CDI has been ADH replacement by means of vasopressin administration. Vasopressin may be administered in different forms, depending on the clinical situation.

It may be given by injection in the form of aqueous vasopressin in acute care settings (duration 1–4 hours). Aqueous vasopressin's short-duration action allows for greater control of fluid balance in rapidly fluctuating situations. General indications for its administration include urinary output exceeding 200 mL/hr for 2 consecutive hours, urinary specific gravity (SG) less than 1.005, and an elevated serum sodium level.

Vasopression may also be given as Pitressin tannate in oil (duration 24–72 hours) or intranasally in the form of Diapid (lypressin) or desmopressin acetate (DDAVP).

Until the polyuria is controlled by vasopressin therapy, careful attention must be paid to replacement of fluid (particularly if the patient has a decreased level of consciousness or other disturbances interfering with the perception of thirst or the ability to drink). However, it is important to recall that a potential complication of vasopressin therapy is water intoxication (excessive retention of water).

If the patient with CDI has some residual capacity to secrete ADH, drugs that increase the release of ADH or enhance its action on the kidney may be used instead of hormonal replacement therapy. Such drugs include chlorpropamide (Diabinese), an oral hypoglycemia agent, and carbamazepine (Tegretol), an anticonvulsant.

Paradoxically, thiazide diuretic agents are sometimes used to decrease the polyuria associated with DI.[59] It is believed that the thiazides act by decreasing the amount of sodium ions that reach the distal tubules of the kidneys. Patients taking thiazides for treatment of DI should be instructed to avoid liberal use of salt because it decreases the effectiveness of the drug.

NURSING INTERVENTIONS

1. Identify patients at risk for hypernatremia (review Table 4-8).

2. Monitor fluid losses and gains. Look for abnormal losses of water or low water intake, and for large gains of sodium as may occur with prescription drugs having a high sodium content. For example, 24 g of carbenicillin disodium (a possible daily dose) contain 142 mEq of sodium.[60] Fleet enema solution also has a high sodium content.

3. Monitor for symptoms of hypernatremia (see Table 4-9). Evaluate these in relation to other factors in the patient's history.

4. Monitor serum sodium levels as frequently as indicated.

5. Prevent hypernatremia in debilitated patients unable to perceive or respond to thirst by offering them fluids at regular intervals. If fluid intake remains inadequate, consult with the physician to plan an alternate route for intake, by either tube feedings or the parenteral route.

6. If tube feedings are used, give sufficient water to keep the serum sodium and the blood urea nitrogen (BUN) levels within normal limits (see Chapter 13).

7. Monitor the patient's response to corrective parenteral fluids by reviewing serial sodium levels and observing any changes in neurological signs. With gradual decrease in the serum sodium level, the neurological signs should improve, not worsen. Be aware that the serum sodium should be decreased gradually (see Treatment; see Case Study 2).

8. For patients with DI:
   A. Monitor parameters outlined in Table 4-11.
   B. Ensure that the alert DI patient with intact thirst mechanism is allowed to drink at will; also, ensure that this individual is near a bathroom as frequent voiding is anticipated until the condition is brought under control.
   C. Ensure that the patient with a decreased level of consciousness, or other disability interfering with drinking, is given adequate fluid; if the patient is unable to take fluids orally, consult with the physician to obtain parenteral fluid orders.

TABLE 4–11.
Assessment for Diabetes Insipidus

---

1. Be aware of patients at risk for DI
   Central DI
   ▶ Head trauma (particularly with fractures at the base of the skull or surgical procedures near the pituitary)
   ▶ Cerebral infections
   ▶ Brain tumors
   Nephrogenic DI
   ▶ Hypokalemia
   ▶ Hypercalcemia
   ▶ Certain drugs (such as lithium and demeclocycline)
2. Maintain an accurate I & O record for at-risk patients.
   ▶ Look for a significantly greater output than intake (a danger signal of impending hypernatremia). Fortunately, many patients keep themselves "in balance" by drinking approximately as much as they urinate. It is helpful to calculate and record cumulative amounts for several days to obtain a more accurate account of the patient's fluid balance status, particularly if onset of polyuria was insidious
3. Be alert for polyuria in at-risk patients.
   ▶ It is frequently necessary to measure hourly urine volumes in such individuals to foster early detection. For example, a frequent directive in the care of postoperative neurosurgical patients is to report a urine volume greater than 200 mL in each of 2 consecutive hours or more than 500 mL in a 2-hour period.
4. Monitor urinary SG in at-risk patients.
   ▶ A persistently dilute urine is a hallmark of DI. (The SG may be as low as 1.005.)
5. Monitor serum sodium levels at least once a day (more often as indicated) in at-risk patients.
   ▶ Look for hypernatremia (serum sodium > 145 mEq/L). Once vasopressin therapy has been initiated, look for hyponatremia (a possible rebound effect).
6. Monitor body weights.
   ▶ Look for weight loss paralleling polyuria. Maintaining a weight chart helps detect excessive fluid loss, particularly when I & O records are in doubt (as may occur in incontinent patients).

DI, diabetes insipidus; SG, specific gravity.

Summary of Hypernatremia

ETIOLOGICAL FACTORS	DEFINING CHARACTERISTICS
Deprivation of water (most common in those unable to perceive or respond to thirst)	Thirst usually occurs early
	Dry, sticky mucous membranes, and dry, swollen tongue
Increased insensible water loss (as in hyperventilation)	Fever may be present
Watery diarrhea	Severe hypernatremia
Ingestion of salt in unusual amounts	▸ Disorientation
	▸ Hallucinations
Excessive parenteral administration of sodium-containing solutions	▸ Lethargy when undisturbed
▸ Hypertonic saline (3% or 5% NaCl)	▸ Irritability when stimulated
▸ Sodium bicarbonate	▸ Focal or grand mal seizures
▸ Isotonic saline	▸ Coma
Profuse sweating with no water replacement	Serum sodium >145 mEq/L
	Serum osmolality >295 mOsm/kg
Near drowning in sea water	Urinary SG >1.015, provided water loss is from nonrenal route
Heatstroke	For diabetes insipidus, see Table 4-10
Diabetes insipidus if water intake is inadequate	

Anticipate performing this intervention in neurological patients, particularly in the early postoperative period.

D. Administer medications for DI with an understanding of their actions.

E. Be aware that a potential complication of vasopressin administration is water intoxication (excessive retention of water causing a low serum sodium level). This is particularly important because it is difficult to regulate vasopressin dosage in patients with rapidly fluctuating clinical states.

F. Educate patients regarding the proper use of prescribed medications and how to monitor and record fluctuations in their fluid I & O and body weight.

Case Studies

1. An 80-year-old woman living in a nursing home had a stroke and developed aphasia and hemiplegia. Because of her neurological deficits, she required a great deal of assistance to eat and drink. Due to lack of attention from the staff, she ingested insufficient water and developed a serum sodium of 188 mEq/L.

Commentary: A serum sodium concentration greater than 150 mEq/L is virtually never seen in an alert patient with a normal thirst mechanism and access to water.[61] This hypernatremic patient represents a common problem in patients with decreased awareness and inability to drink. One author stated that hypernatremic dehydration constitutes a "sentinel health event" in patients without documented rapid free-water loss. A *sentinel health event* is defined as an illness or death that should be preventable, given adequate care, or should at least cause those caring for the patient to ask why the event occurred.[62] In the absence of free-water loss, hypernatremic dehydration probably indicates fluid deprivation (a form of neglect).

2. A 60-year old woman with a serum sodium level of 185 mEq/L was transferred from a nursing home to an acute care facility. Aggressive IV therapy with large volumes of 5% dextrose in water was instituted, and her serum sodium dropped to 145 mEq/L in 5 hours. She became unresponsive; a lumbar puncture revealed an opening pressure of 32 cm of water (normal is 10–20 cm of water).

Commentary: This patient had been hypernatremic for some time, allowing her brain to adapt to the hyperosmolal state by increasing brain osmolality. (In hypernatremia, brain volume declines initially and then begins to adapt toward normal within 24 hours.)[63] Once this cerebral adaptation has occurred, any rapid lowering of the serum sodium level creates an osmotic gradient, allowing water to move into the brain, increasing brain size and causing cerebral edema. This is precisely what happened in the above case; had the serum sodium been decreased gradually, cerebral edema would not have occurred.

3. Over a 16-hour period, a young child was inadvertently given 800 mL of 5% NaCl solution (containing 855 mEq of sodium/L) instead of the prescribed 5% dextrose in half-strength saline (containing 77 mEq of sodium/L). She developed lethargy, convulsions, and coma before the error was discovered. Despite resuscitative efforts, the child died. *Commentary:* Instead of a hypotonic sodium fluid, this child received a grossly hypertonic sodium solution, causing fatal brain damage. This terrible event would never have occurred had the fluid been checked properly before being administered.

4. A 55-year-old comatose woman with a basal skull fracture was transferred to a medical center from a small suburban hospital. Her urine output was noted to be 200 mL/hr and her serum sodium was 170 mEq/L. Urine osmolality was 80 mOsm/kg (extremely dilute, reflecting excessive water loss in the urine) and the serum osmolality was 360 mOsm/kg (reflecting the hypernatremia). A diagnosis of central DI was made and vasopressin tannate in oil was administered. In 3 days the serum sodium level had fallen to 130 mEq/L. *Commentary:* This patient was not hydrated adequately at the outset and thus developed hypernatremia. The staff should have been alert for CDI because of the nature of the injury (basal skull fracture). In the acute phase of CDI, most physicians prescribe aqueous vasopressin because its short duration of action allows for greater control of fluid balance in rapidly fluctuating states. Recall that vasopressin tannate in oil has a duration of 24 to 72 hours and thus makes control difficult in rapidly fluctuating situations.

5. A 65-year-old man had received diuretics to manage his hypertension for the last 6 months. During a visit to his physician, he reported that he was more thirsty than usual and frequently had to get up at night to urinate (nocturia). Laboratory analysis found his serum potassium to be 2.4 mEq/L. He was hospitalized for evaluation; it was found that he could concentrate his urine to only 300 mOsm/kg on fluid restriction (instead of the expected 1200–1400 mOsm/kg in normal renal function). After correction of the hypokalemia, his renal concentrating ability and urine volume eventually returned to normal. *Commentary:* This patient had acquired nephrogenic DI due to hypokalemia. Many patients with potassium depletion complain of polyuria; it is caused by a reduced ability to concentrate the urine due to

decreased responsiveness to ADH. This resistance to ADH may be due to an interference with the generation and action of cyclic AMP.[64] Although the nephrogenic DI associated with hypokalemia is usually reversible, recall that more severe changes are possible with prolonged hypokalemia. Lesions may occur in the epithelial cells of the proximal tubule; in addition, interstitial fibrosis is occasionally observed.[65] The interstitial lesions may be irreversible. Because of these and other potential complications of hypokalemia, the imbalance should be prevented or at least detected early.

SODIUM AND HEAT STRESS

Physiological disturbances related to heat stress range from mild to severe. The discussion below describes the relationship between sodium and the major types of heat-related disorders.

HEAT SYNCOPE

Heat syncope is associated with postural hypotension, which occurs when blood is diverted to peripheral tissues for cooling. Diminished venous return to the heart and reduction of cardiac output lead to cerebral ischemia, which accounts for the syncope. This condition is most likely to occur in persons deficient in salt and water, particularly if cardiovascular disease is present. Thus, patients receiving diuretics are at increased risk. Treatment other than rest in a cool environment generally is not needed.[66]

HEAT EDEMA

Shortly after entering a hot climate, slight swelling of the hands and feet is very common among unacclimatized individuals (those not accustomed to the heat). Most often occurring in women, the edema disappears as heat tolerance is gained. Likely causes are salt and water retention from salt supplementation, increased aldosterone production, and oliguria after heat-induced vasodilation.[67] Fortunately, this is a self-limiting condition that does not require treatment.

HEAT CRAMPS

As the name implies, *heat cramps* are characterized by painful muscle contractions in persons exposed to heat stress. More specifically, heat cramps are painful, intermittent contractions of skeletal muscles after strenuous activity in a hot environment. (Of interest, they most often occur in individuals in excellent physical condi-

tion who are accustomed to working in a hot environment.) Such individuals are able to produce large quantities of sweat in response to strenuous exercise and
heat stress.

Precipitating factors are strenuous exercise, hemodilution (due to large water intake with no salt), and
cooling of the muscle. Because patients with heat
cramps are hyponatremic, it is believed that the mechanism for heat cramp production is sodium depletion in
the muscle.[68] Typically, heat cramps occur toward the
end of a strenuous period, on relaxation or taking a
cool shower. (Cooling of the involved muscle cells apparently slows sodium transport and depolarizes the
cells.)[69]

Ingestion of salt before or during exercise is usually
an effective prophylaxis for heat cramps. To replace salt
lost in sweat, salt can be added to foods as a seasoning
or liquids having salt as a component can be consumed. Once heat cramps have occurred, treatment involves salt ingestion, either orally or IV. For severe, un-
relenting cramps, oral or IV salt solutions quickly
relieve all signs.[70]

HEAT EXHAUSTION

Heat exhaustion is a common yet vague clinical entity.
Although pure forms are uncommon, heat exhaustion
can be divided into two major forms, that associated
primarily with sodium depletion (hyponatremia) and
that associated with dehydration (water deficit with
hypernatremia).

Heat Exhaustion Due Primarily to Salt Depletion

Heat exhaustion due to salt depletion occurs when large
volumes of sweat from heat-stressed individuals are replaced by adequate volumes of water but too little salt.
This condition differs from heat cramps in two ways:
first, it tends to occur in individuals who are *not* accustomed to heat stress, and second, it involves systemic
effects beyond skeletal muscle cramps. Among these
are fatigue, weakness, giddiness, frontal headache,
anorexia, nausea, vomiting, and diarrhea.[71] Because
water is consumed to replace the lost sweat, marked
weight loss may not occur. Treatment consists of administering salted liquids by mouth. If necessary, isotonic saline (0.9% NaCl) may be given IV.

Heat Exhaustion Due to Water Depletion

This form of heat exhaustion is caused when sweat
losses are not replaced by the individual working under
heat stress, resulting in a negative water balance. As a
rule, this set of circumstances is experienced by indi-

viduals for whom the water supply is limited (eg, sol-
diers or laborers who are unable to gain access to
water). Clinically, there is intense thirst, fatigue, weakness, discomfort, and impaired judgment.[72] Body temperature is almost always elevated, although not to the
level associated with heatstroke. The person with *heat
exhaustion due to water depletion* usually has a temperature that is normal or lower than 102° F (39° C),
whereas the person with heatstroke usually has a much
higher temperature. Left untreated, heat exhaustion
condition may terminate in heatstroke.[73]

Treatment consists of water replacement. However,
as discussed earlier in the chapter, rapid correction of
severe hypernatremia must be guarded against to avoid
initiating convulsive seizures. It has been recommended
that the serum osmolality be decreased at a rate no
faster than 2 to 4 mOsm/hr.[74] If possible, water should
be given orally. However, if the patient is vomiting or
unconscious, the solution of choice is 5% dextrose in
water; when the serum sodium has fallen to 150 mEq/L,
hypotonic saline (0.45% NaCl) can be substituted for
water.[75]

HEATSTROKE

Heatstroke is likely with elevation of body temperature
beyond a critical point (in the range of 106–108° F).[76]
Symptoms include delirium, dizziness, abdominal distress, and eventually loss of consciousness. Symptoms
are related in part to reduced circulatory volume
brought about by excessive sweating. Others are directly related to the effects of hyperthermia on the
brain and other body tissues. Autopsies on individuals
who died from heatstroke have shown hemorrhages
and parenchymatous cellular degeneration throughout
the body.

Two forms of heatstroke are often described, classical and exercise-induced. Classical heatstroke occurs
primarily in invalids or in the elderly during a sustained heat wave. In contrast, exertion-induced heatstroke usually occurs in well-conditioned athletes or
workers whose physical means to dissipate heat are exceeded by endogenous heat production. Examples include football players, marathon runners, and military
recruits.

Most important in the treatment of heatstroke is
lowering body temperature to a safe level. Several
methods have been proposed, tested, and in varying
degrees accepted to accomplish safe heat reduction.
These include cold water immersion with skin massage,[77] compressed air/warm water sprays,[78] and strate-
gically placed ice packs.[79]

Placement of IV lines and tracheal intubation are
necessary, as is placement of a rectal thermistore to

measure core temperature. Hypotension is likely to be present as blood is shunted to the periphery for cooling. Excessive fluid replacement should be guarded against because pulmonary edema could result as cooling promotes return of peripheral blood to the central circulation. Sodium levels are variable, and often depend on conditions leading to heatstroke. The most important laboratory measurements at time of admission are arterial blood gases, serum electrolyte concentrations, and complete blood count. Treatment is based on results and other clinical findings.

PREVENTIVE MEASURES AND RATIONALES

Heat disorders can often be prevented, or at least minimized, by some relatively simple measures.

1. Before engaging in sustained strenuous activity, undergo acclimatization to a hot environment.
   ► Exposure to heat for several hours each day while performing a reasonably heavy workload will increase tolerance to heat in 1 to 3 weeks.[80] Acclimatized individuals attain an increased maximum rate of sweating, increased plasma volume, and decreased loss of salt in the sweat and urine. The latter two effects are related to an increased production of aldosterone. (Although the sodium content of sweat in these individuals is less than that in nonacclimatized persons, it can still be the source of significant sodium loss.)
2. To offset the body's loss of water and salt in sweat, drink cool liquids at regular intervals while undergoing heat stress.
   ► First, consider fluids that are inappropriate for replacing losses. Alcohol is certainly contraindicated because it has diuretic effects but, more important, because it can alter judgment about heat exposure. Further, a brief period of moderate or heavy alcohol intake often appears to cause loss of acclimatization.[81] Coffee and tea are not recommended for sole use in fluid replacement as these beverages have diuretic properties and predispose to further fluid loss.
   ► Depending on individual need, fluid replacement can be in the form of water, a sodium chloride solution, or a balanced electrolyte solution. *Water is often sufficient* when the subject has taken in a normal diet supplying ample sodium, potassium, and other electrolytes. However, sustained losses of sweat over prolonged periods may necessitate electrolyte replacement in addition to water. A solution of sodium chloride (4 tsp of salt to a gallon of water) for oral consumption may suffice to prevent heat cramps.[82] Care must be taken

to avoid excessive salt and insufficient water intake because this practice predisposes to water-depletion heat exhaustion that can culminate in heatstroke.[83]

► A few oral electrolyte-rehydrating fluids are available commercially and usually contain varying quantities of carbohydrates in the form of simple sugars or glucose polymers. Advantages of carbohydrates in replacement fluids are improved endurance during strenuous exertion (due to muscle glycogen sparing) and pleasant taste (perhaps ensuring that they will be consumed in greater quantity than plain water or electrolyte solutions). However, a potential difficulty with carbohydrates is their effect on gastric emptying time, that is, the higher the solution's carbohydrate content or osmolality, the more likely gastric emptying is to be inhibited, thereby reducing the rate of fluid absorption into the system. Some authors believe that fluids with a high carbohydrate concentration slow gastric emptying and produce satiety, thus discouraging further intake of needed fluids.[84]

> To compare the effects of drinking distilled water with those of carbohydrate-electrolyte solution* on physiological disturbances during prolonged strenuous exercise in the heat, Carter and Gisolfi[85] studied seven males during and after vigorous bouts of cycle exercise. The authors concluded that the carbohydrate-electrolyte beverage used in their study maintained plasma volume at a level higher than water during exercise, supplied an energy source, and rehydrated subjects faster than water during recovery.

► The number of people participating in marathons and triathlons has greatly increased over the past decade. Electrolyte disturbances are more likely to occur during events that last a prolonged period in the heat. During triathlon events in high environmental temperatures, volume depletion and hyponatremia are likely if the athlete replaces sweat losses with water (although in inadequate amounts) but no salt. As Hiller[86] reported, it is common for endurance athletes to be both volume depleted and hyponatremic after races, such as triathlons, lasting longer than 8 hours. In these situations, the exercise-induced hyponatremia is a combination of massive unreplaced sodium losses associated with partially replaced massive water losses. Hiller[87] recommends that

---

*Composed of 4.85% polycose, 2.65% fructose, 9.2 mM Na^+, 5.0 mM K^+, 2.1 mM Ca^+, 2.1 mM Mg, 9.6 mM Cl^-, 250 mOsm/L

endurance athletes practice programmed replacement of hourly fluid losses (such as 500 mL of fluid for each 1-lb weight loss), and that they use some form of sodium replacement during events lasting longer than 4 hours. He further recommends that they prepare by increasing their salt intake during the period before the event during which they become acclimatized. If sodium-containing fluids are needed to treat athletes after the events, 5% dextrose in normal saline may be used for races lasting longer than 4 hours and 5% dextrose in either normal or half-normal saline for events lasting less than 4 hours.[88]

3. Strenuous activity on hot days should be curtailed as much as possible.

   ▶ Periods of prolonged exercise, such as training programs or athletic events, should take place during the cooler parts of the day (before 8 am and after 5 pm). Care should be taken to avoid direct solar heat radiation during the hottest hours of the day (11 am to 2 pm).

4. When possible, loose, porous clothing should be worn to allow for heat dissipation.

   ▶ A hat and light-colored clothing are helpful in decreasing the amount of heat absorbed from direct sunlight, although workers in specific jobs may need different types of clothing. For example, those working with radiant heat should wear reflective garments. Unfortunately, the nature of some work requires that special protective clothing be worn, further predisposing to heat injury. For example, welders and others exposed to sparks should wear self-extinguishing materials like "green cotton," that is, cotton treated with flame retardant.[89]

   ▶ Firefighters must wear heavy protective clothing (often rubberized) that predisposes them to increased heat stress. Engaging in strenuous activity while dressed in impervious plastic sweat clothing is potentially disastrous. The belief that this activity can safely result in weight loss in overweight athletes is erroneous.

5. During extreme high temperatures, individuals without air conditioners or fans should make use of "cooling centers" that are usually available in most communities.

   ▶ Unfortunately, many elderly inner-city residents are hesitant to leave their homes for cooling centers during heat waves because of a fear of burglaries or vandalism.

6. Adequate fluids should be provided for confused or otherwise debilitated patients unable to respond to thirst.

7. Coaches and trainers in athletic programs and supervisors in the workplace should be aware of the warning signs of heat disorders and the measures to deal with them.

8. Participants and planners of competitive sports events should consider the following points:

   A. Competitors should train in the heat before the big event to promote acclimatization.

   B. Competitors should avoid fluid restriction before the start of the event. Pre-event dehydration results in a reduction of the body's sweating and, therefore, cooling abilities.

   C. Fluid stations should be readily available at strategic locations to allow the competitors to replace needed fluids.

   D. Competitors and race officials should be aware that events lasting longer than 4 hours are more likely to produce fluid and electrolyte problems than are those lasting less than 4 hours.

   E. Trained spotters should be placed at regular locations during the event to identify competitors with early signs of heat injury. Cooling and fluid replacement should be initiated on the spot. Athletes should use the "buddy system" and assume mutual responsibility for each other's well being during the event.

REFERENCES

1. Goldberger E: A Primer of Water, Electrolyte and Acid–Base Syndromes, 7th ed, p 353. Philadelphia, Lea & Febiger, 1986

2. Maxwell M, Kleeman C, Narins R: Clinical Disorders of Fluid and Electrolyte Metabolism, 4th ed, p 462. New York, McGraw-Hill, 1987

3. Katz M: Hyperglycemia-induced hyponatremia: Calculation of expected serum sodium depression. N Engl J Med 40:10, 1966

4. Sterns R: Severe symptomatic hyponatremia, treatment and outcome: A study of 64 cases. Ann Intern Med 107:656, 1987

5. Ibid

6. Kokko J, Tannen R: Fluids and Electrolytes, 2nd ed, p 1000. Philadelphia, WB Saunders, 1990

7. Ibid, p 76

8. Maxwell et al, p 465

9. Rose B: Clinical Physiology of Acid–Base and Electrolyte Disorders, 3rd ed, p 611. New York, McGraw-Hill, 1989

10. Weissman P, Shenkman L, Gregerman R: Chlorpropamide hyponatremia: Drug-induced inappropriate antidiuretic hormone activity. N Engl J Med 284:65, 1971

11. Rose, p 611

12. Kokko, Tannen, p 168

13. Ibid

14. Wijdicks et al: Hyponatremia and cerebral infarction in patients with ruptured intracranial aneurysms: Is fluid restriction harmful? Ann Neurol 17:137, 1985

15. Illowsky B, Kirch D: Polydipsia and hyponatremia in psychiatric patients. Am J Psychiatry 145:675, 1988
16. Hariprasad et al: Hyponatremia in psychogenic polydipsia. Arch Intern Med 140:1639, 1980
17. Kokko, Tannen, p 165
18. Mwambingu F: Water intoxication and oxytocin. Br Med J 290:113, 1985
19. Chung et al: Postoperative hyponatremia. Arch Intern Med 146:333, 1986
20. Kokko, Tannen, p 164
21. Rose, p 612
22. Ibid
23. Kokko, Tannen, p 169
24. Hahn R: Relations between irrigant absorption rate and hyponatremia during transurethral resection of the prostate. Acta Anaesthesiol Scand 32:53, 1988
25. Vitting et al: Frequency of hyponatremia and non-osmolar vasopressin release in the acquired immunodeficiency syndrome. JAMA 263:973, 1990
26. Agarwal et al: Hyponatremia in patients with the acquired immunodeficiency syndrome. Nephron 53:317, 1989
27. Arieff A, Guisado R, Lazarowitz V: Effects on the central nervous system of hypernatremia and hyponatremic states. Kidney Int 10:104, 1976
28. Vanatta J, Fogelman M: Moyer's Fluid Balance: A Clinical Manual, 4th ed, p 44. Chicago, Year Book Medical Publishers, 1988
29. Kokko, Tannen, p 166
30. Rose, p 618
31. Ibid, p 619
32. Pennington J: Bowes & Church's Food Values of Portions Commonly Used, 15th ed, p 177, 1989
33. Vanatta, Fogelman, p 45
34. Ibid
35. Ibid
36. Rose, p 641
37. Ibid, p 653
38. Ibid, p 642
39. Maxwell et al, p 923
40. Kokko, Tannen, p 180
41. Ross E, Christie S: Hypernatremia. Medicine 48:441, 1969
42. Schrier R: Renal and Electrolyte Disorders, 3rd ed, p 60. Boston, Little, Brown, 1986
43. Rose, p 646
44. Ibid
45. Maxwell et al, p 1084
46. Vanatta, Fogelman, p 49
47. Ibid, p 50
48. Ibid
49. Ibid
50. Maxwell et al, p 1179
51. Ibid
52. Shires GT: Fluids, Electrolytes, and Acid Bases, p 6. New York, Churchill Livingstone, 1988
53. Schwartz S, Shires T, Spencer F: Principles of Surgery, 5th ed, p 75. New York, McGraw-Hill, 1989
54. Vanatta, Fogelman, p 49
55. Schrier, p 32
56. Votey S, Peters A, Hoffman J: Disorders of water metabolism: Hyponatremia and hypernatremia. Emerg Med Clin North Am 7:749, 1989
57. Kokko, Tannen, p 1010
58. Votey et al, p 749
59. Maxwell et al, p 495
60. Goldberger, p 102
61. Rose, p 642
62. Himmelstein D, Jones A, Woolhander S: Hypernatremic dehydration in nursing home patients: An indicator of neglect. J Am Geriatr Soc 31:466, 1983
63. Rose, p 652
64. Ibid, p 647
65. Schrier, p 233
66. Knochel J, Reed G: Disorders of heat regulation. In: Maxwell M, Kleeman C, Narins R (eds): Clinical Disorders of Fluid and Electrolyte Metabolism, 4th ed, p 1206. New York, McGraw-Hill, 1987
67. Ibid
68. Ibid, p 1207
69. Ibid
70. Ibid
71. Ibid
72. Ibid
73. Scott J: Heat-related illnesses: When are they a true emergency? Postgraduate Medicine 85(8): 154, 1989
74. Knochel, Reed, p 1208
75. Ibid
76. Guyton A: Textbook of Medical Physiology, 7th ed, p 859, Philadelphia, WB Saunders, 1986
77. Costrini A: Emergency treatment of exertional heatstroke and comparison of whole body cooling techniques. Medicine and Science in Sports and Exercise 22(1): 15, 1990
78. Wyndham C, Strydom B, Cooke H: Methods of cooling subjects with hyperpyrexia. J App Physiol 14:771, 1959
79. Kielblock A, VanRensberg J, Franz R: Body cooling as a method for reducing hyperpyrexia. South African Medical Journal 69:378, 1986
80. Guyton, p 859
81. Knochel, Reed, p 1209
82. LaDou J: Occupational Medicine, p 111. Norwalk, Appleton Lange, 1990
83. Knochel, Reed, p 1213
84. Goldberger E: A Primer of Water, Electrolyte and Acid–Base Syndromes, 7th ed, p 35. Philadelphia, Lea & Febiger, 1986
85. Carter J, Gisolfi C: Fluid replacement during and after exercise in the heat. Med Sci Sports Exerc 21:532, 1989
86. Hiller W: Dehydration and hyponatremia during triathlons. Med Sci Sports Exerc 21:S219, 1989
87. Ibid
88. Ibid
89. Eisma T: Cool under fire: Wearers of heat-protective clothing must avoid heat stress. Occup Health Saf November: 26, 1989

5

Potassium Imbalances

Disturbances in potassium balance are common because they are associated with a number of disease and injury states. Unfortunately, they may also be induced by the administration of a variety of medications as well as by therapies such as hyperalimentation and chemotherapy.

It is important to review some pertinent facts about potassium before proceeding to discussions of hypokalemia and hyperkalemia.

POTASSIUM BALANCE

Potassium is the major *intracellular* electrolyte; in fact, 98% of the body's potassium is inside the cells. The remaining 2% is in the extracellular fluid (ECF): this 2% is all-important in neuromuscular function. Potassium is constantly moving in and out of cells according to the body's needs, under the influence of the sodium–potassium pump.

The normal serum potassium concentration ranges from 3.5 to 5.0 mEq/L; even minor variations are significant. Normal renal function is necessary for maintenance of potassium balance as 80% of the potassium excreted daily from the body is by way of the kidneys. The other 20% is lost through the bowel and sweat glands.

Potassium must be replaced daily; approximately 40 to 60 mEq/day suffice in the adult if there are no abnormal losses occurring. Dietary intake in the average adult is 50 to 100 mEq/day.

Potassium influences both skeletal and cardiac muscle activity. For example, alterations in its concentration change myocardial irritability and rhythm. Electrocardiogram (ECG) changes produced by serum potassium level variations are illustrated in Figure 5-1. Although the correlation between serum potassium level and ECG changes is not sufficiently precise to predict serum potassium measurements, serial ECG may reveal whether a patient's serum level is moving toward hypokalemia or hyperkalemia.[1] Other changes associated with deficit or excess of potassium are de-

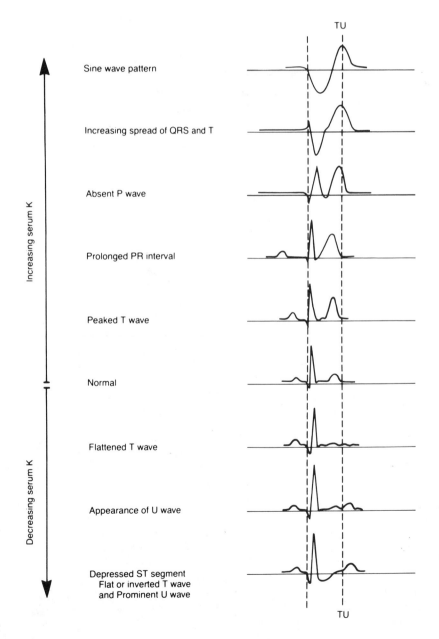

FIGURE 5–1.
Electrocardiographic manifestations of hypokalemia and hyperkalemia. Either extreme in the serum potassium level may lead to ventricular fibrillation; ventricular standstill or complete heart block is more common in hyperkalemia. (Wolfson AB [ed]: Endocrine and Metabolic Emergencies, Emerg Med Clin North Am 783, 1980; with permission.)

scribed in the sections dealing with defining characteristics of these imbalances.

Alterations in acid–base balance have a significant effect on potassium distribution. The mechanism involves shifts of hydrogen ions (H^+) and potassium ions (K^+) between the cells and ECF. Hypokalemia can cause alkalosis and alkalosis can cause hypokalemia. For example, hydrogen ions move out of the cells in alkalotic states to help correct the high pH and potassium ions move in (to maintain electroneutrality). Hyperkalemia can cause acidosis and acidosis can cause hyperkalemia. For example, in acidotic states, some of the excess hydrogen ions enter the cells to help correct plasma pH. In so doing, potassium ions are released from the cells to maintain electroneutrality.

Knowledge of the facts above helps in the detection of abnormal potassium states when pH disturbances are present. In such situations it is possible that the serum potassium levels will appear normal even when total body deficits or excesses are present.

HYPOKALEMIA

Hypokalemia refers to a below-normal serum potassium concentration. It usually indicates a real deficit in total potassium stores; however, it may occur in patients having normal potassium stores when alkalosis is present (because alkalosis causes a temporary shift of serum potassium into the cells). As noted earlier, hypokalemia is a common disturbance with a number of etiologies. Frequently, a combination of factors predisposes to hypokalemia.

ETIOLOGICAL FACTORS

Etiological factors associated with hypokalemia are listed in Table 5-1 and discussed below.

Gastrointestinal Losses

Gastrointestinal (GI) losses of potassium are probably the most common cause of potassium depletion. Vomiting and gastric suction frequently lead to hypokalemia, partly because of actual potassium loss in gastric fluid, but largely because of increased renal potassium loss associated with metabolic alkalosis. (Recall that loss of acidic gastric fluid causes metabolic alkalosis; then, the kidneys attempt to conserve hydrogen ions to correct the pH disturbances. In this process, potassium ions are lost in greater amounts.)

Relatively large amounts of potassium are contained in intestinal fluids; for example, diarrheal fluid may contain as much as 30 mEq/L. Therefore, potassium deficit occurs frequently with diarrhea, prolonged intes-

TABLE 5–1.
Etiological Factors Associated With Hypokalemia

Gastrointestinal loss
▶ Diarrhea
▶ Laxative abuse
▶ Prolonged gastric suction
▶ Protracted vomiting
▶ Villous adenoma

Renal loss
▶ Diuretic therapy (K-losing diuretics)
▶ Hyperaldosteronism or excessive glucocorticoids
▶ Sodium penicillin, carbenicillin, or amphotericin B
▶ Steroid administration
▶ European licorice abuse

Sweat losses
▶ Potassium loss can be significant in the heavily perspiring individual acclimated to heat

Shift into cells
▶ Hyperalimentation
▶ Alkalosis
▶ Excessive secretion or administration of insulin

Poor intake
▶ Anorexia nervosa
▶ Alcoholism
▶ Debilitation

tinal suction, recent ileostomy, and villose adenoma. A dramatic cause of diarrheal potassium loss occurs with villous adenomas, with which up to 1 to 3 L of potassium-rich fluid (as high as 80 mEq/L) may be lost.[2]

Renal Losses

Hyperaldosteronism increases renal potassium wasting and can lead to severe potassium depletion. Primary hyperaldosteronism is relatively rare, occurring in patients with adrenal adenomas and adrenal hyperplasia. Secondary hyperaldosteronism is a common occurrence in patients with cirrhosis, nephrotic syndrome, congestive heart failure, and malignant hypertension.

Potassium-losing diuretics, such as the thiazides, furosemide, and ethacrynic acid, can certainly induce hypokalemia, particularly when given in high doses to patients with poor potassium intake. Approximately 20% to 30% of patients taking 50 mg of hydrochlorothiazide (HCTZ) daily develop hypokalemia.[3] Combined use of thiazides and furosemide greatly increases the likelihood of serious hypokalemia. Surreptitious use of diuretics to control weight is an increasing problem in these days of easy drug availability.

Other drugs associated with increased renal losses of potassium include high-dose sodium penicillins, especially carbenicillin.[4] Amphotericin B is also commonly associated with increased renal losses of potassium. In fact, half of the patients treated with amphotericin B develop hypokalemia.[5]

High serum glucocorticoid levels, as occur in Cushing's syndrome, or excessive steroid administration, for conditions such as arthritis or asthma, can cause potassium depletion.

European licorice contains glycyrrhizinic acid, a substance that has a pharmacological action similar to mineralocorticoid; thus, excessive intake of this substance can cause hypokalemia.

The osmotic diuresis associated with glucosuria causes real potassium wasting, which is presumably associated with increased fluid delivery to the distal tubular potassium secretory site.

Sweat Losses

Potassium deficit related to heavy perspiration is most likely to occur in persons who are acclimated to heat since sweat glands in these individuals tend to excrete more potassium than in those who are not acclimated to heat stress. The mechanism involved is presumably the result of an aldosterone-related effect attempting to conserve sodium (the primary electrolyte in sweat). Sweat losses exceeding 10 L/day have been reported in individuals exercising in a hot climate.

Shift into Cells

In alkalosis, hydrogen ions shift out of the cells to help correct the pH defect; potassium ions from the ECF move into the cells to maintain electroneutrality. Entry of potassium into skeletal muscle and hepatic cells is promoted by insulin. Thus, patients with persistent insulin hypersecretion may experience hypokalemia. This is often seen in individuals receiving high-carbohydrate parenteral fluids (as in hyperalimentation). Later in the chapter insulin administration will be discussed as a therapeutic measure for temporary relief of life-threatening hyperkalemia.

Poor Intake

Patients unable or unwilling to eat a normal diet for a prolonged period are candidates for hypokalemia. However, strict fasting usually induces only a moderate depletion of total body potassium if there are normal homeostatic mechanisms. Usually poor intake is coupled with other problems in individuals with low serum potassium levels. For example, in addition to poor intake, individuals with anorexia nervosa frequently abuse diuretics and laxatives and induce vomiting to maintain a low body weight. Also alcoholics frequently have other factors predisposing to hypokalemia (such as vomiting, diarrhea, and magnesium deficiency). Refeeding a malnourished patient can lead to serious hy-

pokalemia if inadequate potassium is supplied because insulin release is stimulated by the feeding and promotes anabolism with entry of potassium into the cells.

DEFINING CHARACTERISTICS

Because potassium is the major cation in intracellular fluid (ICF), it is understandable that potassium deficit can result in widespread derangements in normal physiological functioning. Some of the more common changes are discussed below. It must be remembered that severe hypokalemia can result in death through cardiac or respiratory arrest. See Table 5-2 for a summary of defining characteristics of hypokalemia. Clini-

TABLE 5–2.
Defining Characteristics of Hypokalemia

Skeletal Muscle

Fatigue

Weakness, perhaps progressing to flaccid quadriparesis[6] (initially most prominent in the legs, especially the quadriceps, and then extending to the arms; involvement of respiratory muscles soon follows)

Cramps, restless legs

Rhabdomyolysis

Cardiovascular System

Ventricular arrhythmias

Increased sensitivity to digitalis (digitalis toxicity occurs at lower digitalis levels when hypokalemia is present)

Hypotension (related to autonomic dysfunction and decreased peripheral resistance)

ECG changes:
▶ ST segment depression
▶ Broad, sometimes inverted, progressively flatter T waves
▶ Enlarging U wave sometimes becomes superimposed on the T wave to give appearance of prolonged Q–T interval

Renal System

Impaired urinary concentrating ability when hypokalemia is prolonged, causing dilute urine, polyuria, nocturia, and polydipsia

Increased ammonia production and hydrogen ion excretion

Gastrointestinal System

Anorexia, nausea, and vomiting

Decreased bowel motility can result in ileus or gastric atony

Metabolic Effects

Slightly elevated blood glucose (due to insulin suppression)

Often associated with metabolic alkalosis (high pH and bicarbonate)

---

cal signs are usually not present until the potassium level falls below 3.0 mEq/L.

Neuromuscular Changes

Potassium levels less than 3.0 mEq/L are often associated with muscular weakness and adynamic ileus. At least two mechanisms are involved; the first involves changes in the resting membrane potential and the other has to do with altered operation of intracellular enzymes. Symptoms such as anorexia, nausea, vomiting, prolonged gastric emptying, gaseous distention, and paralytic ileus are due to weakness of the smooth muscles of the GI tract and impairment of the response to parasympathetic stimulation. Orthostatic hypotension may occur as a result of autonomic insufficiency produced by hypokalemia. In summary, hypokalemia affects cardiac, striated, and smooth muscle.

Cardiac Changes

The major cardiac effects of hypokalemia include abnormalities of electrophysiology and contractility. The most important cardiac derangement associated with hypokalemia is the potential for a variety of atrial and ventricular arrhythmias, particularly in patients with ischemic myocardial disease and those receiving digitalis preparations. Cardiac sensitivity to digitalis preparations is heightened by hypokalemia (see Figure 5-1 and Table 5-2).

Hormonal Changes

Hypokalemia has been shown to suppress insulin release and can cause mild hyperglycemia. Fortunately, correction of the hypokalemia usually restores the blood sugar to normal. Hypokalemia also suppresses aldosterone secretion.

Renal Changes

Inability to maximally concentrate urine is frequently associated with prolonged potassium depletion. This, in turn, results in dilute urine, polyuria, nocturia, and polydipsia. The reduced ability to concentrate urine is the result of a decreased responsiveness to antidiuretic hormone (ADH).[7] The resistance to ADH appears to be due to interference with the generation and action of cyclic adenosine monophosphate (AMP).[8]

For reasons that remain unclear, a number of patients with hypokalemia have increased renal phosphate excretion and develop hypophosphatemia.[11]

Other Changes

A condition called *rhabdomyolysis* (disintegration of striated muscle fibers with excretion of myoglobin in the urine) can occur with potassium depletion. Possible causes of this condition are changes in intracellular metabolism and vasoconstriction.[9]

TREATMENT

The best treatment for hypokalemia is prevention. For patients at risk, a diet with ample potassium content should be provided. Table 5-3 lists some foods with high potassium content. However, once hypokalemia has developed, dietary potassium intake may be ineffective replacement because most potassium in foods is complexed to anions that metabolize into bicarbonate.[10] Therefore, patients with significant hypokalemia associated with metabolic alkalosis (bicarbonate excess) should be given potassium chloride (KC1).[11] Because KC1 is efficiently absorbed through the GI tract, no more should be given orally than would be given intravenously (IV) over 2 to 3 hours.[12]

When dietary intake is inadequate, the physician may prescribe one of the commercially prepared potassium substitutes (available in liquids, effervescent tablets, capsules, or slow-release tablets). Also available for potassium supplementation are potassium-containing salt substitutes. Many of these contain 50 to 60 mEq of potassium per teaspoon (see Table 5-4). When possible, treatment of hypokalemia by oral replacement is favored because this route allows the serum potassium to rise slowly in equilibration with the intracellular compartment.

Usual maintenance requirements for potassium are 40 to 60 mEq/day in patients with no abnormal routes of potassium loss or other above-average needs for replacement (such as hyperalimentation). When potassium cannot be consumed in adequate amounts in the diet, and when oral potassium supplements are not feasible, the IV route is indicated for replacement. The IV route is mandatory for patients with severe hypokalemia (such as 2.0 mEq/L or less).

Although KC1 is usually used to replace potassium deficits, the physician may prescribe potassium acetate or potassium phosphate. Potassium acetate can be used to treat patients with potassium loss associated with metabolic acidosis (as in renal tubular acidosis and potassium-losing nephritis); the acetate is metabolized to bicarbonate and thus helps correct the acidosis. Potassium phosphate is used when the patient has deficits of both potassium and phosphate.

According to one source, it takes approximately 40 to 60 mEq of potassium to elevate the serum potassium by 1 mEq/L.[13] Another source states that, if the serum potassium is less than 3 mEq/L, an infusion of 200 to 400 mEq of potassium is generally necessary to raise the serum potassium by 1 mEq/L; if the serum potassium is between 3.0 and 4.5 mEq/L, 100 to 200 mEq

TABLE 5–3.
Some Foods With High Potassium Content

FOOD	POTASSIUM (mg)	POTASSIUM (mEq APPROXIMATE)
Fruits		
Apricots, raw, 3 medium	313	8.0
Bananas, raw, 1 medium	451	11.6
Cantaloupe, raw, 1 cup pieces	494	12.7
Dates, dried, 10	541	13.9
Orange, 1 medium	250	6.4
Raisins, dried, seedless, ⅔ cup	751	19.3
Vegetables		
Avocado, raw, Florida, 1 medium	1484	38.1
Carrot, raw, 1 medium	233	6.0
Potato, baked, without skin, 1 medium	610	15.6
Tomato, raw, 1	254	6.5
Beverages		
Apricot nectar, canned, 8 fl oz	286	7.3
Orange juice, canned, 8 fl oz	436	11.2
Milk, 1% fat, 8 fl oz	381	9.8

(Pennington J, Church H: Bowes and Church's Food Values of Portions Commonly Used, 15th ed. Philadelphia, JB Lippincott, 1989)

TABLE 5–4.
Potassium and Sodium Content of Some Salt Substitutes

PRODUCT	POTASSIUM (mg/tsp)	SODIUM (mg/tsp)
Morton Lite salt	1500 (38 mEq)	1100
Morton salt substitute	2800 (72 mEq)	—
Morton seasoned salt substitute	2100 (54mEq)	—
No Salt salt alternative	2500 (64 mEq)	5
No Salt salt alternative, seasoned	1330 (34 mEq)	2
Table salt (reference)	—	2300

(Pennington J, Church H: Bowes and Church's Food Values of Portions Commonly Used, 15th ed, p 186. Philadelphia, JB Lippincott, 1989)

will raise the serum potassium by 1 mEq/L.[14] These are very rough estimates that may be markedly affected by several factors. A safe approach is to make an initial estimate of the needed rate of potassium administration and assess serum potassium and heart function at frequent intervals, adjusting the dose accordingly.

NURSING INTERVENTIONS

1. Be aware of patients at risk for hypokalemia (see Table 5-1) and monitor for its occurrence (see Table 5-2). Since hypokalemia can be life-threatening, it is important to detect it early.

2. Assess digitalized patients at risk for hypokalemia especially closely for symptoms of digitalis toxicity because hypokalemia potentiates the action of digitalis. Be aware that the physician usually prefers to keep the serum potassium level in the high normal range in digitalized patients.[15]
3. Take measures to prevent hypokalemia when possible.
   A. Prevention may take the form of encouraging extra potassium intake for at-risk patients (when the diet allows). Some foods high in potassium (and relatively low in sodium) are listed in Table 5-3. Of course, one must always consider dietary restrictions imposed by other conditions (such as diabetes mellitus).
   B. When hypokalemia is due to abuse of laxatives or diuretics, education of the patient may help alleviate the problem. Part of the nursing history and assessment should be directed at identifying problems amenable to prevention through education.

4. Administer oral potassium supplements when prescribed, keeping the points summarized in Table 5-5 in mind.
5. Be aware that patients may not need potassium supplements if they are using salt substitutes because these substances usually contain significant amounts of potassium (see Table 5-4). Educate patients regarding the use of salt substitutes, keeping the following facts in mind:
   A. Salt substitutes may contain from 50 to 60 mEq of potassium per teaspoon. While they are often viewed as helpful for those taking potassium-losing diuretics (such as furosemide or thiazides), they can be dangerous for patients taking potassium-conserving diuretics (such as spironolactone, triamterene, and amiloride).
   B. As with any potassium-containing substance, there is a danger of hyperkalemia with excessive use, particularly if renal function is impaired.
6. Be thoroughly familiar with the critical facts related to administering potassium IV (see Table 5-6).

TABLE 5–5.
Nursing Considerations in Administering Oral Potassium Supplements

1. Dilute liquid and effervescent supplements as indicated by the manufacturers' directions to avoid GI irritation and a saline laxative effect. (A commonly recommended amount is 4 oz of juice or water for each 20-mEq dose.) Some manufacturers recommend instructing patients to sip the diluted solution slowly, over a 5- to 10-minute period, to minimize GI irritation. Also, instruct patients not to swallow effervescent products until they have stopped fizzing and are totally dissolved.
2. Administer slow-release tablets with a full glass of water to help them dissolve in the GI tract.
3. Administer potassium supplements immediately after meals or with food to help minimize GI irritation.
4. Observe patients taking slow-release KCl tablets for GI bleeding as these tablets may cause intestinal and gastric ulceration. (Usually these products are reserved for patients who cannot tolerate liquid or effervescent preparations, often because of taste.)
5. Do not crush potassium tablets unless the manufacturer's directions specifically state that it is appropriate. For example, directions furnished for K-Tab[16] and Slow-K[17] state that the tablets should be swallowed whole, without crushing, chewing, or sucking of the tablets. In contrast, directions for Ten-K[18]

state that, since each crystal of the KCl has a polymeric coating, the tablet can be halved or crushed if the patient has difficulty swallowing the tablet.
6. Be aware that the most common adverse reactions to oral potassium salts are nausea, vomiting, abdominal discomfort, and diarrhea. These symptoms are likely due to GI irritation and are usually managed by diluting the preparation further, reducing the dose, or by administering it with meals.
7. Be aware that hyperkalemia can result from overdosage of these supplements. Monitor patients for signs of hyperkalemia. Single doses should not exceed 40 mEq[19]; preferably, no more than 20 mEq should be given per dose.
8. Be aware that potassium supplements are contraindicated in patients receiving potassium-sparing diuretics (ie, spironolactone [Aldactone], triamterene [Dyrenium], and amiloride [Midamor]). Dosages of potassium supplements should be decreased when the patient is using generous portions of potassium-containing salt substitutes.
9. Be aware that there are numerous forms of potassium supplements available commercially and that their concentrations are highly variable. Check the physician's order carefully against the preparation's label because some trade names are quite similar.

TABLE 5–6.
Critical Points in Administering Potassium IV

1. Never administer concentrated potassium solutions from ampules without first diluting them as directed by the manufacturer. The usual concentration is 40 mEq/L of infusion solution, with 80 mEq/L as the maximum desired concentration.

2. In general, concentrations greater than 60 mEq/L should not be given in peripheral veins since venous pain and sclerosing may occur.[20] Some recommend giving no more than 40 mEq/L to prevent damage to peripheral veins.[21,22] Certainly concentrated solutions of KCl (>8 mEq/100 mL) can cause pain and irritation of peripheral veins, and can lead rapidly to postinfusion phlebitis.[23]

3. Never give potassium solutions by IV push; doing so will very likely cause cardiac arrest.

4. Exercise great care when adding KCl to infusion solutions, especially in flexible containers. Thoroughly mix KCl with the solution after adding it to parenteral containers. Squeeze the medicine ports of plastic bottles while they are in the upright position and then mix thoroughly by inversion and agitation.

5. Do not add KCl to a container in the hanging position! Doing so will likely result in pooling of the KCl with a resultant high concentration bolus of the drug being administered. This may have serious and even fatal results.[24]

6. Monitor rate of flow very carefully; watch urinary output. There should be clear-cut clinical indications for therapy with potassium solutions before they are admin-

istered to patients with anuria or oliguria; if used for such patients, the rate should be conservative and the patient carefully monitored.[25] For patients with any degree of renal insufficiency or heart block, Zull[26] recommends cutting the infusion rate in half (eg, 5–10 mEq/hr instead of 10–20 mEq/hr).

7. Consider acceptable rates in relation to the patient's need for potassium replacement. Acceptable administration rates and concentrations of potassium solutions are not uniformly defined. Indeed, there is much variation among hospitals, and even among services within hospitals. However, the following guidelines should be considered:

   ▶ For usual situations, administer potassium at a rate not exceeding 10 mEq/hr.[27,28] (Others recommend rates not exceeding 10–20 mEq/hr[29,30]; still another recommends limiting rate to no more than 10 mEq/hr through peripheral veins and no more than 20 mEq/hr through central veins.[31])

   ▶ For extreme hypokalemia, rates should be no more than 40 mEq/hr (while constantly monitoring ECG).[32,33] (Others recommend up to 30–60 mEq/hr in life-threatening situations,[34] or up to 80 mEq/hr on very rare occasions.[35])

8. Take great care to avoid accidental administration of the solution in subcutaneous tissue because it is extremely irritating and can cause serious tissue loss requiring prolonged hospitalization and perhaps even skin grafting.

---

7. Be aware that any patient experiencing life-threatening symptoms, such as arrhythmias or paralysis, requires urgent potassium replacement. See factors related to emergency IV potassium administration summarized in Table 5-7.

Case Studies

1. A 40-year-old woman was admitted to the hospital with complaints of progressive muscle weakness. She had been taking a thiazide diuretic for several weeks and had recently developed vomiting and diarrhea. Postural hypotension was noted to be present (110/70 when supine and 90/60 when upright). Skin turgor was reduced. Laboratory data included the following:

$$Plasma\ K = 2\ mEq/L$$
$$HCO_3 = 40\ mEq/L$$
$$Cl = 70\ mEq/L$$

Commentary: This patient had increased losses of potassium from the GI tract as well as in the urine. Her major presenting symptom, diffuse progressive muscle weakness, is common in hypokalemia. In addition to hypokalemia, signs of fluid volume deficit (FVD) were present (reduced skin turgor and postural hypotension). Recall that postural hypotension can also be a sign of hypokalemia. On questioning, it was found that she was taking a friend's diuretic to induce weight loss. Note the presence of hypochloremic alkalosis (below-normal chloride and greatly elevated bicarbonate).

2. A 65-year-old man with a draining intestinal fistula was receiving a total parenteral nutrition (TPN) solution at the rate of 120 mL/hr. The total potassium intake was 100 mEq/day. On a routine ECG, flattened T waves, ST segment depression, and arrhythmias were detected. A blood sample was then

TABLE 5–7.
Nursing Considerations in Emergency IV Potassium Administration

1. In emergency situations, doses of potassium, and the amount of fluid in which the potassium salts are administered, vary with the patient's clinical status. As a rule, to minimize venous irritation and to promote safety, it is preferable to administer potassium in as dilute a solution as possible.
   ▸ In extreme situations (such as K < 2.0 mEq/L and ECG abnormalities or neuromuscular complications) in which fluid restriction is not a problem, the physician may prescribe as much as 40 mEq/hr by way of a solution that contains no more than 60 mEq/L.[36] When the serum K concentration reaches 2.5 mEq/L and the ECG manifestations of hypokalemia are absent, the rate should be slowed to no more than 10 mEq/hr, using a solution that contains no more than 30 mEq/L.[37]
   ▸ Sometimes, in patients unable to tolerate large fluid loads, more concentrated potassium solutions are used, such as 10 or 20 mEq/100 mL[38] or 80 to 120 mEq/250 mL.[39] Suggestions offered by Rapp[40] for administering concentrated solutions include the following:
      A. If a central line is in place, use it for the infusion (as rapid blood flow here will dilute the KCl solution). Monitor ECG carefully.
      B. If a central line is not available, and fluid restriction is not a problem, piggyback the concentrated KCl solution into the running primary line to help dilute the solution and minimize irritation of the peripheral vein. (NOTE: Although piggybacking may be helpful, it seems more reasonable in this situation to administer the potassium as a dilute solution.)
      C. If the above steps don't work, consider use of a small amount of lidocaine (requires a medical order). The lidocaine is sometimes added to the KCl solution or is injected through the tubing over a 1-minute period immediately before the infusion is begun. (Note: Although lidocaine may help relieve venous pain, it probably does *not* prevent venous irritation and phlebitis.)
   ▸ During rapid potassium replacement (particularly >20 mEq/hr), the ECG should be closely monitored.

2. It is common practice to administer concentrated KCl solutions through central veins.[41–44] The rationale for recommending the central route is that these solutions are extremely irritating to peripheral veins, although not to central veins because of their large blood flow. It should be noted that some authors caution against using central veins for concentrated KCl solutions because cardiac conduction problems may be induced.[45,46] Instead of peripheral or central veins, they suggest using other large veins (eg, the femoral vein).

3. In the treatment of severe hypokalemia, KCl is usually added to nondextrose solutions to avoid the small temporary reduction in serum potassium level that is associated with dextrose infusion.

4. Even in emergency situations, the maximum daily administration should be closely monitored and limited. Usually, no more than 100 to 200 mEq/day are recommended.[47]

5. Because the rapid administration of potassium is potentially dangerous even in severely hypokalemic patients, it should be used only in life-threatening situations. The aim of potassium replacement in severe deficits is to eliminate life-threatening symptoms (such as arrhythmias or paralysis), and not to return the serum level quickly to normal.
   ▸ Complete heart block has been described when potassium was administered at the rate of 80 mEq/hr.[48]
   ▸ Remember that IV-administered potassium may take 8 to 48 hours before it is incorporated into the cells.[49]
   ▸ A rapid increase in the plasma K concentration from a very low level may cause symptoms similar to true hyperkalemia, even when the serum concentration is within normal limits.[50]

drawn that revealed a plasma potassium level of 2.5 mEq/L. The rate of TPN infusion was tapered promptly while serum glucose levels were monitored closely and an IV infusion of KCl was initiated in a peripheral vein at the rate of 10 mEq/hr. After alleviation of the signs of hypokalemia, the TPN infusion was slowly reinstituted with adequate potassium added.

Commentary: Potassium requirements in the patient receiving TPN are variable, often ranging between 30 and 200 mEq/day.[51] Most often there is greater than usual potassium need since, during nutritional repletion, potassium will be deposited in the newly synthesized cells, causing serum levels to fall abruptly if potassium is not supplied in sufficient amounts. This patient's needs were even greater than usual

---

Summary of Hypokalemia

ETIOLOGICAL FACTORS	DEFINING CHARACTERISTICS
Diarrhea	Fatigue
Vomiting or gastric suction	Anorexia, nausea, and vomiting
Potassium-losing diuretics (such as furosemide and thiazides)	Muscle weakness
	Decreased bowel motility (intestinal ileus)
Steroid administration	Cardiac arrhythmias
Carbenicillin, sodium penicillin, amphotericin B	Increased sensitivity to digitalis toxicity
Hyperaldosteronism	Polyuria, nocturia, dilute urine (if hypokalemia is prolonged)
Hyperalimentation	Mild hyperglycemia
Poor intake, as in anorexia nervosa, alcoholism, potassium-free parenteral fluids	Postural hypotension
	Serum K <3.5 mEq/L
Osmotic diuresis (as occurs in uncontrolled diabetes mellitus or mannitol administration)	Paresthesias or tender muscles

Renal tubular acidosis	ECG changes
	  Flattened T waves
	  ST segment depression

Cushing's syndrome	

---

because intestinal fistulas result in significant potassium loss.

3. A 31-year-old woman with a history of acute leukemia was admitted to an acute care facility with fever. On admission, her serum potassium level was 4.1 mEq/L. To deal with the infection, she was started on ticarcillin disodium, 3 g intravenous piggyback (IVPB) every 4 hours, and tobramycin, 90 mg, IVPB, every 8 hours. Isotonic saline was administered at a rate of 40 ml/hr. On the third day of her hospitalization, her serum potassium was noted to have fallen to 2.8 mEq/L. She complained of weakness, fatigue, anorexia, and constipation. Potassium was replaced by the parenteral route until oral supplements could be tolerated.

Commentary: As noted earlier in this chapter, sodium penicillin is associated with increased renal losses of potassium, particularly when volume depletion is present.

HYPERKALEMIA

Hyperkalemia refers to a greater-than-normal serum potassium concentration. It seldom occurs in patients with normal renal function. Like hypokalemia, it is often due to iatrogenic (treatment-induced) causes. While less common than hypokalemia, it is often more dangerous because cardiac arrest is more frequently associated with high serum potassium levels.

ETIOLOGICAL FACTORS

Etiological factors associated with hyperkalemia are listed in Table 5-8 and are discussed below. Some of the causes of hyperkalemia are simple and straightforward (such as direct gain exceeding the kidney's excretory rate). Others are related to shifts of potassium out of the cells into the plasma, or to decreased production of aldosterone, which causes potassium retention. Note the potassium-elevating influence exerted by several commonly used drugs, particularly when there are preexisting abnormalities in potassium metabolism.

Pseudohyperkalemia

A number of causes of factitious ("pseudo") hyperkalemia exist. When the blood sample is allowed to hemolyze, potassium leaks from ruptured erythrocytes into the serum. In a recent study, 61 (19.8%) of 308 patients were found to have single elevated serum potassium measurements on samples that were noted to be grossly hemolyzed.[52] Other causes of pseudohyperkalemia include marked leukocytosis or thrombocytosis, drawing blood above a site where potassium is infusing, and obtaining a sample from an extremity in which repeated clenching and unclenching of the fist has been performed.

Although the effect of fist clenching has been recognized for many years,[53] it continues to be a problem. Don et al[54] reported a case in which a man was admitted for evaluation of hyperkalemia. Blood drawn from

TABLE 5–8.
Etiological Factors Associated With Hyperkalemia

Pseudohyperkalemia
▶ Hemolysis of blood sample
▶ Thrombocytosis
▶ Leukocytosis
▶ Prolonged tight application of tourniquet; fist clenching and unclenching immediately before or during blood drawing

Decreased potassium excretion
▶ Oliguric renal failure
▶ Potassium-conserving diuretics, such as spironolactone (Aldactone), triamterene (Dyrenium), and amiloride (Midamor)
▶ Deficiency of adrenal steroids, as in hypoaldosteronism and Addison's disease
▶ Nonsteroidal antiinflammatory drugs (especially indomethacin and piroxican)

High potassium intake
▶ Improper use of oral potassium supplements
▶ Excessive use of salt substitutes
▶ Rapid IV administration of potassium solutions
▶ Rapid transfusion of aged blood
▶ High-dose potassium penicillin salts

Shift of potassium out of cells
▶ Acidosis, metabolic or respiratory
▶ Tissue damage, as in crush injuries and burns
▶ Malignant cell lysis after chemotherapy, particularly lymphoma and leukemia
▶ Hyperglycemia with insulin deficiency
▶ Beta-adrenergic blockers
▶ Profound digitalis toxicity

Other causes
▶ Captopril
▶ Cyclosporin
▶ Heparin

this individual in an outpatient setting (using a tourniquet with repeated fist clenching and unclenching) had a serum potassium concentration of 6.9 mmol/L. In the hospital, blood drawn from an indwelling catheter (without use of a tourniquet and fist clenching) had a normal value of 4.1 mmol/L. (It increased to 5.1 mmol/L within 1 minute after application of a tourniquet and repeated fist clenching.) The researchers concluded that it is advisable to avoid fist clenching altogether when obtaining samples for potassium testing, and to rely on venous stasis alone, if needed, as an aid in performing phlebotomy.

Failure to be aware of factitious causes of hyperkalemia can result in aggressive treatment of the nonexistent hyperkalemia with serious lowering of serum potassium levels. Some clinicians favor obtaining an ECG when the reported value exceeds 6.0 mEq/L. Absence of ECG evidence for hyperkalemia is usually consistent with a factitious reading because higher lev-

els of hyperkalemia, 7 to 10 mEq/L, are almost always accompanied by ECG abnormalities.[55,56] However, on rare occasions, severe hyperkalemia can present without typical ECG manifestations.

Decreased Renal Excretion

A major cause of hyperkalemia is decreased renal excretion of potassium. This is understandable when one considers that the kidney is the major route of potassium excretion. Significant hyperkalemia, therefore, is commonly seen in untreated patients with renal failure, particularly when potassium is being liberated from cells during infectious processes or exogenous sources of potassium are excessive (as in diet or medications).

A deficiency of adrenal steroids causes sodium loss and potassium retention; thus, hypoaldosteronism and Addison's disease predispose to hyperkalemia. Between 40% and 65% of patients with chronic adrenal insufficiency manifest hyperkalemia on initial diagnosis.[57] Hyporeninemic hypoaldosteronism (type IV renal tubular acidosis) is a common renal cause of hyperkalemia. This condition is usually seen in elderly persons with mild renal insufficiency, many of whom are diabetic as well.[58]

Potassium-conserving diuretics, such as spironolactone (Aldactone), triamterene (Dyrenium), and amiloride (Midamor), are commonly implicated as causes of hyperkalemia (particularly when there is renal dysfunction, potassium supplementation, or concomitant use of other drugs predisposing to potassium retention). Serious and even fatal complications have been associated with these drugs.[59]

Hyperkalemia occurs with a variety of nonsteroidal antiinflammatory drugs (NSAID) in association with renal insufficiency. However, only indomethacin (Indocin) and piroxican (Feldene) have been reported to produce clinically significant hyperkalemia in patients without underlying renal disease.[60] It appears that hyperkalemia is related to reduced plasma and urinary aldosterone levels.[61]

High Potassium Intake

Although sustained hyperkalemia is rarely observed after potassium ingestion in individuals with normal renal function, it can occur with massive oral potassium ingestion or by rapid IV potassium administration.

A case was recently reported in which a young physician took potassium in the form of a potassium-containing salt substitute to ward off hypokalemia after diuretic use and a bout of diarrhea.[62] On admission to a hospital, her plasma potassium concentration was 8.4 mmol/L. An ECG revealed signs of severe hyperkalemia (peaked T waves, absent P wave, and a broadened QRS complex). She experienced cardiorespiratory arrest and was resuscitated. After treatment, the hyperkalemia resolved; however, posthypoxic brain damage occurred.

Although excessive potassium intake by the oral route is less dangerous than the IV route (because GI absorption may be limited by either vomiting or diarrhea from the large potassium load), the above case illustrates that care is required with potassium administration in all situations. Cases are on record in which both intentional and accidental oral potassium overdosages have resulted in fatalities.[63,64]

Although potassium-containing salt substitutes are often recommended for patients requiring sodium restriction, they are contraindicated for patients on potassium-restricted diets or those with renal disease who have diminished capacity to excrete potassium. Note in Table 5-4 that the potassium content in most salt substitutes is quite high.

Because it is possible to exceed the renal tolerance of any patient with rapid IV potassium administration, extreme caution is required when administering potassium solutions. See Tables 5-6 and 5-7. As described in Chapter 11, the serum concentration of potassium increases as storage time of blood increases. Therefore, aged blood should not be given to patients with impaired renal function. Even the potassium content of high protein oral nutrient supplements can be a problem in some patients.

Shift of Potassium out of Cells

In the presence of acidosis, potassium leaks out of the cells into the ECF, resulting in hyperkalemia. (This occurs as hydrogen ions enter the cells to help correct the ECF *p*H.) An elevated extracellular potassium level should be anticipated when extensive tissue trauma has occurred, as can happen in crushing injuries or severe infections. Similarly, it can occur with lysis of malignant cells after administration of chemotherapy, particularly in lymphomas, leukemia, and myeloma.

Hyperglycemia with insulin deficiency can produce hyperkalemia. Recall that in normal individuals, hyperglycemia stimulates insulin release and promotes movement of extracellular potassium into the cells. However, in diabetics, the insulin response is lacking. Therefore, the hyperglycemia and resultant hypertonicity promotes potassium movement from the cells to the ECF, and it is not unusual to find a somewhat elevated plasma potassium level in a hyperglycemic diabetic before treatment. As described above, acidosis contributes to this shift of potassium out of the cells.

Beta-adrenergic blockers (such as propranolol) increase the risk of hyperkalemia by interfering with entry of potassium into the cells. The increase in plasma potassium concentration is usually modest (0.2–0.5 mEq/L) and corrects on discontinuation of the drug.[65]

Dangerous hyperkalemia is rarely due to beta-blockers alone,[66] but these blockers can exacerbate hyperkalemia in patients with other risk factors.[67] For example, dialysis patients treated with propranolol (Inderal) exhibit an approximately 1.0 mEq/L increase in predialysis serum potassium levels.[68]

Digoxin has produced fatal hyperkalemia when taken in large amounts.[69] Although digitalis toxicity is aggravated by hypokalemia, severe digitalis intoxication poisons the Na/K ATPase pump, resulting in potassium release from the cells and hyperkalemia.[70]

Other Causes

One study found captopril (an angiotensin-converting enzyme inhibitor) to be one of the drugs most frequently implicated in producing hyperkalemia.[71] Significant hyperkalemia has been reported in association with captopril in patients with renal insufficiency, presumably due to captopril's inhibitory effect on aldosterone secretion.[72]

Cyclosporin can cause hyperkalemia through a combination of mechanisms. For example, it can decrease potassium excretion, decrease prostaglandin production, and lower plasma renin and aldosterone levels.[73] Cyclosporin-induced hyperkalemia does not seem to be related either to dosage or duration of therapy.[74]

Because chronic heparin administration blocks a step in aldosterone synthesis, it can occasionally cause hyperkalemia.[75] Elevated serum potassium levels have been produced with heparin doses of 20,000 units/day.[76] Other factors that predispose to hyperkalemia may be required for overt abnormalities in potassium regulation to become apparent, however, as there are infrequent reports of heparin-induced hyperkalemia, despite widespread use of this drug.[77] However, in a recent study, heparin usage was present in a substantial percentage of patients having other conditions favoring hyperkalemia.[78]

DEFINING CHARACTERISTICS

Clinically, the most important effect of hyperkalemia is its effect on the myocardium. In addition, it affects neuromuscular and hormonal functioning. These effects are listed in Table 5-9.

Cardiac Effects

Cardiac effects of an elevated serum potassium level are usually not significant below a concentration of 7 mEq/L but they are almost always present when the level is 8 mEq/L or greater. As the plasma potassium concentration is increased, disturbances in cardiac conduction occur. The earliest changes, often appearing at a serum potassium level greater than 6 mEq/L,

TABLE 5–9.
Defining Characteristics of Hyperkalemia

Cardiac effects
▶ Tall, peaked T wave in precordial leads
▶ Widened QRS complex
▶ Prolonged P–R interval
▶ Decreased amplitude and disappearance of the P wave
▶ Sine wave (blending of QRS into T wave)
▶ Ventricular arrhythmias
▶ Cardiac arrest

Neuromuscular effects
▶ Vague muscular weakness (usually first sign)
▶ Flaccid muscle paralysis (first noticed in the legs, later in the trunk and arms; facial and respiration muscles affected last; muscles supplied by cranial nerves usually spared)
▶ Paresthesias of face, tongue, feet, and hands is common and is the result of stimulation of pain receptors
▶ Central nervous system not affected; patient often remains alert and apprehensive in spite of other changes until cardiac arrest occurs

Gastrointestinal effects
▶ Nausea
▶ Intermittent intestinal colic or diarrhea

Laboratory data
▶ Serum K^+ >5.0 mEq/L
▶ Often associated with acidosis

are peaked narrow T waves and a shortened Q–T interval. If the serum potassium level continues to rise, the P–R interval becomes prolonged and is followed by disappearance of the P waves. Finally, there is decomposition and prolongation of the QRS complex. Ventricular arrhythmias and cardiac arrest may occur at any point in this progression (see Fig. 5-1).

Hyperkalemia slows the heart rate, may cause atrioventricular (AV) block, and prolongs depolarization.[79] Factors exaggerating ECG changes of hyperkalemia are low serum sodium and calcium levels, as well as acidosis and a high serum magnesium concentration. These changes are counteracted by an increased serum calcium level, explaining why calcium infusion is an emergency treatment for serious hyperkalemia. Medications that may aggravate hyperkalemia include procainamide, propranolol, and heparin.[80]

In profound hyperkalemia, the heart becomes dilated and flaccid due to decreased strength of contraction (related to a decreased number of active muscle units). Detrimental myocardial effects of hyperkalemia are more pronounced when the serum potassium elevates rapidly.

Neuromuscular Effects

Severe hyperkalemia causes muscle weakness and even paralysis related to a depolarization block in muscle.

Similarly, ventricular conduction is slowed. Although hyperkalemia has marked effects on the peripheral neuromuscular system, it has little effect on the central nervous system.[81] Rapidly ascending muscular weakness leading to flaccid quadriplegia has been reported in patients with very high serum potassium levels (as occurs in renal failure or Addison's disease). Paralysis of respiratory muscles and those required for phonation can also occur.

Gastrointestinal Changes

Gastrointestinal symptoms, such as nausea, intermittent intestinal colic, or diarrhea, usually occur in hyperkalemic patients. Uremic enteritis often occurs.[82] These changes have been attributed to smooth-muscle hyperactivity.

TREATMENT

Restriction of Potassium Intake and Drugs Potentiating Hyperkalemia

In nonacute situations, adequate treatment may be limited to restriction of dietary potassium and discontinuance of agents predisposing to hyperkalemia (including potassium-sparing diuretics, potassium supplements, and potassium-containing salt substitutes). Other drugs that have a predisposing effect to hyperkalemia include nonsteroidal antiinflammatory agents, captopril, and beta-adrenergic blockers. (See previous discussion of possible etiological factors for hyperkalemia.)

Removal of Potassium

Sodium Polystyrene Sulfonate

Sodium polystyrene sulfonate is a cation exchange resin that removes potassium from the body by exchanging sodium for potassium in the intestinal tract. Although it is an effective method for managing developing hyperkalemia, because of its relatively slow onset, it should not be the sole treatment for severe hyperkalemia.

Sodium polystyrene sulfonate can be given orally (15–30 g), or rectally (50 g) as a retention enema.[83] Because the drug is constipating, it is usually given orally with an osmotic agent, such as sorbitol. When given as a retention enema, an inflated rectal catheter may be needed to ensure retention of the dissolved resin for 30 to 60 minutes. An enema removes potassium within 30 to 60 minutes, whereas oral doses require 1 to 2 hours.[84] Oral doses can be repeated every 4 to 6 hours as needed, and enemas can be repeated every 2 to 4 hours as indicated.[85] Each enema can lower the plasma potassium concentration by as much as 0.5 to 1.0 mEq/L.[86] For every mEq of potassium bound by the resin, consider 1 to 2 mEq of sodium is released for absorption.[87] The patient's tolerance for sodium, therefore, must be considered. For example, severe congestive heart failure limits the amount of resin that can be safely administered.

Dialysis

Dialysis can remove potassium effectively but should be reserved for situations in which more conservative methods do not suffice. Although peritoneal dialysis can be started relatively quickly, it is not as effective as hemodialysis. (For example, using 2-L exchanges cycled every 45 minutes, peritoneal dialysis can remove approximately 10 to 15 mEq of potassium per hour, as compared to 25 to 30 mEq/hr for hemodialysis.[88]) A major limitation of hemodialysis is the time needed to prepare the patient for the procedure.

One study reported on the successful initiation of hemodialysis during cardiopulmonary resuscitation (CPR) of a young uremic male who suffered cardiac arrest due to lethal hyperkalemia.[89] Despite 55 minutes of CPR and conventional treatment for hyperkalemia, cardiac arrest persisted. Hemodialysis was initiated during CPR and the patient recovered uneventfully.

Emergency Measures

Three generally accepted stop-gap measures for treating severe hyperkalemia include IV administration of (1) calcium gluconate, (2) hypertonic dextrose and insulin, and (3) sodium bicarbonate. Although controversy exists as to which of these methods should be instituted first, they all seem to have a place in the emergency management of hyperkalemia.[90-92]

Calcium Gluconate

Calcium gluconate is administered only to patients who need immediate myocardial protection against the toxic effects of severe hyperkalemia. Although calcium gluconate does not lower the serum potassium level, it does temporarily protect the heart. This protective effect begins within 1 or 2 minutes but lasts only 30 to 60 minutes. However, this action allows time for one of the measures described below (administration of either insulin and hypertonic dextrose or sodium bicarbonate) to force serum potassium into the cells. The usual dose is 10 mL of a 10% calcium gluconate solution administered slowly over 2 to 3 minutes.[93] The ECG should be continuously monitored during administration; the appearance of bradycardia is an indication to stop the infusion. (Extra caution is required if the patient has undergone digitalization as parenteral administration of calcium sensitizes the heart to digitalis and may precipitate toxicity.)

Glucose and Insulin

Insulin facilitates potassium movement into the cells, thus reducing the plasma potassium level. Glucose administration in nondiabetic patients may cause a marked increase in insulin release from the pancreas and produce the desired plasma potassium-lowering effect.[94] However, because patients who are acutely ill may not have the desired response, variable amounts of glucose and insulin are often given simultaneously to patients with hyperkalemia. For example, some favor the infusion of 10 units of regular insulin with an ampule of 50% glucose (25 g) over a 5-minute period.[95] Others do not agree with the IV administration of 50% dextrose because of its hypertonicity and recommend an infusion of 500 mL of a 10% dextrose solution with 15 to 20 units of regular insulin over 1 hour.[96] Although the potassium-lowering effect of insulin and glucose is delayed about 30 minutes, the effect may persist for 4 to 6 hours.[97]

Sodium Bicarbonate

Sodium bicarbonate infusion temporarily shifts potassium into the cells, and is especially helpful if the patient has metabolic acidosis. The effect begins within a few minutes and may last up to 2 hours. The typical dose is 45 mEq of $NaHCO_3$ (one ampule of a 7.5% $NaHCO_3$ solution) infused slowly over a 5-minute period; if necessary, the dose can be repeated within 30 minutes, or $NaHCO_3$ can be added to an IV infusion fluid.[98] The sodium in the $NaHCO_3$ preparation may antagonize potassium's effect at the cell membrane, thereby furnishing an additional benefit. Because of the sodium content, however, the patient should be monitored for volume overload (particularly since many hyperkalemic patients have underlying renal insufficiency).

NURSING INTERVENTIONS

1. Be aware of patients at risk for hyperkalemia (see Table 5-8) and monitor for its occurrence (see Table 5-9). Since hyperkalemia is life-threatening, it is imperative to detect it early.
2. Take measures to prevent hyperkalemia when possible by following guidelines for administering potassium safely, both IV and orally.
   A. Follow rules for safe administration of potassium. Review Tables 5-5, 5-6, and 5-7.
   B. Avoid administration of potassium-conserving diuretics, potassium supplements, or salt substitutes to patients with renal insufficiency. Review Table 5-4.
   C. Caution patients to use salt substitutes sparingly if they are taking other supplementary forms of potassium or are taking potassium-conserving

diuretics (such as spironolactone, triamterene, and amiloride).

D. Caution hyperkalemic patients to avoid foods high in potassium content. These include chocolate, coffee, cocoa, tea, dried fruits, dried beans, whole-grain breads, and milk desserts.[99] Meat and eggs also contain substantial amounts of potassium. Review Table 5-3. (Foods with minimal potassium content include butter, margarine, cranberry juice or sauce, ginger ale, gumdrops or jellybeans, lollypops, root beer, sugar, or honey.)[100]

3. Recall that there are a number of causes of factitious hyperkalemia, including the following:

A. Use of a tight tourniquet and heavy exercise of the extremity when obtaining the blood sample (can elevate the serum potassium level as much as 2.7 mEq/L)

B. Hemolysis of the blood sample

C. Leukocytosis in range of 70,000 per cubic millimeter (as in leukemia)

D. Platelet counts greater than 1 million per cubic millimeter

4. To avoid false reports of hyperkalemia, take the following precautions:

A. Avoid prolonged use of tourniquet while drawing blood sample.

B. Do not allow patient to exercise extremity immediately before drawing blood sample.

C. Take blood sample to the laboratory as soon as possible (serum must be separated from cells within 1 hour after collection).

D. Avoid drawing blood specimen from a site above an infusion of potassium solution (or any solution for that matter). See section on obtaining blood samples in Chapter 2.

5. Be familiar with usual treatment regimens for hyperkalemia and factors related to their safe implementation.

Case Studies

1. A 60-year-old man visited his family physician complaining of chronic tiredness and increased skin pigmentation. On examination, his blood pressure was found to be low (98/60). Blood tests revealed a plasma potassium level of 6.8 mEq/L and a plasma

---

Summary of Hyperkalemia

ETIOLOGICAL FACTORS	DEFINING CHARACTERISTICS
Pseudohyperkalemia ▸ Fist clenching during phlebotomy ▸ Hemolysis of sample ▸ Leukocytosis ▸ Thrombocytosis	Vague muscular weakness is usually first sign
	Cardiac arrhythmias, bradycardia, and heart block can occur
Decreased potassium excretion ▸ Oliguric renal failure ▸ Potassium-conserving diuretics ▸ Hypoaldosteronism	Paresthesias of face, tongue, feet, and hands
	Flaccid muscle paralysis (spreads from legs to trunk and arms; respiratory muscles may be affected)
High potassium intake, especially in presence of renal insufficiency ▸ Improper use of oral potassium supplements ▸ Rapid or excessive administration of IV potassium ▸ Rapid transfusion of aged blood ▸ High-dose potassium penicillin ▸ Foods high in potassium (such as dried apricots)	Gastrointestinal symptoms such as nausea, intermittent intestinal colic, or diarrhea may occur

	ECG changes
	  Tall, peaked T waves; widened QRS complex progressing to sine waves
	  Serum K$^+$ >5.0 mEq/L

Shift of potassium out of cells ▸ Acidosis ▸ Tissue trauma ▸ Malignant cell lysis	

sodium level of 132 mEq/L. The BUN was 20 mg/dL and the serum creatinine was 1.2 mg/dL.

Commentary: This patient was diagnosed as having adrenal insufficiency. Recall that aldosterone regulates sodium and potassium balance by causing sodium retention and potassium excretion. Thus, a deficit of aldosterone results in potassium retention and elevation of the plasma potassium level. Note that the patient has normal renal function, as evidenced by the BUN and creatinine levels. Increased skin pigmentation is common in adrenal insufficiency.

2. A 30-year-old man with chronic renal failure developed vomiting and diarrhea. Because he became very weak, his family brought him to the emergency room. In addition to severe muscle weakness he was noted to have decreased skin turgor. An ECG revealed tall, peaked T waves and widening of the QRS complex. Blood tests revealed a plasma potassium level of 9.4 and a creatinine level of 2.9 mg/dL.

Commentary: Due to fluid volume depletion after the bout of vomiting and diarrhea, this patient developed decreased renal perfusion and a reduced ability to excrete potassium. Because of the life-threatening situation (evidenced by the high plasma potassium level and the EKG changes), he was treated with calcium gluconate and sodium bicarbonate. A dextrose and saline solution was administered to achieve volume replacement. After volume repletion, kidney perfusion improved and the patient was again able to excrete potassium. Remember that patients with chronic renal failure can become seriously ill when volume depletion and thus decreased renal perfusion occur.

3. A 65-year-old woman was admitted to the emergency room complaining of abdominal cramping and numbness in her extremities. Laboratory data revealed a BUN of 96 and a creatinine of 3.9 mg/dL. The serum potassium was 8.6 mEq/L. She was given a retention enema of Kayexalate (sodium polystyrene sulfonate) in 20% sorbitol. Fifty mL of 50% dextrose and 10 units of regular insulin were given intravenously. An infusion of 5% dextrose and 0.45% NaCl containing two ampules of sodium bicarbonate was started at a rate of 25 mL/hr. By the next day, the serum potassium was reduced to 5.0 mEq/L.

Commentary: Kayexalate is an ion-exchange resin that causes sodium to be exchanged for potassium in the intestine, resulting in potassium excretion by this route. Hypertonic dextrose and insulin favor cellular uptake of potassium, and sodium bicarbonate, by alkalinizing the plasma, also causes potassium to shift temporarily into the cells.

REFERENCES

1. Ansari A: Hypokalemia and hyperkalemia: Diagnosis by electrocardiography. Primary Cardiology 14(4): 17, 1988
2. Zull D: Disorders of potassium metabolism. Emerg Med Clin North Am 7(4):771, 1989
3. Ibid
4. Maxwell M, Kleeman C, Narins R: Clinical Disorders of Fluid and Electrolyte Metabolism, 4th ed, p 529. New York, McGraw-Hill, 1987
5. Rose B: Clinical Physiology of Acid–Base and Electrolyte Disorders, 3rd ed., p 732. New York, McGraw-Hill, 1989
6. Valtier B, Mion G, Pham L, Brochard L: Severe hypokalemic paralysis from an unusual cause mimicks the Guillain-Barré syndrome. Intensive Care Med 15:534, 1989
7. Rose, p 738
8. Ibid
9. Schrier R: Renal and Electrolyte Disorders, 3rd ed, p 228. Boston, Little, Brown, 1986
10. Zull, p 785
11. Ibid
12. Ibid
13. Wilson R (ed): Principles and Techniques of Critical Care, section K, p 24. Kalamazoo, MI, Upjohn, 1976
14. Maxwell et al, p 956
15. Dunagen W, Ridner M: Manual of Medical Therapeutics, 26th ed, p 119. Boston, Little, Brown, 1989
16. Physicians' Desk Reference, 44th ed, p 538. Oradel, NJ, Medical Economics, 1990
17. Ibid, p 2180
18. Ibid, p 2181
19. Seligman M (ed): Drug Therapy Review. A Publication of the Massachusetts General Hospital Pharmacy 1(8), 1986
20. Rose, p 746
21. Vanatta J, Fogelman M: Moyer's Fluid Balance, 4th ed. p 122. Chicago, Year Book Medical Publishers, 1988
22. Kokko J, Tannen R: Fluids and Electrolytes, 2nd ed, p 225. Philadelphia, WB Saunders, 1990
23. Rapp R: Use of lidocaine to reduce pain associated with potassium chloride. Clin Pharm 6:98, 1987
24. Trissel L: Handbook of Injectable Drugs, 3rd ed, p 397. Bethesda, MD, American Society of Hospital Pharmacists, 1983
25. Vanatta, Fogelman, p 120
26. Zull, p 785
27. Kokko, Tannen, p 225
28. Gahart B: A Handbook of Intravenous Medications, 6th ed, p 454. St. Louis, CV Mosby, 1990
29. Rose, p 746
30. Maxwell et al, p 536
31. Askanazi J, Starker P, Weissman C: Fluid and Electrolyte Management in Critical Care, p 71. Boston, Butterworths, 1986
32. Kokko, Tannen, p 225

33. Berk J, Sampliner J: Handbook of Critical Care, 2nd ed, p 41. Boston, Little, Brown, 1982
34. Zull, p 785
35. Vanatta, Fogelman, p 122
36. Dunagen, Ridner, p 61
37. Ibid
38. Zull, p 785
39. Goldberger E: A Primer of Water, Electrolytes and Acid–Base Syndromes, 7th ed, p 287. Philadelphia, Lea & Febiger, 1986
40. Rapp, p 98
41. Goldberger, p 287
42. Berk, p 41
43. Vanatta, Fogelman, p 122
44. Cullen D: Potassium chloride therapy (letter). JAMA 247(2):2778, 1982
45. Kokko, Tannen, p 225
46. Rose, p 746
47. Dunagen, Ridner, p 61
48. Rose, p 746
49. Askanazi et al, p 71
50. Zull, p 785
51. Alpers D, Clouse R, Stenson W: Manual of Nutritional Therapeutics, 2nd ed, p 238. Boston, Little, Brown, 1988
52. Rimmer J, Horn J, Gennari J: Hyperkalemia as a complication of drug therapy. Arch Intern Med 147:867, 1987
53. Skinner S: A cause of erroneous potassium levels. Lancet 1:478, 1961
54. Don et al: Pseudohyperkalemia caused fist clenching during phlebotomy. N Engl J Med 322:1290, 1990
55. Ansari, p 2455
56. Kokko, Tannen, p 251
57. Ibid, p 262
58. Zull, p 788
59. Schwartz A, Cannon-Babb M: Hyperkalemia due to drugs in diabetic patients. Am Fam Pract 39(1): 225, 1989
60. Rimmer et al, p 869
61. Schwartz, Cannon-Babb, p 226
62. van der Loeff H, van Schijndel S, Thijs L: Cardiac arrest due to oral potassium intake. Intensive Care Med 15:58, 1988
63. Illingsworth R, Proudfoot A: Rapid poisoning with slow-release potassium. Br Med J 281:485, 1980
64. Wetli C, Davis J: Fatal hyperkalemia from accidental overdose of potassium chloride. JAMA 240:1339, 1978
65. Schwartz, Cannon-Babb, p 227
66. Zull, p 788
67. Rimmer et al, p 869
68. Kokko, Tannen, p 268
69. Schwartz, Cannon-Babb, p 228
70. Zull, p 788
71. Rimmer et al, p 869
72. Ibid
73. Kokko, Tannen, p 268
74. Schwartz, Cannon-Babb, p 229
75. Zull, p 789
76. Kokko, Tannen, p 268
77. Ibid
78. Rimmer et al, p 869
79. Huerta B, Lemberg L: Potassium imbalances in the coronary unit. Heart Lung 14:193, 1985
80. Ibid
81. Schrier, p 239
82. Vanatta, Fogelman, p 125
83. Dunagen, Ridner, p 64
84. Kokko, Tannen, p 255
85. Rose, p 781
86. Ibid
87. Ibid
88. Kokko, Tannen, p 256
89. Lin J, Huang C: Successful initiation of hemodialysis during cardiopulmonary resuscitation due to lethal hyperkalemia. Crit Care Med 18(3):342, 1990
90. Iqbal Z, Friedman E: Preferred therapy of hyperkalemia in renal insufficiency: Survey of nephrology training-program directors. N Engl J Med 320(1):60, 1989
91. Batle et al: More on therapy for hyperkalemia in renal insufficiency (letter). N Engl J Med 320(2):1496, 1989
92. Spital A: Bicarbonate in the treatment of severe hyperkalemia. Am J Med 85:511, 1989
93. Rose, p 779
94. Ibid
95. Dunagen, Ridner, p 63
96. Zull, p 791
97. Ibid
98. Rose, p 780
99. Goldberger, p 256
100. Ibid

6

Calcium Imbalances

Because many factors affect calcium regulation, there are a multitude of causes of altered calcium balance. Both hypocalcemia and hypercalcemia are relatively common imbalances, particularly in the acutely ill. For example, in one study, 64% of the patients in the intensive care unit were found to be hypocalcemic.[1] The opposite imbalance, hypercalcemia, is often seen in patients with malignant disease. To facilitate understanding of calcium disturbances, a review of factors affecting calcium balance follows.

CALCIUM BALANCE

DISTRIBUTION AND FUNCTION

Over 99% of the body's calcium is concentrated in the skeletal system, where it is a major component of strong, durable bones and teeth. About 1% of skeletal calcium is rapidly exchangeable with blood calcium; the rest is more stable and only slowly exchanged. The small amount of calcium located outside the bone circulates in the serum partly bound to protein and partly ionized. Because it is a necessary ingredient of cell cement, calcium helps hold body cells together. In addition, calcium exerts a sedative action on nerve cells and plays a major role in the transmission of nerve impulses. It helps regulate muscle contraction and relaxation, including normal heart beat. Calcium is instrumental in activating enzymes that stimulate many essential chemical reactions in the body and plays a role in blood coagulation. Dietary calcium is absorbed primarily from the proximal small intestine and is excreted in the urine.[2]

SERUM CONCENTRATION

The test most frequently performed in clinical settings to measure serum calcium is "total calcium," with results normally ranging from 8.5 to 10.5 mg/dL. The total calcium in serum is the sum of the ionized (47%) and nonionized (53%) calcium components. The nonionized portion consists of calcium bound to albumin (40%) and the portion chelated to anions, which includes citrate and phosphate (13%).

Many laboratories now have the capability to directly measure the ionized calcium level (normally ranging from 4.0 to 5.0 mg/dL). This is highly desirable, especially in critically ill patients, because it is the ionized calcium that is physiologically active and clinically important.

When only the total serum calcium level is available, the reading must be evaluated in relation to the serum albumin concentration. In the noncritically ill, it is estimated that a decrease in the serum albumin of 1.0 g/dL (10 g/L) will decrease the total calcium by 0.8 mg/dL (0.2 mmol/L).[3] For example, if the patient's serum albumin is below normal by 1 g/dL (eg, 2.5 g/dL rather than 3.5 g/dL), the measured total serum calcium concentration of 8.0 mg/dL should be adjusted upward to 8.8 mg/dL. In this situation, the ionized calcium level would be estimated at about half of the adjusted value (4.4 mg/dL). The direct relationship between albumin and total calcium often leads clinicians to ignore a low total serum calcium level in the presence of a similarly low serum albumin level.

The above estimation is not valid when situations are present that affect *p*H (and thus the percentage of ionized calcium). When the arterial *p*H increases (alkalosis), more calcium becomes bound to protein. Although the total serum calcium remains unchanged, the ionized portion decreases. Thus, symptoms of hypocalcemia often occur in the presence of alkalosis. Acidosis (low *p*H) has the opposite effect; that is, less calcium is bound to protein and therefore more exists in the ionized form. Signs of hypocalcemia will develop only rarely in the presence of acidosis, even when the total serum calcium level is lower than normal.

The estimation described above is not valid when situations are present that affect the quantity of substances available to bind with calcium, such as increased free fatty acids (common in stressed patients). Other factors that can acutely lower ionized calcium levels are increased levels of lactate, bicarbonate, citrate, and phosphate, and some substances in radiographic contrast media.[4] As indicated above, it is often recommended that ionized calcium levels (rather than total calcium) be measured in critically ill patients because of the usually complex nature of their conditions.[5]

REGULATION

Many biochemical and hormonal factors act to maintain normal calcium balance. Among the most important are parathyroid hormone, calcitonin, and calcitriol (an active metabolite of vitamin D).

Parathyroid hormone (PTH) promotes a transfer of calcium from the bone to plasma (raising the plasma calcium level). The bones and teeth are ready sources for replenishment of low plasma calcium levels. Parathyroid hormone also augments the intestinal absorption of calcium and enhances net renal calcium reabsorption. Calcitonin (produced by the thyroid) is a physiological antagonist of PTH. It promotes transfer of calcium from plasma to the bones, lowering the plasma calcium level. Calcitonin secretion is directly stimulated by a high serum calcium concentration.

Calcitriol promotes calcium absorption from the intestine, aids in PTH-induced mobilization of bone calcium, and limits calcium excretion when hypocalcemia is present. Calcitriol is the most active form of vitamin D_3. Its main action is to enhance the availability of calcium and phosphate for new bone formation and the prevention of symptomatic hypocalcemia and hypomagnesemia.

CALCIUM DEFICIENCY–ASSOCIATED DISEASES

Osteoporosis

Osteoporosis is associated with prolonged low intake of calcium. This disease strikes millions of Americans, mostly women. It is characterized by loss of bone mass, causing bones to become porous, brittle and, therefore, susceptible to fracture. Although serum calcium levels are usually normal in these individuals, *total* body calcium stores are greatly diminished. Bone loss begins at an earlier age in women than in men and is accelerated by menopause. However, men also develop negative calcium balance in later years. A dual process is involved in osteoporosis: increased bone resorption and inadequate bone formation. Menopause leads to rapid bone loss in women because estrogen deficiency reduces calcium absorption and increases excretion; as a result, bone loss far outpaces bone deposition.

Risk of developing serious bone problems is greater in women who (1) are white or Asian, (2) are thin and small-framed, (3) are cigarette smokers, (4) have sedentary lifestyles, (5) frequently diet and have low calcium intakes, (6) take medications for thyroid disorders or for convulsive disorders, and (7) have had their ovaries removed.[6]

Inactivity predisposes to bone loss by reducing the efficiency of calcium use. Conversely, regular physical exercise (such as running, walking, or bicycling) slows the rate of bone loss and improves calcium balance. See nursing interventions 6 to 8 for hypocalcemia later in this chapter and Chapter 26 for further discussion of osteoporosis.

Hypertension

Several authors suggest that a low calcium intake increases blood pressure, and that increasing calcium intake may protect against hypertension.[7,8] In a study reported by Belizan et al,[9] 30 healthy young adults who received calcium supplements of 1000 mg/day experienced a reduction in blood pressure compared to 27 subjects who received placebos. According to another source, mild hypertension can be lowered (2–3 mmHg) by the use of 1000 mg of calcium per day.[10]

HYPOCALCEMIA

ETIOLOGICAL FACTORS

Hypoparathyroidism

Primary hypoparathyroidism causes hypocalcemia, as does surgical hypoparathyroidism; however, the latter is a more common cause. Hypocalcemia reportedly occurs in up to 70% of patients undergoing parathyroidectomy, particularly when a severe hyperparathyroid state was present before surgery.[11] The postoperative tetany may be due to rapid calcium uptake by osteoblasts.[12]

Transient hypocalcemia reportedly occurs in 5% to 10% of patients undergoing thyroidectomy.[13] After total thyroidectomy, symptoms may be related to impaired blood supply to the remaining parathyroid tissue. Another possibility is the release of calcitonin (a calcium-lowering hormone) from the thyroid gland.

Hypocalcemia can also occur after radical neck dissection and is most likely in the first 24 to 48 hours. Probably the mechanism is ischemia to the parathyroid tissue after dissection and hemostatic maneuvers.

Acute Pancreatitis

Inflammation of the pancreas causes release of proteolytic and lipolytic enzymes; it is believed that calcium ions combine with the fatty acids released by lipolysis, forming soaps. It has also been suggested that hypocalcemia may be related to excessive secretion of glucagon from the inflamed pancreas, resulting in increased secretion of calcitonin.[14] Recent studies indicated that PTH secretion is inadequate in patients with acute pancreatitis, thus preventing uptake of calcium from bones to correct the hypocalcemia. In any event, hypocalcemia is a common problem, occurring in as many as 10% to 80% of patients with acute pancreatitis.[15] See Chapter 17.

Hypomagnesemia

Hypomagnesemia (<1 mg/dL) can cause hypocalcemia.[16] Mechanisms probably include impaired PTH release and end-organ resistance to this hormone. In magnesium-deficiency states, the regulatory mechanisms for maintaining serum calcium in the normal range are evidently impaired. One study reported that 22% of the hypocalcemia patients in their sample also had hypomagnesemia.[17]

Hyperphosphatemia

Hyperphosphatemia usually causes a reciprocal drop in the serum calcium level. Because hyperphosphatemia is associated with renal failure, hypocalcemia is common in renal patients. Hyperphosphatemia and hypocalcemia may also be seen during overtreatment of hypercalcemia with phosphate, or during hyperalimentation.

Sometimes phosphate salts are given to decrease elevated serum calcium levels. Phosphate reduces the calcium level by several means, although the exact mechanisms are not well understood.[12] One mechanism involves the formation of a colloidal calcium phosphate complex within the extracellular fluid (ECF); this complex is taken up by macrophages in the liver and may be deposited in soft tissues.

Alkalosis

As described earlier, alkalosis can induce a decreased ionized serum calcium concentration as a result of increased binding of Ca^{++} to albumin. Although the total calcium concentration remains normal in this situation, tetany (presumably caused by the fall in ionized calcium) can occur if the blood *pH* rises above 7.6.[18]

Inadequate Vitamin D

Inadequate consumption of vitamin D or insufficient exposure to the sun (ultraviolet radiation) can cause reduced calcium absorption and thus lead to hypocalcemia. Deficiency of vitamin D occurs in malabsorptive states such as steatorrhea due to pancreatic insufficiency, biliary obstruction, or small-bowel disease.

Malabsorption Syndromes

Calcium absorption occurs primarily in the proximal small intestine and is regulated by PTH and circulating vitamin D. Hypocalcemia may occur after small bowel resection, partial gastrectomy with gastrojejunostomy, jejunoileal bypass, and Crohn's disease. When effective intestinal surface area is lost, there are fewer available sites for calcium absorption. Contributing to hypocalcemia is the concurrent presence of hypomagnesemia, which is also common in patients with malabsorption problems. As described above, hypomagnesemia apparently impairs PTH secretion and end-organ response to this hormone.

Infusion of Citrated Blood

Citrate is present in excess in bank blood preserved with citrate-phosphate-dextrose (CPD), which is used to preserve the life of blood and to act as an anticoagulant. Recall that citrate is negatively charged and calcium is positively charged, resulting in an attraction between these ions. Therefore, transient hypocalcemia can occur with massive administration of citrated blood (as in exchange transfusions in neonates), since citrate can combine with ionized calcium and temporarily remove it from the circulation (sometimes referred to as "chelation"). Normally, citrate is oxidized to bicarbonate by the liver. However, when infused rapidly, or in the presence of shock or liver damage, the excess citrate ions may bind calcium ions, dropping the ionized level in serum. Also at risk for citrate-induced ionized calcium deficit during massive transfusion are small children, elderly or osteoporotic patients, and those who have been bedridden for 8 to 10 weeks or longer; all of these tend to have inadequate stores of bone calcium and thus are less able to compensate for declined ionized calcium levels.[19]

Chernow et al[20] reported a significant fall in total serum calcium (from 9.49 ± 0.11 to 7.6 ± 0.11 mg/dL) in 21 patients after transfusion with packed red blood cells. One source recommends that calcium be administered to patients receiving large quantities of whole blood or packed cells rapidly (3–5 units of whole blood or 5–8 units of packed cells in 4 hours or less).[21] Citrate intoxication affects myocardial function, causing bradycardia, arrhythmias, and hypotension; it is particularly dangerous in patients with preexisting myocardial disease.[22] A less troublesome problem induced by citrate is circumoral paresthesia, which is fairly common during hemapheresis procedures.

Drugs

Many medications can predispose to hypocalcemia. Some are listed in Table 6-1 with a brief description of the underlying mechanisms.

Alcoholism

Alcohol abuse can cause hypocalcemia for several reasons (such as direct effect of ethanol, intestinal malabsorption, low levels of 25-(OH)-D$_3$, hypomagnesemia, hypoalbuminemia, and pancreatitis).[24] The most serious of these is probably hypomagnesemia. Magnesium replacement increases responsiveness to PTH and correction of the hypocalcemia.[25]

Neonatal Hypocalcemia

During the first 3 days of life, hypocalcemia may occur in neonates and may be related to functional immaturity of the parathyroid glands. Those most at risk are infants born to insulin-dependent diabetic mothers, and those with asphyxia at birth.[26] After the first 3 days of life, hypocalcemia may be caused by milk with a high phosphate (in relation to calcium) content.[27]

Other Factors

Ionized hypocalcemia is found in patients with gram-negative sepsis. Possible causes are acquired parathyroid gland insufficiency, dietary vitamin D deficiency, or renal hydroxylase insufficiency.[28] Medullary thyroid carcinoma may produce hypocalcemia if calcitonin (a calcium-lowering hormone) is secreted by the tumor. As discussed earlier, conditions associated with low serum albumin levels (such as cirrhosis of the liver and the nephrotic syndrome) are frequently associated with a low total serum calcium concentration. Often, the ionized calcium concentration is normal and there are no symptoms of hypocalcemia. However, in patients with nephrotic syndrome, the ionized level may be low.[29]

DEFINING CHARACTERISTICS

Clinical manifestations of hypocalcemia vary widely among patients and depend on severity, duration, and

TABLE 6–1.
Drugs With Calcium-Lowering Effects

DRUG	MECHANISM
Loop diuretics (such as furosemide)	Increases renal excretion of calcium
Anticonvulsants (especially Dilantin and phenobarbital)	Inhibits gastrointestinal calcium absorption and increases vitamin D metabolism
Citrate-buffered blood and blood products	Presumably binds ionized Ca^{++} with citrate
Phosphates (orally, IV, or enema)	Phosphate combines with calcium
Mithramycin	Decreases calcium mobilization from bone
Calcitonin	Decreases calcium mobilization from bone
Drugs that lower serum Mg level (such as Cisplatin and Gentamycin)	By inducing hypomagnesemia, may decrease calcium mobilization from bone
EDTA (disodium edetate)	Physically combines with calcium for excretion
Alcohol (chronic abuse)	Multiple factors (see text)
Certain radiographic contrast media [23]	Those containing chelating agents combine with calcium

rate of development.[30] The presence of hypomagnesemia and hypokalemia concurrently can potentiate the neurological and cardiac abnormalities associated with hypocalcemia.

Neuromuscular Manifestations

Tetany, the most characteristic manifestation of hypocalcemia, refers to the entire symptom complex induced by increased neural excitability. Findings may include sensations of tingling around the mouth (circumoral paresthesia), and in the hands and feet, as well as spasms of the muscles of the extremities and face. Although laryngeal spasms may occur, they only rarely result in asphyxia.[31]

When hypocalcemic patients lack overt signs of tetany, neuromuscular excitability (latent tetany) can be elicited in two ways. One involves inflating a blood pressure cuff on the upper arm to above systolic pressure for about 3 minutes and observing for carpal spasm (Trousseau's sign, see Fig. 2-15). Another involves tapping over the facial nerve just anterior to the ear and observing for ipsilateral facial muscle contraction (Chvostek's sign, see Fig. 2-14).

Central Nervous System Manifestations

Severe hypocalcemia can cause convulsions, and, in fact, these may be the initial manifestation.[32] Other central nervous system signs may include irritability, depression, memory impairment, delusions, and hallucinations.

Cardiovascular Manifestations

Altered cardiovascular hemodynamics may be the most significant effect of hypocalcemia in some patients, which is understandable when the important role calcium ions play in the contraction of cardiac muscle is considered.

In persons with cardiomyopathies, hypocalcemia can precipitate congestive heart failure which is unresponsive to inotropic drugs until the hypocalcemia is corrected.[33] Often these patients are predisposed to both hypocalcemia and hypomagnesemia after using potent loop diuretics and digoxin.

In patients with hypocalcemia due to citrated blood transfusions, the cardiac index, stroke volume, and left ventricular stroke work values have been found to be much lower than during normocalcemia.[34] Hypocalcemia prolongs the Q–T interval, although it is not necessarily diagnostic of this imbalance.

Other Changes

In chronic hypocalcemia, the skin may be dry and scaling, and nails brittle, and the hair dry and easily shed; cataracts are common. Chronic hypocalcemia in children can retard growth and lower the IQ.

TREATMENT

As noted above, there are numerous etiological factors associated with hypocalcemia. Ideally, treatment is directed at alleviating the cause. If this is impractical or ineffective, the following general measures should be considered. If tolerated, adequate oral calcium intake should be provided as either carbonate, gluconate, or citrate salts. In general, 1 or 2 g of elemental calcium daily, in four divided doses, is sufficient.[35] In some cases, long-term management may require the use of vitamin D preparations. These should be used with caution if severe hyperphosphatemia is present, because the danger of calcium phosphate precipitation in the soft tissues exists. If hyperphosphatemia is present, oral phosphate-binding medications (such as aluminum hydroxide) may be indicated.

Emergency Measures

Acute symptomatic hypocalcemia is a medical emergency, requiring prompt administration of intravenous (IV) calcium. Parenteral calcium salts include calcium gluconate, calcium chloride, and calcium gluceptate. Although calcium chloride produces a significantly higher ionized calcium than an equimolar amount of calcium gluconate, it is not used as often because it is more irritating to the vein and can cause tissue sloughing if allowed to infiltrate. For severe hypocalcemia symptoms, 10 mL of 10% calcium gluconate, administered slowly IV, may be prescribed with ECG-control[36]; this should be given at a rate not exceeding 2 mL/min.[37] Sometimes a calcium salt is added to an infusion bottle and run in over several hours, depending on the dosage. A too rapid IV administration of calcium can cause cardiac arrest, preceded by bradycardia. The diluted method of calcium administration is generally recommended because it is less likely to produce venous irritation than is undiluted calcium given by IV push.[38] Patients receiving a continuous calcium infusion should be on a cardiac monitor; additionally, their serum calcium level should be followed closely.[39] Because of the previously discussed relationship between magnesium and calcium, calcium replacement may be ineffective in restoring serum calcium levels until the magnesium deficit is corrected. Intravenous calcium administration is particularly dangerous, and should be undertaken only with great caution, in patients receiving digitalis preparations because hypercalcemia predisposes to digitalis cardiotoxicity and arrhythmias.

An infusion of calcium gluconate may be needed to correct the postoperative hypocalcemia that can occur in the first 24 to 48 hours after neck surgery (such as thyroidectomy, radical neck dissection, or parathyroidectomy). The flow rate is titrated according to clinical signs and serum calcium levels. Fortunately, the hypocalcemia is often transient and mild.[40]

In general, approximately 1000 mg/day of calcium gluconate are required to raise the total serum calcium level by 1 mg/dL.[41] When oral calcium supplements can be tolerated, the oral route is preferred over the IV route because it is safer.

When the serum calcium level approaches normal, the 24-hour urine calcium content must be monitored to prevent hypercalciuria (more than 300 mg of calcium in the urine over 24 hours) and thus avoid predisposing to renal stone formation.[42]

NURSING INTERVENTIONS

1. Be aware of patients at risk for hypocalcemia and monitor for its occurrence (see Summary of Hypocalcemia). Also, review previous sections for explanations of etiological factors and defining characteristics.
2. Be prepared to adopt seizure precautions when hypocalcemia is severe.
3. Monitor condition of airway closely as laryngeal stridor can occur.
4. Take safety precautions if confusion is present.
5. Be aware of factors related to the safe administration of calcium replacement salts (see Treatment).
6. Educate individuals in high-risk groups for osteoporosis (especially postmenopausal women not on estrogen therapy) about the need for dietary calcium intake. If adequate amounts are not consumed in the diet (as is often the case), calcium supplements should be considered. There is some controversy surrounding calcium requirements in older persons; many investigators do not think the requirements need to be changed (from 800 mg to 1200–1500 mg/day), whereas others favor the change to reduce the risk of osteoporosis.[43]
   A. Most sources recommend that the calcium intake for older persons be 1000 to 1500 mg each day. The best way for healthy individuals to ensure an adequate calcium intake is to eat a wide variety of foods from the four food groups daily. (Table 6-2 lists some foods high in calcium.)
   B. As stated above, calcium supplements may be necessary for individuals unable to consume sufficient calcium in their diets, such as those who do not tolerate milk or dairy products well. Table 6-3 lists some commercial sources for calcium supplementation and their elemental content. Note that most of these are calcium carbonate preparations, which furnish about 40% absorbable calcium. In contrast, other salts furnish a lower percentage of absorbable calcium, such as calcium citrate (21%), calcium gluconate (9%), and calcium glubionate (6.5%). The variation in absorption among calcium salts has made it common practice to refer to the ele-

TABLE 6–2.
Calcium Content in Common Foods

FOOD	CALCIUM (mg)	SODIUM (mg)	PROTEIN (g)	CALORIES (APPROXIMATE)
Whole milk, 8 oz	290	122	8	150
Lowfat milk (2%), 8 oz	298	122	8	122
Lowfat milk (1%), 8 oz	300	122	8	89
Skim milk, 8 oz	303	128	8	89
Lowfat yogurt, with fruit added, 8 oz	345	133	10	240
Mozzarella cheese, part skim, 1 oz	183	132	7	72
Parmesan cheese, grated, 2 tbs	140	186	4	46
Oysters, raw, 5 to 8 medium	94	73	8	66
Pink salmon, *with bones*, canned, ¼ cup	122	242	13	88
Tofu, 3½ oz	128	7	8	72
Ice cream, vanilla, 1 cup	208	82	6	290
Broccoli, 1 large stalk, cooked, about ⅔ cup	88	10	3	26
Raisins, ¼ cup	48	24	2	232

(Copyright 1989, American Journal of Nursing Co. Adapted from Geriatric Nursing, April 1989, vol. 10, no. 2. Used with permission. All rights reserved)

TABLE 6–3.
Calcium-Containing Products for Oral Use

PRODUCT	ELEMENTAL Ca CONTENT* (mg/TABLET)	ANION	VITAMIN D CONTENT (IU/TABLET)
Alka 2	200	Carbonate	
Alka-Mints	340	Carbonate	
Biocal	250, 500	Carbonate	
Calcet	153	Carbonate, gluconate, lactate	100
Calsup	300, 600	Carbonate	±200
Ca Plus	280	Protein complex	
Calciday	667	Carbonate	
Caltrate	600	Carbonate	±125
Dical-D	350	Phosphate	400
Neocalglucon	115 (per 5 mL)	Glubionate	
Os-Cal	250, 500	Carbonate	
Oystercal	250, 375, 500	Carbonate	
Titralac	200 400 (per 5 mL)	Carbonate	
Tums	200	Carbonate	

*   *The contents of anhydrous calcium salts as elemental calcium are as follows: glubionate 6.5%; gluconate, 9%; lactate, 13%; dibasic phosphate, 23%; carbonate, 40%.*
(Adapted from Alpers D, Clouse R, Stenson W: Manual of Nutritional Therapeutics, 2nd ed, p 89. Boston: Little, Brown, 1988)

mental content rather than to the total content (much of which is not available for use by the body). For example, a 500-mg dose of calcium carbonate furnishes 200 mg of elemental calcium (40% of 500 mg is 200 mg), whereas a 500-mg dose of calcium gluconate furnishes only 33 mg (6.5% of 500 is 33 mg). Calcium citrate and calcium lactate are more soluble than the others and may be absorbed better in elderly individuals.[44] Apparently calcium is best absorbed when taken in divided doses rather than all at once.

C. Some postmenopausal women are advised by their physicians to take estrogen. When estrogen cannot be taken, calcitonin may be prescribed for 12 to 18 months as an alternative for women with type I osteoporosis.[45]

D. Individuals with a tendency to form renal stones should be encouraged to consult their physicians before greatly increasing their calcium intake. For such individuals, the physician must determine a safe calcium dosage range; this is usually determined by studying urinary calcium levels. Also, these individuals should drink no less than 2 to 3 q of fluid a day to protect against stone formation.

7. Inform individuals at risk for osteoporosis about the value of regular physical exercise in decreasing bone loss. Walking is tolerated well by all age groups and is an excellent form of exercise, as is bicycling. (See Chapter 26 for further discussion of exercise and osteoporosis.)

8. To prevent osteoporosis in later years, educate young women about the need for a normal diet ensuring adequate calcium intake. Also, discuss the calcium loss associated with alcohol and nicotine use. Smoking lowers estrogen levels and interferes with the body's absorption of calcium; women who smoke are at greater risk of developing osteoporosis.[46]

Case Studies

1. A 46-year-old woman with end-stage renal disease was admitted with a secondary diagnosis of seizure activity and multiinfarct dementia. She required dialysis twice a week. On admission, laboratory data revealed the following:

Na^+ = 138 mEq/L	BUN = 41 mg/dL
	Serum
K = 5.8 mEq/L	creatinine = 8.2 mg/dL
Ca = 7.0 mg/dL	Albumin = 3.0 g
PO_4 = 7.1 mEq/L	HCO_3 = 13.5 mEq/L

Summary of Hypocalcemia

ETIOLOGICAL FACTORS	DEFINING CHARACTERISTICS
Surgical hypoparathyroidism (may follow thyroid surgery or radical neck surgery for cancer)	Numbness, tingling of fingers, circumoral region, and toes
Malabsorption	Cramps in muscles of extremities
Vitamin D deficiency	Hyperactive deep-tendon reflexes (such as patellar and triceps)
Acute pancreatitis	Trousseau's sign
Excessive administration of citrated blood	Chvostek's sign
Primary hypoparathyroidism	Mental changes, such as confusion and alterations in mood and memory
Alkalotic states (decreased ionized calcium)	Convulsions (usually generalized but may be focal)
Hyperphosphatemia	Spasm of laryngeal muscles
Medullary carcinoma of thyroid	Cardiac manifestations; ECG shows prolonged Q–T interval
Hypoalbuminemia (as in cirrhosis, nephrotic syndrome, and starvation)	Spasms of muscles in abdomen (can simulate acute abdominal emergency)
Hypomagnesemia	Total serum calcium level below 8.5 mg/dL, or ionized level below normal (<50%)
Decreased ultraviolet exposure	Sulkowitch's test showing light precipitation (see Table 2-4)

Commentary: Note the low serum calcium level and the presence of hypoalbuminemia. With correction for the low serum albumin level, the serum calcium would be nearer to normal. (Recall that for every gram the serum albumin is below the normal level of 4–5 g, 0.8 mg must be added to the reported calcium level; since the albumin level is 1 or 2 g below normal, 0.8 or 1.6 must be added to the reported calcium level, making it from 7.8–8.6 mg/dL.) Although the total calcium level was below normal, the ionized fraction of the calcium was normal; thus, symptoms of hypocalcemia were not present. Note that this patient has metabolic acidosis (evidenced by the low serum bicarbonate level); both hypoalbuminemia and acidosis favor increased calcium ionization. Rapid correction, or overcorrection, of acidosis in a renal patient predisposes to precipitation of hypocalcemic symptoms. Hyperphosphatemia was present, a major factor in explaining the hypocalcemia. Among the medications prescribed for this patient were Basaljel (to bind the excess phosphate) and Os-Cal (a calcium supplement). Seizure activity was managed by the administration of Dilantin and phenobarbital (seizures were related to the cerebral infarcts, not to hypocalcemia).

2. A hysterical young woman was admitted to the emergency department after an automobile accident in which she fractured her arm. She complained of circumoral paresthesia and then fainted. Arterial blood gas findings included a pH of 7.55 (alkalosis) and a $PaCO_2$ of 20 mmHg (normally 40 mmHg).

Commentary: Hyperventilation secondary to hysteria is a common cause of tetany in the hospital emergency department. In this situation, the tetany resulted from a reduction in the plasma ionized calcium level consequent to respiratory alkalosis. Fainting was due to cerebral ischemia caused by the low $PaCO_2$ (recall that a low $PaCO_2$ causes cerebral vasoconstriction). The total serum calcium level was probably normal, although the ionized fraction decreased. Correction of the hyperventilation (and thus of respiratory alkalosis) will restore the ionized calcium level to normal and alleviate symptoms.

HYPERCALCEMIA

The prevalence of hypercalcemia in the hospital inpatient population ranges from 0.6% to 3.6%.[47] When severe, hypercalcemia is a dangerous imbalance; in fact, hypercalcemic crisis can have a mortality rate as high as 50% if not treated promptly.[48]

ETIOLOGICAL FACTORS

Approximately 98% of patients with hypercalcemia have one of the following three conditions: malignancy, hyperparathyroidism, or thiazide-diuretic use.[49] Hypercalcemia of malignancy is the most common cause and is usually related to increased bone resorption associated with the presence of neoplastic tissue. See Chapter 24 for a discussion of tumors associated with hypercalcemia.

Due to increased PTH, hyperparathyroidism causes increased bony release of calcium, augmented intestinal calcium absorption, and renal reabsorption of calcium. A single adenoma of the parathyroid gland is the most common cause.[50]

About 20% of hypercalcemia cases are associated with thiazide diuretic use.[51] These drugs, by potentiating the action of PTH on the kidneys, can produce a small-to-moderate increase in serum calcium. Furthermore, they can potentiate the hypercalcemic action of other conditions predisposing to hypercalcemia.

Milk–alkali syndrome can occur in peptic ulcer patients treated for a prolonged period with milk and alkaline antacids, particularly calcium carbonate.[52] Patients who take large quantities of calcium-containing antacids may present with marked hypercalcemia.[53] Other drugs predisposing to hypercalcemia are listed in Table 6-4.

Bone mineral is lost during immobilization, sometimes causing elevation of total calcium in the bloodstream. The hypercalcemia associated with immobilization is the result of an imbalance between the rates of bone formation and bone resorption. This process is more conspicuous in patients with Paget's disease or in those in whom bone turnover is increased (such as adolescents during a growth spurt). Factors leading to hypercalcemia during immobilization are still largely unexplained.[54]

DEFINING CHARACTERISTICS

The magnitude of the serum calcium elevation and the length of time over which it developed have major significance for clinical findings, as does the underlying cause of hypercalcemia. For example, acute hypercalcemia is more symptomatic than chronic hypercalcemia. Also, malignancies can present with severe hypercalcemia (>15 mg/dL) more commonly than other conditions.[55]

In some patients mild hypercalcemia is found on routine examinations; others may present in hypercalcemic crisis. As a rule, symptoms of hypercalcemia are proportional to the degree the serum calcium level is elevated, although this is not always the case.

Neuromuscular Changes

Hypercalcemia reduces neuromuscular excitability because it acts as a sedative at the myoneural junction. Symptoms such as muscular weakness and depressed deep tendon reflexes may occur.

TABLE 6–4.
Drugs With Calcium-Elevating Effects

DRUG	MECHANISM
Thiazide diuretics	Decrease renal calcium excretion
Lithium	Decreases renal calcium excretion
Prolonged megadoses of vitamins A and D	Vitamin A likely increases calcium mobilization from bone; vitamin D increases GI calcium absorption and mobilization of calcium from bone
Tamoxifen for breast cancer therapy	Increases mobilization of calcium from bone
Androgens or estrogens for breast cancer therapy	Increases mobilization of calcium from bone
Theophylline	Perhaps increases effect of endogenous parathyroid hormone
Milk with soluble alkali (especially calcium carbonate)	Multiple mechanisms

Gastrointestinal Symptoms

Constipation, anorexia, nausea and vomiting are common symptoms of hypercalcemia. Constipation results from decreased gastrointestinal (GI) motility caused by calcium's action on smooth muscle and nerve conduction, as well as from dehydration.[56] Delayed gastric emptying, nausea, and vomiting are also related to altered GI motility. Patients with hypercalcemia are predisposed to duodenal ulcer disease because of increased gastric acid secretion, promoted by calcium on the parietal cells of the stomach. Duodenal ulcer disease reportedly occurs in 10% to 20% of patients with hypercalcemia.[57] Another potential GI complication of severe hypercalcemia is pancreatitis (occurring in as many as 35% of patients with acute hypercalcemic crisis).[58] This is probably related to deposition of calcium in the pancreatic ducts.

Behavior Changes

Behavior changes may range from subtle alterations in personality to acute psychosis, and may include confusion, impairment of memory, and bizarre behavior. Although the cause of these symptoms is not known, it has been suggested that increased calcium in the cerebrospinal fluid is involved.[59] The more severe symptoms tend to occur when the serum calcium level is approximately 16 mg/dL or higher. In a study of eight hypercalcemic cancer inpatients over 66 patient days, Mahon[60] found that the most evident changes were those affecting mental status. For example, many subjects could not remember their home phone numbers or perform simple mathematical computations. Some displayed inappropriate behaviors, such as pulling out a Foley catheter while the balloon was inflated. When serum calcium levels decreased toward normal values, the mental symptoms subsided.

Renal Changes

Disturbed renal tubular function produced by the hypercalcemia can cause polyuria and polydipsia. More specifically, this disturbed function is a form of nephrogenic diabetes insipidus that is usually reversible within 1 to 12 weeks after correction of the imbalance. The concentrating defect may become clinically apparent when the plasma calcium concentration exceeds 11 mg/dL.[61] Renal colic may occur as a result of kidney stones, which may form from the excess calcium presented to the kidneys for excretion. Hypercalcemia may also produce acute renal failure, which may or may not be reversible.[62]

Cardiovascular Changes

Calcium is important in cardiac function; it exerts a positive inotropic effect on the heart and reduces heart rate in a way similar to the effect of cardiac glycosides. As described earlier, calcium administration to patients receiving digitalis must be done with extreme care because it can precipitate severe arrhythmias (with shortening of the Q–T interval on ECG).

The relationship between blood pressure and calcium metabolism is complex and difficult to understand. However, it appears that individuals with normal cardiovascular function can adjust to relatively large changes in Ca^{++} without changes in blood pressure.[63]

TREATMENT

Treatment for hypercalcemia is directed at reducing the serum calcium level by increasing urinary calcium excretion, inhibiting bone resorption, blocking intestinal calcium absorption, or enhancing formation of calcium complexes. Treatment should also be directed at correcting the underlying cause of hypercalcemia when possible.

General Conservative Measures

When hypercalcemia is not life-threatening, treatment may be limited to simple actions such as ensuring an adequate fluid intake to avoid volume depletion and eliminating drugs that can contribute to hypercalcemia (such as thiazide diuretics, vitamin D preparations, or calcium-containing antacids). Whenever possible, the patient should be encouraged to be active (as immobility predisposes to hypercalcemia).

Emergency Measures

Because most patients with severe hypercalcemia are volume depleted, isotonic saline (0.9% NaCl) may be ordered initially at a rate of 300 to 500 mL/hr until the intravascular volume has been restored.[64] At that point, a slowed saline infusion is maintained to promote renal calcium excretion. (Recall that sodium inhibits tubular reabsorption of calcium.) Cardiovascular and renal function should be assessed before rapid saline infusion because fluid overload and congestive heart failure are potential complications. In patients with adequate renal and cardiac function, administration of alternating 0.45% and 0.9% NaCl at infusion rates as high as 300 to 500 mL/hr to achieve diuresis may be ordered.[65] Furosemide should be used as necessary to prevent volume overload and to enhance calcium excretion. (For example, 10–40 mg every 2 to 4 hours may be prescribed to maintain urine output at 200–300 mL/hr.)[66] It may be necessary to monitor the central venous pressure (CVP) to detect fluid overload, particularly in the elderly or those with marginal cardiac reserve. Breath sounds at least should be monitored at regular intervals. Hourly intake-output (I&0) records should be maintained. With the large urinary output will come losses of potassium and magnesium that must be corrected as indicated by laboratory data.

When the use of saline and furosemide described above is ineffective or contraindicated, different measures may be instituted. Among these are the administration of calcitonin, mithramycin, phosphate salts, or diphosphonates. In some situations, either peritoneal or hemodialysis may be indicated.

By inhibiting bone resorption, salmon calcitonin may temporarily lower the serum calcium level by 1 to 3 mg/dL in patients with severe hypercalcemia due to excessive bone resorption (such as occurs with carcinoma, multiple myeloma, or primary hyperparathyroidism).[67] This therapy is effective within 2 hours after initial dose is administered, its peak effect is reached at 24 to 48 hours, and its acting duration is 4 to 7 days in most cases.[68] The customary starting dose is 4 Medical Research Council (MRC) units per kilogram subcutaneously every 12 hours.[69] Calcitonin is a safe drug, but its hypocalcemic effect is mild and many individuals become unresponsive to it after 6 to 10 days of treatment.[70]

Mithramycin (a cytotoxic antibiotic) lowers serum calcium by inhibiting osteoclastic bone resorption and by decreasing bone turnover. This drug is usually effective in hypercalcemia caused primarily by increased bone resorption (such as occurs with many malignancies and hyperparathyroidism). Because mithramycin is potentially nephrotoxic, it should be used cautiously in patients with impaired renal function. Due to the potential for nephrotoxicity and hepatotoxicity, mithramycin's long-term use is limited. Liver enzymes and renal function should be monitored during therapy with this drug. Side effects can include anorexia, nausea, vomiting, bone marrow suppression, and thrombocytopenia.

Phosphate Salts

Phosphate salts reduce serum calcium concentration by several mechanisms. For example, phosphate inhibits bone resorption. Also, oral phosphate therapy inhibits intestinal calcium absorption by forming poorly soluble calcium salts. However, the following point should be considered. Increasing the serum phosphate concentration alters the extracellular calcium–phosphate equilibrium to promote calcium deposition into bone and soft tissue (metastatic calcification). Due to the risk of soft-tissue calcification, phosphate therapy should be limited primarily to patients with low serum phosphate levels (<3.0 mg/dL) and adequate renal function. The serum phosphate levels should be kept between 4 and 5 mg/dL and the calcium–phosphate product less than 70.[71] Phosphate salts may be administered orally as Phospho-Soda or Neutra-Phos, or by a 100-mL Fleet retention enema twice daily.[72] Intravenous phosphate therapy should be used with extreme caution in the treatment of hypercalcemia because it can cause severe calcification in various tissues, including the vein in which it is given. Because extraskeletal calcification is potentially fatal, one author disapproves of the IV administration of phosphates to treat hypercalcemia.[73]

Glucocorticoids

Glucocorticoids can reduce the serum calcium level by inhibiting calcium absorption in the intestine, and by inhibiting osteoclastic bone resorption.[74] Steroid therapy may be initiated with hydrocortisone, 5 mg per kilogram of body weight per day, for 2 to 3 days; later, the dose is reduced to a maintenance level.[75] A draw-back to glucocorticoids is that clinically significant reductions in serum calcium may not occur for 5 to 10 days after therapy is initiated.[76] Due to the slow onset of action, glucocorticoids are combined with other therapeutic measures when used to treat patients with severe hypercalcemia.

Diphosphonates

The diphosphonates are a relatively new group of compounds that retard bone turnover and are thus helpful in the management of hypercalcemia.[77] Diphosphonates can be administered by oral or IV routes.[78] According to one source, etidronate disodium (EHDP), in a dosage of 7.5 mg per kilogram of body weight per day in 200 mL of 0.9% NaCl given IV over 2 hours, is effective in lowering the serum calcium in 50%–75% of patients.[79] Although the precise causative mechanism is not known, mild hyperphosphatemia can occur from the administration of diphosphonate.[80]

NURSING INTERVENTIONS

1. Be aware of patients at risk for hypercalcemia and monitor for its presence. See Summary of Hypercalcemia and review above sections on etiological factors and defining characteristics.
2. Increase patient mobilization when feasible; recall that immobilization favors hypercalcemia. Hospitalized patients at risk for hypercalcemia should be ambulated as soon as possible; outpatients should be told the importance of frequently moving about.
3. Encourage the oral intake of sufficient fluids to keep the patient well hydrated. Sodium-containing fluids should be given, unless contraindicated by other conditions, since sodium favors calcium excretion. One should always consider the patient's "likes" and "dislikes" when encouraging oral fluids. Patients at home should be instructed to drink 3 to 4 qts of fluid per day, if possible.
4. Discourage excessive consumption of milk products and other high-calcium foods. Depending on the cause of hypercalcemia, dietary restrictions do not necessarily need to be stringent. Consult with physician and dietitian as indicated.
5. Encourage adequate bulk in the diet to offset the tendency to constipation.
6. Take safety precautions if confusion or other mental symptoms of hypercalcemia are present. Explain to the patient and family that the mental changes associated with hypercalcemia are reversible with treatment (see Case Study 1).
7. Be aware that cardiac arrest can occur in patients with severe hypercalcemia; be prepared to deal with this emergency situation.

8. Be aware that bones may fracture more easily in patients with chronic hypercalcemia as bone resorption has been excessive, weakening the bony structure. Transfer patients cautiously.
9. Educate home-bound oncology patients with a predisposition for hypercalcemia, and their families regarding symptoms that occur with this condition. Instruct them to report symptoms to the health care providers before they become severe. In a study reported by Mahon,[81] symptoms that most frequently caused readmission of cancer patients were constipation, confusion, anorexia, increasing bone pain, weight loss, and weakness. In a study of 22 hospitalized and 18 ambulatory cancer patients, Coward[82] reported that 90% were unaware that hypercalcemia might be a complication of their cancer. Furthermore, only one of the patients knew the symptoms of cancer-induced hypercalcemia. Almost 70% of the patients did not recall being told of measures that might prevent hypercalcemia.
10. Be alert for signs of digitalis toxicity when hypercalcemia occurs in digitalized patients.
11. Be familiar with the treatment modalities for hypercalcemia and associated nursing functions (see Treatment in this chapter and Table 24-4 in Chapter 24).
12. Help prevent formation of calcium renal stones in patients with long-standing hypercalcemia or immobilization by
    A. Forcing fluids to maintain a dilute urine, thus avoiding supersaturation of precipitates
    B. Encouraging fluids that yield an acid-ash (such as prune or cranberry juice) as a urinary pH less than 6.5 favors calcium solubility. (Be aware that dietary modifications do not usually alter urinary pH significantly; therefore, pharmacological acidifying agents [such as ascorbic acid, potassium acid phosphate, or methionine] may be prescribed by the physician to ensure a uniformly low pH.)
    C. Preventing urinary stasis by turning the immobilized patient frequently, elevating the head of the bed, and having the patient sit up if this can be tolerated
    D. Encouraging weight-bearing and ambulation as soon as possible

Case Studies

1. A 76-year-old woman, described as poorly nourished, was admitted through the emergency department. According to her family, she had become progressively confused and weaker over the past 2 to 3 weeks and was incontinent of large amounts of urine; also, she had vomited frequently and was

Summary of Hypercalcemia

ETIOLOGICAL FACTORS	DEFINING CHARACTERISTICS
Hyperparathyroidism	Muscular weakness
Malignant neoplastic disease:	Tiredness, listlessness, lethargy
▸ Solid tumors with metastases (breast, prostate, and malignant melanomas)	Constipation
▸ Solid tumors without bony metastases (lung, head and neck, and renal)	Anorexia, nausea, and vomiting
▸ Hematologic tumors (lymphoma, acute leukemia, and myeloma)	Decreased memory span, decreased attention span, and confusion
Thiazide diuretics	Polyuria and polydipsia
Prolonged immobilization	Renal stones
Large doses of vitamin D	Neurotic behavior progressing to frank psychoses possible (reversible with correction of hypercalcemia)
Overuse of calcium-containing antacids or calcium supplements	Cardiac arrest possible in severe hypercalcemia
Milk–alkali syndrome	ECG showing shortened Q–T interval
	Bone changes seen on X-ray in chronic hypercalcemia
	Serum calcium > 10.5 mg/dL
	Sulkowitch's test showing dense precipitation (see Table 2-4)

constipated. On assessment she was found to be responsive to painful stimuli only. Skin turgor was poor. A fracture in her left hip was confirmed by film. Bowel sounds were hypoactive. The blood pressure was 96/50, pulse 136, and respirations 28. While in the emergency department, the patient suffered cardiac arrest three times and was successfully resuscitated. The serum calcium was found to be 18.6 mg/dL. A solution of 0.45% NaCl containing KC1 was infused at a rate of 200 mL/hr. Lasix 20 mg was given IV push every 6 hours. By the 36th hour, her serum calcium was 16.1 mg/dL. However, rales were heard in bases of both lungs and periods of shortness of breath developed. Also, she was noted to have 2+ pitting peripheral edema. The IV fluids were cut back to 75 mL/hr. Mithramycin was administered. By the 5th day, the serum calcium was 13.4 mg/dL and the patient was more alert, although responding inappropriately. She remained incontinent of urine and complained of pain. Constipation was relieved by enemas. On the 6th day, mithramycin was repeated and she was begun on Neutra-Phos, 500 mg four times daily. On the 7th day, she was alert and oriented most of the time. Her lungs were clear and there was no edema. When encouraged, she took oral fluids and

foods. Also, she was able to void in the bedpan and was only occasionally incontinent. Active bowel sounds were heard in all four quadrants. The serum calcium was 8.1 mg/dL. She was diagnosed as having carcinoma of the ovary with metastases to the bone; radiation therapy and chemotherapy were administered. She was discharged on Neutra-Phos, 500 mg four times daily.

Commentary: This patient displayed classic symptoms of hypercalcemia; they included weakness, confusion, vomiting, constipation, polyuria, and, worst of all, cardiac arrest. The treatment regimen was also close to a textbook picture in that saline fluids were given rapidly in conjunction with IV Lasix. Because of her advanced age, she had difficulty tolerating fluids at a rate of 200 mL/hr, as evidenced by the rales and shortness of breath. Mithramycin was needed to help correct the hypercalcemia, as was Neutra-Phos. Over a period of days, the hypercalcemia was slowly corrected; note that her mental status improved as the serum calcium level diminished.

2. A 40-year-old woman with cancer of the cervix and vulva had documented bone and lung metastases and was cared for at home. However, when she

became lethargic and developed inappropriate behavior, her family brought her to the emergency room. Other symptoms included severe weakness, nausea, and vomiting, no bowel movement for 5 days, inability to eat and drink for 2 days, and poor skin turgor. Bowel sounds were hypoactive in all four quadrants. Abnormalities noted on laboratory data included a serum calcium level of 16.4 mg/dL and a serum potassium of 2.8 mEq/L. Initial orders (first 24 hours) included the following:

1. Add 40 mEq of KCl to a liter of 0.9% NaCl solution and infuse at a rate of 250 mL/hr; alternate with a solution of 0.45% NaCl with 40 mEq of KCl at a rate of 250 mL/hr.
2. Lasix 20 mg, IV push every 6 hours
3. Neutra-Phos 500 mg, by mouth four times daily

Commentary: After 3 days, the serum calcium was 12.2 mg/dL and the serum potassium was 3.7 mEq/L. The patient remained confused. On the 6th day, mithramycin was administered. Saline infusions and furosemide were continued. By the 7th day, the serum calcium was down to 9.5 mg/dL. On the 9th day, she was discharged home on Neutra-Phos 500 mg three times daily, with a serum calcium level of 8.9 mg/dL. At the time of discharge, she was responding appropriately and was oriented to her surroundings.

REFERENCES

1. Chernow et al: Hypocalcemia in critically ill patients. Crit Care Med 10:848, 1982
2. Olinger M: Disorders of calcium and magnesium. Emerg Med Clin North Am 7(4): 796, 1989
3. Ibid, p 798
4. Ibid
5. Zaloga G, Willey S, Chernow B: Altered calcium binding in severe illness: A common cause for misinterpretation of serum calcium levels in critically ill patients (Abstr). Crit Care Med 14(4): 406, 1986
6. Calcium: A Summary of Current Research for the Health Care Professional, p 12. Rosemont, IL, National Dairy Council, 1984
7. Belizan et al: Preliminary evidence of the effect of calcium supplementation on blood pressure in normal pregnant women. Am J Obstet Gynecol 146: 175, 1983
8. McCarron D, Morris C, Cole C: Dietary calcium in human hypertension. Science 217:267, 1982
9. Belizan et al: Reduction of blood pressure with calcium supplementation in young adults. JAMA 249: 1161, 1983
10. McCarron D, Morris C: Blood pressure response to oral calcium in persons with mild to moderate hypertension. Ann Intern Med 103(6, part 1): 825, 1985
11. Condon R, Nyhus L: Manual of Surgical Therapeutics, 7th ed, p 269. Boston, Little, Brown, 1988
12. Ibid
13. Ibid
14. Goldberger E: A Primer of Water, Electrolyte and Acid–Base Syndromes, 7th ed, p 309. Philadelphia, Lea & Febiger, 1986
15. Ryzen E, Rude R: Low intracellular magnesium in patients with acute pancreatitis and hypocalcemia. West J Med 152:145, 1990
16. Maxwell M, Kleeman C, Narins R: Clinical Disorders of Fluid & Electrolyte Metabolism, 4th ed, p 773. New York, McGraw-Hill, 1987
17. Whong S: Predictors of clinical hypomagnesemia. Arch Intern Med 144:1794, 1984
18. Kokko J, Tannen R: Fluids and Electrolytes, 2nd ed, p 357. Philadelphia: WB Saunders, 1990
19. Condon, Nyhus, p 259
20. Chernow et al, p 851
21. Condon, Nyhus, p 258
22. Ibid
23. Mallette L, Gomez L: Systematic hypocalcemia after clinical injections of radiographic contrast media: Amelioration by omission of calcium chelating agents. Radiology 147:677, 1983
24. Maxwell et al, p 776
25. Ibid
26. Ibid
27. Ibid
28. Zaloga G, Chernow B: Pathogen mechanisms for hypocalcemia during gram negative sepsis (Abstr). Crit Care Med 14(4): 405, 1986
29. Maxwell et al, p 776
30. Dunagan W, Ridner M: Manual of Medical Therapeutics, 26th ed. Boston, Little, Brown, 1989
31. Olinger, p 800
32. Ibid
33. Ibid
34. Maxwell et al, p 777
35. Kokko, Tannen, p 617
36. Condon, Nyhus, p 270
37. Goldberger, p 255
38. McFadden E, Zaloga G: Calcium regulation. Crit Care Q 6:16
39. Olinger, p 805
40. Dunagan, Ridner, p 430
41. McFadden, Zaloga, p 17
42. McFadden E, Zaloga G, Chernow B: Hypocalcemia: A medical emergency. Am J Nurs 83:230, 1983
43. Chernoff R, Lipschitz D: Enteral feeding and the geriatric patients. In: Rombeau J, Caldwell M (eds): Enteral and Tube Feeding, 2nd ed, p 389. Philadelphia: WB Saunders, 1990
44. Todd B: Calcium: Should we supplement? p 97. Geriat Nurs March/April, 1989
45. Dunagan, Ridner, p 433
46. Osteoporosis: Some bare bone facts. Health Views, p 5. St. Louis, Washington University Medical Center, December 1985
47. Maxwell et al, p 761
48. McFadden, Zaloga, p 12
49. Olinger, p 804

50. Ibid
51. Dent et al: The incidence and cause of hypercalcemia. Postgrad Med J 63:745, 1987
52. Goldberger, p 321
53. Olinger, p 804
54. Maxwell et al, p 764
55. Ibid, p 768
56. Ibid, p 770
57. Hellstrom J: Hyperparathyroidism and gastroduodenal ulcer. Acta Chem Scand 116:207, 1959
58. Maxwell et al, p 770
59. Ibid, p 768
60. Mahon S: Symptoms as clues to calcium levels. Am J Nurs 87(3): 354, 1987
61. Rose B: Clinical Physiology of Acid–Base and Electrolyte Disorders, 3rd ed, p 646. New York, McGraw-Hill, 1989
62. Maxwell et al, p 499
63. Olinger, p 805
64. Dunagan, Ridner, p 426
65. Ibid
66. Olinger, p 806
67. Dunagan, Ridner, p 426
68. Wisneski L: Salmon calcitonin in the acute management of hypercalcemia. Calcif Tissue Int (Suppl) 46:S26, 1990
69. Kokko, Tannen, p 602
70. Olinger, p 807
71. Strewler et al: Nonparathyroid hypercalcemia. Adv Intern Med 32:235, 1987
72. Dunagan, Ridner, p 427
73. Stevenson J: Current management of malignant hypercalcemia. Drugs 36:229, 1988
74. Maxwell et al, p 771
75. Ibid
76. Dunagan, Ridner, p 426
77. Maxwell et al, p 772
78. Ibid
79. Dunagan, Ridner, p 427
80. Kokko, Tannen, p 573
81. Mahon, p 354
82. Coward D: Hypercalcemia knowledge assessment in patients at risk of developing cancer-induced hypercalcemia. Oncology Nursing Forum 15(4): 471, 1988

7

Magnesium Imbalances

MAGNESIUM BALANCE

Of the body's magnesium approximately 67% is contained in the bone, 31% in the cells, and 1% in the extracellular compartment.[1] The normal serum magnesium level is 1.3 to 2.1 mEq/L. (This value can be converted to mg/dL by multiplying by 1.2, or to millimoles by dividing by 2, thus expressing normal serum magnesium as 1.6–2.5 mg/dL or 0.65–1.1 mmol/L respectively.) Its high concentration in bone relates magnesium closely to calcium and phosphorus. However, because it is a major intracellular ion, it is also closely related to potassium.

Next to potassium, magnesium is the most abundant intracellular cation. It activates many intracellular enzyme systems and plays a role in both carbohydrate and protein metabolism.

Control of magnesium is not well understood; however, many of the factors that regulate calcium balance influence magnesium as well. A curious relationship exists between magnesium and calcium; although low serum levels of these electrolytes produce similar effects (that is, decreased neuromuscular irritability), their actions sometimes antagonize each other.[2] For example, magnesium narcosis can be antagonized by parenteral calcium administration. Magnesium balance is also affected by many of the same agents and diseases that influence potassium balance. Although factors controlling magnesium balance are not well known, both parathyroid hormone (PTH) and corticosteroids have been implicated.

An average diet supplies approximately 20 to 30 mEq/day, whereas the daily requirements are about 18 to 30 mEq/day.[3] Dietary magnesium is absorbed primarily in the jejunum and ileum.[4] When the body is deficient in magnesium, the percentage of absorbed magnesium from the diet may sharply increase from the usual 30% to 40%.[5]

The kidneys are the primary route of magnesium excretion. Fortunately, the kidneys are capable of conserving magnesium efficiently in times of need; in fact, they can reduce renal losses to as low as 1.0 mEq/day.[6] The thick ascending limb of Henle's loop is the major site of magnesium reabsorption. Therefore, diuretics (such as furosemide) that act in this region can cause large magnesium losses.

Variations in the serum magnesium level affect the irritability of nerve tissue. These effects are manifested on the central nervous system, on peripheral nerves, and on the myoneural junction. In brief, hypomagnesemia increases irritability whereas hypermagnesemia depresses neural functions.

Magnesium exerts effects on the cardiovascular system, acting peripherally to produce vasodilatation. Magnesium can produce a drop in blood pressure and can cause cardiac arrest in diastole.[7] Imbalances in magnesium predispose to ventricular arrhythmias.[8]

HYPOMAGNESEMIA

Hypomagnesemia is a common imbalance in critically ill patients. For example, a recent study found that 61% of patients admitted to two postoperative intensive care units had lower than normal serum magnesium levels.[9] Similarly, 65% of patients with normal renal function in a medical intensive care unit population were found to have lower than normal serum magnesium levels.[10] However, some authors suggest that hypomagnesemia is the most underdiagnosed electrolyte deficiency in current medical practice,[11] perhaps because it is easily mistaken for potassium deficit, a condition with which it is often associated. In general, a change in the serum concentration of one ion causes the other to deviate in the same direction.[12]

Magnesium deficit also occurs in less acutely ill individuals, such as those experiencing withdrawal from alcohol and those receiving nourishment (as in tube feedings or total parenteral nutrition) after a period of starvation. Several clinical situations are associated with hypomagnesemia; some of the more common etiological factors are described below.

ETIOLOGICAL FACTORS

Gastrointestinal Losses

An important route for magnesium loss is the gastrointestinal (GI) tract. Losses may take the form of drainage from nasogastric suction, diarrhea, or fistulas. Because fluid from the lower GI tract is richer in magnesium (10–14mEq/L) than is fluid from the upper tract (1–2 mEq/L), losses from diarrhea and intestinal fistulas are more likely to induce magnesium deficit than are those from gastric suction.[13] One should be aware that, although magnesium losses are relatively low in nasogastric suction, hypomagnesemia will occur if losses are prolonged and parenteral fluids are magnesium free.

Because the distal small bowel is the major site of magnesium absorption, any disruption in small bowel function, as occurs in intestinal resection or inflammatory bowel disease, can lead to hypomagnesemia. One study reported that 15 of 42 patients with malabsorption syndromes had subnormal serum magnesium levels[14]; the degree of hypomagnesemia showed a rough correlation with the degree of steatorrhea. In the presence of steatorrhea, it is believed that magnesium ions are excreted in the stool in the form of magnesium soaps.

Alcoholism

Chronic alcoholism is the most common cause of hypomagnesemia in the United States. One study found that 30% of all alcoholics and 86% of patients with delirium tremens had hypomagnesemia during the first 1 to 2 days of hospitalization.[15] Although there are no convincing data to indicate that hypomagnesemia causes delirium tremens, it is likely that magnesium deficiency aggravates alcohol withdrawal.[16] For this reason, it is recommended that the serum magnesium level be measured every 2 or 3 days in hospitalized alcoholic patients undergoing withdrawal.[17] Although the serum magnesium level may be normal on admission, it can fall as a result of metabolic changes associated with therapy (such as the intracellular shift of magnesium associated with intravenous (IV) glucose administration).

Decreased dietary intake of magnesium is a major factor in the development of hypomagnesemia in alcoholics. Other factors include increased GI losses (due to episodic emesis and diarrhea) and intestinal malabsorption. In addition, alcohol ingestion is believed to increase magnesium excretion in the urine.

Refeeding After Starvation

In the catabolic state, the protein structure of cells is metabolized as energy sources; as a result, intracellular ions are lost, and total body concentrations of these ions (magnesium, potassium, and phosphate) are decreased.[18] Conversely, during nutritional repletion, these electrolytes are taken from the serum and deposited into newly synthesized cells. Thus, if the enteral or parenteral feeding formula is deficient in magnesium content, serious hypomagnesemia will occur. Serum levels of these primarily intracellular ions should be measured at regular intervals during the administration of IV total parenteral nutrition and even during enteral feedings, especially in patients who have undergone a period of starvation. See Chapters 12 and 13 for further discussions of this topic.

Drugs Disrupting Magnesium Homeostasis

The loop diuretics (furosemide, bumetanide, and ethacrynic acid) increase urinary magnesium excretion. Although the loop diuretics are the most potent magnesuric diuretics, long-term use of thiazide diuretics may also lead to mild hypomagnesemia.[19]

Although the exact mechanism is not clear, it has been demonstrated that aminoglycosides (such as gentamycin, tobramycin, and kanamycin) are associated with urinary magnesium wasting. For example, one study found that of 55 patients receiving aminoglycoside antibiotics, 38% developed hypomagnesemia associated with renal magnesium wasting.[20] Amphotericin B (an antifungal agent) can also cause hypomagnesemia.[21]

Cisplatinum (Cisplatin) administration is associated with hypomagnesemia secondary to increased urinary excretion of magnesium; this potentially nephrotoxic chemotherapy agent causes hypomagnesemia in a dose-related manner.[22] Cyclosporin usage in bone marrow and renal transplant patients may produce a significant drop in the serum magnesium concentration, perhaps by increasing urine wastage of magnesium.[23]

Recall that citrate is a preservative added to collected blood to prolong its longevity. Rapid administration of citrated blood (eg, faster than 1.5 mL/kg/min) can temporarily drop the ionized magnesium level because citrate chelates circulating magnesium ions (and calcium ions).[24] This is most likely to occur when citrate clearance is diminished by renal or hepatic disease or by hypothermia.[25]

Other Factors

Magnesium deficiency is often seen in patients with diabetic ketoacidosis. It is primarily the result of increased renal excretion of magnesium during osmotic diuresis (caused by the high glucose load) and of the shifting of magnesium into cells that occurs with insulin therapy. See Chapter 21.

Some causes of renal disease, such as glomerulonephritis, pyelonephritis, and renal tubular acidosis, may produce hypomagnesemia by impairing renal magnesium reabsorption. However, remember that, with *advanced* renal disease (glomerular filtration rate [GFR] less than 10–25 mL/hr), *hyper*magnesemia usually results from impaired renal magnesium excretion.[26]

Pancreatitis may cause hypomagnesemia in much the same way that it causes hypocalcemia (see Chap. 17 for a discussion of this topic). In addition, any condition associated with hypercalcemia, such as excessive doses of vitamin D or calcium supplements, may result in renal magnesium loss.[27] It should be noted that magnesium and calcium share a common route of absorption in the intestinal tract and appear to have a mutually suppressive effect; thus, if calcium intake is unusually high, calcium will be absorbed in preference to magnesium, and vice versa.

Magnesium deficiency has also been described in burn patients and is possibly related to loss of magnesium during débridement and bathing of denuded skin. Other conditions believed to predispose to hypomagnesemia are sepsis and hypothermia.[28]

Administration of magnesium-free, sodium-rich IV fluids to induce extracellular fluid expansion can cause hypomagnesemia. In fact, any condition predisposing to excessive calcium or sodium in the urine can augment renal excretion of magnesium since magnesium is normally reabsorbed in the kidney with calcium and sodium.[29]

DEFINING CHARACTERISTICS

Defining characteristics resulting from magnesium deficiency are largely confined to the neuromuscular system. Some of the effects of hypomagnesemia are due directly to the low serum magnesium level, whereas others are due to secondary changes in potassium and calcium metabolism. Hypomagnesemia can cause hypocalcemia because it interferes with the calcium-elevating effects of PTH; it may also cause hypokalemia.

Manifestations of magnesium deficiency do not usually occur until the serum magnesium level is less than 1 mEq/L.

Neuromuscular Changes

Neuromuscular hyperexcitability with muscular weakness, tremors, and athetoid movements may be seen. Other manifestations may include tetany, generalized tonic–clonic or focal seizures, laryngeal stridor, and positive Chvostek's and Trousseau's signs. It has been suggested that hypomagnesemia may increase acetylcholine action at the nerve ending, resulting in lowering of the threshold of the muscle membrane.[30] The neuromuscular symptoms of hypomagnesemia are similar to those occurring in hypocalcemia and result mainly from increased neuronal excitability. Because severe hypomagnesemia may ultimately result in hypocalcemia and hypokalemia, it is possible that the symptoms may be partly due to these disturbances. Vague but nonspecific GI symptoms have been described. For example, dysphagia may develop.[31]

Cardiovascular Effects

Magnesium deficiency predisposes to cardiac arrhythmias, such as premature ventricular contractions, supraventricular tachycardia, and ventricular fibrillation. In fact, tachyarrhythmias are a well-documented complication of magnesium depletion. Because standard antiarrhythmic drugs and defibrillation may be ineffective in controlling ventricular arrhythmias associated with magnesium deficiency, refractory arrhythmias should be treated with IV magnesium salts.[29] ECG changes observed in hypomagnesemia include P–R and Q–T interval prolongation, widened QRS complex, ST segment depression, and T wave inversion.[32] In a study of 20 patients with severe hypomagnesemia, Kingston et al[33] failed to demonstrate changes in ECG readings.

Increased susceptibility to digitalis toxicity is associated with low serum magnesium levels. An experiment with animals found that the uptake of digoxin by myocardial cells was enhanced by magnesium depletion.[34] One report found that hypomagnesemia was present twice as often in digitalis-toxic patients (21%) as in nontoxic patients (10%).[35] This is important because patients receiving digoxin are also likely to be on diuretic therapy, which predisposes to renal loss of magnesium.

Magnesium depletion has been suggested as a factor associated with alcoholic cardiomyopathy.[36] Some sources report that hypomagnesemia is associated with vasomotor changes such as painful, cold hands and feet.[37]

Central Nervous System Changes

Because decreased serum magnesium increases irritability of nerve tissue, convulsions may occur.[38] Disorientation is common.[39] Other changes may include ataxia, vertigo, depression, and psychosis.[40]

Associated Imbalances

As mentioned earlier, hypomagnesemia is often associated with *hypokalemia*. This occurs because, in the presence of magnesium deficiency, the kidneys tend to excrete more potassium.

In addition, hypomagnesemia is often associated with *hypocalcemia*. Apparently this occurs because magnesium deficiency impairs PTH secretion and causes end-organ resistance to PTH.[41]

TREATMENT

Mild magnesium deficiency can be corrected by diet alone. Principal dietary sources of magnesium are green vegetables, meat, sea foods, dairy products, and cereals.[42] When necessary, magnesium salts in tablet form (such as magnesium oxide) can be given orally to replace continuous excessive losses. However, diarrhea is a side effect that can interfere with the usefulness of oral magnesium preparations.

Magnesium may be given IV or by deep intramuscular injection when indicated. Parenteral magnesium is especially helpful in individuals with symptomatic hypomagnesemia or malabsorption. Before magnesium administration, renal function should be assessed as the kidneys are primarily responsible for the elimination of magnesium. When renal function is impaired in those receiving daily doses of magnesium, blood levels should be monitored.[43] During parenteral magnesium replacement, serum magnesium levels should be monitored, as should deep tendon reflexes. Marked depression of deep tendon reflexes signals too high a serum magnesium level and is an indication that no further magnesium should be administered. (Reports of serum levels at which loss of the patellar reflex occurs are variable; some state it is decreased at 4–7 mEq/L and lost at 10–15 mEq/L.[44] Others state it is lost at 7 to 10 mEq/L, occurring before the respiratory depression expected at 10–15 mEq/L.[45]) The IV route is indicated in patients manifesting dangerous signs of hypomagnesemia, such as increased neuromuscular excitability or cardiac dysrhythmias.[46] To treat hypomagnesemic patients having seizures or tetany, 1 to 2 g of magnesium sulfate (2–4 mL of a 50% solution containing 8–16 mEq of magnesium) may be prescribed IV over a 15-minute period.[47] Further therapy may be given as 1 g of magnesium sulfate (2 mL of a 50% solution) intramuscularly every 4 to 6 hours, depending on the clinical status and laboratory data.[48]

A report of severe hypermagnesemia resulting from improperly written or executed orders for IV magnesium sulfate pointed out the need for extreme caution in administering magnesium.[49] Three cases of severe hypermagnesemia were attributed to the inadvertent use of 50-mL vials of 50% magnesium sulfate. In two cases, the orders called for "one amp" of 50% magnesium sulfate by slow IV infusion. Although the prescriber intended that a 2-mL ampule be given, a 50-mL ampule was substituted. In the third case, the order was for a 50-mL vial of 50% dextrose. Instead, a 50-mL vial of magnesium sulfate was mistakenly used. The author emphasized the need to recognize the potency of currently available electrolyte solutions and the importance of physicians writing precise orders pertaining to their use. Certainly, orders containing terms such as "amp" or "vial" without further specification should not be written by physicians or accepted by nurses. The third case emphasizes the need to read product labels carefully before use. Never rely solely on the size, shape,

TABLE 7–1.
Nursing Considerations in Administering IV Magnesium

1. Check the order for IV magnesium. Be sure that it stipulates the concentration of the solution to be used, as well as the number of milliliters to be infused. Do not accept orders for "amps" or "vials" without further specifications.
2. Use IV magnesium with great caution in patients with impaired renal function. (Recall that the primary route of magnesium excretion is via the kidneys; thus, it is easy to induce hypermagnesemia when renal impairment is present.)
3. Monitor urine output at regular intervals. It should be maintained at a level of at least 100 mL every 4 hours.[50] (An output less than this volume raises the question of adequate urinary elimination of magnesium.)
4. Check deep tendon reflexes (such as patellar "knee-jerk" reflex) before each dose of magnesium, or periodically during continuous infusion of the drug. If reflexes are absent, do not give additional magnesium, and notify the physician. (Because deep tendon reflexes are decreased before adverse respiratory and cardiac effects occur, the presence of knee-jerks can usually be relied on to indicate that life-threatening hypermagnesemia is not present.)

5. Be aware that doses of other central nervous system depressants (such as barbiturates, narcotics, hypnotics, and systemic anesthetics) should be reduced when given concurrently with magnesium preparations. Monitor the level of consciousness.
6. Be aware that therapeutic doses of magnesium can produce flushing and sweating because magnesium acts peripherally to produce vasodilation. Inform the patient that this might occur to minimize concern. These effects are more likely to occur with too rapid administration.
7. Closely assess patients receiving large doses of magnesium:
   ▸ Check blood pressure, pulse, and respirations every 15 minutes and monitor the serum magnesium level at regular intervals. Look for a sharp fall in blood pressure or respiratory distress; both are signs of excessive magnesium. See Table 7-3.
   ▸ If the patient displays signs of severe hypermagnesemia, stop IV administration of magnesium and run in the IV solution from the primary line (as appropriate) to keep the vein open. Notify the physician and be prepared to administer artificial ventilation and IV calcium (if prescribed).

---

or label design of the container for product identification. General nursing considerations related to administering magnesium salts are listed in Table 7-1.

NURSING INTERVENTIONS

1. Be aware of patients at risk for hypomagnesemia and monitor for its presence. See Summary of Hypomagnesemia and review above sections for a discussion of etiological factors and defining characteristics.
2. Assess digitalized patients at risk for hypomagnesemia especially closely for symptoms of digitalis toxicity since a deficit of magnesium predisposes to toxicity.
3. Be prepared to take seizure precautions when hypomagnesemia is severe.
4. Monitor condition of airway as laryngeal stridor can occur.
5. Take safety precautions if confusion is present.
6. Be familiar with magnesium replacement salts and factors related to their safe administration. Review Treatment above and Table 7-1 for nursing consid-

erations in administering magnesium solutions parenterally.
7. Be aware that magnesium-depleted patients may experience difficulty in swallowing. (Dysphagia is probably related to the athetoid or choreiform movements associated with magnesium deficit.) If difficulty in swallowing is suspected, test the ability to swallow with water before offering oral medications.
8. When magnesium deficit is due to abuse of diuretics or laxatives, educating the patient may help alleviate the problem. Part of the nursing assessment should be directed toward identifying problems amenable to prevention through education.
9. Be aware that most commonly used IV fluids have either no magnesium or a relatively small amount. For example, D_5W, isotonic saline, and lactated Ringer's solution have no magnesium. Prolonged use of magnesium-free parenteral fluids, with no oral intake of magnesium and abnormal losses of magnesium by the GI or renal route, will eventually lead to hypomagnesemia. When indicated, discuss need for magnesium replacement with physician.

10. For patients experiencing abnormal magnesium losses who are able to consume a general diet, encourage the intake of magnesium-rich foods (such as green vegetables, meat, sea food, dairy products, and cereal).

Case Studies

1. A 65-year-old emaciated woman with carcinoma of the stomach was started on a total parenteral nutrition (TPN) protocol because she was unable to eat or tolerate enteral tube feedings. On the 7th day, when electrolytes were checked for the first time, the serum magnesium was found to be 0.8 mEq/L. She was lethargic and had coarse tremors, most notable in the arms. Total parenteral nutrition was stopped and 12 mL of 50% magnesium sulfate was added to a liter of 10% glucose in water and infused over 3 hours. Additional magnesium was administered over the next 2 days. Total parenteral nutrition was slowly restarted with adequate magnesium supplementation.

Commentary: Serum electrolytes should be measured regularly during TPN: in fact, they should be measured daily for the first 5 days. The purpose is to detect abnormalities before they become severe. Requirements for the intracellular ions—potassium, magnesium, and phosphate—vary with calorie and nitrogen intake and the nutritional state of the patient. As the anabolic state is achieved with TPN, these ions are incorporated into the newly synthesized cells. In this way, extracellular deficits will develop if inadequate amounts are provided in the nutrient solution.

2. A 50-year-old man with a history of chronic alcoholism was admitted for treatment. He had been on a diet of only alcoholic beverages for a week and then was "on the wagon" for a few days. Because of nausea, he ate very little. On examination, he was noted to have hyperactive knee jerks. Laboratory findings included a serum magnesium level of 0.7 mEq/L.

Commentary: Hypomagnesemia is a frequent occurrence in alcoholic patients. Contributing to poor

---

Summary of Hypomagnesemia

ETIOLOGICAL FACTORS	DEFINING CHARACTERISTICS
Chronic alcoholism, particularly during withdrawal	Neuromuscular irritability:
Intestinal malabsorption syndromes	▸ Increased reflexes
Diarrhea	▸ Coarse tremors
Nasogastric suction	▸ Positive Chvostek's and Trousseau's signs (see Figs. 2-14, 2-15)
Aggressive refeeding after starvation (as in TPN) without adequate Mg replacement	▸ Convulsions
Prolonged administration of magnesium-free maintenance IV fluids	Cardiac manifestations:
Diabetic ketoacidosis	▸ Tachyarrhythmias
Hyperaldosteronism (either primary, or secondary, as in congestive heart failure or cirrhosis)	▸ Increased susceptibility to digitalis toxicity
Drugs:	▸ ECG changes in severe cases: P–R and Q–T interval prolongation, widened QRS complex, ST segment depression, and T wave inversion
▸ Diuretics	
▸ Aminoglycoside antibiotics (such as gentamicin)	Mental changes:
▸ Cisplatin	▸ Disorientation in memory
▸ Excessive doses of vitamin D or calcium supplements	▸ Mood changes
▸ Citrate preservative in blood products	▸ Intense confusion
Pancreatitis	▸ Hallucinations
Others:	Serum magnesium level <1.3 mEq/L or 1.6 mg/dL (usually symptoms don't appear until serum magnesium is <1 mEq/L)
▸ Burns, sepsis, and hypothermia	Hypocalcemia and hypokalemia frequently occur with severe hypomagnesemia

dietary intake of magnesium as a major cause of magnesium deficiency is the increased renal loss of this electrolyte associated with excessive alcohol intake.

3. A 40-year-old man developed a high-output intestinal fistula after treatment for an intestinal obstruction. For 2 weeks he received only isotonic saline (0.9% NaCl) and 5% dextrose in water with added KCl. He developed choreiform movements of the arms and muscle twitching. In addition, he was noted to be confused. Laboratory findings included

$$Serum\ Na = 140\ mEq/L$$
$$K = 3.3\ mEq/L$$
$$Mg = 0.7\ mEq/L$$

Commentary: Although the serum sodium level is normal, the magnesium is far below normal and there is some degree of hypokalemia, despite addition of KCl to the IV fluids. Recall that intestinal fluid contains approximately 10 to 12 mEq/L of magnesium. These losses were not replaced since the IV fluids were magnesium free. With a negative magnesium balance, there is often an associated loss of potassium even with adequate intake.

HYPERMAGNESEMIA

ETIOLOGICAL FACTORS

Renal Failure

Although hypermagnesemia is generally uncommon, it may be seen quite frequently in patients with advanced renal failure (GFR < 30 mL/min).[51] This is understandable when it is recalled that magnesium is primarily excreted by the kidneys, and, thus, diminished renal function results in abnormal renal magnesium retention. Renal patients' predisposition to hypermagnesemia can be aggravated if they are given magnesium to control convulsions or if they inadvertently receive one of the many commercial antacids or laxatives containing variable amounts of magnesium salts (see Table 7-2). Despite its relatively low prevalence, hypermagnesemia probably occurs more frequently than it should because clinicians are often unaware of the magnesium content of various preparations.[52]

Renal patients may also receive an exogenous magnesium load during hemodialysis, because of either inadvertent use of hard water or an error in manufacture of the concentrate used for preparing the dialysate.

Elderly persons are at greater risk for hypermagnesemia because they have age-related reduced renal function and tend to consume more magnesium-containing preparations (such as antacids or mineral supplements) than younger individuals.

TABLE 7–2.
Some Commonly Used Medications Containing Magnesium

ANTACIDS	LAXATIVES
Aludrox	Citrate of Magnesia
Camalox	Milk of Magnesia
Creamalin	
Delcid	
Di-Gel	
Gelusil	
Maalox	
Mylanta	
Riopan	
Silain-Gel	
Simeco	
Trisagel	

Other Factors

Overly vigorous treatment with magnesium salts can cause hypermagnesemia in patients with normal renal function, as can conventional doses in those with renal impairment. Magnesium sulfate is sometimes administered to treat eclampsia or to delay delivery. In either case, excessive magnesium administration can cause both maternal and fetal hypermagnesemia. In a recent study of the use of magnesium sulfate as a tocolytic agent in 111 women, investigators reported that side effects were common but were rarely severe enough to cause cessation of therapy.[53] They cautioned that, because 90% of parenterally administered magnesium sulfate is cleared by the maternal kidneys, the drug should be administered with extreme caution in women with impaired renal function.

Transient elevations in serum magnesium levels can occur during periods of extracellular fluid volume depletion, as in adrenal insufficiency or after diuretic abuse. Hypermagnesemia can also be related to untreated diabetic ketoacidosis when catabolism causes release of cellular magnesium that cannot be excreted due to the oliguria associated with fluid volume depletion.

An elevated magnesium level can be artifactual (false) when blood specimens are drawn with an excessively tight tourniquet or allowed to hemolyze.

DEFINING CHARACTERISTICS

The clinical manifestations of hypermagnesemia largely reflect the ion's action on the nervous and

TABLE 7-3.
Clinical Indicators of Hypermagnesemia in Approximate Relationship to Degree of Serum Elevation*

SERUM MG LEVEL (mEq/L)	CLINICAL INDICATORS
3–5	Peripheral vasodilatation with facial flushing, sense of warmth, and tendency for hypotension; nausea and vomiting
4–7	Drowsiness; decreased deep tendon reflexes; muscle weakness
5–10	More severe hypotension and bradycardia
7–10	Loss of patellar reflex
10	Respiratory depression
10–15	Respiratory paralysis; coma
15–20	Cardiac arrest

* These are only general ranges; precise levels at which signs and symptoms are expected to develop are not uniformly defined. Reports in the literature vary widely in regard to symptoms and the level at which they appear (see text).

cardiovascular systems. Because magnesium is not routinely measured with other electrolytes, one must maintain a high index of suspicion for hypermagnesemia in at-risk patients.

Table 7-3 lists some rough relationships between the serum levels of magnesium and expected symptoms. However, it should be emphasized that authorities do not agree on precise serum magnesium levels and correlation with clinical signs and symptoms. In fact, quite variable reports may be found in the literature. For example, some authors indicate that deep tendon reflexes are usually lost when the serum magnesium concentration exceeds 6 mEq/L[54]; others describe this as occurring at a level of 10 to 15 mEq/L.[55] Most authors seem to agree that deep tendon reflexes become hypoactive before respiratory depression occurs, making this an important area for assessment. Despite the wide variations in reports of levels at which symptoms occur, it is clear that the patients at risk for hypermagnesemia (especially those receiving magnesium infusions) must be closely monitored for potential problems. See Chapter 23 for a discussion of the use of magnesium sulfate as an anticonvulsant for patients with preeclampsia.

TREATMENT

The best treatment for hypermagnesemia is prevention. This can be accomplished by avoiding administration of magnesium to patients with renal failure and by administering magnesium salts carefully to seriously ill patients.

In the presence of hypermagnesemia, any parenteral or oral magnesium salt should be discontinued. This may be all that is needed if the deep tendon reflexes are still present. However, in the presence of respiratory depression or defective cardiac conduction, emergency measures such as ventilatory support and IV calcium administration are indicated. As little as 5 to 10 mEq of calcium may readily reverse a potentially lethal respiratory depression or cardiac arrhythmia.[56] (Recall that calcium acts as a direct antagonist to magnesium.)

Hemodialysis with a magnesium-free dialysate is an effective treatment that should produce a safe serum magnesium level within 4 to 6 hours.[57]

NURSING INTERVENTIONS

1. Be aware of patients at risk for hypermagnesemia and assess for its presence. See Summary of Hypermagnesemia and preceding sections explaining etiological factors and defining characteristics.

   When hypermagnesemia is suspected, assess the following parameters:

   ▸ Vital signs: Look for low blood pressure and shallow respirations with periods of apnea.
   ▸ Patellar reflexes: If absent, notify physician since this usually implies a serum magnesium level greater than 7 mEq/L. If allowed to progress, cardiac or respiratory arrest could occur.
   ▸ Level of consciousness: Look for drowsiness, lethargy, and coma.

2. Do not give magnesium-containing medications to patients with renal failure or compromised renal function. (Be particularly careful in following "standing orders" for bowel preparation for radiography because some of these include the use of magnesium citrate.)

3. Caution patients with renal disease to check with their health care providers before taking over-the-counter medications. See Table 7-2 for a list of some commonly used medications containing magnesium.

4. Be aware of factors related to safe parenteral administration of magnesium salts. Review Table 7-1.

Case Studies

1. A 43-year-old woman was awaiting a kidney transplant when an order was written for a barium enema. Routine orders for bowel preparation in the institution included the administration of magnesium citrate as a laxative. Without considering the need to modify directives for a renal patient, the preparation was administered. Shortly after administration of

---

Summary of Hypermagnesemia

ETIOLOGICAL FACTORS	DEFINING CHARACTERISTICS
Renal failure (particularly when magnesium-containing medications are administered)	Early signs:
	▸ Flushing and a sense of skin warmth (due to peripheral vasodilatation)
Excessive magnesium administration during treatment of eclampsia or to delay labor	▸ Mild hypotension (due to blockage of superficial ganglia as well as direct effect on smooth muscle)
Untreated diabetic ketoacidosis	▸ Nausea and vomiting
Extracellular fluid volume depletion (as in adrenal insufficiency or after diuretic abuse)	Drowsiness, hypoactive reflexes, and muscular weakness
Hemodialysis with excessively hard water or with a dialysate inadvertently high in magnesium content	More severe hypotension as serum concentration of magnesium increases
	Depressed respirations
	Absent deep tendon reflexes, respiratory paralysis, and coma
	Cardiac abnormalities:
	▸ Sinus bradycardia, prolonged P–R, QRS, and Q–T intervals
	▸ Heart block and cardiac arrest in diastole

---

magnesium citrate, the patient became very lethargic and developed muscular weakness.

Commentary: Magnesium salts should never be given to patients with acute or chronic renal disease because diseased kidneys are incapable of eliminating magnesium. Blindly following standing orders caused serious problems for this patient. Hemodialysis was performed on an emergency basis.

2. A 62-year-old woman with chronic glomerulonephritis took Maalox (a magnesium-containing antacid) to alleviate gastric discomfort. She developed lethargy and difficulty in breathing. On admission to an acute care facility, her serum magnesium level was found to be 7.8 mEq/L (normal is 1.5–2.5 mEq/L). Ten mEq of calcium gluconate were administered to alleviate respiratory depression. Hemodialysis was initiated.

Commentary: As above, magnesium-containing medications are contraindicated in patients with acute or chronic renal disease. Part of patient education should be directed at the need to avoid such preparations.

REFERENCES

1. Kokko J, Tannen R: Fluids and Electrolytes, 2nd ed, p 631. Philadelphia, WB Saunders, 1990
2. Vanatta J, Fogelman M: Moyer's Fluid Balance, 4th ed, p 129. Chicago, Year Book Medical Publishers, 1988
3. Maxwell M, Kleeman C, Narins R: Clinical Disorders of Fluid and Electrolyte Metabolism, 4th ed, p 302. New York, McGraw-Hill, 1987
4. Kokko, Tannen, p 632
5. Ibid
6. Schrier R: Renal and Electrolyte Disorders, 3rd ed, p 334. Boston, Little, Brown, 1986
7. Goldberger E: A Primer of Water, Electrolyte and Acid–Base Syndromes, 7th ed, p 342. Philadelphia, Lea & Febiger, 1986
8. Schrier, p 344
9. Chernow et al: Hypomagnesemia in patients in postoperative intensive care. Chest 95(2): 391, 1989
10. Ryzen et al: Magnesium deficiency in a medical ICU population. Crit Care Med 13(1): 19, 1985
11. Whang R: Magnesium deficiency: Pathogenesis, prevalence and clinical implications. Am J Med 82(suppl 3A): 24, 1987
12. Kokko, Tannen, p 634
13. Chernow et al: Hypomagnesemia: Implications for the critical care specialist. Crit Care Med 10:193, 1982
14. Booth et al: Incidence of hypomagnesemia in intestinal malabsorption. Br Med J 2:141, 1963
15. Sullivan et al: Magnesium metabolism in alcoholism. Am J Clin Nutr 63:297, 1963
16. Zaloga G, Chernow B: Magnesium metabolism in critical illness. Crit Care Q 6:24, 1983
17. Ibid

18. Silberman H, Eisenberg D: Parenteral and Enteral Nutrition for the Hospitalized Patient, p 200. East Norwalk, CT, Appleton-Century-Crofts, 1982
19. Kokko, Tannen, p 641
20. Zaloga et al: Hypomagnesemia is a common complication of aminoglycoside therapy. Clin Res 31: 261A, 1983
21. Dunagen W, Ridner M: Manual of Medical Therapeutics, 26th ed, p 252. Boston, Little, Brown, 1989
22. Kokko, Tannen, p 641
23. Ibid, p 825
24. Zaloga, Chernow, p 24
25. Ibid
26. Ibid, p 23
27. Chernow et al, p 193
28. Ibid, p 194
29. Ibid, p 193
30. Schrier, p 347
31. Goldberger, p 344
32. Chernow et al, p 194
33. Kingston M, Al-siba B, Skooge W: Clinical manifestations of hypomagnesemia. Crit Care Med 14(11): 950, 1985
34. Goldman et al: The effect on myocardial ^{3}H-digoxin of magnesium deficiency. Proc Soc Exp Biol Med 136:747, 1971
35. Beller et al: Correlation of serum magnesium levels and cardiac digitalis intoxication. Am J Cardiol 33:225, 1974
36. Chernow et al, p 195
37. Goldberger, p 342
38. Vanatta, Fogelman, p 131
39. Ibid
40. Maxwell et al, p 838
41. Swenson S, Lewis J, Selby K: Magnesium metabolism in man with special reference to jejunoileal bypass for obesity. Am J Surg 127:250, 1974
42. Kokko, Tannen, p 638
43. Maxwell et al, p 844
44. Kokko, Tannen, p 642
45. Rivlin M, Morrison J, Bates G: Manual of Clinical Problems in Obstetrics and Gynecology, 3rd ed, p 32. Boston, Little, Brown, 1990
46. Maxwell et al, p 844
47. Dunagen, Ridner, p 429
48. Ibid
49. Hoffman et al: An amp by any other name: the hazards of intravenous magnesium dosing (letter). JAMA 261:557, 1989
50. Gahart B: A Handbook of Intravenous Medications, 6th ed, p 328. St. Louis, CV Mosby, 1990
51. Maxwell et al, p 904
52. Kokko, Tannen, p 970
53. Dudley D, Gagnon D, Varner M: Long-term tocolysis with intravenous magnesium sulfate. Obstet Gynecol 73:373, 1989
54. Maxwell et al, p 846
55. Kokko, Tannen, p 642
56. Schrier, p 352
57. Alfrey et al: Hypermagnesemia after renal homotransplantation. Ann Intern Med 73:367, 1970

8

Phosphorous Imbalances

Until recently, little attention was given to phosphate disturbances in clinical settings. However, increasing recognition of the frequency of phosphate disturbances and increased use of therapeutic interventions that profoundly affect overall phosphate balance have roused a greater interest in phosphorus metabolism.

PHOSPHORUS BALANCE

Phosphorus is a critical constituent of all the body's tissues. It is essential to the function of muscle, red blood cells, and the nervous system, and to the intermediary metabolism of carbohydrate, protein, and fat.

Normal serum phosphate level ranges from 2.5 to 4.5 mg/dL (0.81–1.45 mmol/L). Levels are greater in children, presumably because of the higher rate of skeletal growth. Serum levels may vary throughout the day; for example, glucose intake, insulin administration, or hyperventilation can lower the serum phosphate by increasing cellular uptake of phosphate.

Adequate dietary intake of phosphorus is ensured by a normal diet as phosphorus is plentiful in many foods, including red meat, fish, poultry, eggs, milk products, and legumes. Most ingested phosphate is absorbed in the jejunum. However, absorption can be impaired by certain medications (such as phosphate-binding antacids) or by malabsorptive disorders. Maintenance of normal phosphate balance requires an efficient renal conservation mechanism because the kidneys are the major route of excretion of phosphorus, being responsible for approximately 90% of the phosphorus excreted daily. During times of low phosphate intake, the kidneys retain more phosphorus.

HYPOPHOSPHATEMIA

Hypophosphatemia refers to a serum phosphate concentration below the lower limit of normal (<2.5 mg/dL); it is considered to be severe when less than 1.0 mg/dL.[1] It may occur in the presence of total body phosphate deficit or may merely reflect a temporary shift of phosphorus into the cells.

ETIOLOGICAL FACTORS

A wide variety of clinical disorders and therapeutic interventions can cause hypophosphatemia. These etiological factors are listed in the Summary of Hypophosphatemia and are discussed briefly below. Essentially, they fall into one of three categories: shift of phosphate from the extracellular fluid (ECF) into the cells, decreased absorption of phosphate from the gastrointestinal (GI) tract, and increased renal phosphate losses.[2] Many of the precipitating causes are treatment related.[3] For example, Halevy and Bulvik[4] reported that medications contributed to hypophosphatemia in 82% of the cases in their study; among the implicated medications were intravenous (IV) glucose, antacids, anabolic steroids, and diuretics.

Glucose Administration

Glucose administration causes endogenous release of insulin, which in turn promotes the transport of both glucose and phosphorus into the cells (primarily of the skeletal muscle and liver). Normally the decline in serum phosphorus does not exceed 0.5 mg/dL[5] although the response is more severe in starving patients. A survey of 100 subjects with hypophosphatemia showed parenteral administration of glucose to be the cause in 45% of the cases.[6] A lesser effect is associated with oral glucose intake.

Nutritional Recovery Syndrome

The nutritional recovery syndrome is sometimes referred to as the "refeeding syndrome." Hypophosphatemia may occur during the administration of calories in normally required amounts to patients with severe protein–calorie malnutrition (such as those with anorexia nervosa, elderly debilitated patients who are unable to eat, or alcoholics). Alcoholics appear to be at particular risk, with hypophosphatemia occurring in up to 50% of hospitalized patients and often corresponds to refeeding.[7] It occurs most commonly with overzealous refeeding of simple carbohydrates. For example, rapid refeeding of starved prisoners of war has been shown to produce the "nutritional recovery syndrome."[8] Substituting skim milk for simple carbohydrates reduced the problem in this population because skim milk is high in phosphorus and potassium, a result that suggests these electrolytes are important during the refeeding period.[9] A prerequisite for the syndrome is that the cells be capable of anabolism; during the anabolic phase there is an influx of phosphorus into the cells (primarily the body's muscle mass).

Hyperalimentation

Development of marked hypophosphatemia in malnourished patients receiving total parenteral nutrition (TPN) without adequate phosphorus replacement has been well documented and may occur within the first 24 hours, although it often becomes evident only after 2 to 3 days of treatment. It is caused by a rapid influx of phosphorus into the body's muscle mass at the initiation of anabolism (tissue building) after a period of catabolism.

Respiratory Alkalosis

Prolonged, intense hyperventilation can depress serum phosphorus to values in the vicinity of 0.5 mg/dL, presumably by inducing respiratory alkalosis. Clinical situations associated with respiratory alkalosis include gram-negative bacteremia, withdrawal from chronic alcoholism, heat stroke, acute salicylate poisoning, primary hyperventilation, and thyrotoxicosis.

Hypophosphatemia associated with alkalosis is secondary to increased cellular phosphate uptake. Although the underlying mechanism is unknown, it is likely that alkalosis stimulates glycolysis, increasing the formation of phosphorylated intermediates and thereby pulling more phosphorus into the cells.[10] This process causes a precipitous fall in the serum phosphorus concentration.

Alcohol Withdrawal

A common cause of severe hypophosphatemia is alcoholism. In fact, hypophosphatemia affects about 50% of patients with alcoholism requiring hospitalization.[11] Malnourished chronic alcoholics given IV glucose may have serum phosphate levels reduced to less than 1.0 mg/dL.[12] Factors contributing to phosphate depletion in alcoholics include poor intake, vomiting, use of antacids, and diarrhea. The fact that some alcoholics develop phosphate depletion in the absence of these factors suggests the presence of other mechanisms, perhaps including the effects of ethanol per se, magnesium deficiency, ketoacidosis, and hypocalcemia.[13]

Pharmacological Phosphate Binding

Antacids are used in uremic patients to bind with dietary phosphorus and prevent its absorption, thus normalizing serum phosphorus concentrations. However, excessive phosphorus binding by aluminum hydroxide, magnesium hydroxide, or aluminum carbonate gels may cause severe hypophosphatemia, particularly when there is poor dietary intake of phosphorus. Phosphate-binding antacids are more likely to produce hypophosphatemia when other conditions associated with this imbalance are present, such as diuretic therapy, renal tubular defects, or hyperparathyroidism.

Diabetic Ketoacidosis

Patients with poorly controlled diabetes who have glycosuria, ketonuria, and polyuria lose phosphate excessively into the urine. Although patients with untreated ketoacidosis may have normal or slightly elevated serum phosphorus levels, administration of insulin and parenteral fluids quickly causes serum phosphorus levels to drop below normal.

Insulin Administration

Because insulin promotes glycolysis, it causes a shift of phosphorus into the cells. In a study reported by Van-Landingham et al,[14] hypophosphatemia was found in 30% of a tube-fed population. This usually occurred in patients who were treated with insulin for hyperglycemia and was assumed to be secondary to intracellular transport of phosphate.

Thermal Burns

Hypophosphatemia is common in patients with extensive burns and usually appears within several days after injury. The mechanism by which it develops is not clear. Because burn patients often hyperventilate, it is possible that respiratory alkalosis occurs and results in acceleration of glycolysis causing hypophosphatemia. It has also been postulated that urinary loss of phosphate may occur during the diuresis of salt and water, or that phosphorus may be taken up by the cells as the burned patient becomes anabolic. Burned patients may remain unexplainably hypophosphatemic for months after their injuries.[15]

Other Factors

A survey of 100 hypophosphatemic patients suggested that diuretics were the cause in 7%.[16] Other possible causes include GI malabsorption syndrome, vitamin D deficiency, acute gout, hypokalemia, hypomagnesemia, and hypocalcemia. Hypomagnesemia fosters hypophosphatemia through increased urinary losses of phosphate. Hypocalcemia can cause phosphaturia through stimulation of parathyroid hormone release.[17]

DEFINING CHARACTERISTICS

Most signs and symptoms of phosphorus deficiency apparently result from deficiency of adenosine triphosphate (ATP), 2,3-diphosphoglycerate (2,3-DPG), or both. Cellular energy resources are impaired by ATP deficiency and oxygen delivery to tissues by 2,3-DPG deficiency.

Nervous System Changes

Cellular deficiencies of ATP and 2,3-DPG can produce a wide range of neurological symptoms which may include irritability, apprehension, weakness, numbness, paresthesias, dysarthria, confusion, obtundation, convulsive seizures, and coma.[18] For the alcoholic patient, consider that the presence of hallucinations is more likely due to delirium tremors than to hypophosphatemic encephalopathy, since hallucinations do not usually accompany the latter.

Cardiomyopathy

There are indications that hypophosphatemia can cause congestive cardiomyopathy. A case was reported in which a woman with severe hypophosphatemia presented with biventricular failure with cardiomegaly; correction of the hypophosphatemia led to rapid improvement. After 6 weeks, there were no signs of heart disease.[19]

Hematological Changes

Hypophosphatemia affects all the blood cells, but changes in the red cells are most pronounced. As stated above, a decline in 2,3-DPG levels in erythrocytes occurs in hypophosphatemia. Recall that 2,3-DPG is an enzyme in red cells that normally interacts with hemoglobin to promote the release of oxygen. Thus, low levels of 2,3-DPG may reduce the delivery of oxygen to peripheral tissues, resulting in tissue anoxia. Hemolytic anemia may occur because the red cells are more fragile and easily destroyed as a result of low ATP levels.

In laboratory animals, hypophosphatemia has been noted to produce depression of the chemotactic, phagocytic, and bacterial activity of granulocytes. These abnormalities are apparently reversible with correction of the hypophosphatemia. It is thought that hypophosphatemia impairs granulocytic function by interfering with ATP synthesis. Obviously, patients with impaired leukocyte function are at greater risk of infection.

Muscle Changes

Muscle damage may develop as the muscle ATP level declines. This is manifested clinically by muscle weakness, release of creatinine phosphokinase (CPK), and, at times, acute rhabdomyolysis (disintegration of striated muscle). Profound muscular weakness has been described in severely hypophosphatemic patients, as has muscular pain. Elevations in CPK levels have been reported in patients with serum phosphate concentrations less than 1 mg/dL for 1 to 2 days.[20] It is possible that muscle cell injury could be the result of disrupted functioning of chemical processes important in maintaining cellular membrane integrity.

Ventilatory Changes

Several authors have reported weakness of the chest muscle in hypophosphatemic patients.[21,22] Ventilatory muscle fatigue may arise from cellular depletion of ATP, impaired cellular oxygenation, and central respiratory depression.[23] Varsano et al recommended that the possibility of hypophosphatemia be considered for each patient who develops acute ventilatory failure or presents a problem of respiratory weaning.[24]

Other Factors

There are indications that phosphorus deficiency may produce an insulin-resistant state, resulting in hyperglycemia.[25] Pronounced hypophosphatemia may also be accompanied by severe metabolic acidosis.

Prolonged hypophosphatemia has reportedly been associated with osteomalacia and pseudofractures. Patients with symptoms resembling ankylosing spondylitis have improved with phosphorus administration.

TREATMENT

Mild-to-Moderate Hypophosphatemia

Treatment of hypophosphatemia varies with the cause and severity of the imbalance. If mild and asymptomatic, it may be adequately managed by treatment of the primary disorder.[26] Because phosphorus is plentiful in the diet, improved nutrition may suffice. However, if hypophosphatemia is likely to persist, therapy may require oral supplementation. Often, milk is recommended for the treatment of chronic phosphate deficiency because it is high in phosphate; it is also an excellent source of calcium and potassium. Of course, if calcium is contraindicated, milk is not recommended. If milk is not tolerated, Neutra-Phos capsules (250 mg of elemental phosphorus and 7 mEq each of Na^+ and K^+ per capsule) or Phospho-Soda 5 mL (each milliliter contains 120 mg of phosphorus and 4.8 mEq Na^+) may be prescribed as needed.[27] The usual dose is two capsules of Neutra-Phos or 5 mL of Phospho-Soda given two or three times daily.[28] Diarrhea is a side effect that may limit dosage of these agents.

Severe Hypophosphatemia

Severe hypophosphatemia is dangerous and requires prompt treatment. Aggressive IV phosphorus repair is usually limited to patients with a serum phosphorus level below 1 mg/dL.[29] Only general guidelines are available for the IV replacement of phosphates. According to one source, 20 mmol of sodium phosphate or potassium phosphate administered every 8 hours IV may be necessary until symptoms abate; for patients weighing less than 60 kg, the rate and amount should be reduced.[30] Recommendations for specific patients vary according to the underlying problem, renal status, and accompanying electrolyte disturbances. Possible dangers of IV phosphorus administration include hypocalcemia and metastatic calcification from hyperphosphatemia. Reportedly, the parenteral administration of phosphate salts will lower ionized calcium if the product of calcium times the phosphorus is greater than 58 mg/dL.[31] The ECF phosphate level should not be elevated above normal during treatment because this can cause precipitation of calcium salts in tissues, lowering of ionized calcium, or both.[32]

Another consideration is that calcium and phosphate should not be administered in the same IV infusion because of the risk of precipitation.[33] Extreme caution is indicated if phosphorus is administered to patients with renal insufficiency and a marked decrease in glomerular filtration rate because of the danger of hyperphosphatemia. In alcoholic patients, it is practical to administer phosphate, potassium, and magnesium in a single solution.[34]

The effect of replacement salts on the serum phosphorus level should be followed closely. Subsequent doses should be adjusted according to clinical status and the new serum phosphorus level. Some premixed balanced electrolyte parenteral solutions contain phosphorus (such as Ionosol T, Isolyte M, and Electrolyte #75). Intravenous replacement products are also available as ampules of sodium or potassium phosphate (to be mixed with compatible IV solutions). The amount of sodium or potassium administered must be considered; for example, potassium phosphate is contraindicated in patients with high potassium levels. Similarly, sodium phosphate should be used cautiously in patients with sodium-retaining states.

Phosphorus replacement in patients receiving total parenteral nutrition (TPN) is discussed in Chapter 12; replacement in patients with diabetic ketoacidosis is discussed in Chapter 21.

NURSING INTERVENTIONS

1. Identify patients at risk for hypophosphatemia. See the Summary of Hypophosphatemia and discussion of etiological factors.
   ▶ Particularly at risk are extremely malnourished patients being started on TPN or large caloric intake by tube feeding (refeeding syndrome in starving patients).
   ▶ Also at great risk are alcoholic patients undergoing withdrawal therapy and initial treatment with IV glucose fluids.
   ▶ Similarly at great risk are patients with diabetic ketoacidosis during the early treatment period with insulin and IV fluids. This is particularly true if serum phosphate levels were low on admission. Fortunately, low-dose insulin therapy has decreased the incidence of rapid phosphate cellular shifts during early treatment (see Chap. 21).
2. Monitor patients at risk for the presence of hypophosphatemia. See Summary of Hypophosphatemia and discussion of defining characteristics.
   ▶ Monitor serum phosphate levels in patients at high risk. Notify physician when levels are low. Hypophosphatemia is profound when serum levels are less than 1.0 mg/dL.
   ▶ Be alert for paresthesias, particularly about the mouth.
   ▶ Be alert for muscle weakness and pain. Test hand grasp strength on a serial basis to monitor for muscle weakness. Monitor for changes in speech that may reflect muscular weakness.
   ▶ Be alert for mental changes associated with hypophosphatemia, such as apprehension, confusion, delirium, and decreased level of consciousness.
   ▶ Be alert for signs of cardiac and ventilatory failure in patients with severe hypophosphatemia.
3. Be aware that severely hypophosphatemic patients are thought to be at greater risk for infection because of changes in white blood cells. As always, take precautions to prevent infections (as in meticulous care of central lines for TPN patients).
4. Administer IV phosphate products cautiously. Be aware that they should be administered slowly in dilute infusion solutions to avoid phosphate intoxication. Dosage should be individualized to the patient's requirements. According to one source, 20 mmol of sodium or potassium phosphate can be given IV over 8 hours in urgent situations and repeated until symptoms abate.[35] For patients weighing less than 60 kg, administration rates or amounts should be reduced.[36] Frequent monitoring of serum phosphorus levels is required to guide therapy.
5. Be aware that phosphorus requirements in TPN are roughly 10 mmol per 1000 calories.[37] As stated above, dosages of phosphorus must be tailored to the patient's individual needs. To accomplish this, serum levels must be monitored on a regular basis. Of note, fat emulsions contain about 10 mmol of phosphate per 500-mL bottle.[38]
6. Be aware of the need to introduce hyperalimentation *gradually* in patients who are malnourished. Gradual introduction of the feeding solution is less apt to be associated with rapid shifts of phosphate into the cells. Monitor rates of TPN flow frequently.
7. Be aware that sudden increase in the serum phosphorus level can cause hypocalcemia. For this reason, serum calcium levels should be monitored. Watch for twitching around the mouth, laryngospasm, positive Chvostek's sign, paresthesias, arrhythmias, and hypotension.
8. Because it is possible to give too much phosphorus when administering phosphate solutions, monitor for signs of hyperphosphatemia and of the salt in which it is administered.

   For example, excessive administration of potassium phosphate could cause paresthesias of the extremities, flaccid paralysis, listlessness, confusion, weakness, arrhythmias, heart block, and ECG abnormalities. Serum potassium or sodium levels (depending on the replacement salt) should be monitored in addition to serum phosphorus levels.
9. Monitor for diarrhea in patients taking oral phosphorus supplements; consult with physician if it persists or becomes severe.
10. Mix powdered oral phosphorus supplements with

Summary of Hypophosphatemia

ETIOLOGICAL FACTORS	DEFINING CHARACTERISTICS
Glucose administration	Paresthesias
Refeeding after starvation	Muscle weakness (perhaps manifested as decreased strength of hand grasp and difficulty speaking)
Hyperalimentation	
Alcohol withdrawal	
Diabetic ketoacidosis	Muscle pain and tenderness
Respiratory alkalosis	Mental changes, such as apprehension, confusion, delirium, and coma
Phosphate-binding antacids	Cardiomyopathy
Recovery phase after severe burns	Acute respiratory failure (perhaps related to chest muscle weakness)
	Seizures
	Decreased tissue oxygenation
	Joint stiffness
	Serum phosphate <2.5 mg/dL

---

chilled or iced water to make them more palatable. Also, palatability may be increased by refrigerating the solution made from the powder. (Any palatable juice or beverage may be used in place of water.)

Case Study

1. A 40-year-old woman with a history of severe diarrhea was admitted for 3 weeks. During this period she was nauseated and ate poorly. Two months earlier she had undergone a bilateral salpingo-oophorectomy for ovarian cancer and a radium implant. A 30-lb weight loss was sustained over the previous 4-months. Weight on admission was 88 pounds. A retroperitoneal small-bowel fistula was found and surgical repair of the fistula and a colostomy were performed. After she suffered a multitude of postoperative complications, TPN was begun. At this time, serum electrolytes were found to be:

Na^+ = 136 mEq/L	PO_4 = 3.4 mg/dL
Cl^- = 93 mEq/L	CO_2 content = 31 mEq/L
K^+ = 3.6 mEq/L	Glucose = 128 mg/dL
Ca^{++} = 8.7 mg/dL	BUN = 8 mg/dL

Eight days later, her condition had markedly deteriorated. A glucose intolerance (blood glucose 270 mg/dL) required the administration of regular insulin, 20 units, every 6 hours. Inflammation was noted at the central line insertion site. At this time, her serum phosphate level was 0.4 mg/dL (normal

is 2.5–4.5 mg/dL). Assessment revealed slurred speech and drooping of the mouth and tongue. The patient appeared restless and anxious and complained of numbness all over.

The next day, muscle twitching and gross abnormal movements were noted. The patient was unable to grasp objects with her hands and was too weak to raise her arms. She complained of pain whenever anything touched her skin. At this time, her serum phosphate level was 0.2 mg/dL. A nutritional consultation was made and IV phosphate administration was started.

Two days later her speech remained slurred, spastic movements continued, and intense sensitivity to touch remained. However, her glucose intolerance had improved. Spot checks decreased from 2% to 0.10% glucose. Slowly, over a period of days, her hand grasps became perceptibly stronger and the muscle pain diminished. Numbness eventually disappeared. Three weeks later, the patient was discharged with a serum phosphate level of 4.5 mg/dL.

Commentary: The fact that this patient had essentially been starving caused her to suffer the nutritional recovery syndrome when overzealous refeeding was initiated with inadequate phosphorus in the TPN solution. Note that the serum phosphorus concentration reached extremely low levels before it was noticed and treated. Typical signs of hypophosphatemia were present. Even after the serum phosphorus concentration was raised to normal levels, it took days for the clinical manifestations to resolve (indicating sustained cellular deficits). This patient was allowed to become critically ill before the cause of her problem was diagnosed and treated.

HYPERPHOSPHATEMIA

ETIOLOGICAL FACTORS

A variety of conditions can lead to hyperphosphatemia. The major one is, of course, renal disease. In a study reported by Betro and Pain,[39] 84 cases of nonuremic hyperphosphatemia were described; according to the authors, no one cause was outstanding in frequency and, in over 50% of the cases, no definite explanation for the abnormality could be found.

Renal Disease

An increase in the serum phosphorus concentration is observed in patients with chronic renal failure when the glomerular filtration rate (GFR) is 30 mL/min or less. Also, hyperphosphatemia is common in acute renal failure.[40]

Chemotherapy for Neoplastic Disease

Large quantities of phosphates may be released into the circulation when chemotherapy is administered for neoplastic disease (particularly acute lymphoblastic leukemia and lymphoma) and are the result of cell destruction and liberation of intracellular phosphates.

High Phosphate Intake

Hyperphosphatemia may develop in infants fed cow's milk, which contains 1220 mg of calcium and 940 mg of phosphorus per liter (as compared to human milk, which contains 340 mg of calcium per liter and 150 mg of phosphorus per liter).[41] Patients taking large quantities of milk for peptic ulcer management may develop increased serum phosphorus levels.

It is possible to impose an excess phosphorus load if phosphate substances are administered incorrectly, either IV, orally, or in the form of phosphate-containing enemas. Substantial absorption of phosphorus can occur from the large bowel when Fleet Phospho-Soda is given as an enema. Use of laxatives containing sodium phosphate may result in accidental phosphate poisoning. Blood transfusions can also be a source of phosphorus because this substance leaks from the blood cells during storage.

Muscle Necrosis (Rhabdomyolysis)

Recall that muscle tissue contains the bulk of soft-tissue phosphate. Therefore, necrosis of muscle is a potent cause of hyperphosphatemia. Situations associated with rhabdomyolysis include direct trauma, viral infections, and heat stroke.

Increased Phosphorus Absorption

Large intake of vitamin D, either therapeutic or self-administered, causes increased phosphorus absorption which, together with impaired renal function, can result in hyperphosphatemia.

Endocrine Disorders

Decreased parathyroid activity (hypoparathyroidism) results in decreased calcium concentration and increased phosphate concentration. Hyperthyroidism may cause hyperphosphatemia, probably related to the osteoporosis that occurs in this condition.[42]

DEFINING CHARACTERISTICS

An elevated serum phosphate level causes little in the way of symptoms. The most important long-term consequence is soft-tissue calcification, which occurs mainly in patients with reduced glomerular filtration rates; the most important short-term consequence is tetany.

Soft-Tissue Calcification

High levels of serum inorganic phosphate are harmful because they promote precipitation of calcium phosphate in nonosseous sites. One such site is the kidney, where precipitation of calcium phosphate can result in progressive renal impairment. Other sites may include the joints, arteries, skin, or cornea. Soft-tissue calcification is seen primarily in patients with chronic renal failure and long-term serum phosphate elevation. An attempt is made to control the hyperphosphatemia and thus keep the calcium and phosphate product below 70. Recall that normal serum levels of calcium (8.5–10.5 mg/dL) and phosphate (2.5–4.5 mg/dL) have a product of approximately 30 to 40.

Hypocalcemia and Tetany

Because of the reciprocal relationship between phosphorus and calcium, a high serum phosphorus level tends to cause a low calcium concentration in the serum. Tetany can result and present as sensations of tingling in the tips of the fingers and around the mouth. These sensations may increase in severity and spread proximally along the limbs and to the face and be followed by numbness. Muscle spasms and pain may occur. Symptoms of tetany are most likely to occur in patients who are hyperphosphatemic because of a high phosphate load, either exogenous or endogenous. Because renal patients often have some degree of acidosis, they are less prone to develop symptoms of hypocalcemia because acidosis favors increased calcium ionization.

Other Effects

One effect of hyperphosphatemia is an increase in red blood cell 2,3-DPG levels. Thus, in patients with chronic renal failure, hyperphosphatemia helps protect against the adverse effects of anemia on tissue oxygenation.

TREATMENT

When possible, treatment is directed at the underlying disorder. If due to excessive phosphate administration in drugs or in milk, the disorder is rather easily remedied by eliminating the products. Dietary restriction of phosphorus intake is also indicated.

Phosphate binding agents such as aluminum hydroxide (Amphogel) and aluminum carbonate (Basaljel) are frequently used to decrease the serum phosphate level in renal patients. In some instances, dialysis is necessary.

NURSING INTERVENTIONS

1. Identify patients at risk for hyperphosphatemia. See the Summary of Hyperphosphatemia and the section on etiological factors.
2. Monitor for signs of tetany, such as tingling sensations in the fingertips and around the mouth, and presence of muscle cramps or positive Chvostek's and Trousseau's signs in at-risk patients. Be aware that these symptoms are probably due to hypocalcemia induced by the high phosphate level and are most likely to occur in patients who have taken in a high phosphate load. They are much less likely to occur in acidotic renal patients with high phosphate and low calcium levels because calcium ionization is increased in the presence of acidosis.
3. Be aware that soft-tissue calcification can be a long-term complication of a chronically elevated serum phosphate level. Calcification may occur in sites such as the kidney, arteries, joints, and cornea. Monitor for signs of these complications.
4. Administer prescribed oral and IV phosphate supplements cautiously and monitor serum phosphate levels periodically during their use.
5. When appropriate, instruct patients that use of

phosphate-containing laxatives may result in acute phosphate poisoning.

6. Be aware that phosphate-containing enemas can result in hyperphosphatemia if used injudiciously, particularly in children and those with slow bowel emptying. Instruct patients accordingly.
7. When a low-phosphorus diet is prescribed, instruct patients to avoid foods high in phosphorus content. Such foods include hard cheese or cream, nuts and nut products, whole grain cereals (such as bran and oatmeal), dried fruits, dried vegetables, special meats such as kidneys and sardines and sweetbreads, and desserts made with milk).[43]

Case Study

A 22-year-old woman was diagnosed as having refractory nephrotic syndrome. At the time of her original diagnosis, she experienced an insidious yet rapid onset of weight gain and lower extremity edema. She also noticed swelling in her wrists and tightness of her clothes and jewelry. She had 4+ proteinuria and her serum albumin was 1.1 g/dL. High-dose steroids were prescribed. When she developed an infection, she was admitted to the hospital. She was treated for the infection and for fluctuations in sodium and potassium levels. She also suffered with diarrhea for several days. It was not until the 11th day of her hospitalization that the serum phosphorus level was measured. Laboratory values included

Na^+ = 121 mEq/L	CO_2 content = 20 mEq/L
K^+ = 4.2 mEq/L	Ca^{++} = 7.0 mg/dL
Cl^- = 91 mEq/L	P = 7.7 mg/dL
Albumin = 1.5 g/dL	

Because she had sustained a 30-pound weight gain in a short period, and because of the low serum sodium level, a fluid restriction of 800 mL/day was initiated. Albumin was administered to raise the plasma oncotic pressure. Calcium carbonate was administered to increase the serum calcium level. On the 15th day of her hospitalization, the serum calcium had increased to 8.0 mg/dL and the serum phosphorus had decreased to 5.5 mg/dL. The serum sodium concentration increased to a level of 139 mEq/L.
Commentary: No symptoms related to hyperphosphatemia were present. Because the patient was hypoalbuminemic, the low serum calcium level was somewhat misleading. (Recall that for each gram the serum albumin level is below normal, the measured total serum calcium level drops by 0.8 mg/dL; therefore, the actual calcium level was closer to 8.6 mg/dL.) Also, since calcium ionization is increased in the presence of hypoalbuminemia and

---

Summary of Hyperphosphatemia

ETIOLOGICAL FACTORS	DEFINING CHARACTERISTICS
Renal failure	Short-term consequences: symptoms of tetany, such as tingling of fingertips and around mouth, numbness, and muscle spasms
Chemotherapy, particularly for acute lymphoblastic leukemia and lymphoma	
Large intake of milk, as in treatment of peptic ulcer	Long-term consequences: precipitation of calcium phosphate in nonosseous sites, such as the kidney, joints, arteries, skin, or cornea
Use of cow's milk in infants	
Excessive intake of phosphate-containing laxatives	Serum phosphate >4.5 mg/dL
Overzealous administration of phosphorus supplements, orally or IV	
Excessive use of Fleet's phosphosoda as enema solution, particularly in children and individuals with slow bowel elimination	
Large vitamin D intake (increases phosphorus absorption)	
Hypoparathyroidism	
Hyperthyroidism	

---

acidosis, no symptoms of hypocalcemia occurred. Note the presence of metabolic acidosis, evidenced by the low carbon dioxide content value of 20 mEq/L (normally about 26 mEq/L).

REFERENCES

1. Maxwell M, Kleeman C, Narins R: Clinical Disorders of Fluid and Electrolyte Metabolism, 4th ed, p 790. New York, McGraw-Hill, 1987
2. Kokko J, Tannen R: Fluids and Electrolytes, 2nd ed. p 972. Philadelphia, WB Saunders, 1990
3. Tucker S, Schimmel E: Postoperative hypophosphatemia: A multifactorial problem. Nutr Rev 47(4): 111, 1989
4. Halevy J, Bulvik S: Severe hypophosphatemia in hospitalized patients. Arch Intern Med 148:153, 1988
5. Knochel J: The pathophysiology and clinical characteristics of severe hypophosphatemia. Ann Intern Med 137:205, 1977
6. Juan D, Elrazak M: Hypophosphatemia in hospitalized patients. JAMA 242:163, 1979
7. Kokko, Tannen, p 972
8. Mollison P: Observations on cases of starvation at Belsen. Br Med J 1:4, 1946
9. Maxwell et al, p 795
10. Ibid
11. Schrier R: Renal and Electrolyte Disorders, 3rd ed, p 302. Boston, Little, Brown, 1986
12. Varsano et al: Hypophosphatemia as a reversible cause of refractory ventilatory failure. Crit Care Med 11:908, 1983
13. Knochel, p 207
14. Vanlandingham et al: Metabolic abnormalities in patients supported with enteral tube feeding. Journal of Parenteral and Enteral Nutrition 5(4): 322, 1981
15. Knochel, p 205
16. Juan, Elrazak, p 972
17. Tucker, Schimmel, p 111
18. Schrier, p 304
19. Ibid, p 306
20. Knochel, p 213
21. Boelens et al: Hypophosphatemia with muscle weakness due to antacids and hemodialysis. Am J Dis Child 120:350, 1970
22. Furlan et al: Acute areflexic paralysis. Arch Neurol 32:706, 1975
23. Varsano et al: Hypophosphatemia as a reversible cause of refractory ventilatory failure. Crit Care Med 11:908, 1983
24. Ibid
25. Hamburger S, Rush D: Hypophosphatemia. Mo Med, 79:87, 1982
26. Dunagan W, Ridner M: Manual of Medical Therapeutics, 26th ed, p 428. Boston, Little, Brown, 1989
27. Ibid
28. Alpers D, Clouse R, Stenson W: Manual of Nutritional Therapeutics, 2nd ed, p 97
29. Lentz R, Brown D, Kjellstrand C: Treatment of severe hypophosphatemia. Ann Intern Med 89:941, 1978

30. Vanatta J, Fogelman M: Moyer's Fluid Balance, 4th ed., p 138. Chicago, Year Book Medical Publishers, 1988
31. Kokko, Tannen, p 666
32. Vanatta, Fogelman, p 138
33. Dunagan, Ridner, p 428
34. Kokko, Tannen, p 666
35. Vanatta, Fogelman, p 138
36. Ibid
37. Pestana C: Fluids and Electrolytes in the Surgical Patient, 4th ed, p 191. Baltimore, Williams & Wilkins, 1989
38. Baker W: Hypophosphatemia. Am J Nurs 85(9): 1001, 1985
39. Betro M, Pain R: Hypophosphatemia and hyperphosphatemia in a hospital population. Br Med J 1(5795):273, 1972
40. Schrier, p 274
41. Ibid, p 273
42. Betro, Pain, p 275
43. Goldberger E: A Primer of Water, Electrolyte and Acid–Base Syndromes, 7th ed, p 209. Philadelphia, Lea & Febiger, 1986

9

Acid–Base Imbalances

This chapter provides a basic explanation of acid–base imbalances. Etiological factors and defining characteristics of each of the four imbalances are presented, followed by brief discussions of their treatment. For the nursing interventions used to deal with these disturbances, the reader should see the later chapters concerning specific situations associated with acid–base imbalances.

Before turning to the four acid–base disturbances, it will be helpful to review how the body regulates acid–base balance.

REGULATION OF ACID–BASE BALANCE

The body has the remarkable ability to maintain plasma *p*H within the narrow normal range of 7.35 to 7.45. It does so by means of chemical buffering mechanisms, by the kidneys, and by the lungs. *p*H is defined as hydrogen ion concentration; the more hydrogen ions, the more acidic the solution. The *p*H range that is compatible with life (6.8–7.8) represents a tenfold difference in hydrogen ion concentration in plasma.

It has been estimated that metabolism normally produces 13,000 mEq/day of hydrogen ions; less than 1% of this amount is excreted by the kidneys. It is obvious, then, that renal shutdown can be present for hours or days before life-threatening acid–base imbalance occurs; yet, cessation of breathing for minutes produces critical acid–base changes.

CHEMICAL BUFFERING MECHANISMS

Chemical buffers are substances that prevent major changes in the *p*H of body fluids by removing or releasing hydrogen ions; they can act within a fraction of a second to prevent excessive changes in hydrogen ion concentration.

The body's major buffer system is the bicarbonate (HCO_3)–carbonic acid (H_2CO_3) buffer system. Normally, there are 20 parts of bicarbonate to 1 part of carbonic acid. If this ratio is upset, the *p*H will change. It is the ratio that is important in maintaining *p*H, not absolute values.

Example: In a normal individual:

$$\frac{HCO_3}{H_2CO_3} = \frac{24 \text{ mEq/L}}{1.2 \text{ mEq/L}} = \frac{20}{1} \, (pH = 7.4)$$

In an individual with chronic obstructive lung disease, one might see:

$$\frac{HCO_3}{H_2CO_3} = \frac{48 \text{ mEq/L}}{2.4 \text{ mEq/L}} = \frac{20}{1} \, (pH = 7.4)$$

Carbon dioxide (CO_2) is a potential acid; when CO_2 is dissolved in water, it becomes carbonic acid: $CO_2 + H_2O = H_2CO_3$. Thus, when carbon dioxide is increased, the carbonic acid content is also increased, and vice versa.

If either bicarbonate or carbonic acid is increased or decreased so that the 20:1 ratio is no longer valid, acid–base imbalance results. Figure 9-1 demonstrates changes in plasma *p*H when the bicarbonate:carbonic acid ratio is altered.

Other less important buffer systems in the extracellular fluid (ECF) include the inorganic phosphates and the plasma proteins. Intracellular buffers include proteins, organic and inorganic phosphates, and, in red blood cells, hemoglobin.

KIDNEYS

The kidneys regulate the bicarbonate level in ECF; they are able to regenerate bicarbonate ions as well as to reabsorb them from the renal tubular cells.

In the presence of respiratory acidosis, and most cases of metabolic acidosis, the kidneys excrete hydro-

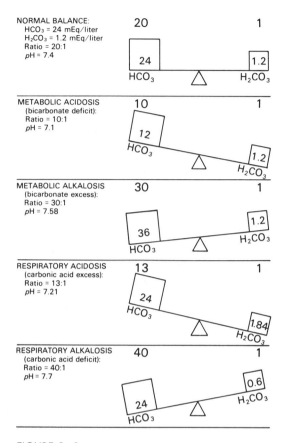

FIGURE 9–1.

Examples of *p*H changes with alterations in the bicarbonate : carbonic acid ratio. (Metheny N: Quick Reference to Fluid Balance, p 144. Philadelphia, JB Lippincott, 1984; with permission.)

gen ions and conserve bicarbonate ions to help restore balance. (The kidneys obviously cannot compensate for the metabolic acidosis created by renal failure.)

In the presence of respiratory and metabolic alkalosis, the kidneys retain hydrogen ions and excrete bicarbonate ions to help restore balance.

As stated earlier, renal compensation for imbalances is slow (a matter of hours or days).

LUNGS

Under the influence of the respiratory center, the lungs control the carbon dioxide (and thus carbonic acid) content of ECF by adjusting ventilation in response to the amount of carbon dioxide and, to a lesser extent, oxygen in the blood.

An acute rise in $PaCO_2$ (partial pressure of CO_2 in arterial blood) is a powerful stimulant to respiration.

The stimulatory effect of increased CO_2 reaches its peak within a few minutes; however, it gradually declines for the next 1 or 2 days to as little as 20% of the initial effect.[1] Therefore, after several days, elevation of blood CO_2 has only a weak effect as a respiratory stimulant.

PaO_2 (partial pressure of O_2 in arterial blood) influences respiration; however, its effect is not nearly as marked as that of $PaCO_2$. Decreased PaO_2 normally will not stimulate alveolar ventilation significantly until it falls to very low levels. For example, a decrease to approximately 60 mmHg has an imperceptible effect on ventilation. However, if the O_2 continues to fall to 40 mmHg to 30 mmHg, alveolar ventilation will increase 1.5 to 1.7-fold.[2]

Also, the lungs compensate for metabolic disturbances by either conserving or retaining carbon dioxide.

1. In the presence of metabolic acidosis, respiration is increased, causing greater elimination of carbon dioxide (to lighten the acid load).
2. In the presence of metabolic alkalosis, respiration is decreased, causing carbon dioxide to be retained (increasing the acid load).

Faulty pulmonary function disrupts acid–base balance. For example, hypoventilation due to chronic obstructive pulmonary disease (COPD) causes excessive carbon dioxide retention and respiratory acidosis; hyperventilation due to hysteria causes excessive elimination of carbon dioxide and respiratory alkalosis. Of course, the lungs are unable to compensate for metabolic *p*H disturbances when there is severe pulmonary dysfunction; in these instances, compensation must be accomplished solely by the kidneys.

MEASUREMENT OF ACID–BASE BALANCE

Before discussion of acid–base measurement, it is useful to review the definition of "acid" and "base." Simply stated, an acid is a substance that can donate hydrogen ions. For example, H_2CO_3 (carbonic acid) $\rightarrow H^+$ (hydrogen ion) $+ HCO_3^-$ (bicarbonate). A base is a substance that can accept hydrogen ions (H^+). For example, $HCO_3^- + H^+ \rightarrow H_2CO_3$.

The best way to evaluate acid–base balance is by measuring arterial blood gases (Table 9-1). Arterial blood gases (ABG) sample blood that has come from various parts of the body (not just one extremity as is the case with venous blood). Also, arterial blood gives information on how well the lungs are oxygenating the blood.

Note in Table 9-1 that only two of the listed measures are actually of gases ($PaCO_2$ and PaO_2). However, reporting the nonrespiratory component (bicarbonate) is essential to understanding the respiratory measures. In review, the $PaCO_2$ is controlled by the lungs and refers to the pressure exerted by dissolved CO_2 gas in blood. Carbon dioxide should be considered as an acid substance because, when dissolved in water, it forms carbonic acid (H_2CO_3). Also, PaO_2 refers to the pressure exerted by dissolved O_2 in the blood.

In the evaluation of acid–base status, the reporting of CO_2 content is often confusing. This measure is usually included with electrolyte determinations. Although listed on the laboratory sheet as "CO_2," it is actually a measure of the sum of bicarbonate (24 mEq/L) and dissolved CO_2 gas (1.2 mEq/L). Note the normal ratio of 20 parts of HCO_3 to 1 part of dissolved CO_2 gas. Thus, in normal situations, the CO_2 content should be 25.2 mEq/L.[3] Because CO_2 content primarily reflects the concentration of bicarbonate, it is largely a measure of the nonrespiratory (or metabolic) component of acid–base balance. Instead of merely using CO_2 as a term, it is important to clarify whether it refers to the gas ($PaCO_2$) or the CO_2 content.

Paramount to evaluation of blood gases is accurate collection of the sample; thus, Table 9-2 lists some guidelines for obtaining samples for arterial blood gas analysis. To assure patient safety and accuracy, only clinicians specially instructed in drawing blood gas samples should perform this maneuver. Listed at the end of the chapter, after discussion of the four primary acid–base imbalances, are guidelines for interpreting blood gases (Table 9-9) and information regarding the calculation of expected compensatory changes (Table 9-10).

METABOLIC ACIDOSIS

Metabolic acidosis (HCO_3 deficit) is a clinical disturbance characterized by a low *p*H (increased hydrogen concentration) and a low plasma bicarbonate concentration. It can be produced by a gain of hydrogen ion or a loss of bicarbonate. In compensation, the lungs hyperventilate to decrease the $PaCO_2$ concentration (movement in the same direction as the primary bicarbonate disturbance).

ANION GAP

Metabolic acidosis can be divided into two forms, depending on the values of the serum anion gap:

$$\text{Anion Gap (AG)} = Na^+ - (Cl^- + HCO_3^-) = 12 \pm 2 \text{ mEq/L}$$

TABLE 9-1.
Arterial Blood Gases

TERM	NORMAL VALUE	DEFINITION—IMPLICATIONS
pH	7.35–7.45	Reflects H^+ concentration; acidity increases as H^+ concentration increases (pH value decreases as acidity increases) ▸ pH < 7.35 (acidosis) ▸ pH > 7.45 (alkalosis)
$PaCO_2$	35–45 mmHg	Partial pressure of CO_2 in arterial blood ▸ When <35 mmHg, hypocapnia is said to be present (respiratory alkalosis) ▸ When >45 mmHg, hypercapnia is said to be present (respiratory acidosis)
PaO_2	80–100 mmHg (decreases with age)	Partial pressure of O_2 in arterial blood ▸ Any reading above 80 mmHg (on room air) is considered acceptable ▸ In adults younger than 60 yr (on room air) <80 mmHg indicates mild hypoxemia <60 mmHg indicates moderate hypoxemia <40 mmHg indicates severe hypoxemia ▸ Somewhat lower levels are accepted as normal in aged persons because there is some loss of ventilatory function with advanced age
Standard HCO_3	22–26 mEq/L	HCO_3 concentration in plasma of blood that has been equilibrated at a $PaCO_2$ of 40 mmHg, and with O_2 to fully saturate the hemoglobin
Base excess (BE)	−2–+2 mEq/L	Reflects metabolic (nonrespiratory) body disturbances, which may be primary or compensatory in nature Always negative in metabolic acidosis (deficit of alkali or excess of fixed acids) Always positive in metabolic alkalosis (excess of alkali or deficit of fixed acids) Arrived at by multiplying the deviation of standard HCO_3 from normal by a factor of 1.2, which represents the buffer action of red blood cells

As the equation demonstrates, sodium represents the major cation in body fluids, and chloride and bicarbonate represent the two major anions. There are other anions in body fluid that are not accounted for in the equation, including anionic proteins, phosphates, sulfates, and organic anions (such as ketones and lactic acid). Normally the sum of these unmeasured anions should be no greater than 12 ± 2 mEq/L. However, in some situations, these anions are markedly increased and the anion gap is greater than expected. These situations are referred to as high anion gap metabolic acidosis. On the other hand, if the primary problem is direct loss of bicarbonate, gain of chloride, or decreased renal ammonia production, the anion gap will be within normal limits (12 ± 2 mEq/L). Table 9-3 lists causes of metabolic acidosis classified as either high or normal anion gap.

HIGH ANION GAP ACIDOSIS

Diabetic ketoacidosis occurs in diabetics with a severe insulin deficiency coupled with excessive secretion of counterregulatory hormones. Due to insulin deficiency, lipolysis is increased, releasing free fatty acids that are delivered to the liver where they are converted to ketones. Accumulation of ketones (anions) causes a reciprocal decrease in bicarbonate and an increase in the anion gap.

Hepatic ketone production is a normal consequence of starvation; yet, the excess ketones are rarely a cause of severe acidosis in healthy nondiabetic persons. However, alcoholics who have gone on a recent drinking binge while eating poorly may suffer significant ketoacidosis. Although ketosis is initiated by starvation, alcohol itself stimulates ketoacid production. Thus, al-

TABLE 9–2.
Arterial Blood Gas Drawing Procedure

Equipment:

1. 5- or 10-mL glass syringe or plastic syringe with vented plunger
2. Sodium heparin, 1000 units/mL
3. Needles (21-, 22-, or 23-gauge short bevel)
4. Container of ice (emesis basin or large disposable cup)
5. Alcohol wipe
6. 2″ × 2″ gauze pad
7. Cork
8. Laboratory requisition

Method:

1. Wash hands and apply gloves.
2. Be sure patient has been in steady state for at least 15 minutes (eg, no recent changes in inspired oxygen).
3. Draw 1 mL of heparin into syringe to wet the barrel; discard excess heparin through needle, taking care that the hub of the needle is left full of heparin and there are no air bubbles.
4. Prepare patient for arterial puncture by explaining procedure and possible discomforts. Emphasize the importance of relaxation and need to keep extremity immobilized during the procedure.
5. Locate radial artery (brachial site may be used; avoid femoral artery if at all possible).
6. Hyperextend site (by placing folded towel under wrist or elbow).
7. Locate maximal pulsation point of artery; cleanse site with alcohol wipe.
8. Puncture artery at site of maximal pulse intensity:
   ▶ This is easiest with the syringe and needle approximately perpendicular to the skin; however, if the needle is inserted at an angle there may be better hemostasis after the needle is removed.
   ▶ Often the needle goes through both sides of the artery and only when the needle is slowly withdrawn does the blood gush up into the syringe in pulsations; if it is necessary to aspirate blood by pulling on the plunger, it is impossible to be sure the blood is arterial rather than venous.
9. Obtain needed volume of blood specified by laboratory.
10. Remove needle and squirt out any air bubbles. At the same time, have second person apply pressure to puncture site with gauze pad (at least 5 minutes; 10 minutes if the patient is on anticoagulants or has bleeding disorder).
11. Stick needle into cork and gently rotate syringe to ensure that the blood mixes with the heparin.
12. Label, place immediately in iced container, and send to laboratory.
    Information needed includes whether patient is receiving oxygen; if so, how much and by what route, and if the patient is on continuous ventilation: tidal volume, respiratory frequency, inspired oxygen concentration, amount of positive end-expiratory pressure, continuous positive airway pressure, and amount of dead space.

(Adapted from Hudak C, Gallo B, Benz J: Critical Care Nursing, 5th ed, p 309. Philadelphia, JB Lippincott.)

TABLE 9–3.
Causes of Metabolic Acidosis Classified as High Anion Gap or Normal Anion Gap

HIGH ANION GAP (GAIN OF UNMEASURED ANIONS)	NORMAL ANION GAP
Diabetic ketoacidosis	Diarrhea
Starvational ketoacidosis	Biliary or pancreatic fistulas
Alcoholic ketoacidosis	Excessive administration of isotonic saline or ammonium chloride
Lactic acidosis	
Renal failure	Ureteroenterostomies
Poisonings:	Renal tubular acidosis
▶ Salicylate	Acetazolamide (Diamox)
▶ Ethylene glycol	
▶ Methyl alcohol	

coholic ketoacidosis can produce concentrations of ketones in the blood that are similar to those seen in severe diabetic ketoacidosis. Alcoholic ketoacidosis is reported to occur in two vastly different populations: chronic alcoholics and young children. In children, alcoholic ketoacidosis typically occurs when a small child who has fasted overnight awakens and samples an alcoholic drink left out by the parents the previous evening.[4]

Lactic acidosis, a common form of metabolic acidosis, is most often associated with states of poor tissue perfusion or hypoxia. In lactic acidosis there is increased production or degradation of lactate, or both, resulting in an accumulation of lactic acid. The normal plasma lactate level is 0.9 to 1.1 mEq/L. In most cases of lactic acidosis, the lactate level is 10 to 30 mEq/L with a reciprocal decrease in bicarbonate and increase in the anion gap.[5]

Recall that the kidneys are responsible for regulating the serum bicarbonate concentration. During renal failure with uremia this capability is compromised, resulting in bicarbonate's replacement with sulfate, phosphate, or various organic acids. Uremic acidosis usually occurs when the glomerular filtration rate (GFR) is reduced to below 20 to 30 mL/min.[6]

Ingestion of toxic substances, such as salicylates, ethylene glycol, and methanol produces metabolites that cause metabolic acidosis with a high anion gap. Excessive salicylate ingestion alters peripheral metabolism, causing overproduction of organic acids. Ethylene glycol is metabolized to glycolic acid and oxalic acids, and methanol is transformed to formaldehyde and formic acid.[7] Abnormal increases in these anions cause a reciprocal decrease in bicarbonate and elevation of the anion gap.

Example: High anion gap (patient with lactic acidosis)

$$Na^+ = 131 \text{ mEq/L} \qquad AG = Na^+ - (HCO_3^- + Cl^-)$$
$$HCO_3^- = 9 \text{ mEq/L} \qquad 131 - (9 + 86)$$
$$= 36 \text{ mEq/L}$$
$$Cl^- = 86 \text{ mEq/L} \qquad (\text{normal is} < 16 \text{ mEq/L})$$

NORMAL ANION GAP ACIDOSIS

Diarrhea causes direct loss of bicarbonate in the stool, ECF volume depletion, and concentration of the remaining serum chloride, resulting in hyperchloremic acidosis. Because no change is caused in the "unmeasured" anions, the anion gap remains within normal limits. The same mechanism is seen in pancreatic and biliary fistulas, through which bicarbonate-rich fluid is lost in external drainage.

Hyperchloremic acidosis often develops in patients with urinary diversion into the sigmoid colon. Apparently it is associated with bicarbonate secretion into the colon in exchange for the reabsorption of urinary chloride. The same changes may occur with urinary diversion to an ileal segment.

Excessive infusion of chloride-containing fluids, such as isotonic sodium chloride (0.9% NaCl) or ammonium chloride, can cause hyperchloremic acidosis. Other causes include renal tubular acidosis and carbonic anhydrase inhibitors. Renal tubular acidosis exists in various forms and can be characterized by either bicarbonate loss in the urine or inability to generate new bicarbonate. As the plasma bicarbonate decreases, the chloride level increases. Carbonic anhydrase inhibitors (such as acetazolamide) cause renal bicarbonate wasting.

Example: Normal anion gap (patient with ureterosigmoidostomy)

$$Na^+ = 134 \text{ mEq/L} \qquad AG = Na^+ - (HCO_3 + Cl^-)$$
$$HCO_3^- = 10 \text{ mEq/L} \qquad 134 - (10 + 115)$$
$$= 9 \text{ mEq/L}$$
$$Cl^- = 115 \text{ mEq/L}$$

DECREASED ANION GAP

When the anion gap is less than normal, the possibility of laboratory error should be considered. Other possible causes include increase in unmeasured cations (as in lithium intoxication) and decreased unmeasured anions (as in hypoalbuminemia). The latter is not surprising because albumin accounts for most of the nonchloride or nonbicarbonate anions in blood.

Metabolic acidosis can be acute or chronic. Expected blood gas changes for uncompensated, partly compensated, and completely compensated metabolic acidosis are presented in Table 9-4.

DEFINING CHARACTERISTICS

Both etiological factors and defining characteristics of metabolic acidosis are given in the Summary of Metabolic Acidosis. An example of blood gases in patients with metabolic acidosis is presented below.

TABLE 9–4.
Expected Directional Changes in Blood Gases in Metabolic Acidosis

IMBALANCE	pH	HCO$_3$	PaCO$_2$	BASE EXCESS
Uncompensated metabolic acidosis	↓	↓	N	↓
Partly compensated metabolic acidosis	↓	↓	↓	↓
Completely compensated metabolic acidosis	N	↓	↓	↓

N, normal.

Summary of Metabolic Acidosis (base bicarbonate deficit)

ETIOLOGICAL FACTORS	DEFINING CHARACTERISTICS
Normal anion gap: ▸ Diarrhea ▸ Intestinal fistulas ▸ Ureterosigmoidostomy ▸ Acidifying drugs (such as ammonium chloride) ▸ Renal tubular acidosis (RTA) High anion gap: ▸ Diabetic ketoacidosis ▸ Starvational ketoacidosis ▸ Alcoholic ketoacidosis ▸ Lactic acidosis ▸ Renal failure ▸ Ingestion of toxins (such as salicylates, ethylene glycol, and methanol)	Headache Confusion Drowsiness Increased respiratory rate and depth (may not become clinically evident until HCO_3 is quite low) Nausea and vomiting Peripheral vasodilatation (may be present, causing warm, flushed skin) Decreased cardiac output when pH falls below 7.1 Arterial blood gases: ▸ Fall in pH (<7.35) ▸ $HCO_3 < 22$ mEq/L (primary) ▸ $PaCO_2 < 35$ mmHg (compensation by lungs) ▸ Base excess (BE) always negative Hyperkalemia frequently present (except in RTA, diarrhea, and use of acetazolamide)

Example: Patient with diabetic ketoacidosis

$pH = 7.05$	
$HCO_3 = 5$ mEq/L	(primary disturbance, excess of ketones)
$PaCO_2 = 12$ mmHg	(represents compensatory hyperventilation)
$BE = -30$ mEq/L	

Acidemia depresses myocardial contractility, lowers the fibrillation threshold, and blunts the pressor response to catecholamines,[8] but it also enhances tissue oxygenation by shifting the oxyhemoglobin dissociation curve to the right.

TREATMENT

Because treatment is directed toward correction of the metabolic defect, it varies considerably with the condition. However, a general discussion of the use of bicarbonate merits discussion at this point because it is somewhat controversial. Those who do not favor its use point out the possible risks of hypernatremia, volume overload, and acute hypokalemia, in addition to decreased oxygen delivery due to shifting of the oxyhemoglobin dissociation curve to the left. Those who are not convinced that bicarbonate administration is without merit point out its long-term clinical use. It seems judicious to use bicarbonate cautiously when clinically indicated, particularly when cardiac instability is likely to occur due to very low pH values. Because the recommended use of bicarbonate varies greatly with the underlying condition, it is best to review specific clinical situations later in the text. For example, cardiac arrest is discussed in Chapter 19 and diabetic ketoacidosis in Chapter 21.

Two potentially beneficial approaches to the treatment of metabolic acidosis are currently under study and include dichloroacetate (DCA) and carbicarb (a mixture of sodium carbonate and sodium bicarbonate).[9] In a recently reported animal study, carbicarb was found to be superior to $NaHCO_3$ for the treatment of hypoxic states in the presence of lactic acidosis.[10]

METABOLIC ALKALOSIS

Metabolic alkalosis (HCO_3 excess) is a clinical disturbance characterized by a high pH (decreased hydrogen concentration) and a high plasma bicarbonate concentration. It can be produced by a gain of bicarbonate or a loss of hydrogen ion. In compensation, the lungs hypoventilate to increase the $PaCO_2$ concentration (movement in the same direction as the primary bicarbonate disturbance).

ETIOLOGICAL FACTORS

Probably the most common cause of metabolic alkalosis is vomiting or gastric suction (results in loss of hydrogen and chloride anions). Metabolic alkalosis occurs frequently in pyloric stenosis since only gastric fluid is lost in this disorder. Recall that gastric fluid has an acid pH (usually 1 to 3); loss of acidic fluid, of course, increases alkalinity of body fluids. (Vomiting related to other conditions sometimes involves loss of both gastric and alkaline upper small-intestinal fluid. When this occurs, the severity of the pH change is tempered.)

Other factors predisposing to metabolic alkalosis include the loss of potassium, such as that caused by certain diuretics (eg, thiazides, furosemide, and ethacrynic acid) and the presence of excessive adrenalcorticoid hormones (as in hyperaldosteronism and Cushing's syndrome). Hypokalemia produces alkalosis in two ways: (1) In the presence of hypokalemia, the kidneys conserve potassium and thus increase hydrogen ion excretion (recall that these ions compete for renal excretion). (2) Cellular potassium moves out into the ECF in an attempt to maintain near normal serum levels (as potassium leaves the cell, hydrogen must enter, to maintain electroneutrality).

Excessive alkali ingestion, as in the use of bicarbonate-containing antacids (eg, Alka-Seltzer) or sodium bicarbonate during cardiopulmonary resuscitation, can also cause metabolic alkalosis.

Abrupt relief of chronically high carbon dioxide level in plasma (eg, assisted ventilation) results in a "lag period" before the chronically high serum bicarbonate level can be corrected by the kidneys.

DEFINING CHARACTERISTICS

Alkalosis is manifested primarily by symptoms related to decreased calcium ionization, such as tingling of the fingers and toes, dizziness, and hypertonic muscles. Respirations are depressed as a compensatory action by the lungs.

Arterial blood gases show an increased pH (>7.45) and an elevated bicarbonate (>26 mEq/L), the primary disorder. To help temper the severity of the imbalance, compensatory hypoventilation occurs (elevating the $PaCO_2$) and is more pronounced in semiconscious, unconscious, or debilitated patients than in alert patients. The former may develop marked hypoxemia as a result of hypoventilation. The base excess is always positive.

Example: Patient with vomiting

$$pH = 7.62$$
$$HCO_3 = 45 \text{ mEq/L}$$
$$PaCO_2 = 48 \text{ mmHg}$$
$$BE = 16 \text{ mEq/L}$$

Other laboratory values are also disrupted in metabolic alkalosis. The serum potassium is often, although not always, below 3.5mEq/L. The serum chloride is relatively lower than sodium, since an elevation in the serum bicarbonate level causes the chloride level to drop. (Recall that as one anion elevates, another tends to drop to maintain electroneutrality.)

The ionized fraction of serum calcium decreases in the presence of alkalosis as more calcium combines with serum proteins. Because it is the ionized fraction of calcium that influences neuromuscular activity, it is understandable why symptoms of hypocalcemia are often the predominant ones of alkalosis.

Urinary chloride is sometimes measured to help determine the cause of metabolic alkalosis. It is usually less than 15 mEq/L when metabolic alkalosis is due to vomiting or gastric suction or diuretic use (late). Conversely, it is usually greater than 20 mEq/L when metabolic alkalosis is due to hyperaldosteronism, Cushing's syndrome, or profound potassium depletion (serum potassium < 2.0 mEq/L).

Metabolic alkalosis can be acute or chronic. Expected directional changes in blood gases for uncompensated, partly compensated, and completely compensated metabolic alkalosis are listed in Table 9-5.

The Summary of Metabolic Alkalosis lists the etiological factors and defining characteristics of metabolic alkalosis.

TREATMENT

Treatment is aimed at reversal of the underlying disorder. Sufficient chloride must be supplied for the kidney to absorb sodium with chloride (allowing the excretion of excess bicarbonate). Treatment also includes restoration of normal fluid volume by administration of sodium chloride fluids (because continued volume depletion serves to maintain the alkalosis).

RESPIRATORY ACIDOSIS

Respiratory acidosis (H_2CO_3 excess) can be either acute or chronic; the acute imbalance is particularly dangerous. When respiratory acidosis is acute, the bicarbonate level remains in the normal range because renal compensation is very slow. Therefore, the high $PaCO_2$ can quickly produce a sharp decrease in plasma pH.

TABLE 9–5.
Expected Directional Changes in Blood Gases in Metabolic Alkalosis

IMBALANCE	pH	HCO₃	PaCO₂	BASE EXCESS
Uncompensated (acute) metabolic alkalosis	↑	↑	N	↑
Partly compensated (subacute) metabolic alkalosis	↑	↑	↑	↑
Completely compensated (chronic) metabolic alkalosis	N	↑	↑	↑

N, normal.

When respiratory acidosis is chronic, as in COPD, the kidneys compensate for the elevated $PaCO_2$ by increasing the bicarbonate level. (Compensatory renal bicarbonate generation takes several hours to several days to develop.)

ETIOLOGICAL FACTORS

Respiratory acidosis is always due to inadequate excretion of carbon dioxide (inadequate ventilation), resulting in elevated plasma carbon dioxide levels and thus carbonic acid levels. In addition to an elevated $PaCO_2$, hypoventilation usually causes a decrease in PaO_2.

Acute respiratory acidosis is associated with certain emergency situations (such as acute pulmonary edema, aspiration of a foreign object, atelectasis, pneumothorax, overdosage of sedatives, and severe pneumonia).

Chronic respiratory acidosis is associated with chronic situations such as emphysema, bronchiectasis, and bronchial asthma. Other etiological factors are listed in the Summary of Respiratory Acidosis.

DEFINING CHARACTERISTICS

Clinical signs vary between acute and chronic respiratory acidosis and are listed in the Summary of Respiratory Acidosis.

Acute Respiratory Acidosis

Sudden hypercapnia (elevated $PaCO_2$) can cause increased pulse and respiratory rate, increased blood pressure, mental cloudiness, and a feeling of fullness in the head ($PaCO_2$ causes cerebrovascular vasodilatation

---

Summary of Metabolic Alkalosis (base bicarbonate excess)

ETIOLOGICAL FACTORS	DEFINING CHARACTERISTICS
Vomiting or gastric suction	Those related to decreased calcium ionization, such as
Hypokalemia	► Dizziness
Hyperaldosteronism	► Tingling of fingers and toes
Cushing's syndrome	► Circumoral paresthesia
Potassium-losing diuretics (eg, thiazides, furosemide, ethacrynic acid)	► Carpopedal spasm
	► Hypertonic muscles
Alkali ingestion (bicarbonate-containing antacids)	Depressed respiration (compensatory action by lungs)
Parenteral NaHCO₃ administration for cardiopulmonary resuscitation	Arterial blood gases:
	► pH > 7.45
Abrupt relief of chronic respiratory acidosis	► Bicarbonate > 26 mEq/L (primary)
	► PaCO₂ > 45 mmHg (compensatory)
	► Base excess (BE) always positive
	Hypokalemia often present
	Serum Cl relatively lower than Na

and increased cerebral blood flow, particularly when higher than 60 mmHg).

Ventricular fibrillation may be the first sign of respiratory acidosis in the anesthetized patient (due to hyperkalemia associated with acidosis). Respiratory acidosis may occur as soon as 15 minutes after the start of anesthesia and is most likely to occur in patients with chronic pulmonary disease. As stated above, arterial blood gas changes occur immediately when ventilation is abruptly altered. The pH may reach a level of 7 or less in a few minutes. The PaCO$_2$ is greater than 45 mmHg, and may reach 120 mmHg or higher. The bicarbonate is normal or only slightly elevated because there has been little time for renal compensation (an exception would be the patient with COPD who has a chronically elevated bicarbonate; in this situation, it would not be high enough to compensate for the sudden increase in PaCO$_2$). The PaO$_2$ is below normal when the patient is breathing room air, and is the result of hypoventilation.

Example:

$$pH = 7.26$$
$$PaCO_2 = 56 \ mmHg$$
$$HCO_3 = 24 \ mEq/L$$

Chronic Respiratory Acidosis

The patient with chronic respiratory acidosis may complain of weakness, dull headache, and the symptoms of the underlying disease process. The arterial blood gases reveal a pH less than 7.35 or within the lower limit of normal (if complete compensation has occurred). The PaCO$_2$ is greater than 45 mmHg (frequently between 50–60 mmHg or greater). Patients with COPD who gradually accumulate carbon dioxide over a prolonged period (days to months) may not develop symptoms of hypercapnia (listed previously under Acute Respiratory Acidosis) because compensatory changes have had time to occur. For example, an emphysematous patient kept alive with oxygen

therapy for more than 1 year was mentally alert although his PaCO$_2$ was 140 mmHg. A rapid rise in the PaCO$_2$ to 140 mmHg in the normal person would surely produce unconsciousness. The patient with chronic respiratory acidosis has had time for partial or complete renal compensation; therefore, the bicarbonate is above normal, as is the base excess.

Example:

$$pH = 7.38$$
$$PaCO_2 = 76 \ mmHg$$
$$HCO_3 = 42 \ mEq/L$$
$$BE = +14 \ mEq/L$$

Remember that, when the PaCO$_2$ is chronically above 50 mmHg, the respiratory center becomes relatively insensitive to carbon dioxide as a respiratory stimulant, leaving hypoxemia as the major drive for respiration. Excessive oxygen administration removes the stimulus of hypoxemia, and the patient develops "carbon dioxide narcosis" unless the situation is quickly reversed.

Expected directional changes in blood gases in uncompensated, partly compensated, and completely compensated respiratory acidosis are listed in Table 9-6.

TREATMENT

Treatment is directed at improving ventilation; exact measures vary with the cause of inadequate ventilation. Pharmacological agents are used as indicated. For example, bronchodilators help reduce bronchial spasm; antibiotics are used for respiratory infections. Pulmonary hygiene measures are employed, when necessary, to rid the respiratory tract of mucus and purulent drainage. Adequate hydration (2–3 L/day) is indicated to keep the mucous membranes moist and thereby facilitate removal of secretions. Supplemental oxygen is used as necessary.

A mechanical respirator, used cautiously, may improve pulmonary ventilation. Remember that over-

TABLE 9–6.
Expected Directional Changes in Blood Gases in Respiratory Acidosis

IMBALANCE	pH	PaCO$_2$	HCO$_3$	BASE EXCESS
Uncompensated respiratory acidosis (acute)	↓	↑	N	N
Partly compensated respiratory acidosis	↓	↑	↑	↑
Completely compensated respiratory acidosis	N	↑	↑	↑

N, normal.

zealous use of a mechanical respirator may cause such rapid excretion of carbon dioxide that the kidneys will be unable to eliminate excess bicarbonate with sufficient rapidity to prevent alkalosis and convulsions. For this reason, the elevated $PaCO_2$ must be decreased slowly.

RESPIRATORY ALKALOSIS

ETIOLOGICAL FACTORS AND DEFINING CHARACTERISTICS

Respiratory alkalosis (H_2CO_3 deficit) is always due to hyperventilation, which causes excessive "blowing off" of carbon dioxide and, hence, a decrease in plasma H_2CO_3 content. Etiological factors associated with respiratory alkalosis and defining characteristics are listed in the Summary of Respiratory Alkalosis.

As with respiratory acidosis, acute and chronic conditions can occur in respiratory alkalosis. In the acute state, the pH is elevated above normal as a result of a low $PaCO_2$ and a normal bicarbonate level. (Recall that the kidneys cannot alter the bicarbonate level quickly.)

Example: Acute respiratory alkalosis

$$pH = 7.52$$
$$PaCO_2 = 30 \text{ mmHg}$$
$$HCO_3 = 24 \text{ mEq/L}$$
$$BE = +2.5 \text{ mEq/L}$$

In the compensated state, the kidneys have had time to lower the bicarbonate level.

Example: Chronic respiratory alkalosis

$$pH = 7.40$$
$$PaCO_2 = 30 \text{ mmHg}$$
$$HCO_3 = 18 \text{ mEq/L}$$
$$BE = -5 \text{ mEq/L}$$

Summary of Respiratory Acidosis (carbonic acid excess)

ETIOLOGICAL FACTORS

Acute respiratory acidosis:
- Acute pulmonary edema
- Aspiration of a foreign body
- Atelectasis
- Pneumothorax, hemothorax
- Overdosage of sedatives or anesthetic
- Position on OR table that interferes with respirations
- Cardiac arrest
- Severe pneumonia
- Laryngospasm
- Mechanical ventilation improperly regulated

Chronic respiratory acidosis:
- Emphysema
- Cystic fibrosis
- Advanced multiple sclerosis
- Bronchiectasis
- Bronchial asthma

Factors favoring hypoventilation:
- Obesity
- Tight abdominal binders or dressings
- Postoperative pain (as in high abdominal or chest incisions)
- Abdominal distention from cirrhosis or bowel obstruction

DEFINING CHARACTERISTICS

Acute respiratory acidosis:
- Feeling of fullness in the head ($PaCO_2$ causes cerebrovascular vasodilatation and increased cerebral blood flow, particularly when higher than 60 mmHg)
- Mental cloudiness
- Dizziness
- Palpitations
- Muscular twitching
- Convulsions
- Warm, flushed skin
- Unconsciousness
- Ventricular fibrillation may be first sign in anesthetized patient (related to hyperkalemia)
- ABGs:
  - pH < 7.35
  - $PaCO_2$ > 45 mmHg (primary)
  - HCO_3 normal or only slightly elevated

Chronic respiratory acidosis:
- Weakness
- Dull headache
- Symptoms of underlying disease process
- ABGs:
  - pH < 7.35 or within lower limits of normal
  - $PaCO_2$ > 45 mmHg (primary)
  - HCO_3 > 26 mEq/L (compensatory)

TABLE 9–7.
Expected Directional Changes in Arterial Blood Gases in Respiratory Alkalosis

IMBALANCE	pH	PaCO$_2$	HCO$_3$	BASE EXCESS
Uncompensated respiratory alkalosis	↑	↓	N	N
Partly compensated respiratory alkalosis	↑	↓	↓	↓
Completely compensated respiratory alkalosis	N	↓	↓	↓

N, normal.

Expected directional changes in blood gases in uncompensated, partly compensated, and completely compensated respiratory alkalosis are listed in Table 9-7.

TREATMENT

If the cause of respiratory alkalosis is anxiety, the patient should be made aware that the abnormal breathing practice is responsible for the symptoms accompanying this condition. Instructing the patient to breath more slowly (to cause accumulation of carbon dioxide) or to breath into a closed system (such as a paper bag) is helpful. Usually a sedative is required to relieve hyperventilation in very anxious patients. (If alkalosis is severe enough to cause fainting, the increased ventilation will cease and respirations will revert to normal.)

Treatment for other causes of respiratory alkalosis is directed at correcting the underlying problem.

MIXED ACID–BASE IMBALANCES

The preceding discussions have described single acid–base imbalances. These single imbalances do indeed occur. However, one should be aware that in some clinical situations the patient may have two or more primary acid–base disturbances simultaneously. Some examples are given in Table 9-8 and at the end of the

TABLE 9–8.
Examples of Combinations of Mixed Acid–Base Disorders

Metabolic acidosis/respiratory acidosis

| Cardiopulmonary arrest | Hypoxemia produces lactic acidosis with decrease in HCO$_3$ |
| | Respiratory arrest causes CO$_2$ retention |

Metabolic acidosis/respiratory alkalosis

| Salicylate intoxication | Salicylate alters peripheral metabolism and causes overproduction of organic acids with resultant decrease in HCO$_3$ |
| | Salicylate stimulates respiratory center and causes decrease in CO$_2$ |

Metabolic acidosis/metabolic alkalosis

| Renal failure with vomiting | Renal failure causes retention of acid metabolites with decrease in HCO$_3$ |
| | Vomiting causes loss of H$^+$ and Cl$^-$ and, thus, increase in HCO$_3$ |

Metabolic alkalosis/respiratory alkalosis

| Vomiting during pregnancy | Vomiting causes loss of H$^+$ and Cl$^-$ and, thus, increase in HCO$_3$ |
| | Progesterone increase during pregnancy stimulates respirations and causes decrease in CO$_2$ |

Metabolic alkalosis/respiratory acidosis

| Vomiting with COPD | Vomiting causes loss of H$^+$ and Cl$^-$ and, thus, increase in HCO$_3$ |
| | Chronic obstructive pulmonary disease is associated with sustained elevation of CO$_2$ |

COPD, chronic obstructive pulmonary disease.

TABLE 9–9.
Systematic Assessment of Arterial Blood Gases

The following steps are recommended to evaluate arterial blood gas values. They are based on the assumption that the average values are

$$pH = 7.4$$
$$PaCO_2 = 40 \text{ mmHg}$$
$$HCO_3 = 24 \text{ mEq/L}$$

I. *First, look at the pH.* It can be high, low, or normal as follows:

$$pH > 7.4 \text{ (alkalosis)}$$
$$pH < 7.4 \text{ (acidosis)}$$
$$pH = 7.4 \text{ (normal)}$$

A normal pH may indicate perfectly normal blood gases, *or* it may be an indication of a *compensated* imbalance. A compensated imbalance is one in which the body has been able to correct the pH by either respiratory or metabolic changes (depending on the primary problem). For example, a patient with primary metabolic acidosis starts out with a low bicarbonate level but a normal carbon dioxide level. Soon afterward, the lungs try to compensate for the imbalance by exhaling large amounts of carbon dioxide (hyperventilation). Another example, a patient with primary respiratory acidosis starts out with a high carbon dioxide level; soon afterward, the kidneys attempt to compensate by retaining bicarbonate. If the compensatory maneuver is able to restore the bicarbonate: carbonic acid ratio back to 20:1, full compensation (and thus normal pH) will be achieved.

II. *The next step is to determine the primary cause of the disturbance.* This is done by evaluating the $PaCO_2$ and HCO_3 in relation to the pH.

pH > 7.4 (alkalosis)

1. *If the $PaCO_2$ is <40 mmHg,* the primary disturbance is respiratory alkalosis. (This situation occurs when a patient hyperventilates and "blows off" too much

carbon dioxide. Recall that carbon dioxide dissolved in water becomes carbonic acid, the acid side of the "carbonic acid : base bicarbonate" buffer system.)

2. *If the HCO_3 is >24 mEq/L,* the primary disturbance is metabolic alkalosis. (This situation occurs when the body gains too much bicarbonate, an alkaline substance. Bicarbonate is the basic, or alkaline side of the "carbonic acid–base : bicarbonate buffer system.")

pH < 7.4 (acidosis)

1. *If the $PaCO_2$ is >40 mmHg,* the primary disturbance is respiratory acidosis. (This situation occurs when a patient hypoventilates and thus retains too much carbon dioxide, an acidic substance.)

2. *If the HCO_3 is <24 mEq/L,* the primary disturbance is metabolic acidosis. (This situation occurs when the body's bicarbonate level drops, either because of direct bicarbonate loss or because of gains of acids such as lactic acid or ketones).

III. *The next step involves determining if compensation has begun.*

This is done by looking at the value other than the primary disorder. If it is moving in the same direction as the primary value, compensation is underway. Consider the following gases:

Example:

	pH	$PaCO_2$	HCO_3
(1)	7.20	60 mmHg	24 mEq/L
(2)	7.40	60 mmHg	37 mEq/L

The first set (1) indicates acute respiratory acidosis without compensation (the $PaCO_2$ is high, the HCO_3 is normal). The second set (2) indicates chronic respiratory acidosis. Note that compensation has taken place; that is, the HCO_3 has elevated to an appropriate level to balance the high $PaCO_2$ and produce a normal pH.

---

chapter. A number of steps and formulas are available to evaluate blood gas changes and help determine if they are purely compensatory in nature or represent a *second* primary imbalance. These are listed here in Tables 9-9 and 9-10.

SAMPLE MIXED ACID–BASE PROBLEMS

Use rules in Tables 9-9 and 9-10 to analyze the following situations:

Respiratory Alkalosis Plus Metabolic Acidosis

Example: A patient has taken an overdose of aspirin. Recall that early in salicylate poisoning, the medulla is stimulated to produce hyperventilation (respiratory alkalosis results). Later, due to disrupted glucose metabolism, metabolic acidosis may result.

$$pH = 7.4$$
$$PaCO_2 = 18 \text{ mmHg}$$
$$HCO_3 = 16 \text{ mEq/L}$$
$$BE = -10 \text{ mEq/L}$$

TABLE 9–10.
Compensatory Changes Related to Primary Acid–Base Disturbances

IMBALANCE	PRIMARY CHANGE	COMPENSATORY CHANGE
Metabolic acidosis (base bicarbonate deficit)	HCO_3 decreased	$1.5(HCO_3) + 8 \pm 2$
Metabolic alkalosis (base bicarbonate excess)	HCO_3 increased	0.6 mmHg increase in $PaCO_2$ for every 1 mEq/L rise in HCO_3
Respiratory acidosis (carbonic acid excess)		
▸ Acute	$PaCO_2$ increased	1.0 mEq/L increase in HCO_3 for every 10 mmHg rise in $PaCO_2$
▸ Chronic	$PaCO_2$ increased	3.5 mEq/L increase in HCO_3 for every 10 mmHg rise in $PaCO_2$
Respiratory alkalosis (carbonic acid deficit)		
▸ Acute	$PaCO_2$ decreased	2.0 mEq/L decrease in HCO_3 for every 10 mmHg fall in $PaCO_2$
▸ Chronic	$PaCO_2$ decreased	5.0 mEq/L decrease in HCO_3 for every 10 mmHg fall in $PaCO_2$

Summary of Respiratory Alkalosis (carbonic acid deficit)

ETIOLOGICAL FACTORS	DEFINING CHARACTERISTICS

ETIOLOGICAL FACTORS

Extreme anxiety (most common cause)

Hypoxemia

High fever

Early salicylate intoxication (stimulates respiratory center)

Gram-negative bacteremia

Central nervous system lesions involving respiratory center

Pulmonary emboli

Thyrotoxicosis

Excessive ventilation by mechanical ventilators

Pregnancy (high progesterone level sensitizes the respiratory center to CO_2; physiological)

DEFINING CHARACTERISTICS

Lightheadedness (a low $PaCO_2$ causes cerebral vasoconstriction and thus decreased cerebral blood flow)

Inability to concentrate

Those of decreased calcium ionization (numbness and tingling of extremities and circumoral paresthesia; more likely to occur if respiratory alkalosis develops rapidly)

Hyperventilation syndrome:
▸ Tinnitus
▸ Palpitations
▸ Sweating
▸ Dry mouth
▸ Tremulousness
▸ Precordial pain (tightness)
▸ Nausea and vomiting
▸ Epigastric pain
▸ Blurred vision
▸ Convulsions and loss of consciousness (may be partly due to cerebral ischemia, caused by cerebral vasoconstriction)

ABGs:
▸ pH > 7.45
▸ $PaCO_2$ < 35 mmHg (primary)
▸ HCO_3 < 22 mEq/L (compensatory)

Note in the above situation that the simultaneous appearance of respiratory alkalosis and metabolic acidosis has produced a normal *p*H. (This is not always the case; one imbalance may be stronger than the other and cause an abnormal *p*H in its favor.)

If the only problem in this situation were respiratory alkalosis, the HCO$_3$ would be expected to be approximately 20 mEq/L. Note that it is lower than expected (indicating metabolic acidosis).

If the only problem were metabolic acidosis, the PaCO$_2$ would be expected to be approximately 32 mEq/L. Note that it is lower than expected (indicating respiratory alkalosis).

Respiratory Acidosis Plus Metabolic Acidosis

Example: A patient has lactic acidosis secondary to cardiac failure, and hypercapnia secondary to pneumonia.

$$pH = 7.10$$
$$PaCO_2 = 50 \text{ mmHg}$$
$$HCO_3 = 15 \text{ mEq/L}$$
$$BE = -6 \text{ mEq/L}$$

Because both primary disturbances produce acidosis, the *p*H is quite low. If the only problem were acute respiratory acidosis, the HCO$_3$ level would elevate to slightly above normal. (Instead, it has decreased.) If the only problem were metabolic acidosis, the PaCO$_2$ would decrease. (Instead, it has elevated.)

REFERENCES

1. Guyton A: Textbook of Medical Physiology, 7th ed, p 507. Philadelphia, WB Saunders, 1986
2. Ibid, p 509
3. Hudak C, Gallo B, Benz J: Critical Care Nursing, 5th ed, p 323. Philadelphia, JB Lippincott, 1990
4. Hoffman R, Goldfrank L: Ethanol-associated metabolic disorders. Endocrine and Metabolic Emergencies 7(4): 943, 1989
5. Kokko J, Tannen R: Fluids and Electrolytes, 2nd ed, p 31. Philadelphia, WB Saunders, 1990
6. Ibid
7. Ibid, p 34
8. Kearns T, Wolfson A: Metabolic acidosis. Endocrine and Metabolic Emergencies 7(4): 823, 1989
9. Ibid
10. Bersin R, Arieff A: Improved hemodynamic function during hypoxia with Carbicarb, a new agent for the management of acidosis. Circulation 77(1): 227, 1988

BIBLIOGRAPHY

Dunagan W, Ridner M: Manual of Medical Therapeutics, 26th ed. Boston, Little, Brown, 1989

Maxwell M, Kleeman C, Narins R: Clinical Disorders of Fluid and Electrolyte Metabolism, 4th ed. New York, McGraw-Hill, 1987

Rose B: Clinical Physiology of Acid–Base and Electrolyte Disorders, 3rd ed. New York, McGraw-Hill, 1989

unit three

PRINCIPLES OF
PARENTERAL FLUID THERAPY

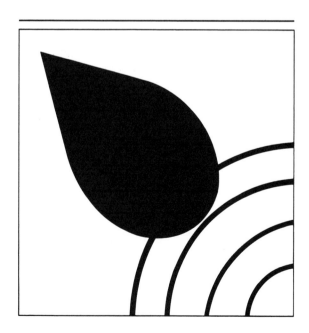

10

Intravenous Therapy

Intravenous (IV) therapy is a major treatment modality for patients in acute and chronic care settings. Further, about 75% of parenteral solutions are administered with one or more additives. Provision of IV nursing care is no longer limited to acute care settings or extended skilled nursing centers. Dramatic growth in the home infusion market has developed since the mid-1980s; annual revenues in the home care market are projected to exceed $2 billion by 1992. Not only has the cost-effectiveness of home infusion services been widely recognized, but other benefits have emerged as well. These include a lower incidence of infection and greater patient comfort due to provision of care in familiar surroundings (devoid of the impersonal atmosphere often characteristic of hospitals).[1] Since the 1940s, nurses have played a major role in the administration of IV therapy. Exact nursing responsibilities are not, however, uniformly defined and tend to vary among geographical areas, health care facilities, and areas of clinical specialization. Many acute care facilities use an organized IV therapy department that is responsible for the provision of all IV therapy procedures. Other IV therapy departments may focus only on the provision of complex procedures, and serving as a resource to the nursing staff. Although nurses specializing in IV nursing often practice in diverse settings, the need for proficiency and competency in all clinical aspects of IV therapy nursing practice is evident.[2]

INTRAVENOUS THERAPY EQUIPMENT

INFUSION SYSTEMS

Three basic types of infusion systems are currently available in the United States; they include the plastic bottle or bag, the closed system, and the open system. Plastic containers have no vacuum and, because they are flexible and collapsible, do not need air to replace fluid flowing from the container. All other systems employ glass bottles that have a partial vacuum and thus require air vents. In the *closed system,* only filtered air is admitted to the container; the air vent, containing the filter, is an integral part of the administration set. In the *open system,* air enters through a plastic tube and collects in the air space in the bottle.

Plastic containers have gained widespread acceptance, largely because they are lighter and more easily stored and discarded than glass bottles. Since the plastic containers have no rubber bushing, coring is eliminated and particulate matter is reduced. Also, since air venting is not required, the risk of airborne contamination and air emboli is reduced.

Accidental puncture of plastic bags can occur; therefore, before use, they should be squeezed and visually examined for evidence of damage. Remember that plastic containers should never be written on with pen, pencil, or marker.

Methods for adding medications to the fluid containers vary with each system. The manufacturer's instructions regarding this procedure must be closely followed.

ADMINISTRATION SETS

All containers require some type of administration set to deliver fluid to the patient. There are numerous varieties of administration sets available commercially and the variety itself may be a source of confusion. Directions provided by manufacturers for use of the sets must be read; one should not presume that an unfamiliar set works exactly as does another made by a different manufacturer. Indeed, as IV therapy equipment is proliferating by leaps and bounds, one must frequently adjust to new kinds of devices. Due to space limitations, only the basic and most commonly used administration sets will be described in this chapter.

Regular or "Macro" Administration Sets

Regular sets (with or without in-line filters) are the basic administration sets used for infusion of primary parenteral fluids. The drop factors of these commercial sets vary according to manufacturer (see Table 10-1). Some sets have a "flashball," which is located between the tubing and the male adaptor. It is probably best not to use a set equipped with a flashball when the infusion is being delivered under pressure (a separation may occur between the flashball and either the Luer connector or the tubing).

Pediatric or "Micro-Drip" Sets

It is often necessary to maintain the flow of a parenteral infusion at a minimal rate. Achieving such rates by gravity flow may be accomplished by the use of special sets, originally designed for pediatric infusions. In a *micro-drip* set, the standard drip tube is replaced by one of much smaller diameter. These sets will deliver 50 to 60 drops/mL, depending on the viscosity of the solution.

Check-Valve Sets

Infusion sets are available with in-line pressure-sensitive check-valves, which provide an efficient and safe method for administering medications and fluids (see Fig. 10-1).

A secondary infusion or a single dose of a medica-

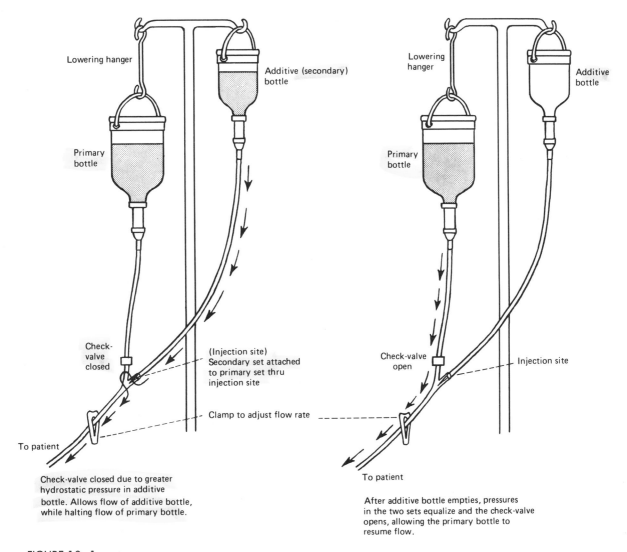

FIGURE 10–1.
Intravenous piggyback setup with back check-valve. (Metheny N, Snively WD: Nurses' Handbook of Fluid Balance, 4th ed, p 168. Philadelphia, JB Lippincott, 1983; with permission.)

tion is delivered "IV piggyback" into the injection site, which is located below the check-valve. The check-valve closes off the primary container during the time of the piggyback infusion and then automatically allows the primary infusion to start when the piggyback infusion is complete. Check-valve action prevents mixing of the two infusions, eliminates the risk of air entering the system when the "piggyback" container empties, and prevents occlusion of the cannula due to interruption of the infusion. To successfully use the check-valve system, it is imperative that the primary container be suspended lower than the secondary piggyback container. This is achieved by using extension

hangers, which are usually contained in the secondary administration set package. *Caution:* The rate of flow is regulated by the *primary* set regulator; the flow-clamp contained in the secondary medication set is considered a *strictly "on–off"* clamp.

Nonpolyvinyl Chloride IV Administration Sets

Due to the absorption of fat emulsions and certain drugs into the walls of polyvinyl chloride (PVC) tubing, nonpolyvinyl chloride IV administration sets are available for gravity infusion and for volumetric pumps.

Volume Control Sets

There are a number of commercial sets designed to administer precisely limited amounts of solution. These sets gained wide use in the 1960s and 1970s for intermittent drug administration and for pediatric IV therapy. However, certain hazards (primarily contamination) associated with the use of these sets were noted by Henry et al[3] in 1982 and as early as 1975 when the National Coordinating Committee on Large Volume Parenterals (NCCLVPs) stated that "the use of volume control sets is discouraged for intermittent drug therapy in adults."[4]

FILTERS

Intravenous filters are designed to prevent the passage of particulate matter, ie, glass, rubber, metal, fungi, bacteria, or drug precipitates, into the vascular system. Filter sizes range from 5 to 0.22 μ and are designed as either an integral part of the administration set or an add-on device. The 0.22-μm filter is considered both an absolute bacteria retentive and an air-eliminating filter.

Consideration must be given to the pounds per square inch (PSI) rating of the filter when used concurrently with a positive pressure electronic infusion device. The filter must withstand the PSI exerted by the infusion pump to prevent filter rupture. To achieve ideal final filtration, the filter should be located adjacent to the cannula site and routine filter change should coincide with the administration set change. There are two schools of thought relevant to the use of 0.22-μm filtration. The Intravenous Therapy Nurses' Society (INS) Standards of Practice recommends that a 0.22-μm bacterial retentive filter be used routinely for the delivery of IV therapy.[5] The Centers for Disease Control (CDC) does not recommend in-line filters as a routine infection control.[6]

It is imperative that the manufacturer's directives be followed carefully when using a filter.

FILTER ASPIRATION NEEDLES

A *filter aspiration needle* is a device attached to the syringe used to draw the IV medication from its container (either a rubber-topped vial or a glass ampule). The filter needle traps particles such as glass, rubber, or metal and, thus, allows the use of a more particulate-free fluid. A new needle is applied before the medication is injected into the IV container (use of the filter needle for this purpose would allow the trapped particles to be injected into the IV fluid).

FLOW CONTROL DEVICES

A variety of accessory flow control devices is available from various manufacturers. Most of these regulate flow rate more precisely than does the standard roller clamp. The devices, however, are less precise than electronic infusion devices. The manufacturer's instructions for use should be closely observed.

ELECTRONIC INFUSION DEVICES

The two basic groups of electronic infusion devices are controllers and pumps. Such devices provide more accurate administration of fluids and drugs than is possible with routine gravity-flow delivery. Their precise flow rate is particularly advantageous in the administration of hyperalimentation fluids, chemotherapy, and other potent medications (such as dopamine, heparin, lidocaine, nitroprusside, and oxytocin).

A controller is an electronic device used to regulate IV flow rates. It relies on gravity rather than exertion of pressure. Intravenous controllers are useful whenever the force of gravity is sufficient to provide the desired flow rate. They are appropriate for a large percentage of infusions that do not require the accuracy of a volumetric pump. (Controllers are limited because drop rate is not a completely accurate reflection of volume infused due to variations in drop size.)

Infusion pumps are classified as being positive pressure devices with most available models producing flow rates in the range of 1 to 999 mL/hr. However, some models can deliver as much as 2000 mL/hr. Micro-pumps, used primarily in neonatal intensive care units (ICU), are programmed to deliver 0.1 to 99.9 mL/hr. If resistance develops, the pump exerts positive pressure to overcome the resistance; it will not, however, exceed preset limits. When the maximum preset limit is reached, the device's occlusion alarm sounds and the infusion ceases. Some models require designated special administration sets, whereas others accept standard administration sets. The three classifications of pumps are (1) syringe pump, (2) volumetric pump, and (3) nonvolumetric pump.

Although most pumps provide single channel delivery, newer innovative designs are currently available that allow for more than one channel (a realistic need for many patients in high acuity settings). One such device is the Omni-Flow 4000 (Abbott Laboratories, Abbott Park, IL); this is a four-channel programmable medication infusion system.

Before using any electronic infusion device, the caregiver must be aware of the distinctive functional characteristics of the selected device.[7]

1. Read the manufacturer's directions carefully before using any infusion pump or controller as there are many variations in available models. (Instruction manuals should be readily available on all units using these devices.) It is best to learn how to safely operate each type of pump or controller under the direction of someone knowledgeable in its use (eg, an in-service program presented by a representative of the manufacturer). It is particularly important to read the manufacturer's recommendations before administering blood with an infusion pump because some models damage red cells and cause hemolysis.

2. Remember that some types of final filters may be damaged by the high pressures exerted by infusion pumps; read the directions furnished by manufacturers of specific filters before using them with infusion pumps. Some filters may cause rate inaccuracies.

INTRAVENOUS CANNULAS

Parenteral solutions and IV medications are introduced into the venous system through a steel needle or a plastic catheter. Metal needles consist of two types, metal cannulas and scalp-vein needles.

Metal Cannula

A *metal cannula* is usually made of stainless steel and is noncorrosive and relatively inert in relation to the tissues. Once the traditional needle, it is seldom used today.

Scalp-Vein Needle

A *scalp-vein needle* is similar to the metal cannula but has two flexible wings attached to the hub (see Fig. 10-2). Two types are available. One has a piece of plastic

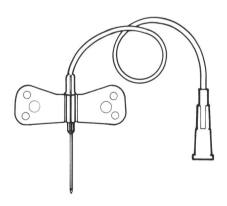

FIGURE 10–2.
Scalp-vein needle (winged infusion set).

tubing permanently attached to a female Luer adapter which, in turn, attaches to the administration set. The other has a short length of plastic tubing with a permanently attached, resealable injection site. The needle with the resealable injection site is often referred to as an "intermittent infusion set" or, more commonly, a "heparin lock." When not in use, patency is maintained by the instillation of a dilute solution of heparin or isotonic saline.

INTRAVENOUS CATHETERS

Essentially there are three types of IV catheters; these include the following:

OVER-THE-NEEDLE PLASTIC CATHETER: A plastic catheter mounted over a needle. After the venipuncture is made, the catheter is guided off the needle and into the vein.

THROUGH-THE-NEEDLE CATHETER: After the venipuncture is performed, a catheter is threaded through the needle into the vein.

INLYING CATHETER: A plastic catheter that is introduced by means of a cut-down, a minor surgical procedure performed by a physician.

Single lumen peripheral catheters are the type most commonly used. A dual-lumen peripheral catheter is now available from Arrow International, Inc. (Reading, Pennsylvania). The unique design of this dual-lumen catheter provides the means to deliver potentially incompatible fluids concurrently.

Note: All the previously described venipuncture devices are intended for one-time use only; they are not to be used for multiple venipuncture attempts. It is also recommended that IV catheters be radiopaque for detection by radiology in the event that the catheter is accidentally severed with resultant catheter emboli.

INTERMITTENT INFUSION SETS

When immediate intravascular accessibility is desired for the intermittent administration of drugs by "IV push" (IVP) or "IV piggyback" (IVPB), an *intermittent infusion device* is indicated.

Such a device may be the same as the previously described scalp-vein needle with the short segment of tubing that ends with a resealable injection port (see Fig. 10-3) or it may be one of the IV catheters that has been converted to an intermittent infusion set by the aseptic attachment of a Luer-locking, resealable injection cap. Patency of either of these devices may be maintained by periodic flushing of the device with a di-

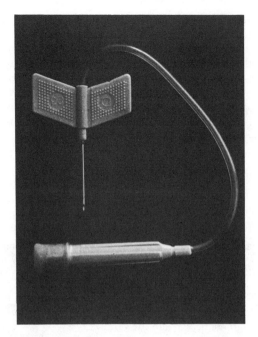

FIGURE 10–3.
Intermittent infusion set.

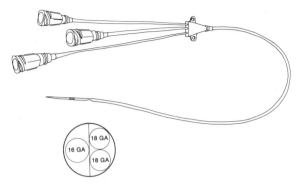

FIGURE 10–4.
Multilumen central venous catheter. (Courtesy of Arrow International Inc, Reading, PA.)

lute heparin solution (usually in strengths of either 10 or 100 units/mL). Many practitioners are currently reporting that they are successfully maintaining patency of these devices simply with sterile normal saline for injection.[8]

If the heparin flush is used, the SASH (saline flush, administration of drug, saline flush, heparinization) method incorporating the following steps should be employed when using the intermittent infusion set:

1. Inject 1 to 2 mL of isotonic saline (0.9% NaCl) to confirm placement of the cannula and to minimize incompatibility risks. (S)
2. Administer prescribed medication/infusion. (A)
3. Flush cannula again with 1 to 2 mL isotonic saline. (S)
4. Instill 1 mL of dilute heparin solution to maintain patency. (H)

CENTRAL VENOUS CATHETERS

It is often necessary to access central veins for the delivery of hyperosmolar infusates, both on a short-term (such as concentrated antibiotics) or long-term basis (such as total parenteral nutrition [TPN]). Innovations in technology have made a variety of sophisticated central venous catheters available to meet this need. With the exception of peripherally inserted central catheters (PICC lines), the responsibility for the placement of central venous catheters is that of the physician. The

basic single-lumen central venous catheter is usually 8 to 12 inches (20–30 cm) in length and is inserted percutaneously. A frequently used central venous catheter is the one designated as a multilumen catheter. Such catheters are bilumen, trilumen, or even quadlumen. Multilumen catheters consist of a catheter stem with separate and distinct lumens running throughout the length of the catheter (see Fig. 10-4). Each lumen is attached to a separate extension (pigtail) to permit easy handling and identification. With these devices, more than one drug can be administered at a time. Problems associated with incompatible solutions are avoided because (due to placement in a central vein) blood volume and its natural turbulence mix the solutions and provide quick dilution. Also, there is only one site to care for.

Tunneled Central Venous Catheters

Indwelling central venous catheters for long-term use (see Fig. 10-5) are being used with increasing frequency in many medical centers to administer TPN solutions, chemotherapeutic agents and other drugs, and blood products; they are also used as vehicles from which to draw blood samples. Examples of these types of catheters include the Broviac and Hickman catheters. Both are made of silicone, and each manufacturer offers single or multilumen options. The Broviac catheter has one dacron cuff; the Hickman has one or two. Fibrous tissue adheres to the dacron cuff in the subcutaneous tunnel and serves as a barrier to infection. The Hickman catheter is a modification of the Broviac catheter; its internal diameter is 1.6 mm as compared with 1.0 mm in the Broviac catheter.

The catheter is implanted in the operating room with the aid of fluoroscopy. A small incision is made in the deltopectoral groove, and the cephalic vein is isolated. A subcutaneous tunnel is then gently formed with a long forceps. When the tip of the forceps has

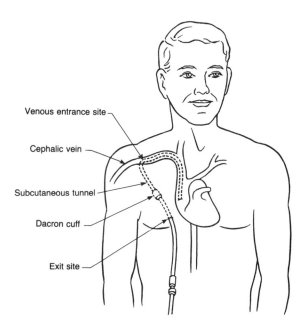

FIGURE 10–5.
Indwelling central venous catheter for prolonged total parenteral nutrition or chemotherapy. (Metheny N, Snively WD: Nurses' Handbook of Fluid Balance, 4th ed, p 155. Philadelphia, JB Lippincott, 1983; with permission.)

reached a point between the nipple and sternum, it is exteriorized through a small incision (no larger than 1 cm). The catheter is then drawn up the tunnel. The dacron cuff is positioned between the two incisions and over an intercostal space. The catheter is then inserted into the vein and threaded into the lower part of the superior vena cava (at the entrance of the right atrium). Dressings are initially applied to both the insertion site and the exit site. Catheters may remain in place for months.

Tunneled catheters may be used for continuous or intermittent therapy. When used for intermittent infusions, a Luer locking injection port is securely and aseptically engaged in the catheter hub. The smallest gauge, shortest length that will accomplish the prescribed therapy, should be used to access the device.[9]

During periods of nonuse, patency of the catheter is maintained by the instillation of heparinized saline solution. The exception to this rule is when a Groshong (Davol, Inc, Cranston, RI) catheter is in place. The unique design of the Groshong catheter allows maintenance of patency only by the instillation of sterile normal saline for injection.

When not in use, tunneled catheters are often compressed with a smooth clamp. Never use a sharp or serrated clamp because of the potential for catheter damage.

Care of the catheter exit site consists of cleaning the site and applying an antimicrobial agent and a sterile occlusive dressing. The catheter should be taped to the patient's chest to minimize the risk of accidental tugging or tension on the catheter. Patients and their families are often taught to care for these catheters in the home setting.

The removal of tunneled/implanted catheters is a medical procedure.[10]

Totally Implanted Central Venous Devices

Many patients reported that the protruding portions of the tunneled catheters were both esthetically and psychologically disturbing. To alleviate these concerns, a totally implantable system for the delivery of IV fluids and drugs was devised and has attained widespread use. Such a system allows repeated access for IVP injections and short- or long-term infusion of drugs, TPN, blood products, or other fluids. Blood sampling may also be achieved. Because the system is totally implanted under the skin, the risk of infectious complications is reduced. Moreover, such a system does not interfere with a patient's normal daily activities. The system consists of two major components: the subcutaneous injection port and a Silastic catheter. The system is usually implanted under local anesthesia in the operating room. Totally implanted systems require minimal routine care and maintenance. Patency of the system during extended periods between use is maintained by periodic flushing with a dilute heparin solution. The system is always accessed with a noncoring needle such as a Huber point needle (see Fig. 10-6).

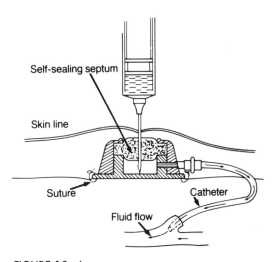

FIGURE 10–6.
How drugs or fluids are administered through the Port-A-Cath System. (Courtesy of Pharmacia Deltech, Inc. St. Paul, MN)

Peripherally Inserted Central Catheters

Although initially developed for neonates, peripherally inserted central catheters (PICC) are used today in a variety of patients requiring venous access for weeks or months of IV therapy. Generally, these catheters are composed of silicone elastomers or polyurethane materials.[11,12] These catheters are currently being placed successfully by specialized IV nurses in a variety of health care settings. Inserted in the basilic, median cubital, or cephalic vein in the antecubital area, the catheter tip may terminate in either the axillary or subclavian vein or the superior vena cava. The prescribed therapy is the final determinant of the catheter tip location.

Peripherally inserted central catheter lines greatly enhance the delivery of IV therapy in any health care setting by sparing the patient multiple "sticks," interruptions in treatment, and vein trauma often associated with traditional short-term peripheral cannula.

Major disadvantages of PICC lines are daily care requirements and effects on activity and body image due to the exit site being in the antecubital space.[13] An occlusive transparent dressing is required over the catheter exit site at all times, not only to serve as a contamination barrier, but to prevent accidental dislodgement of the nonsutured catheter. Be aware that the small lumen size of some PICC lines precludes their use for obtaining blood specimens, blood transfusion therapy, or both.

Caution: One should always refer to state regulations for specific regional guidelines governing the insertion of PICC lines.

INITIATING PERIPHERAL IV THERAPY

SITE SELECTION

Certain factors must be considered when selecting a vein for the initiation of IV therapy; these include the following:

▶ Suitable location
▶ Purpose of infusion
▶ Expected duration of therapy
▶ Condition of veins
▶ Restrictions imposed by patient's current clinical status and past medical history
▶ Dominant extremity

Although most superficial veins are accessible for venipuncture, some are not practical for extended IV therapy.

Antecubital Veins

The median cephalic and median basilic veins are located in the antecubital fossa and are readily accessible for venipuncture because of their prominent size. However, because of their location over an area of joint flexion, there is the potential for needle dislodgment, infiltration, or mechanical phlebitis due to unrestricted motion of the extremity. Also, damage to these veins during venipuncture results in limited access to veins in the lower arm and hand.

Because of the close proximity of arteries and veins in the antecubital fossa, special care must be employed to prevent an undesired intraarterial injection of medications. If a patient complains of severe pain in the hand or arm on initiation of an infusion, suspect arteriospasm due to inadvertent intraarterial injection. The infusion should be stopped immediately. Exercise caution since aberrant arteries in the antecubital area have been found to exist in one person out of ten.[14] Fortunately, arteries can generally be detected by the presence of pulsation, a thicker and tougher vessel wall, and the appearance of bright red blood.

Hand Veins

The early use of veins in the dorsal aspect of the hand (see Fig. 10-7) is important if parenteral therapy is to be prolonged; successive venipunctures can then be made in the proximal veins. Use of the dorsal metacarpal veins is, of course, dependent on their condition. In certain elderly patients, they may be a poor choice because blood extravasation occurs more readily in small, thin veins, and adequate securing of the needle may be impossible due to the presence of thin skin and lack of supportive tissue. Because of the small blood volume in these veins, they should not be used for the infusion of hypertonic or otherwise irritating solutions.

Forearm Veins

The cephalic vein is located along the radial border of the forearm and is an excellent site for venipuncture. The accessory cephalic vein and the cephalic vein both readily accommodate large needles and thus provide excellent routes for transfusions (see Fig. 10-8). The basilic vein is often overlooked during a course of IV therapy because of its inconspicuous position. Visualization of the basilic vein can be readily achieved by flexing the elbow and bending the arm up. The median antebrachial vein, when prominent, offers another route for IV therapy. Often, though, this vein does not present as a well-defined vessel.

Scalp Veins

Use of scalp veins for parenteral infusion is unique to pediatric IV therapy. Superficial veins located in the

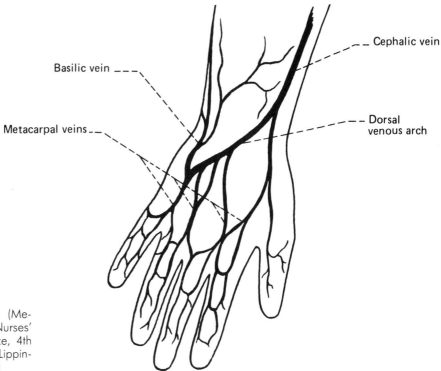

FIGURE 10–7.
Superficial veins of hand. (Metheny N, Snively WD: Nurses' Handbook of Fluid Balance, 4th ed, p 137. Philadelphia, JB Lippincott, 1983; with permission.)

Cephalic vein

Basilic vein

Dorsal venous arch

Metacarpal veins

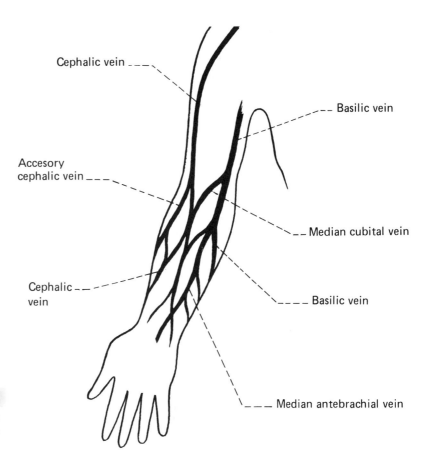

FIGURE 10–8.
Superficial veins of the forearm. (Metheny N, Snively WD: Nurses' Handbook of Fluid Balance, 4th ed, p 138. Philadelphia, JB Lippincott, 1983; with permission.)

Cephalic vein

Basilic vein

Accesory cephalic vein

Median cubital vein

Cephalic vein

Basilic vein

Median antebrachial vein

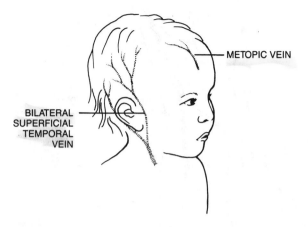

FIGURE 10–9.
Scalp veins in infant.

head may be used in infants through the toddler stage. Generally readily accessible for venipuncture are the metopic vein, which descends down the middle of the forehead, and the bilateral superficial-temporal veins located in front of the pinna of the ear. (see Fig. 10-9).[15]

Other suitable pediatric peripheral IV sites include the hand, foot or antecubital fossa.[16]

Veins of the Lower Extremity

Objections to use of veins in the lower extremities of adults arise from the danger of pulmonary embolism due to a thrombus extending from the superficial veins into the deep veins. There is also concern that, because of the stagnant blood in varicosities, a pooling of infused medications could cause an untoward reaction when a toxic concentration reaches the circulating blood. Many institutions have a policy prohibiting venipuncture in a lower extremity. Before using these veins, the policy of the institution should be reviewed.

General Considerations

▶ When feasible it is best to use veins in the non-dominant upper extremity.
▶ When multiple punctures are anticipated, it is best to make the first venipuncture distally and work proximally with subsequent punctures.
▶ Avoid venipuncture in the affected arm of patients with axillary dissection, as in radical mastectomy (embarrassed circulation affects the flow of the infusion, causing increased edema).
▶ Avoid checking the blood pressure on the arm receiving an infusion because the cuff interferes with fluid flow, forces blood back into the needle, and may cause formation of a clot.
▶ If a lower extremity *must* be used for venipuncture, ascertain that such use is supported by written fa-

cility policy and monitor the site closely throughout the infusion.
▶ Restraints should not be placed over a venipuncture site because such action would obstruct blood flow. Also, restraints should not be applied directly to the extremity when the infusion is being delivered by a volumetric infusion pump. If the extremity must be immobilized, an armboard should be used with the restraint applied to the armboard *only*.
▶ An *armboard should be used* when the venipuncture site is located in an area of flexion (such as the wrist or antecubital fossa).
▶ Maintain sufficient height of the solution container during transportation or ambulation of a patient to provide a constant flow rate. When the patient is ambulating, the arm in which the infusion is located should be placed lightly across the waist and the IV pole should be guided with the uninvolved extremity.
▶ The patient should be advised to avoid actions that would involve elevation of the extremity with the venipuncture; such actions might include, for example, arranging hair, shaving, brushing teeth, and using the telephone.

SELECTION OF CANNULA

Factors influencing selection of the venipuncture device include the following:

▶ Purpose of the infusion
▶ Expected duration of therapy
▶ Patient's age and clinical condition
▶ Condition, size, and availability of veins

DISTENTION OF VEINS

After a suitable site has been located, the next step is to distend the vein, usually by means of a tourniquet. A tourniquet also helps to steady the vein when it is placed no higher than 2 inches above the site of injection. It should be tight enough to impede venous flow while maintaining arterial flow, but it should never be too tight (a common error).

Distention of the vein may also be achieved by placing the extremity in a dependent position for several minutes. Sometimes light tapping with the fingers over the proposed site will aid distention; however, if the tapping is too forceful, the vein will constrict due to the painful stimuli. Exercising the muscles distal to the proposed site of venipuncture is sometimes beneficial; however, this should be avoided when a blood specimen is being drawn for measurement of serum electrolyte levels because a false reading may result (see Chapter 2).

SKIN PREPARATION

Seventy percent alcohol is frequently used to prepare the injection site. The most effective method of cleansing the skin is scrubbing with friction for a full minute with a "clean to dirty" circular motion. Unfortunately, skin preparation too often consists of a quick, light wipe with the sponge, which fails to significantly reduce the bacteria count. Povidone–iodine solution is highly desirable for cleansing the injection site because it provides effective bactericidal, fungicidal, and sporicidal activity. (The patient should be questioned about a possible allergy to iodine before its use.) Scientific evidence does not support the need to shave hair from the injection site to reduce bacterial flora. The microabrasions incurred in shaving may actually predispose the patient to infection. With a very hirsute patient, clipping the hair with scissors will facilitate the cohesiveness of the dressing tape.

CANNULA INSERTION TECHNIQUES

Winged Infusion Set

A *winged infusion set,* sometimes called a butterfly or small-vein set, is frequently used for venipunctures. Generally, the bevel of the needle should be facing upward during insertion. However, the introduction of a large needle into a small vein may require the bevel to face downward; otherwise, the needle will pierce the posterior wall of the vein when the tourniquet is removed.

With the tourniquet in place, the needle should pierce the skin to one side of, and approximately one half to one inch below, the point where the needle will enter the vein. As the needle enters the skin, it should be at about a 45-degree angle; after the skin is entered, the needle angle is decreased. Although it seems more logical to enter the vein from above with one quick thrust, there may be less flattening of the vein and decreased risk of perforating the posterior aspect of the vein wall when a lateral approach is used. The free hand is used to palpate the vein while the needle is being introduced. An experienced operator may feel a snap as the needle enters the vein; after this, less resistance is offered to the needle. At this point, one should proceed very slowly with insertion of the needle, threading it into the lumen approximately one half to three fourths of an inch. The tourniquet is then released. Frequently a thin stream of blood is seen in the tubing when the needle enters the vein. If in doubt, pinch the tubing just above the needle and release it; usually this will cause a flashback of blood into the tubing.

Fluid should be allowed to flow and the area adjacent to the site should be observed for swelling. The presence of swelling indicates that the needle is not in the vein and fluid is entering the subcutaneous area. The infusion should be discontinued immediately when swelling is noted or if the venipuncture attempt was unsuccessful. The venipuncture must then be made in another area. A tourniquet should not be reapplied immediately to the same extremity; if applied too soon, a hematoma will develop and the patient will experience unnecessary pain and discomfort.

After successful venipuncture, the next step involves anchoring the device securely. Place a strip of tape horizontally over the wings; then place a strip of tape vertically over each wing. *Caution:* Do not allow tape to cover actual insertion site.

Plastic Catheter Mounted Over a Needle

A venipuncture is performed in the usual manner, with the needle inserted far enough to ensure entry of the catheter into the vein. After the catheter is slid into the vein to the desired length, the needle is carefully removed. Never partially withdraw the needle from the catheter and reinsert it into the catheter; such action could result in a catheter embolus. Securely anchor the catheter hub/tubing connection to the skin with tape.

Plastic Catheter Inserted Through a Needle

After performance of a normal venipuncture, the catheter is inserted into the vein through the needle. If venipuncture is not successful, pull out the needle and catheter together. The catheter should not be pulled out first because the sharp edges of the needle could sever it as it is being withdrawn, resulting in catheter embolism. (The manufacturer's directions should be followed closely.)

DRESSING TO VENIPUNCTURE SITE

After the cannula has initially been securely anchored, an antimicrobial agent should be applied to the site followed by the application of a dry sterile dressing. The dressing should be labeled with the following information:

Type, gauge, and length of cannula
Date and time of insertion
Name or initials of person performing venipuncture

A tension loop in the administration set tubing will prevent unwarranted tension on the cannula.

MAINTENANCE OF VENIPUNCTURE SITE

Frequent observations should be made for evidence of infiltration, cannula occlusion, phlebitis, site infection, and accuracy of flow rate. To minimize the risk of IV therapy-associated nosocomial infection, it is recommended that:

► Parenteral fluid containers be changed every 24 hours[17,18]
► Peripheral and central primary and secondary sets be changed every 48 hours[19]
► Primary intermittent administration sets be changed every 24 hours[20]
► Administration sets used for TPN be changed every 24 hours[21]
► Any administration set be changed immediately on suspected contamination or when the integrity of the product has been compromised
► Gauze dressings be changed every 48 hours on peripheral and central cannula sites and immediately if the integrity of the dressing is compromised[22]
► Transparent semipermeable membrane dressings be changed at established intervals and immediately if the integrity of the dressing is compromised[23]

SITE ROTATION

Many practitioners believe that plastic cannulas are about twice as likely to produce venous complications as metal needles. It has been suggested that, because metal needles infiltrate more quickly than plastic devices, they are changed more frequently, decreasing the occurrence of phlebitis. It is known that the longer the IV device remains in place, the higher the rate of positive cultures; this emphasizes the importance of regular site rotation.

According to CDC recommendations, a peripheral venipuncture device should not be left in place longer than 72 hours and preferably should be changed at 48-hour intervals.[24] This agency further notes, however, that this guideline may need to be modified when the patient has few suitable veins. In the event that site rotation is unachievable, explicit documentation noting the reason for noncompliance with this recommendation should be made. Further, concise charting is required daily to describe the appearance of the existing site. Close monitoring of the site should follow and the observations should be noted in the patient's chart.

The Revised Intravenous Nursing Standards of Practice issued by the INS in 1990 recommends that a peripheral venous cannula be removed every 48 hours and immediately on suspected contamination or complication.[25]

DETERMINING FLOW RATE

Physician's Orders

The physician should prescribe the flow rate as well as the type of solution to be given. The nurse initiating

the infusion, or involved in its maintenance, must be aware of the composition of the prescribed fluid, its usual flow rate, its desired effects, and complications associated with its use.

Factors Affecting Desired Flow Rate

The following are some of the factors considered in determining the best flow rate for the infusion:

► Composition of the fluids (see Table 11-1)
► Body surface area
► Age
► Clinical status with special emphasis on renal and cardiac function
► Tolerance to infusion

The desired rate for the infusion varies with the type of fluid being infused. For example, isotonic solutions may be infused more rapidly than very hypertonic solutions.

The patient's need for fluids influences the desired rate of administration; for example, a patient in hypovolemic shock needs aggressive fluid administration. The infusion rate, in this instance, is much more rapid than usual. Because the heart and kidneys both play a major role in the use of fluids introduced IV, the presence of cardiac or renal damage can greatly alter the desired infusion rate. If the pumping action of the heart is inadequate, rapid infusion of fluids could result in dangerous fluid excess. Failure of the kidneys to excrete unneeded water and electrolytes can also result in excessive amounts of these substances in the body. Geriatric patients almost always have some degree of cardiac and renal impairment; therefore, fluids are administered more slowly to them than to young adults.

One of the best guides to safe flow rate is the patient's tolerance to the infusion. Remember that different persons respond differently to parenteral fluid infusions just as they do to other medications. For this reason, patients must be closely monitored for adverse reactions throughout infusions of parenteral solutions. Reactions associated with different parenteral fluids are addressed briefly in Chapter 11 and more explicitly in the early chapters dealing with specific imbalances.

Variations of Drop Size with Different Commercial Sets

Most nurses think in terms of "drops per minute" when considering fluid flow rate. Remember that commercial parenteral administration sets vary in the number of drops delivering 1mL (Table 10-1). Unless one knows which administration set is to be used, it is more practical to consider the number of milliliters to be infused in 1 minute. From this figure, the number of drops per

TABLE 10–1.
Variation in Size of Drop in Commercial Administration Sets*

COMPANY	"REGULAR" SET
Abbott Lab	15
Travenol Lab	10
McGaw Lab	15

* *Approximate number of drops needed to deliver 1 mL.*

minute can be computed by the following formula when the drop size of the administration is learned:

$$\text{Drop factor} \times \text{mL/min} = \text{drops/min}$$

For example, to deliver 3 mL/min using a set with 10 drops to 1 mL, a flow rate of 30 drops/min would be necessary. To administer the same amount using a set with 15 drops to 1 mL, a flow rate of 45 drops/min would be necessary. Drop size can vary somewhat according to the viscosity of the fluid being infused. Other factors affecting drop size include room temperature and height of the bottle; however, for practical purposes, the calibration of the IV set (gtt/min) should be accepted as valid. (Manufacturers list the drop factors on the administration set packages.)

Calculation of Flow Rate

When one knows the amount of fluid to be administered in a prescribed time span, plus the drop factor of the administration set, the appropriate flow rate (in drops/min) can be easily calculated by using the following mathematical formula:

$$\text{drops/min} = \frac{\text{total volume infused (mL)} \times \text{drop factor (drops/mL)}}{\text{total time of infusion in minutes}}$$

Sample Problem: Infuse 1000 mL of 5% dextrose in water (D/W) in 2 hours (assume an administration set with 10 drops to 1 mL is to be used)

Total volume	=	1000 mL
Drops/mL	=	10
Total time of infusion in minutes	=	120

$$\frac{1000 \times 10}{120} = \text{approximately 80 drops/min}$$

Flow rates can also be determined by a calculator supplied by the manufacturer of the administration set. To facilitate monitoring of the infusion, it is helpful to use a "time strip" that indicates the desired hourly levels of the infusion container. Many authorities advocate using an IV flow sheet during the patient's IV therapy regimen.

FACTORS INFLUENCING GRAVITY FLOW RATE

Be aware that once the flow rate of an infusion has been appropriately regulated there are certain factors that can alter it.

Change in Position of Cannula

A change in the cannula position may place the bevel against or away from the venous wall. Adequate flow rate will diminish if the cannula is pushed against the venous wall; conversely, the flow will increase when the cannula moves away from the venous wall.

Height of the Parenteral Solution Container

Because infusions flow in by gravity, a change in the height of the infusion container in relation to the patient can increase or decrease the flow rate (the greater the distance between the patient and the container, the faster the rate).

Patency of the Cannula

A small clot may occlude the cannula lumen and cause the flow rate to decrease or totally cease. Clot formation may occur when an increase in venous pressure in the infusion extremity forces blood into the cannula; this phenomenon might be caused by lying on the infusion arm, constriction from a blood pressure cuff or an improperly placed restraint, and the improper placement of the parenteral solution containers when a continuous-flow administration set is being used. *Positive pressure, such as irrigation with isotonic saline, should never be employed to relieve clot formation;* the dislodged clot could cause an infarction and, if infected, spread the infection to other parts of the body. Gentle aspiration may be attempted for removing fresh clots from an occluded cannula. If strong resistance is encountered during the aspiration procedure, or if the clot is of long-standing duration, the site should be discontinued with gentle withdrawal of the occluded cannula.

Venous Spasm

A cold or irritating solution may retard flow rate by producing venous spasm. A warm pack placed proximal to the infusion site will relieve this condition.

Plugged Air Vent

A plugged air vent can cause an infusion to stop. Thus, patency of the air vent should be checked when there is no other apparent cause for a stopped infusion.

Condition of Final Filter

Final filters can cause decreased flow rates should particulate matter block the filtering surface or an air lock develop.

Crying in Infants

Crying raises venous pressure and, thus, slows the rate of flow.

Presence of a Local Complication

The presence of phlebitis, thrombophlebitis, or an undetected infiltration commonly slows flow rate.

Inappropriate Flow Rate Adjustment

Flow rates of infusions have been dramatically altered by patients or their visitors manipulating the flow clamp or the infusion pump. This possibility should not be overlooked.

INCOMPATIBILITIES

Although pharmacy admixture services are commonplace today, in select circumstances the nurse may be required to add medications to parenteral solutions. With the fast-growing number of medications and types of parenteral fluids available for use, the number of possible combinations is astronomical. It is impossible for the nurse to know, without help, which medications can be safely mixed with each parenteral solution: assistance must come from several sources, including the pharmacist, drug inserts, compatibility charts, and current admixture reference books.

The nurse should observe the following guidelines when preparing an admixture:

1. Thoroughly review the literature provided by the manufacturer of the parenteral solution; most companies have prepared charts noting the compatibility of various medications with their solutions.
2. Review the literature (drug insert) provided by the drug manufacturer.
3. When possible, keep the number of additives to a minimum since the complex interaction between numerous additives can result in a visual, chemical, or therapeutic incompatibility.
4. If doubt exists regarding a possible incompatibility, seek assistance from the hospital pharmacist.
5. Visually check appearance of completed admixture for evidence of incompatibility. A physical incompatibility may be manifested by a haze, color change, or effervescence. *Note:* Chemical incompatibilities are more difficult to detect because they do not always produce a visible change.
6. If a precipitate forms when a medication is added to an IV fluid, the solution should be discarded unless the directions accompanying the medication state otherwise. The IV administration of a solution containing insoluble matter may result in embolism or other damage to the heart, liver, and kidneys.
7. An administration set with a final filter should be used whenever possible to trap undetected precipitates.
8. The degree of solubility of an additive varies with the *p*H, and most incompatibilities are related to changes in *p*H. Solutions of a high *p*H seem to be incompatible with those of a low *p*H. (A chart listing the *p*H of certain drugs and parenteral solutions can help predict potential incompatibilities.)
9. Sodium bicarbonate and calcium salts should never be mixed since they form an insoluble precipitate (calcium carbonate).
10. Valium should not be mixed with any parenteral solution since a precipitate may form. It is also incompatible with any other drug in syringe or solution.[26]
11. It is best not to mix multiple vitamin complexes with potassium penicillin G because the acidic ascorbic acid lowers the *p*H and can cause degradation of the antibiotic.[27]
12. It is best not to mix heparin with antibiotics because heparin may affect the stability of certain antibiotics.[28]
13. Hydrocortisone should not be mixed with tetracycline, since a precipitate will form.[29]
14. It is best not to administer sodium bicarbonate and epinephrine jointly because sodium bicarbonate tends to neutralize epinephrine: they may be administered intermittently through the same tubing if it is flushed first.[30]

COMPLICATIONS OF IV FLUID ADMINISTRATION

Unfortunately, IV therapy predisposes to numerous hazards; these include both local and systemic complications. Local complications occur most frequently; however, systemic complications are more serious—in fact, they may be life-threatening. Because of the potential for problems, the nurse must understand the risks and employ all available measures to prevent their occurrence.

LOCAL COMPLICATIONS

Infiltration

Dislodgment of an IV needle and local infiltration of the solution into subcutaneous tissues are not uncommon, especially when a small, thin-walled vein is used and the patient is active. Infiltration is characterized by the following:

▶ Edema at the site of injection. Compare the infusion area with the identical area in the opposite extremity; otherwise swelling may not be readily noticeable. Temperature of the skin around the insertion site is cooler than the rest of the skin because the IV fluid is cooler than the body.

▶ Pain or discomfort in the area of infiltration. The degree of discomfort depends on the solution or the presence of additives.

▶ Significant decrease in the flow rate, or a halt in flow when the infiltration is extensive. Hypertonic carbohydrate solutions, potassium solutions, and solutions with a *p*H varying greatly from that of the body (such as sixth molar sodium lactate or ammonium chloride) often cause great pain if they infiltrate into the subcutaneous tissues; in this way, venospasm can result. Tissue slough may result from the local irritation.

To detect infiltration in a questionable IV site, the following procedure has proven effective:

1. Locate the vein in which the parenteral solution is infused.
2. Place two fingers on the vein, about 3 to 4 inches above the injection site. Placement of the fingers will depend on the length of the needle or catheter that is in place.
3. While applying digital pressure to the vein, observe the drip chamber of the IV administration set:
   A. Cessation of flow of the solution into the drip chamber during the time that digital pressure is being applied signifies that the needle is in the vein.
   B. If there is *no* alteration in the flow of the solution into the drip chamber during the time the vein is occluded, one must conclude that the needle is in the tissues. (When infiltration is present, the solution continues to flow into the subcutaneous tissue.)

Note: Under no circumstances should an IV solution (with or without medications) be allowed to continue to infuse after infiltration of the site has been confirmed. The site should be discontinued at once.

Although close monitoring of an infusion will not always prevent the occurrence of an infiltration, early detection will greatly reduce the severity of this common complication. Following is a summary of factors that frequently contribute to infiltration:

▶ Lack of proper patient education concerning care of the extremity receiving the infusion
▶ Hyperactive patient
▶ Insecure anchoring of the venipuncture cannula
▶ Improper technique of person initiating therapy (such as pushing bevel of needle through the posterior wall of the vein)
▶ Poor selection of venipuncture site (such as over an area of flexion)
▶ Inappropriate handling of extremity or equipment during ambulation and transportation to ancillary departments

Hematoma

Extravasation of blood into the tissues may be the result of penetration of the posterior wall of the vein during an unsuccessful venipuncture attempt or the application of a tourniquet to the extremity immediately after an unsuccessful venipuncture attempt. Hematomas often result when inadequate time is spent applying pressure to the venipuncture site after the IV device is removed. Band-aids are not considered pressure dressings and should not be used until all bleeding from a discontinued site has ceased. After the device is removed, the patient should be instructed not to rub or scratch the area.

Phlebitis

Phlebitis is defined as inflammation of a vein and is evidenced by heat, redness, swelling, and discomfort adjacent to the venipuncture site. The incidence of infusion-related phlebitis increases with the length of time the cannula is in place.

Phlebitis may be further classified as being:

Chemical (due to *p*H of solution or drug being administered)
Mechanical (due to unwarranted movement of the cannula in the lumen of the vein)
Septic (due to contamination)

Thrombophlebitis

The term *thrombophlebitis* denotes the presence of a thrombosis plus inflammation in the vein. It is evidenced by the previously listed signs of phlebitis plus hardness and tenderness of the veins. As the thrombus increases in size, the flow rate of the infusion will decrease due to the narrowing of the lumen of the vein. There is always the inherent danger of embolism when a thrombosis exists. To minimize the risk of phlebitis/thrombophlebitis, the following guidelines should be observed:

1. Use veins with ample blood volume, particularly when irritating fluids are administered.
2. Use a cannula that is smaller than the vein to provide for greater hemodilution of the solution/medications.
3. Start venipuncture at the distal end of the extremity to allow for successive punctures proximal to previous sites.
4. Avoid venipunctures in the lower extremities and in areas of flexion.
5. For very slow infusions, do not use small veins with inadequate circulating blood; this tends to cause prolonged irritation and increase inflammation.
6. Inspect all solution containers and administration equipment carefully for evidence of contamination.
7. Wash hands and carefully prepare venipuncture site before insertion of cannula.
8. Use an antimicrobial agent at the venipuncture site.
9. Only experienced, qualified personnel should initiate, monitor, and discontinue IV therapy.
10. Securely anchor the cannula to prevent movement.
11. Admixtures should be aseptically prepared under a laminar flow hood.
12. Avoid administering particulate matter by diluting and preparing medications according to manufacturer's recommendations and by using a 0.22-μm filter as indicated.
13. Do not allow a container of solution to infuse longer than 24 hours.
14. Change administration sets and site dressings according to CDC recommendations (every 24–48 hours, depending on the site) and label date and time of change.
15. Rotate venipuncture site every 48 to 72 hours.
16. Always use an armboard if IV site is located in an area of flexion.
17. Provide adequate patient teaching with regard to restrictions, precautions, and proper means of ambulation relative to IV therapy.

SYSTEMIC COMPLICATIONS

Pyrogenic Reaction

The presence of pyrogenic substances (foreign proteins capable of producing fever) in either the infusion solution or the administration setup can induce a febrile reaction. Such a reaction is characterized by the following:

▶ An abrupt temperature elevation (from 100°–106° F [37.7°–41° C] accompanied by severe chills (reaction usually begins about 30 minutes after the start of the infusion)
▶ Backache
▶ Headache
▶ General malaise
▶ Nausea and vomiting
▶ Vascular collapse with hypotension and cyanosis, which may occur when the reaction is severe

The severity of the reaction depends on the amount of pyrogens infused, the flow rate, and the patient's susceptibility. Patients having fever or liver disease are more susceptible than others.

If these symptoms listed above occur, the nurse should stop the infusion at once, check the vital signs, and notify the physician. The solution, administration set, and the venipuncture device (aseptically capped) should be saved so that they can be cultured if necessary.

The widespread use of commercially prepared solutions and administration sets has dramatically decreased the number of pyrogenic reactions. It must be remembered, however, that contaminants can enter the solution flask after the seal is broken. It is, therefore, a wise practice to indicate on the bottle the date and time that the seal was broken. According to the CDC, parenteral solutions should be in use no longer than 24 hours. This is extremely important to remember when patients are receiving KVO (keep vein open) infusions at very slow rates.

Any evidence of cloudiness or other particulate matter in a previously clear solution is an indication to discard it.

Before initiating an infusion, squeeze plastic containers to detect leaks and inspect glass containers against light for cracks or bright reflections that penetrate into the wall of the bottle; if either is present, the solution is no longer sterile and must be discarded. Administration sets should also be routinely inspected for cracks or discolorations before use.

If it is necessary for the nurse to prepare an admixture, careful aseptic technique must be used throughout the procedure. Because traffic generates airborne contamination, the procedure should be done in an isolated area such as a medication or treatment room.

Administration sets should be changed at least every 24 to 48 hours as previously recommended. The administration set should be changed after the administration of blood or other protein-containing solutions because these substances become a growth medium for bacteria.

Air Emboli

Although they are an infrequent occurrence, air emboli are associated with a 40% to 50% mortality and an almost equally high morbidity.[31,32] Cannulation of central veins is far more likely to be associated with air embolism than is cannulation of peripheral veins. The exact quantity of IV air that can lead to death in humans is unknown but appears to be related to the rate of entry. It is known that a much larger amount of air can be tolerated in the venous system than in the arterial system. Ordway[33] extrapolated data from animal studies and concluded that the average lethal dose of air IV in humans would be from 70 to 150 mL/sec. Yeakel[34] reported a fatal episode after the sudden IV administration of 100 mL of air.

Be aware that air can enter the central circulation at a rate of 100 mL/sec through a 12.7- to 15.2-cm (5–6-inch), 14-gauge catheter.[35] Measures the nurse should take to prevent the occurrence of air embolism in specific areas are discussed below.

Central Veins

A time of high risk for air emboli is during the insertion of a central line. Precautionary measures include, but are not limited to, having the patient perform the Valsalva maneuver (forced expiration with the mouth closed) and placing the patient in a Trendelenburg position. During tubing changes the patient should again be placed in the Trendelenburg position (unless otherwise contraindicated) and advised to perform the Valsalva maneuver.[36] If the Trendelenburg position cannot be used, place the patient in a flat, supine position.

Recall that there is a low pressure in the central veins that can pull air in during tubing changes or when connections in the administration apparatus are not air-tight. This low pressure is particularly pronounced in the hypovolemic patient; hypovolemia generates an increased "sucking force" in the central veins. Also, during the inspiratory phase of respiration, the intrathoracic pressure is below that of the atmosphere, making it possible for air to be drawn into the cannulated vein. The Valsalva maneuver increases the intrathoracic pressure as well as the mean pressure in the central veins, decreasing the danger of air being sucked in.

Be sure the connection between the catheter hub and the tubing is secure. Adequate taping of the tubing and catheter lessens the possibility of accidental disconnection. This is of particular importance when the patient is elevated from a flat to a sitting or standing position, since the danger of air embolism is greater when the patient is upright.

Air can enter the central venous system during removal of a central line or up to several days after removal through a subcutaneous track formation. The risk is intensified with catheters that have been in place for long periods. The patient should be placed in the Trendelenburg position and instructed to perform the Valsalva maneuver while the catheter is removed in a continuous smooth motion. Firm pressure should be applied to the discontinued site until all bleeding has ceased. Once hemostasis has been achieved, a sterile, air-impermeable dressing should be applied for 48 to 72 hours. Povidone-iodine ointment applied to the insertion site and covered with a gauze dressing is not appropriate.[37] As the ointment is absorbed into the gauze, the dressing becomes nonocclusive.

Peripheral Veins

Do not elevate the extremity receiving the infusion above the level of the heart because this results in venous collapse and negative venous pressure. Negative pressure in the vein receiving the infusion can draw in air if there are any defects in the apparatus or if the solution flask empties.

Allow the infusion tubing to drop below the level of the extremity. This may help prevent air from entering the vein if the infusion flask empties unobserved.

Keep the clamp used to regulate the flow rate below the level of the heart. If the clamp regulating flow is placed above the level of the heart and is adjusted so that it only partially occludes the tubing, any existing defect in the tubing between the clamp and the level of the heart will allow air to enter the system.[38] On the other hand, if the clamp is placed below the level of the heart, a defect between the drip chamber and the clamp will cause leakage of fluid rather than entry of air (because of the greater pressure in the vein than in the tubing).[39]

All Infusions

Tightly secure all connections in the administration setup to prevent air from being drawn in. If a stopcock is part of the IV setup, the outlets not in use should be completely shut off. Avoid tightening connections so much that forceps are needed to loosen them (this can cause cracking of the tubing or plastic IV device and create an entry site for air).

Inspect plastic bottles and tubing for cracks or other defects.

Discontinue an infusion before the bottle and tubing are completely empty.

Completely clamp off the first bottle to empty in a Y-type setup (parallel hookup); otherwise, air will be drawn into the vein from the empty bottle. The potential for air emboli exists when fluids from two vented containers run simultaneously through the same needle. The use of administration sets with check-values for piggybacking fluids prevents this problem (see discussion of piggybacking earlier in this chapter).

Read and follow the manufacturer's directions for safe use of infusion pumps since some types can pump air into the vein if the infusion bottle is allowed to empty.

The presence of an air embolism is manifested by the following:

Dyspnea and cyanosis
Hypotension
Weak, rapid pulse
Loud, continuous churning sound over the precordium (not always present)
Loss of consciousness

The occurrence of these symptoms in a patient receiving an infusion should lead one to suspect air embolism.

If an air embolism occurs, administration tubing should be promptly clamped. The patient should be immediately turned on his left side with his head down and the lower extremities elevated (left lateral and modified Trendelenburg position). This allows the air to rise into the right atrium and away from the pulmonary outflow tract. Oxygen is administered by mask to achieve a high oxygen concentration.

Note: The nurse should be aware that the presence of air in the administration set, no matter how small a bubble, frequently causes apprehension in patients receiving IV fluids. This apprehension in most situations extends to the patient's family.

Pulmonary Embolism

Pulmonary embolism occurs when a substance, usually a blood clot, becomes free-floating and is propelled by the venous circulation to the right side of the heart and on into the pulmonary artery. Obstruction of the main artery results in circulatory and cardiac disturbances. Recurrent small emboli may eventually result in pulmonary hypertension and right heart failure.[40]

Pulmonary embolism may result from the unwise irrigation of an occluded cannula. Application of positive pressure to an occluded cannula may dislodge the clot into the circulation, possibly resulting in an infarction. Also, the irrigating solution may embolize small, infected cannula thrombi, resulting in septicemia. Most IV therapists favor removal rather than irrigation of occluded catheters.

A catheter emboli can result from improper technique during venipuncture. Under no circumstances should the needle or stylet be redirected into the catheter of an over-the-needle catheter; when using a through-the-needle catheter, the catheter is never to be pulled back through the needle. In the event that a catheter emboli occurs, the physician should be notified immediately so that specialized retrieval interventions can be initiated. For retrievals to be successful, catheters must be radiopaque.

Circulatory Overload

Overloading the circulatory system with excessive IV fluids may cause a rise in the blood pressure and central venous pressure, venous distention, coughing, shortness of breath, increased respiratory rate, and pulmonary edema with severe dyspnea and cyanosis. One should be particularly alert for circulatory overload in patients with cardiac decompensation. If the above symptoms occur, the infusion should be slowed to a "keep-open" rate and the physician notified immediately. The patient can be raised to a sitting position to facilitate breathing, and warming measures (blankets) can be applied to promote peripheral circulation and relieve stress on the central veins. Patients prone to circulatory overload may require central venous pressure or pulmonary capillary wedge pressure monitoring during infusions.

UNIVERSAL PRECAUTIONS

According to the CDC, health care providers should consider all patients as potential sources of transmissible diseases. Therefore, "universal precautions" should be observed for the routine use of appropriate barrier precautions to prevent skin and mucous membrane contact with blood or body fluids of *all* patients.[41] Gloves are considered the minimal barrier for health care workers and should be worn for all invasive procedures or any procedure with the potential for blood contact. In IV nursing, this includes venipuncture, assisting with central vein cannulation, tubing change, and discontinuation of a central or peripheral venipuncture site. Sharp items, including but not limited to needles and catheter stylets, should be placed in a puncture-proof container. Needles should not be recapped.

HYPODERMOCLYSIS

Hypodermoclysis, the administration of a solution subcutaneously, most often in the lateral aspects of the thighs, compares unfavorably with the IV route and is not commonly used. The types of fluids that can be given subcutaneously are few, since they must closely resemble the electrolyte content and tonicity of extracellular fluid (ECF) if they are to be absorbed. Some of the fluids generally considered reasonably safe for subcutaneous administration include the following:

Isotonic saline (0.9% NaCl)
Half-isotonic saline (0.45% NaCl) with 2.5% dextrose
Lactated Ringer's solution
Half-strength lactated Ringer's solution with 2.5% dextrose

Probably the only advantage of hypodermoclysis over the IV route is that it is easier to initiate. Several sources in the literature report a renewed interest in hypodermoclysis for the short-term support of elderly patients in extended care facilities lacking personnel skilled in IV therapy techniques.

The infusion rate depends on how well the fluid is absorbed from the injection site. When the fluid is absorbed well, 250 to 500 mL can be given at one site in 1 hour to an adult, but after a short while, the fluid is not this readily absorbed and the tissues become hard and swollen. To hasten absorption, hyaluronidase (Wydase) may be injected into the rubber portion of the tubing near each injection site. One hundred fifty units (75 units to each site) will hasten the absorption of 1 L of solution. If an order for hyaluronidase is not included with the fluid order, a call to the physician could be advantageous.

The patient should be checked often when this route is used; a large amount of swelling can develop unless the flow rate is adjusted carefully. A small, sterile gauze pad should be placed under the needle hub and another should cover the injection site. After removal of the needle, a light sterile dressing should be applied.

Comment: Fluids are not absorbed well from the subcutaneous tissue when blood volume is severely reduced because of accompanying peripheral collapse. The fluids that can be given safely are quite limited and, ironically, the patients for whom hypodermoclysis is most often used (infants, the aged, and the obese) are the ones most likely to be harmed by them.

REFERENCES

1. Niederpruem M: Factors affecting compliance in the home I.V. antibiotic therapy client. Journal of Intravenous Nursing 12(3): 13, 1989
2. Revised Intravenous Nursing Standards of Practice, Intravenous Nurses Society. Journal of Intravenous Nursing (suppl): 53, 1990
3. Henry R: Problems in the use of volume control sets for intravenous fluids. Am J Hosp Pharm 29:485, 1982
4. National Coordinating Committee on Large Volume Parenterals. Recommended methods for compounding IV admixtures. Am J Hosp Pharm 32:261, 1975
5. Revised Intravenous Nursing Standards of Practice, p S57
6. Guidelines for Prevention of Intravascular Infection, Hospital Infection Control, p 28P. Atlanta, Centers for Disease Control, February 1982
7. Plumer A: Principles: Practice of Intravenous Nursing, 4th ed, p 156. Boston, Little, Brown, 1987
8. Shearer J: Normal saline flush versus dilute heparin flush. Journal of the National Intravenous Therapy Association 10(6): 425, 1987
9. Revised Intravenous Nursing Standards of Practice, p S60
10. Ibid, p S47
11. Masoorli S, Angeles T: PICC lines: The latest home care challenge. RN 90(1): 44, 1990
12. Goodwin M: The Seldenger method for PICC insertion. Journal of Intravenous Nursing 12(4): 238, 1989
13. Camp-Sorrell D: Advanced central venous access. Journal of Intravenous Nursing 13(6): 361, 1990
14. Plumer, p 173
15. Teitell B: Unique features of pediatric intravenous therapy. In: Plumer A (ed): Principles and Practice of Intravenous Therapy, p 507. Boston, Little, Brown, 1987
16. Ibid
17. Revised Intravenous Nursing Standards of Practice, p S50
18. Guidelines for Prevention of Intravascular Infections, Hospital Infection Control, p 280. Atlanta, Centers for Disease Control, February 1982
19. Revised Intravenous Nursing Standards of Practice, p S54
20. Ibid
21. Ibid
22. Ibid, p S41
23. Ibid
24. Guidelines for Prevention of Intravascular Infections, Hospital Infection Control, p 28N. Atlanta, Centers for Disease Control, February 1982
25. Revised Intravenous Nursing Standards of Practice, p S46
26. Gahart B: Intravenous Medications, 7th ed, p 200. St. Louis, CV Mosby, 1991
27. Frenier E: Problems of intravenous incompatibilities. American Journal of IV Therapy & Clinical Nutrition 3:23, 1976
28. Ibid
29. Ibid
30. Ibid
31. Kashuk I, Penn I: Airway embolism after central venous catheterization. Surg Gynecol Obstet 159: 249, 1984
32. McConnell E: Preventing air embolism in patients with central venous catheters. Nursing Life, 6:47, 1986
33. Ordway C: Air embolism via CVP catheter without positive pressure. Ann Surg 179:479, 1974
34. Yeakel A: Lethal air embolism from plastic blood storage containers. JAMA 204:267, 1969
35. Flanagan et al: Air embolus: A lethal complication of subclavian venipuncture. N Engl J Med 281:388, 1969

36. Thielen J: Air emboli: A potentially lethal complication of central venous lines. Focus on Critical Care 17(5): 374, 1990
37. Hanley F, Click R, Trancredi R: Delayed air embolism after removal of venous catheters. Ann Intern Med 101:401, 1984
38. Gottlieb J, Ericsson J, Sweet R: Venous air embolism: A review. Anesth Analg 44:776, 1965
39. Ibid
40. Mavor G, Galloway J: The ileofemoral venous segment as a source of pulmonary emboli. Lancet 1:873, 1967
41. Centers for Disease Control. Update: Universal precautions for prevention of transmission of human immunodeficiency virus, hepatitis B virus, and other blood borne pathogens in health care settings. Morbidity and Mortality Weekly Report 37(24): 377, 1988

11

Parenteral Fluids

The nurse's role in parenteral fluid therapy is crucial because it is the nurse who usually initiates fluids and, almost invariably, is responsible for monitoring the patient's response. One must be knowledgeable about the contents of parenteral fluids, their purposes, and the contraindications and complications associated with their uses.

Before discussing the types of parenteral fluids avail-

able, and the factors to be considered with their administration, it is helpful to review some basic facts.

There are essentially three major purposes of parenteral fluid therapy. They include provision of (1) fluids to meet daily maintenance needs, (2) fluids to replace ongoing losses, and (3) electrolytes to correct any existing disturbances. Each of these purposes is briefly discussed below.

PURPOSES OF FLUID THERAPY

PROVISION OF USUAL MAINTENANCE NEEDS

As noted in Table 2-1, the average healthy adult requires approximately 2600 mL/day of fluid to replace fluid lost in urine, stool, exhalation, and radiation from the skin. Many patients require parenteral fluids for only a few days while they are temporarily unable to ingest food and fluid during a limited illness or after surgery. In these patients, the typical fluid prescription for maintenance needs ranges between 2000 and 3000 mL/day.

Of course, the body needs more than water for maintenance. Electrolytes are also needed. The typical adult needs approximately 100 to 150 mEq of sodium, and approximately 40 mEq of potassium, each day.[1] An example of a 24-hour fluid prescription to meet these needs is 2 L of 0.45% NaCl with 20 mEq of KCl added to each liter. Because each liter of 0.45% NaCl contains 77 mEq of sodium, 2 L would provide 154 mEq (easily meeting the daily sodium requirement of most adults). Addition of 20 mEq of KCl to each liter of fluid would provide the typically needed 40 mEq of potassium per day.

Because 0.45% NaCl is a hypotonic solution, it provides some free water to aid in the renal excretion of solutes. Free water can also be supplied in the form of 5% dextrose in water. Calories are needed in parenteral fluids to minimize protein catabolism and prevent ketosis of starvation. Thus, the above example would more likely be 2 L of 5% dextrose in 0.45% NaCl (rather than 0.45% NaCl alone). Because each liter of a 5% dextrose solution provides 50 g of carbohydrate with approximately 170 calories, 2 L would provide 100 g of carbohydrate with 340 calories. Although this is a small fraction of the daily caloric need, it is far better than none in terms of warding off ketosis of starvation. As discussed in Chapter 12, sophisticated solutions are available to meet the nutritional needs of patients requiring prolonged parenteral therapy or of those needing a large caloric intake due to hypermetabolism (as occurs with trauma or burns).

Maintenance needs for sodium and potassium were briefly discussed above. Remember that calcium, magnesium, and phosphorus may be necessary after 1 week of parenteral therapy.[2]

Although 2000 to 3000 mL/day of water for the average healthy adult is a useful figure to keep in mind, it is important to realize that it may need to be adjusted downward for smaller adults. Further, children need entirely different volumes, based on their body size and age. To avoid the possibility of fluid volume error, some clinicians favor the use of fluid volume replacement based on body surface area. For example, a commonly recommended formula calls for 1500 mL/day of fluid per square meter (m^2) of body surface area (BSA). (Nomograms exist that aid in the calculation of BSA from height and weight.) The formula is adjusted upward if the individual has a fluid volume deficit (FVD). For example, for a patient with a moderate FVD, 2400 mL/m^2 of BSA (providing for both maintenance and volume replacement) may be prescribed.

The above discussion of needed fluid volume is predicated on the assumption that the patient has normal renal function. If this is not the case, fluid volume as well as sodium and potassium replacement must be adjusted according to severity of the renal impairment. For example, an oliguric renal failure patient might logically receive the same amount of fluid as the sum of urinary output and estimated insensible losses.

REPLACEMENT OF ABNORMAL FLUID LOSSES

If the patient is losing fluid by an abnormal route (such as gastric suction, vomiting, or diarrhea), more than maintenance fluids must be provided to prevent FVD. In addition, the parenteral fluids' electrolyte content will need to be modified to correct imbalances. The need for a carefully kept intake and output (I&O) record is evident to identify lost water and electrolytes. It is also important to record elevated body temperature because this increases fluid needs. Free water needs are increased in individuals with unusual insensible water losses, such as those who are hyperventilating or are exposed to low environmental humidity. Water needs are also greater in patients with decreased renal concentrating ability because relatively more water is required to eliminate wastes. Finally, fluid requirements are greatly increased by shock, multiple trauma, and sepsis (either because of direct fluid loss or pooling of fluid in the capillaries or interstitial space).

Correction of Existing Electrolyte Disturbances

Providing maintenance fluid and electrolyte needs is complicated if the patient has electrolyte disturbances that need correcting. The task becomes one of safely providing needed electrolytes in conjunction with maintenance needs. (For discussion of fluid therapy for specific electrolyte disturbances, see Chapters 3–9.)

ASSESSMENT OF PATIENTS RECEIVING PARENTERAL FLUID THERAPY

Before parenteral fluid therapy is initiated for a patient with a real or potential fluid balance problem, renal status must be evaluated. There is danger of causing other imbalances if the kidneys are not functioning adequately. For example, administration of potassium-containing fluids to a patient with inadequate renal function can induce serious hyperkalemia.

If the patient with a severe FVD is oliguric, it is necessary to determine if the depressed renal function is due to prerenal azotemia secondary to decreased renal perfusion or, more seriously, to actual renal parenchymal damage (acute tubular necrosis) after prolonged untreated FVD. To differentiate between these conditions, a fluid load is infused over a short period and the patient is observed closely. If urine output improves, the problem was simple FVD; if urine flow is not reestablished, the problem is likely renal insufficiency. A fluid challenge test to distinguish simple FVD from a deficit complicated by acute tubular necrosis (ATN) is described in Chapter 3. These two conditions must be differentiated because prompt treatment of prerenal azotemia can prevent ATN. Treatment of a patient with adequate renal function is simplified greatly. So long as sufficient water and electrolytes are provided, healthy kidneys can select needed substances and maintain normal fluid and electrolyte balances.

Although physicians are responsible for writing fluid orders, nurses share in the responsibility for safe fluid replacement therapy. A major nursing responsibility is the provision of precise I&O records and daily weight charts. The accuracy of this information is crucial to correct formulation of fluid replacement regimens. In addition, nurses must share the responsibility for detecting undesirable trends in these data.

Parameters to be considered in assessment include the following:

▶ Comparison of I&O measurements
▶ Daily or more frequent body weights
▶ Vital signs
▶ Skin turgor
▶ Central venous pressure (CVP)
▶ Urinary specific gravity
▶ Laboratory values

The reader is referred to Chapter 2 for a review of these indices and to later chapters dealing with specific clinical conditions. Chapters 3 through 9 also present specific information regarding assessment of patients receiving parenteral fluids.

To summarize, giving the right amount of fluid depends on calculating measurable fluid losses, estimating insensible and third-space losses, factoring in the functional ability of key homeostatic organs, and revising fluid prescriptions according to current indicators of the patient's fluid and electrolyte status. Thus, standing fluid orders are never acceptable. For typical patients, fluid orders are readjusted every 24 hours. However, this is not sufficient for many critically ill patients whose fluid status is subject to rapid change. For these patients, it may be necessary to readjust fluid directives every 8 hours (or even more frequently).

Finally, as discussed in Chapter 10, care should be taken to ensure that fluids are delivered at the rate and volume prescribed. This requires careful and frequent monitoring of infusions. All fluids given parenterally must be recorded, including, for example, "keep-vein-open" (KVO) solutions and start-up solutions. Sometimes the intended minimal volume for KVO solutions is greatly exceeded, particularly if a macro-drip set is used instead of a micro-drip set. Failure to record these fluids can seriously confound understanding of I&O records and weight charts.

WATER AND ELECTROLYTE SOLUTIONS

Table 11-1 lists some commercially available water and electrolyte solutions. Examples of these fluids are discussed below.

DEXTROSE SOLUTIONS

Five percent dextrose in water (D_5W) is a roughly isotonic fluid given to provide free water. (Distilled water without additives cannot be infused IV because it would cause hemolysis of red blood cells as it entered the vein.)

The dextrose in D_5W is metabolized to carbon dioxide and water, leaving a solution physiologically equivalent to distilled water but without the hemolysis. Water given IV as D_5W is distributed evenly into every body compartment. For each liter of free water given IV, only approximately 80 mL remains in the intravascular space.[3] Thus, D_5W is used to replace deficits of total body water but is never used alone to expand the ECF volume. Too much D_5W can seriously dilute serum sodium, especially in a patient who has excess antidiuretic hormone (ADH) activity.

Dextrose and water solutions are also available in 2.5%, 10%, 20%, and 50% concentrations. Theoretically, because each gram of carbohydrate supplies 4

TABLE 11–1.
Contents of Selected Water and Electrolyte Solutions With Comments About Their Use

SOLUTION	COMMENTS
5% dextrose in water (D_5W): No electrolytes 50 g of dextrose	Supplies approximately 170 cal/L and free water to aid in renal excretion of solutes Should not be used in excessive volumes in patients with increased ADH activity or to replace fluids in hypovolemic patients
0.9% NaCl (isotonic saline): Na^+ 154 mEq/L Cl^- 154 mEq/L	Not desirable as a routine maintenance solution because it provides only Na^+ and Cl^-, which are provided in excessive amounts
0.45% NaCl (½-strength saline): Na^+ 77 mEq/L Cl^- 77 mEq/L	A hypotonic solution that provides Na^+, Cl^-, and free water Na^+ and Cl^- provided in fluid allows kidneys to select and retain needed amounts Free water desirable as aid to kidneys in elimination of solutes
0.33% NaCl (⅓-strength saline): Na^+ 56 mEq/L Cl^- 56 mEq/L	A hypotonic solution that provides Na^+, Cl^-, and free water Often used to treat hypernatremia (because this solution contains a small amount of Na^+, it dilutes the plasma sodium while not allowing it to drop too rapidly.)
3% NaCl: Na^+ 513 mEq/L Cl^- 513 mEq/L	Grossly hypertonic solutions used only to treat severe hyponatremia See Table 4-5 for summary of important nursing considerations in administration
5% NaCl: Na^+ 855 mEq/L Cl^- 855 mEq/L	Dangerous solutions
Lactated Ringer's solution: Na^+ 130 mEq/L K^+ 4 mEq/L Ca^{++} 3 mEq/L Cl^- 109 mEq/L Lactate (metabolized to bicarbonate) 28 mEq/L	A roughly isotonic solution that contains multiple electrolytes in approximately the same concentrations as found in plasma (Note that this solution is lacking in Mg and PO_4.) Used in the treatment of hypovolemia, burns, and fluid lost as bile or diarrhea Useful in treating mild metabolic acidosis
Other isotonic multiple electrolyte solutions: Plasma-Lyte 148 (Baxter) Isolyte S (McGaw) Normosol R (Abbott) Na^+ 140 mEq/L K^+ 5 mEq/L Mg^{++} 3 mEq/L Cl^- 98 mEq/L HCO_3 50 mEq/L (or equivalent)	Isotonic solution that can be used to replace ECF loss Because of relatively high bicarbonate content, can be used to correct mild acidosis
Hypotonic multiple electrolyte solutions: Plasma-Lyte 56 (Baxter) Normosol M (Abbott) Na^+ 40 mEq/L K^+ 13 mEq/L Mg^{++} 3 mEq/L Cl^- 40 mEq/L HCO_3 16 mEq/L (or equivalent)	Hypotonic solution that supplies free water as well as electrolytes
Sodium lactate solution, ⅙ M: Na^+ 167 mEq/L Cl^- 167 mEq/L	A roughly isotonic solution used to correct severe metabolic adidosis (lactate is metabolized to bicarbonate in 1–2 hr by the liver.) Not used in patients with liver disease (lactate cannot be converted to bicarbonate in such individuals); also, not used in patients with oxygen lack (unable to adequately convert lactate to bicarbonate)
Sodium bicarbonate, 5%: Na^+ 595 mEq/L Cl^- 595 mEq/L	A very hypertonic solution used to correct severe metabolic acidosis Should be cautiously administered at a slow rate, under careful volume control Should be administered only with extreme caution to salt-retaining patients (eg, those with cardiac, renal, or liver damage)
Ammonium chloride, 2.14%:	Acidifying solution used to correct severe metabolic alkalosis Due to high ammonium content, must be administered cautiously to patients with compromised hepatic function

calories, the 50 g in a liter of D₅W should supply 200 calories, and the 100 g in a liter of D₁₀W should supply 400 calories. However, because dextrose in parenteral solution provides only 3.4 calories per gram, a liter of D_5W provides 170 calories and a liter of $D_{10}W$ provides 340 calories. Although 50 or 100 g of dextrose is a small portion of an adult's daily caloric requirements, either amount is often enough to stave off the ketosis of starvation, which is why dextrose is often added to electrolyte solutions until the patient can assume oral intake. (Electrolytes have no calories.) As discussed in Chapter 12, a typical total parenteral nutrition (TPN) solution for central vein administration consists of 500 mL of 50% dextrose mixed with 500 mL of amino acid solution (for a net 25% dextrose solution). Because concentrated solutions of dextrose can cause hyperglycemia, they must be infused slowly.

As noted earlier in the chapter, dextrose is often added by commercial sources to electrolyte solutions to provide calories (for example, 5% dextrose in 0.9% NaCl, 5% dextrose in 0.45% NaCl, and 5% dextrose in lactated Ringer's solution).

SODIUM CHLORIDE SOLUTIONS

Isotonic Saline

Also called normal saline, a liter of isotonic saline (0.9% NaCl) contains 154 mEq of sodium and 154 mEq of chloride. Total cations (Na^+) and anions (Cl^-) amount to 308 mEq/L, an isotonic concentration. Solutions are considered roughly isotonic if the total electrolyte content (ie, anions plus cations) approximates 310 mEq/L; hypotonic if the total is less than 250 mEq/L; and hypertonic if electrolyte content exceeds 376 mEq/L. (These are arbitrary figures but are useful as a basis for comparing solutions.)

Although 0.9% sodium chloride is isotonic, it is not considered physiological. That is because extracellular fluid (ECF) normally contains 140 mEq/L of sodium and 103 mEq/L of chloride, amounts that are smaller and in different proportions than those in isotonic saline. Isotonic saline, therefore, imposes an appreciable load of chloride on the kidneys; if it cannot be excreted, hyperchloremic acidosis may follow.[4]

When infused IV, isotonic saline is distributed in the ECF compartment; none enters the intracellular fluid. One liter of isotonic saline adds 1 L to the ECF, theoretically expanding the plasma volume in the average adult by one fourth of a liter and the interstitial volume by three fourths of a liter.[5]

Isotonic saline is ideal for correcting ECF deficits in patients who have hyponatremia, hypochloremia, and metabolic alkalosis (such as patients with excessive vomiting or gastric suction loss). Because of its high

sodium content, however, the solution is used cautiously in patients whose renal or other regulatory mechanisms are compromised.

Half-Strength Saline (0.45% NaCl)

As its name implies, a liter of half-strength saline provides half the electrolytes found in a liter of isotonic saline: 77 mEq each of sodium and chloride. If this hypotonic solution is understood as a mixture of 500 mL of isotonic saline and 500 mL of free water, it is obvious why it is a good choice to provide some sodium to adjust serum levels plus free water to replace insensible losses. As pointed out earlier in the chapter, it is frequently used as a basic fluid for maintenance needs. It is also used to treat hypovolemic patients who have hypernatremia; that is, those who have more of a water than a solute deficit.

Other even more hypotonic sodium chloride solutions are available commercially. Examples of these are 0.11% NaCl (furnishing about 19 mEq/L each of sodium and chloride), 0.2% (34 mEq/L of each), 0.225% (39 mEq/L of each), and 0.33% (56 mEq/L of each). Excessive use of these hypotonic solutions can cause dilutional hyponatremia, especially in people who tend to retain water.

Hypertonic Saline

On rare occasions, hypertonic saline solutions (3% or 5% sodium chloride) are used to treat severe symptomatic hyponatremia. Small volumes are infused slowly and with great caution to avoid inducing a severe volume overload, and, with it, pulmonary edema. Patients with cardiovascular compromise or severe volume overload may need a diuretic to help remove hypotonic fluid as soon as the concentrated saline solution is infused.

Hypertonic saline should be used only in intensive care units because it requires frequent monitoring of blood pressure, central venous pressure, lung sounds, and serum sodium levels. The 3% solution provides 513 mEq/L of sodium and chloride; the 5% solution, 855 mEq/L of each. The reader is referred to Table 4-5 for a summary of important nursing considerations in the administration of hypertonic saline solutions.

BALANCED ELECTROLYTE SOLUTIONS

Numerous balanced electrolyte solutions are available commercially in a wide array of electrolyte combinations. Some are designed for maintenance needs, whereas others are formulated to replace specific body fluids. Each manufacturer usually affixes its own trade name to these solutions, making it necessary to refer to the label to review the specific content. One of the most frequently prescribed balanced solutions, lactated Ringer's, carries the same name regardless of the supplier.

Lactated Ringer's Solution

A liter of this commonly used fluid provides 130 mEq of sodium, 4 mEq of potassium, 3 mEq of calcium, 28 mEq of lactate, and 109 mEq of chloride. Lactated Ringer's solution (LR) contains 137 mEq/L each of cations and anions, for a total concentration of 274 mEq/L. This substitute for isotonic saline was developed to expand plasma volume while providing bicarbonate ions, as well as less chloride than isotonic saline.

Considered a near-physiological solution, the electrolyte content of LR is quite similar to that of plasma. It is often used to correct isotonic fluid volume deficits (as in hypovolemia due to third-space fluid shift after major trauma or surgery). Its chief, but minor, disadvantage is its slight hypoosmolarity; it furnishes 100 to 150 mL/L of free water.[6,7]

Because LR contains lactate that normally is quickly metabolized into bicarbonate, the solution can be used to treat many forms of metabolic acidosis. It can be dangerous to give LR to a patient who has lactic acidosis, however, because failure to convert lactate to bicarbonate can only make matters worse. Acetated Ringer's solution is a better choice for such patients. In that solution, lactate has been replaced with acetate, which can be metabolized by muscles and other peripheral tissues rather than by the liver.

POTASSIUM SOLUTIONS

Premixed potassium-replacement solutions are available in a variety of strengths furnishing from 10 to 40 mEq/L of potassium. Concentrated potassium solutions are available in ampules for addition to parenteral fluids (such as D_5W, 0.9% NaCl, or 0.45% NaCl). Of course, concentrated solutions from ampules are not meant for direct IV injection, which can result in fatal cardiac arrhythmias. See Table 5-6 for a list of critical points in administering potassium IV and Table 5-7 for a review of nursing considerations in emergency IV potassium administration.

MAGNESIUM ADMINISTRATION

Magnesium is not present in most routine IV solutions. However, it is found in some of the balanced electrolyte solutions (see Table 11-1). Magnesium is also available in concentrated form in ampules for addition to parenteral fluids when deemed necessary. The reader

is referred to Table 7-1 for a review of nursing considerations in administering IV magnesium solutions.

SOLUTIONS TO CORRECT ACID–BASE DISORDERS

Alkalinizing Solutions

Alkalinizing solutions (such as sodium lactate or sodium bicarbonate) are available to correct severe metabolic acidosis. A one sixth molar solution of sodium lactate supplies 167 mEq/L each of sodium and lactate; lactate is metabolized by the liver to bicarbonate. Sodium bicarbonate is available as a 5% solution, furnishing 595 mEq/L each of sodium and bicarbonate.[8] Some clinicians elect to mix their own solutions by adding one or more ampules of 7.5% $NaHCO_3$ (44.6 mEq/ampule) to existing parenteral fluids. As described in Chapter 9, controversy exists about when bicarbonate replacement is indicated in the treatment of acidosis. However, because severe acidosis can cause myocardial depression, it is generally recommended that parenteral bicarbonate be used to treat patients with acute metabolic acidosis and a lower pH than 7.2.[9] Bicarbonate therapy must be instituted cautiously because over-alkalinization can induce tetany, seizures, and cardiac arrhythmias. To avoid problems, bicarbonate therapy should cease when the pH reaches 7.2.[10] The use of sodium bicarbonate during cardiorespiratory arrest is discussed in Chapter 19.

Acidifying Solutions

When metabolic alkalosis is due to chloride deficiency, the use of isotonic saline (0.9% NaCl) may suffice as treatment. If hypokalemia is a contributing factor, potassium replacement is indicated.

Sometimes an ammonium chloride solution is prescribed, such as 2.14% ammonium chloride, supplying 400 mEq/L each of chloride and ammonium. However, this fluid is contraindicated with hepatic or renal insufficiency. Under no circumstance should more than 300 mEq/day of ammonium be given.[11]

In some situations, an isotonic solution of hydrochloric acid (150 mEq each of H^+ and Cl^- in 1 L of distilled water) is prescribed.[12] Because it is very corrosive, it is generally infused in a central line. Frequent monitoring of blood gases, pH, and serum electrolytes is indicated for patients receiving treatment for severe alkalosis.

COLLOIDS

In addition to the water and electrolyte solutions described above, patients with fluid and electrolyte disturbances may occasionally require treatment with colloids. Colloids are fluids containing proteins or starch molecules that remain uniformly distributed in fluid and do not form a true solution. Examples of colloids are albumin, plasma protein fraction, dextran, and hetastarch. After IV administration, colloid molecules remain in the vascular space for several days in patients with normal capillary endothelium. By increasing the osmotic pressure within the bloodstream, colloids draw in fluid to increase the intravascular volume.

ALBUMIN AND PLASMA PROTEIN FRACTION

Albumin and plasma protein fraction (PPF) are prepared from donor plasma. Because these products are subjected to an extended heating period during preparation, they do not transmit viral disease.[13] Normal human serum albumin (NHSA) is available as a 5% or 25% solution,* and plasma protein fraction is available as a 5% solution.† Five percent albumin solution is osmotically and oncotically equivalent to plasma, whereas the 25% solution is five times greater than that of plasma.[14]

Albumin provides about 80% of the plasma colloid osmotic pressure (COP) in normal adults.[15] Indications for use of 5% albumin solution can include restoration or maintenance of blood volume, emergency treatment of shock owing to acute blood loss after trauma or surgery, and treatment of hypovolemic shock caused by plasma rather than whole blood loss.[16] Indications for PPF use are similar to those for 5% albumin. However, the rapid administration of PPF (greater than 10 mL/min) has been associated with severe hypotensive episodes believed to be secondary to the presence of a vasoactive contaminant.[17] Although this reaction is rare, many institutions do not use PPF for bypass surgery, or at all.[18] When PPF is used, it should be administered slowly and the patient's vital signs monitored carefully.

In patients in whom there is clinical evidence of both edema and hypovolemia, the 25% albumin solution may expand the vascular volume by translocating fluid from the interstitial to the vascular space.[19] A 25% albumin solution may also be helpful in the treatment of patients with hypoproteinemic conditions, particularly when edema is present. Occasionally one still encounters references to "salt-poor" albumin. Actually, this is a misnomer. The name salt-poor originated from albumin products first produced during World War II

when a high sodium concentration (300 mEq/L) was necessary to preserve albumin solutions used by the military in hot climates. Thus, products with lesser concentrations of salt were designated salt-poor. However, with the development of better stabilizers, all albumin products were subsequently manufactured with lower amounts of sodium (130–160 mEq/L); since November 1977, all albumin products are required to contain this amount of sodium.[20]

In summary, indications for the use of albumin may include the following[21]:

▶ Nonhemorrhagic shock (total protein < 5.2 g/dL)
▶ Burns after the first 24 hours if hypoproteinemia develops
▶ Ascites (if hypotension develops after paracentesis)
▶ Acute/chronic hepatic failure (albumin should be used in combination with a diuretic to induce diuresis in fluid-overloaded patients) or when it is necessary to raise the blood pressure in acutely hypotensive patients
▶ Protein losing nephropathy/enteropathy (albumin should be used in combination with a diuretic to induce diuresis in fluid-overloaded patients)

Albumin will not correct chronic hypoalbuminemia and should not be used for this purpose. In addition, the only use for albumin in wound healing may be to reduce peripheral edema in a hypoproteinemic patient.[22] Under normal circumstances, administered albumin has a half-life of about 11 days.[23]

Reported side effects of albumin and plasma protein fraction include urticaria, flushing, chills, fever, and headache.[24] A history of allergic reactions to these products is a contraindication to their use. Albumin and plasma protein fraction should be used with caution in patients likely to develop fluid overload.

It is not necessary to do compatibility testing for albumin and plasma protein fractions because there are no ABO blood group antigens or antibodies present. The desired dosage varies greatly according to the reason for administration. For this reason, 5% albumin solutions are available in 250-mL, 500-mL, and 1000-mL bottles, and 25% albumin solutions are available in 20-mL, 50-mL, and 100-mL containers. Neither albumin nor plasma protein fraction must be given through a filter.[25] As discussed earlier, it is recommended that the infusion rate of PPF not exceed 10 mL/min.[26]

DEXTRAN AND HETASTARCH

Other colloid substitutes used for volume expansion include dextran and hetastarch (hydroxyethyl starch). These substances are not derived from donor plasma and are thus relatively nontoxic and inexpensive. They

---

*These include Albuminar-5 and Albuminar-25, Albutein 5% & 25%, Buminate 5% & 25%, Plasbumin-5 and Plasbumin-25.
† These include Plasmanate, Plasma Plex, Plasmatein, and Protenate.

also require no compatibility testing and are free of the risk of transfusion-related diseases.[27]

Dextrans

Dextrans are polysaccharides that behave as colloids; they are available as low-molecular-weight dextran (dextran 40)* and high-molecular-weight dextran (dextran 70).† Dextran 70 is more effective than dextran 40 as a substitute for plasma because its molecular weight (70,000) more closely resembles that of albumin (50,000–250,000).[28] Dextran 70 is available as a 6% solution of dextran in isotonic saline; the administration rate is variable, depending on the indication for its use, present blood volume, and patient response. Dextran 40 is available as a 10% dextran solution in either isotonic saline or D_5W and has some advantages over dextran 70.[29] For example, resuscitation of patients with dextran 40 increases microcirculatory flow because of reduced red cell sludging.[30]

The incidence of anaphylactoid reaction after dextran infusion has been estimated at 5.3%.[31] Initial signs include subjective discomfort quickly followed by severe abdominal discomfort, vomiting, and diarrhea.[32] Other reactions include angioneurotic edema and urticaria. Because dextrans are contained in some foods and parenteral drugs, the patient may have been sensitized although no prior dextran infusions were received.[33]

Another complication associated with dextran is interference with blood coagulation, which increases the risk for bleeding. To minimize this risk, the recommended dose approved for clinical use in the United States is limited to 20 mL/kg of body weight over a 24-hour period.[34]

If it is necessary to draw blood for typing and cross-matching, it should be done before dextran is started. If this is not possible, the laboratory should be notified that dextran is in use.

During the administration of dextran, it is important to monitor pulse, blood pressure, central venous pressure, and urine output every 5 to 15 minutes for the first hour and then hourly thereafter as indicated.[35] Because it expands the plasma volume, dextran should be used cautiously in patients with heart or renal disease, and in others prone to fluid retention (such as those taking steroids). Dextran is contraindicated in patients with severe bleeding disorders, known hypersensitivity to dextran, severe congestive heart failure, and renal failure.

These include 10% dextran 40, 10% Gentran 40, 10% LMD, and Rheomacrodex 10%.
†*These include 6% dextran 70, 6% dextran 75, 6% Gentran 70, and Macrodex 6%.*

Hetastarch

Hetastarch (hydroxyethyl starch) is a synthetic colloid made from starch. It is available commercially under the trade name Hespan as a 6% solution, diluted in isotonic saline, in 500-mL containers.

The plasma volume expansion properties of hetastarch approximate those of 5% human albumin. Clinically, hetastarch continues to expand the plasma volume for an interval ranging from 24 to 36 hours.[36] Like dextran, hetastarch is not a substitute for blood in patients requiring blood components.

The properties that make hetastarch desirable as a plasma volume expander are the ones that contribute to some of its potential hazards (circulatory overload, dilutional hypoproteinemia, and lowering of the hematocrit). Because of its plasma volume expansion properties, hetastarch should be used cautiously in patients with heart and renal disease or other conditions predisposing to fluid retention. It is contraindicated in patients with severe bleeding disorders, severe congestive heart failure, and anuric or oliguric renal failure.[37]

Like dextran, hetastarch may alter the coagulation mechanism. More specifically, hetastarch may result in transient prolongation of prothrombin, partial thromboplastin, and clotting times. Because it is primarily eliminated by the kidney, hetastarch should not be used in patients with renal failure. During administration of hetastarch, monitor pulse, blood pressure, CVP, and urine output every 5 to 15 minutes for the first hour and then hourly thereafter as indicated.[38] Also, be alert for an allergic reaction, although the incidence of anaphylactoid reaction is small ($<1\%$ in a clinical study encompassing 16,045 infusions).[39]

When administered for its plasma volume expansion properties, the total dosage and rate of infusion of hetastarch depend on the amount of blood or plasma lost. For adults, the amount usually infused is 500 to 1000 mL. Hespan doses greater than 1500 mL for the typical adult patient are not usually required.[40] One of the main advantages of hetastarch is its cost (about half that of human plasma).[41]

FLUID AND ELECTROLYTE DISTURBANCES ASSOCIATED WITH BLOOD TRANSFUSIONS

Principal indications for blood transfusion are to correct diminished oxygen-carrying capacity of the blood, to replace hemostatic components, or to replenish or expand the circulating intravascular volume. Although blood transfusion can be life saving when indicated, it should not be undertaken lightly because there are a number of inherent risks with the transfusion process. Among these are immune mediated reactions to the transfused substances, infections (such as malaria, hepatitis, and acquired immunodeficiency syndrome), and fluid/electrolyte/acid–base disturbances. Only the latter is discussed in this chapter.

Chemical and physical changes in blood are brought about by preservatives and prolonged storage. These changes in stored blood can cause electrolyte problems and other related complications.

HYPERKALEMIA

Continual destruction of red blood cells occurs when blood is stored; the plasma potassium level increases to 12, 18, and 22 mEq/L at, respectively, 1, 2, and 3 weeks of storage.[42] Potassium is released from the destroyed red blood cells and is also transferred from intact red blood cells into the surrounding plasma. This leakage of potassium is related to loss of cell membrane integrity resulting from hypoxia.

When the stored blood is infused into the recipient, the blood cells are reoxygenated and take up the leaked potassium; however, before this occurs, there can be a transient hyperkalemia if blood administration is extremely rapid. Hyperkalemia is accentuated in patients with metabolic acidosis, renal dysfunction, or both.

Note that *hypo*kalemia can occur as the red blood cells are reoxygenated and take up the potassium they previously leaked out during storage.

HYPOCALCEMIA

Citrate-phosphate-dextrose (CPD)–preserved bank blood contains excessive citrate ions. In some situations, the excess citrate may combine with ionized calcium in the recipient's blood, producing a deficiency of ionized calcium. (Recall that it is ionized calcium that controls neuromuscular irritability.) However, the excess citrate usually causes no difficulty because the liver rapidly converts it to bicarbonate. Another safeguard to protect the body from hypocalcemia is the rapid mobilization of calcium from bone when needed.

Although calcium deficiency caused by administration of citrated blood is rare, it can occur in the following patients:

1. Infants receiving exchange transfusions
2. Adults with severe liver disease
3. Patients with inadequate bone stores (such as young children, elderly or osteoporotic patients, those with bony tumors, or those who have been bedridden for 8 to 10 weeks)[43]
4. Normal adults given rapid transfusions

In the past it was believed that an adult could tolerate the excess citrate in a unit of blood given at a rate of 6 units/hour.[44] However, there are indications that patients with preexisting myocardial disease may experience a fall of cardiac output secondary to reduction in ionized calcium after citrated blood transfusions.[45] Citrate intoxication can cause bradycardia, arrhythmias, and hypotension. If transfusion rates in 4 hours or less are as high as 3 to 5 units of whole blood, or 5 to 8 units of packed red blood cells, calcium gluconate administration is indicated.[46] If the patient is fully digitalized, the dose of calcium should be decreased because calcium and digitalis are synergistic.

ACID–BASE CHANGES

The *p*H of 2- to 3-week-old bank blood falls to approximately 6.9 (due to leakage of lactate and pyruvate into the plasma as a result of red cell hypoxia during storage).[47] The decreased *p*H of stored blood usually has no markedly adverse effects on healthy adults because it is diluted by the patient's own blood. However, development of metabolic acidosis is theoretically possible if aged blood is transfused rapidly.

Also, rapid transfusion of citrate preserved blood in patients with preexisting acidosis (such as premature infants with respiratory problems) can make the acidosis more severe. Patients with preexisting acidosis who are to receive rapid transfusions (such as 1 unit of blood every 20 minutes or faster) may require the administration of sodium bicarbonate. It is not necessary to treat acidosis unless the *p*H is less than 7.25 since the citrate preservative will be metabolized to bicarbonate after 12 to 18 hours.[48]

Although an initial metabolic acidosis may occur during rapid transfusion, metabolic alkalosis may eventually result due to metabolism of citrate to bicarbonate. (Each unit of CPD blood eventually generates 22.8 mEq of bicarbonate.)[49] The alkalosis rarely requires treatment.

It is wise to monitor the patient's *p*H during multiple blood transfusions to detect acid–base imbalances requiring therapy.

HYPERAMMONEMIA

Ammonia concentration in stored blood increases to 280, 420, and 520 μg/dL after 1, 2, and 3 weeks of storage, respectively.[50] Normal patients can tolerate the extra ammonia with no difficulty; however, patients with severe liver disease should be given blood not more than 5 to 7 days old, or red blood cells that have been resuspended in serum albumin or Ringer's acetate solution before infusion.[51]

FLUID VOLUME OVERLOAD

Fluid volume overload and congestive heart failure are frequent complications of blood transfusions. The onset of circulatory overload is usually gradual, with symptoms becoming more severe as the transfusion continues. Symptoms include cough, shortness of breath, neck vein distention, and pulmonary congestion. Many physicians request monitoring of CVP during rapid blood administration. (The procedure for CVP measurement is described in Chapter 2.) More extensive hemodynamic monitoring may be required for patients with cardiac disease.

Individuals with compromised cardiovascular status should be monitored especially closely for fluid volume overload. Instead of whole blood, packed red blood cells (PRBC) are frequently used for such patients to reduce the volume of the infusion (recall that packed cells are obtained by centrifuging whole blood and drawing off approximately 200–225 mL of plasma). Although PRBC have a reduced plasma volume, it is necessary to use a slow infusion rate for high risk patients. At times it may be necessary to ask the blood bank to split a unit of PRBC into two containers and administer each half unit over 4 hours. Prophylactic diuretic therapy (such as 10–20 mg IV furosemide) may also be helpful in the management of these patients.[52]

CRYSTALLOID VERSUS COLLOID RESUSCITATION

In review, crystalloids are electrolyte solutions with the potential to form crystals capable of diffusing through capillary endothelium and becoming distributed throughout the components' extracellular compartment. Because the vascular fluid makes up 25% of the ECF, only 25% of any administered crystalloid will remain in the vascular space. In contrast, colloids remain in the vascular space for several days in patients with normal capillary endothelium. However, in the presence of damaged capillaries, colloids leak out into the tissues.

The long-standing controversy continues regarding which type of therapy (crystalloid versus colloid) is superior in the fluid resuscitation of hypovolemic critically ill patients. When the patient requires the oxygen-carrying capacity of red blood cells, or the hemostatic properties imparted by platelets or coagulation proteins, the appropriate blood obviously should be administered. However, when the choice involves replacement of the circulating volume under circumstances in which there is no documented need for blood, the controversy as to which type of fluid to choose for volume expansion arises (water and electrolyte solutions, such as lactated Ringers or isotonic sodium chloride; or colloids, such as albumin or hetastarch). Rationales for both types of fluids are discussed below.

It is generally agreed that, although colloid solutions are more expensive, they act more promptly than crystalloids to restore hemodynamic stability; it is also generally agreed that crystalloid solutions are more readily available and handier to use, but that much larger volumes are needed to achieve the needed response. In fact, it is necessary to give three to four times as much crystalloid solution to achieve the same plasma volume expansion as albumin.[53] This could induce salt overload, peripheral edema, weight gain, and reduced oncotic pressure. Theoretically, based on Starling's law of fluid movement across a semipermeable membrane, excessive volumes of crystalloids might accumulate in the pulmonary interstitium because of a reduction in the colloid oncotic pressure–pulmonary capillary wedge pressure gradient. However, authorities disagree as to the clinical significance of this phenomenon. Some point out that colloids may also extravasate into the interstitial space if there are damaged capillaries (endothelial leakiness). Protein-rich interstitial fluid can accumulate in the lungs and other tissues, causing adult respiratory distress syndrome and organ failure.[54]

Proponents of crystalloids emphasize that clinical and experimental studies generally indicate that balanced salt solutions are satisfactory for volume replacement, and that they are far less expensive than colloids.[55] For example, Lowe et al[56] reported no difference with regard to survival or incidence of pulmonary problems in randomized trials of crystalloid versus colloid therapy in acutely ill patients. Virgiolo et al[57] found crystalloids easier to use than colloids. In 1988, the cost of 25 grams of normal serum human albumin or 250 mL of plasma protein fraction in one American hospital was $88, compared with $22 for a liter of lactated Ringer's solution.[58] Proponents of crystalloids cite a number of studies that support their beliefs.

Proponents of colloids believe that these fluids are a better alternative to massive infusions of saline solutions in shock and other acute illness because they restore plasma volume without the excessive salt and water administration that leads to pulmonary edema from overexpanded interstitial fluid.[59] Prospective clinical trials conducted over several years in a surgical emergency department by Shoemaker et al[60] indicated that colloid fluids were associated with reduced resuscitation time, reduced mean arterial pressure time deficit, and fewer resuscitation-related complications.

As indicated above, medical research findings exist to support both schools of thought, and the controversy is likely to continue. A recent nursing study compared crystalloid therapy to colloid therapy in postoperative cardiac patients.[61] Differences in hemodynamic stability and fluid requirements were examined in patients randomly assigned to receive either normal saline (crystalloid solution, N = 10) or hetastarch (colloid solution, N = 11) after coronary artery bypass or valve operation. It was found that the patients who received colloids had reduced fluid requirements, superior hemodynamic performance, and shortened intensive care stay when compared with those given crystalloid resuscitation.

The patient's underlying clinical problem also has a substantial influence on the type of fluid resuscitation that should be administered in a given situation. The reader is referred to specific clinical chapters for further discussion of fluid resuscitation recommendations.

REFERENCES

1. Pestana C: Fluids and Electrolytes in the Surgical patient, 4th ed, p 8 and 9. Baltimore, Williams & Wilkins, 1989
2. Dunagan W, Ridner M: Manual of Medical Therapeutics, 26th ed, p 53. Boston, Little, Brown, 1989
3. Sommer M: Fluid resuscitation following multiple trauma. Crit Care Nurs 10(10):74, 1990
4. Shires GT (ed): Fluids, Electrolytes and Acid–Bases, p 17. New York, Churchill Livingstone, 1988
5. Smith E, Brain E: Fluids and Electrolytes: A Conceptual Approach, p 155. New York, Churchill Livingstone, 1980
6. Shires, p 17
7. Maxwell M, Kleeman C, Narins R: Clinical Disorders of Fluid and Electrolyte Metabolism, 4th ed, p 908. New York, McGraw-Hill, 1987
8. Pestana, p 20
9. Dunagan, Ridner, p 65
10. Ibid, p 66
11. Ibid, p 70
12. Rose B: Clinical Physiology of Acid–Base and Electrolyte Disorders, 3rd ed, p 495. New York, McGraw-Hill, 1989
13. Pisciotto P (ed): Blood Transfusion Therapy, 3rd ed, p 34. Arlington, VA, American Association of Blood Banks, 1989
14. Ibid, p 14
15. Falk J, Rackow E, Weil M: Colloid and crystalloid fluid resuscitation. In: Shoemaker W, Ayres S, Grenvik A, Holbrook P, Thompson W (eds): Textbook of Critical Care, 2nd ed, p 1061. Philadelphia: WB Saunders, 1989
16. Rutman R, Miller W: Transfusion Therapy: Principles and Procedures, 2nd ed, p 43. Rockville, MD, Aspen, 1985
17. Ibid, p 44
18. Ibid, p 306
19. Falk et al, p 1061
20. Finlayson J: The birth and demise of "salt-poor" albumin. Am J Hosp Pharm 35:898, 1978
21. Pisciotto, p 35
22. Ibid

23. Kokko J, Tannen R: Fluids and Electrolytes, 2nd ed, p 1004. Philadelphia, WB Saunders, 1990
24. Pisciotto, p 35
25. Ibid, p 35
26. Pestano, p 51
27. Pisciotto, p 36
28. Pestano, p 52
29. Falk et al, p 1063
30. Ibid
31. Thompson W: Rational use of albumin and plasma substitutes. Johns Hopkins Med J 136:220, 1975
32. Falk et al, p 1064
33. Ibid
34. Ibid
35. Gahart, p 174
36. Falk et al, p 1062
37. Gahart, p 175
38. Ibid
39. Ring J, Messner K: Incidence and severity of anaphylactoid reaction to colloid volume substitutes. Lancet i:466, 1977
40. Physicians' Desk Reference, 44th ed, p 197. Oradell NJ, Medical Economics Company, 1990
41. Pestana, p 53
42. Pisciotto, p 5
43. Condon R, Nyhus L: Manual of Surgical Therapeutics, 7th ed, p 259. Boston, Little, Brown, 1988
44. Ibid, p 258
45. Ibid
46. Ibid
47. Pisciotto, p 9
48. Condon, Nyhus, p 260
49. Rutman, Miller, p 291
50. Pisciotto, p 5
51. Condon, Nyhus, p 260
52. Dunagan, Ridner, p 356
53. Walker A, Condon R: Peritonitis and intraabdominal abscesses. In: Schwartz S, Shires G, Spencer F (eds): Principles of Surgery, 5th ed, p 1471. New York, McGraw-Hill, 1989
54. Ibid
55. Shires G, Canizaro P, Carrico J Shock: In: Schwartz S, Shires G, Spencer F (eds): Principles of Surgery, 5th ed, p 158. New York, McGraw-Hill, 1989
56. Lowe et al: Crystalloid vs colloid in the etiology of pulmonary failure after trauma: A randomized trial in man. Surgery 81:676, 1977
57. Virgilio et al: Crystalloid vs colloid resuscitation: Is one better? Surgery 85:129, 1979
58. Casey M: Hypovolemic shock following multiple trauma. In: Sommers M (ed): Difficult Diagnoses in Critical Care Nursing. Rockville, MD, Aspen, 1989
59. Shoemaker W: Fluids and electrolytes in the acutely ill adult. In: Shoemaker et al (eds): Textbook of Critical Care, 2nd ed, p 1138. Philadelphia, WB Saunders, 1989
60. Shoemaker et al: Comparison of the relative effectiveness of colloids and crystalloids in emergency resuscitation. Am J Surg 142:73, 1981
61. Ley et al: Crystalloid versus colloid fluid therapy after cardiac surgery. Heart Lung 19:31, 1990

12

---

*Parenteral Nutrition**

This chapter reviews the effects of parenteral nutrition on fluid and electrolyte balance and describes the nurse's role in caring for patients with imbalances and other metabolic abnormalities caused by this treatment. As a basis for discussion, the indications for parenteral nutrition, characteristics of parenteral nutrients, and nutritional assessment are briefly reviewed.

---

* The opinions or assertions contained herein are the private views of the author and are not to be construed as official or as reflecting the views of the Department of the Army or the Department of Defense.

INDICATIONS FOR PARENTERAL NUTRITION

It is possible to supply all of a patient's essential nutrients and establish positive nitrogen balance via the parenteral route. Parenteral nutrition (sometimes referred to as total parenteral nutrition [TPN]) is often used for patients with hypermetabolic states such as trauma, sepsis, and thermal injury. It may also be indicated for conditions requiring "resting" of the intestines (such as Crohn's disease or intestinal fistulas). In general, TPN is of limited value when the gastrointestinal (GI) tract is expected to be usable within 7 to

10 days in a well-nourished patient with minimal stress and trauma or in the immediate postoperative or post-stress period.[1] Whenever possible, enteral feedings should be favored over parenteral feedings because the enteral route is more physiologically normal.

NUTRITIONAL ASSESSMENT

Determining the patient's nutritional status by practical, objective measures remains a scientific challenge. The markedly undernourished patient can usually be identified by observation alone. However, clinical history and physical examination are needed to determine the nutritional status of other patients. Parameters to consider in obtaining the patient's history and performing the physical examination are listed in Tables 12-1 and 12-2. Because signs and symptoms associated with nutritional deficiencies suggest biochemical changes at the cellular level, they should prompt immediate provision of nutritional support.

The nurse should be aware of the patient's estimated nutritional requirements. Traditionally, dietitians have provided estimates of these requirements. See Table 12-3 for a summary of calculation of nutrient requirements. In patients with wounds, excessive ostomy

TABLE 12–1.
Clinical History

I. Medical history
  A. Analyze body weight changes
    1. Compare usual weight with current and ideal weight to determine weight loss or gain (use standard tables of weights based on sex and body frame size for comparison)
    2. Consider state of hydration when interpreting weight
       a. If fluid resuscitation has occurred, weight will be falsely elevated
       b. If dehydration or unusual body fluid losses have occurred, weight will be falsely decreased
  B. Determine if any increased metabolic needs exist over basal energy expenditure
    1. Postoperative period increases needs for nutrients by 2% to 5%
    2. Peritonitis increases need for nutrients by greater than 5%
    3. Severe infection, long-bone fractures, and other trauma increase need for nutrients by 10%
    4. Burns may increase need for nutrients by 40% to 70%
  C. Identify any chronic diseases that may affect nutrient intake or metabolic needs
    1. Malabsorption syndromes may lead to deficiencies in protein, vitamins, and trace minerals
    2. Dyspnea associated with chronic obstructive pulmonary disease may cause patients with this condition to consume inadequate nutrients
  D. Identify past surgical history that may alter current nutrient intake and use
    1. Gastrojejunostomy, esophagogastrectomy, gastrectomy
    2. Surgical intervention for morbid obesity (gastro-jejunal bypass, stapling procedures, balloon procedures)

  E. Identify increased losses
    1. Draining wounds, fistulas, abscesses, effusions
    2. Chronic blood loss
    3. Dialysis
  F. Consider other factors
    1. Pregnancy, recent childbirth
    2. Recent major surgery
    3. Recent acute illness
    4. Prolonged comatose state
    5. Age
    6. Current level of physical activity
    7. Drug, alcohol, tobacco use
    8. Use of medications on a chronic basis
    9. Use of over-the-counter medications (eg, antacids and laxatives that may lead to depletion of vitamins and minerals)
II. Social history
  A. Consider factors that may affect nutrient intake
    1. Income
    2. Education
    3. Ethnic background
    4. Religion
    5. Who purchases food and prepares meals
    6. Environment during mealtime
III. Dietary history
  A. Consider factors that may alter food intake
    1. Intolerance to certain foods
    2. Fad diets
    3. Dietary modifications secondary to chronic diseases
       a. Sodium restriction for cardiac disease
       b. Protein, electrolyte restriction for renal, liver disease
    4. Poor appetite
    5. Poor dentition or ill-fitting dentures
    6. Chewing and swallowing difficulties
    7. Alterations in smell and taste
    8. Frequent NPO orders for tests, radiographs, bowel preparation
    9. Inability to feed self

(Adapted from Curtis S: Nutritional Assessment. In: Caldwell-Kennedy C, Guenter P [eds]: Nutritional Support Nursing: Core Curriculum. Silver Spring, MD, American Society for Parenteral and Enteral Nutrition, 1988)

TABLE 12–2.
Physical Assessment

I. Hair changes associated with protein-calorie malnutrition
A. Lackluster
B. Thinness, sparseness
C. Pigmentation changes
D. Easy pluckability (inspect comb, pillow, and bed for hair)

II. Lip changes
A. Angular stomatitis
  1. Associated with deficiencies of one or more B vitamins
  2. Cracks, redness at corners of mouth
  3. May result in scars when healed
B. Cheilosis
  1. Associated with riboflavin and niacin deficiency
  2. Vertical cracks in lips

III. Tongue changes
A. Most changes associated with deficiencies of one or more B vitamins
B. May change color (eg, become purplish red or beefy red)
C. Fissures
D. May be painful and hypersensitive, with burning
E. Atrophy of taste buds; tongue may appear smooth and pale

IV. Skin changes
A. Consider general characteristics of skin (dryness and flakiness may be associated with deficiency of vitamin A, essential fatty acids)
B. Petechiae
  1. Hemorrhagic spots on skin at pressure points
  2. May occur in presence of liver disease or during anticoagulation
  3. Associated with deficiencies of vitamins C and K

(Adapted from Curtis S: Nutritional Assessment. In: Caldwell-Kennedy C, Guenter P [eds]: Nutritional Support Nursing: Core Curriculum. Silver Spring, MD, American Society for Parenteral and Enteral Nutrition, 1988)

losses, or decubitus ulcers, the need for extra vitamins and zinc should be evaluated. Likewise, patients with a history of alcohol or tobacco use may require additional B vitamins and ascorbic acid.

The potential metabolic consequences of drug–nutrient interactions should be considered during the initial nutritional and daily patient assessment. All daily requirements for sodium, potassium, calcium, phosphorus, and magnesium are generally supplied in the TPN solution. However, when drugs that provide additional minerals are given, the electrolyte content of the TPN solution must be altered accordingly. For example, the magnesium content of the TPN solution may need changing to accommodate the renal failure patient's need for a magnesium-containing antacid. Patients receiving diuretics will likely need increased amounts of magnesium, potassium, sodium, and zinc

added to the TPN solution to cover urinary losses of these substances. Individuals who continue to consume alcohol or use tobacco may require additional calories and vitamin supplementation.

Hospitalized patients often have an altered metabolic milieu that induces or exacerbates malnutrition. Stress and infection exaggerate the alterations in protein, carbohydrate, and mineral metabolism associated with starvation. For example, infection increases nitrogen loss, decreases synthesis of albumin and transferrin, increases blood sugar by augmenting gluconeogenesis and causing insulin resistance, and increases losses of magnesium, potassium, and phosphorus.[4] Return to normal metabolic responses may occur only after resolution of the underlying medical condition. Although nutritional support is a critical adjunctive therapy, it must be planned in relation to the interaction between the nutrients being delivered in the parenteral nutrition and the altered metabolism of endogenous nutrients, electrolytes, and minerals.

Findings identified from the history, physical examination, and the estimation of the patient's nutritional requirements should guide the plan for medical and nursing interventions.

NUTRIENT REQUIREMENTS

PROTEIN

Proteins have varied and essential roles as enzymes, cellular components, immunoglobulins, and visceral muscle. Synthesis and degradation of protein is a dynamic process that allows the body's protein needs to be met during normal and stressed metabolic circumstances. During brief starvation, protein (nitrogen) excretion is increased in the urine. Negative nitrogen balance generally indicates inadequate caloric intake to meet energy requirements. (Nitrogen balance is the difference between nitrogen intake and output.)

Gluconeogenesis (the conversion of protein to glucose to meet energy requirements) occurs during starvation; unfortunately, the metabolic processes involved with gluconeogenesis consume a significant amount of the energy produced by this biological response. Protein is wasted in the urine and/or the urea pool is increased (as reflected by an elevated serum blood urea nitrogen). If starvation is prolonged or the patient experiences stress or infection, the body will try to conserve body mass by decreasing protein loss.

Provision of adequate glucose calories is essential to prevent burning of infused proteins (in the form of amino acids) for energy. The caloric value obtained from amino acids is not considered in the TPN regi-

TABLE 12–3.
Calculation of Nutrient Requirements

For the depleted patient, use the ideal body weight to compute nutritional requirements. Use the current weight for patients at ideal weight or higher. Optimal weight gain during nutritional support is 0.5 to 1.0 kg (1.1–2.2 lbs) per week. This can be achieved by giving additional 500 kcal/day in addition to calculated caloric requirements. Ideal body weight for height can be calculated by the following formulas:

Ideal male weight = 50 kg (1st 5 ft) + 2.7 kg/inch over 5 feet
Ideal female weight = 45.5 kg (1st 5 ft) + 1.8 kg/inch over 5 feet

Caloric requirements

The Harris-Benedict equation with additives, as recommended by Long et al,[2] can be used to calculate caloric requirements:

Men = [66.47 + (13.75 W) + (5.0 H) − (6.76 A)] × (AF) × (IF)
Women = [65.10 + (9.56 W) + (1.8 H) − (4.68 A)] × (AF) × (IF)

Where W = weight in kg, H = height in cm, A = age in years, AF = activity factor, IF = injury factor.

Activity factor, use		Injury factor, use	
A. Confined to bed	1.20	A. Minor operation	1.20
B. Out of bed	1.30	B. Skeletal trauma	1.35
		C. Major sepsis	1.60
		D. Severe thermal burn	2.10
		E. Closed head injury	1.60
		F. Intravenous steroids	1.30–1.60

Protein requirements

Range is 0.8 to 2.0 g/kg body weight:

Normal	0.8–1.0 g/kg body weight
Moderate Stress	1.0–1.5 g/kg body weight
Severe Stress	1.5–2.0 g/kg body weight

Consider using 0.8 g protein/kg initially until nitrogen balance data can be obtained. Protein calories should not be included in calculations of total caloric intake.

Fat requirements

Approximately 30% of nonprotein calories should be given as fat. A minimum of 4% of nonprotein calories must be given as fat to meet linoleic acid requirements and avoid essential fatty acid deficiency.

Trace elements and vitamin requirements

Trace elements and vitamins are added to total parenteral nutrition solutions in accordance with current guidelines.[3]

men because it is assumed that the amino acids will be incorporated into the cells.

The proportion and quantity of each amino acid within a parenteral formulation can be manipulated to suit specific disease states. For example, solutions containing branched-chain amino acids may be used for patients with hepatic encephalopathy. Special formulations may also be helpful for trauma and stress patients.

GLUCOSE

Glucose (dextrose) is the primary carbohydrate used in parenteral nutrition solutions. It is the preferred source of readily available energy for cellular activity. The dextrose used in TPN solutions is hydrated with a caloric yield of 3.4 kcal/g. (The osmolality and caloric content of various dextrose solutions are given in Table

TABLE 12–4.
Caloric Content and Osmolality of Dextrose Solutions*

DEXTROSE CONCENTRATIONS (%)	kcal/mL	OSMOLALITY
5.0	0.17	252
7.5	0.25	378
10.0	0.34	505
12.5	0.42	631
15.0	0.51	758
20.0	0.68	1010
25.0	0.85	1263
30.0	1.02	1515

* Each gram of glucose (dextrose) provides 3.4 kcal.

12-4.) It is important to deliver most of the patient's calories as dextrose and fat to prevent gluconeogenesis. Recall that gluconeogenesis (conversion of protein to carbohydrate) uses metabolic energy, thus decreasing the net benefit of the calories provided from the glucose in the TPN solution. Glucose is also necessary for normal metabolism of fat.

FAT

Fat is a required nutrient that supplies essential fatty acids needed to maintain the structural integrity of cellular membranes. It is an excellent source of calories. Compared with protein and carbohydrates, which yield 4 kcal/g, fat yields 9 kcal/g. Fat emulsions best tolerated for parenteral administration are those containing a base of either soybean or safflower oil. These emulsions are available as 10% and 20% emulsions and provide 1.1 and 2.0 kcal/mL, respectively.

For proper fat oxidation, adequate glucose intake must be assured. Incomplete fat oxidation results in the production of ketone bodies and can produce acidosis. This is not generally a problem once the patient is receiving glucose from the TPN solution. Although precise requirements are controversial, provision of 30% to 60% of the daily nonprotein calories as fat emulsions is believed to spare protein.[5]

VITAMINS

Water-soluble vitamins are stored in small amounts or not at all, and constant supplementation during parenteral nutrition is required to prevent deficiency syndromes. Fat soluble vitamins (A, D, E, and K) are provided according to individual need.

MINERALS

Mineral requirements during parenteral nutrition vary widely with the patient's underlying disease process and current clinical status. For example, daily sodium requirements may range from 50 to 250 mEq, potassium from 30 to 200 mEq, magnesium from 10 to 30 mEq, calcium from 10 to 20 mEq, and phosphorus from 10 to 40 mmol.[6] Variations in need for potassium and phosphorus are closely related to changes in cellular flux during glucose infusion and from reversal of the catabolic state to an anabolic state. Because deficiency states of trace elements (zinc, chromium, copper, manganese, iodine, selenium, and molybdenum) are possible in TPN patients (particularly those receiving long-term infusions), it is necessary to consider these substances as supplements. Most centers routinely add zinc, copper, chromium, manganese, and iodine to TPN solutions; some centers also provide iron, selenium, and occasionally molybdenum for patients requiring long-term TPN.[7]

NUTRIENT SOLUTIONS

TYPICAL TPN SOLUTION

An example of a typical TPN solution is presented in Table 12-5. However, remember that individual needs may necessitate varying any or all of the components. The solution is prepared by a pharmacist under a laminar-flow hood to maintain strict sterility. Usually,

TABLE 12–5.
Example of a Typical 1-L Total Parenteral Nutrition Solution for Adults

Dextrose, 25%	(500 mL of 50% dextrose solution)
Amino acids, 4.25%	(500 mL of 8.5% amino acid solution)

Electrolytes (includes electrolyte content of amino acid solution)[8]

Sodium	35 mEq
Potassium	30 mEq
Chloride	35 mEq
Magnesium	5 mEq
Calcium	5 mEq
Phosphate	15 mmol
Acetate	70 mEq

Vitamins
  MVI-12 (10 mL/day)

Trace element solution
  1–5 mL/day

Other additives as indicated

500 mL of a 50% dextrose solution is added to 500 mL of an 8.5% amino acid solution for a final concentration of 25% dextrose and 4.25% amino acids. Electrolytes, trace elements, vitamins, and other substances are added according to need.

FAT EMULSIONS

Fat emulsions made from soybean or safflower oil (or a combination of the two) are available as 10% and 20% emulsions providing 1.1 and 2.0 kcal/mL, respectively. The only advantage of a 20% solution is its lower fluid volume for a given caloric yield. Because fat emulsions have a low osmotic pressure (260–340 mOsm/L), they are suitable for either central or peripheral administration.

METABOLIC DERANGEMENTS ASSOCIATED WITH TPN

GLUCOSE ABNORMALITIES

Hyperglycemia

Hyperglycemia is the most common metabolic derangement caused by TPN. For example, one prospective study of 100 patients receiving parenteral nutrition found that 47 had serum glucose concentrations greater than 300 mg/dL.[9] Causes of hyperglycemia include too rapid or uneven administration of the high dextrose solution, increased levels of stress hormones associated with a number of illness and injury states, or both. To prevent hyperglycemia from becoming severe, infuse the TPN solution cautiously while closely monitoring for glucose intolerance. Also, remember that the development or worsening of a glucose intolerance may be a harbinger of sepsis or other complicating condition (such as myocardial infarction).

Uncontrolled hyperglycemia can lead to hyperosmotic hyperglycemia nonketotic coma (HHNC). Fortunately, due to frequent monitoring for glucosuria and hyperglycemia, this complication is less frequent than in the past. See Chapter 21 for a detailed discussion of HHNC.

Hypoglycemia

Hypoglycemia is a possible complication of TPN if the infusion is abruptly discontinued, especially after the infusion rate has been recently increased. Presumably, the high glucose infusion stimulates hyperinsulinism; abrupt discontinuance of the high glucose fluid may temporarily allow the serum glucose level to fall precipitously. Safe discontinuance of TPN therapy is discussed later in the chapter.

FLUID AND ELECTROLYTE, ACID–BASE, AND TRACE ELEMENT DISTURBANCES

Virtually any fluid and electrolyte or metabolic disturbance may occur during parenteral nutrition. Essentially, expected abnormalities fall into two categories. First, the electrolytes or nutrients in the parenteral solution may lead to toxicity when they exceed the body's normal metabolic and excretory capacity; second, the addition of too little of an essential element or nutrient can result in a deficiency state.[10]

Of great importance during parenteral nutrition therapy are the major intracellular ions (potassium, phosphate, and magnesium). During nutritional repletion, these ions, derived from the serum, are incorporated in newly synthesized cells.[11] Failure to supplement these ions adequately can lead to hypokalemia, hypophosphatemia, and hypomagnesemia.

Potassium Imbalances

Potassium abnormalities are common in patients receiving parenteral nutrition. A study of 100 patients found 18 had a serum potassium level less than 3 mEq/L.[12] Hypokalemia in patients receiving parenteral nutrition is related to a shift of potassium from the extracellular to the intracellular compartment during stimulation of potassium transport by endogenously produced insulin or exogenously administered insulin. Serum potassium levels must be monitored closely during the initiation of TPN because there is no direct way to predict which patients will have significant shifting of potassium into the cells. Patients who receive insulin for hyperglycemia need to be monitored especially closely for hypokalemia (see Chapter 5). If hypokalemia is present, TPN should be delayed until the deficiency is corrected.

Of course, excessive addition of potassium to the TPN solution, or excessive intake from other sources without cutting back the amount added to the solution, can lead to hyperkalemia (particularly in patients with impaired ability to eliminate excess potassium).

Phosphate Imbalances

Hypophosphatemia is another common imbalance in patients receiving parenteral nutrition. It is most likely to occur when large volumes of hypertonic dextrose are administered, particularly with insulin, in severely malnourished patients. The intracellular consumption of phosphate during protein synthesis may produce a striking deficit in the serum phosphate level if adequate phosphate supplements are not given. A number of severe metabolic abnormalities are associated with hypophosphatemia (see Chapter 8).

Although rare, hyperphosphatemia is possible if excessive phosphate is added to the TPN solution (particularly in patients who have impaired renal ability to excrete phosphate).

Magnesium Imbalances

Hypomagnesemia is less common than hypokalemia or hypophosphatemia in patients receiving parenteral nutrition. When it occurs, it may be due to intracellular shifting, inadequate replacement, or excess supplementation of calcium (which causes increased renal magnesium excretion). Other causes of hypomagnesemia and clinical signs are described in Chapter 7. Hypermagnesemia can occur if excessive magnesium is supplied in the parenteral formula of patients with renal failure.

Calcium Imbalances

Because most patients receiving parenteral nutrition are malnourished, it is likely that their total serum calcium levels will be below normal. Recall that about half of serum calcium is bound to albumin; therefore, a decrease in serum albumin causes a drop in the total serum calcium level. However, because ionization of calcium usually remains normal in hypoalbuminemic patients, no symptoms are likely. See Chapter 6 for a more detailed discussion of this topic. Another possible cause of hypocalcemia is hypomagnesemia.

Hypercalcemia can occur in patients receiving parenteral nutrition for extended periods. Possible causes are metabolic bone disease associated with long-term parenteral nutrition, or excessive vitamin D supplements.

Acid–Base Imbalances

Either metabolic acidosis or alkalosis can occur in TPN patients. These imbalances are largely a consequence of the basic underlying disease and the TPN solution composition. For example, complete metabolism of the sulfur-containing amino acids (methionine, cysteine, and cystine) results in production of hydrogen ions.[13] Metabolic alkalosis can result from excessive acetate in the TPN solution (because acetate is converted to bicarbonate). Respiratory acidosis can result from excessive carbohydrate infusion (causing increased CO_2 production). In the latter case, patients with respiratory dysfunction may have difficulty eliminating the high CO_2 load.

Trace Element Imbalances

There have been numerous reports of zinc deficiency in patients receiving parenteral nutrition without zinc supplementation. One reason is that massive losses of zinc can occur in the urine of patients with catabolic illnesses. Also, tissue demand for zinc during anabolism quickly depletes plasma stores. Thus, it is conceivable that patients with normal serum zinc levels can develop a deficiency of zinc during rapid accretion of tissue even when supplements are given. Clinically significant zinc deficiency may occur within the first few weeks of parenteral nutrition. Signs of hypozincemia may include diarrhea, delayed wound healing, alopecia, mental changes, abnormalities in taste and smell, and a characteristic dermatitis. As with other additives to parenteral nutrition solutions, it is possible to cause toxicity if too much zinc is added (particularly in patients with renal failure).

Copper deficiency states (such as hypochromic anemia and neutropenia) have been observed in patients receiving parenteral nutrition. Most often, deficiency states are not observed until many months of treatment have elapsed; however, subnormal serum copper values may occur within weeks in some patients if copper intake is inadequate. On the other hand, copper excess can result if too much copper is added to the parenteral solution.

Chromium deficiency can occur in patients receiving long-term parenteral nutrition and cause glucose intolerance (as chromium is necessary for proper use of glucose). This glucose intolerance is reversible with chromium replacement. Other signs of chromium deficiency include mental confusion and a peripheral sensory neuropathy.

Selenium deficiency can occur during long-term parenteral nutrition therapy with solutions lacking this element, but clinical manifestations (primarily cardiomyopathy) are uncommon. Although rare, molybdenum deficiency states may also occur during long-term parenteral nutrition; one patient reportedly developed tachycardia, tachypnea, and several neurological abnormalities. Clinical signs associated with these deficits usually resolve with supplementation of the needed substances.

DELIVERY OF PARENTERAL NUTRITION

Successful parenteral nutrition delivery requires a structured care plan that provides the rationale for associated nursing care. Parenteral nutrition can be infused centrally or peripherally. Both methods are briefly described below, as are general nursing considerations related to the delivery of parenteral nutrition.

PARENTERAL NUTRITION—CENTRAL VENOUS DELIVERY

Sample orders for central TPN are presented in Table 12-6. Infusion of a TPN solution must begin slowly

TABLE 12–6.
Sample Parenteral Nutrition Orders

ORDERS	RATIONALE
1. Immediate chest radiograph before initiation of TPN to ensure placement of catheter in superior vena cava	1. This placement site, with its high blood flow, allows adequate dilution of the hyperosmolar TPN solution.
2. Standard parenteral nutrition solution with standard electrolytes and minerals	2. Although it is possible to vary TPN solutions for patients with specific diseases (eg, renal or hepatic failure), most patients receive standard TPN solutions.
3. Strict intake and output measurements and daily body weights	3. Intake and output and body weight measurements have proven to be reliable and essential parameters to detect fluid overload or dehydration. Expected weight gain with optimal parenteral regimen is 1 to 2 lb/week.
4. Obtain serum electrolytes, BUN, and glucose levels daily for first week of TPN. Obtain serum calcium, phosphorus, and magnesium levels until blood levels stabilize. Monitor liver enzymes every 3–4 days	4. To monitor biochemical response to TPN and detect developing deficiencies or excessive delivery of nutrients
5. Perform urinary glucose spot checks every 6 hours (use Testape or enzyme-based tapes). Do not use Clinitest tablets. If elevated to level of +3 or higher, obtain blood sugar levels.	5. Glucosuria may be a harbinger of early sepsis, or inadequate endogenous insulin, and dictates immediate attention to avoid dehydration, hyperosmotic, nonketotic coma, or unrecognized sepsis. False-positive reaction with Clinitest (amino acids act as reducing substances)
6. A 24-hour urine for urine urea nitrogen is to be collected daily from 2400 to 2400 hours. All specimens should be kept on ice. Lab slips must identify the hours collected and total volume.	6. For calculation of nitrogen balance
7. Vitamin K, 10 mg intramuscularly, after insertion of central venous catheter; then vitamin K 10 mg intramuscularly every Monday.	7. TPN solution does not contain Vitamin K

TPN, total parenteral nutrition; BUN, blood urea nitrogen.

and gradually be increased as tolerated. For example, on day 1 the rate might be 42 mL/hr for a total of 1008 mL (42 mL × 24 hr). On day 2, the rate might be increased to 85 mL/hr (for a total of 2040 mL). On day 3 the rate might be increased to 125 mL/hr if the patient requires more than 2 L of solution to meet caloric or fluid requirements or both.

During TPN initiation, the solution should infuse continuously over the 24-hour period. Patients on long-term TPN (ie, greater than 30 days) should be considered for intermittent administration. During the early phase of TPN administration, when the rate of flow is quite slow, the patient's daily fluid requirement should be given via the peripheral venous route.

If glucosuria (+2 or greater) occurs during the initiation of parenteral nutrition, the infusion rate should not be advanced. After the glucosuria abates, the rate may be slowly increased. If holding the infusion rate fails to relieve the glucosuria, the physician will likely prescribe regular insulin to be added to the TPN formula (dosage determined by the patient's blood glucose level and medical condition). Careful blood and urine glucose monitoring is especially critical during the early TPN therapy period. Blood glucose should be kept below 250 mg/dL and the urine glucose less than +2.

PARENTERAL NUTRITION: PERIPHERAL VENOUS DELIVERY

Parenteral nutrition by the peripheral venous system may be indicated in situations in which it is anticipated that the patient's inability to receive adequate oral or enteral intake will resolve in 3 to 7 days. The final concentration of glucose for peripheral delivery should not exceed 10%.

The parenteral nutrition formula for peripheral delivery can be started at higher flow rates (ie, 125 mL/hr) than for central venous formulas. Fat emulsions must be used to achieve adequate caloric intake. Generally, the calorie:nitrogen ratio of the peripheral formula will be less than 150:1. Fat emulsions should be delivered for 24 hours to enhance the calorie:nitrogen ratio with peripheral parenteral nutrition. Monitoring the patient receiving parenteral nutrition via a peripheral vein is the same as for a patient receiving parenteral nutrition via a central venous catheter.

FAT EMULSION DELIVERY

As stated earlier, fat emulsions may be administered to provide approximately 30% to 60% of the nonprotein calories in TPN patients. Fat emulsions are commercially available in concentrations of 10% and 20%. They can be delivered via a central venous catheter or a peripheral venous catheter with an intravenous (IV) Y-connector when a three-in-one solution is not being used. Fat emulsions should infuse over 12 hours except when the patient is on peripheral TPN or has fluid volume problems necessitating 24-hour delivery.

When giving IV fat emulsion in conjunction with TPN therapy, it is customary to obtain a baseline plasma triglyceride level. Then, while advancing the infusion, plasma triglycerides are measured before each increase in dosage rate. Platelet counts should be done weekly.

DISCONTINUATION OF TPN THERAPY

Total parenteral nutrition therapy should not be discontinued until the patient is taking adequate enteral nutrition (ie, two thirds of maintenance calories). It is generally recommended that the TPN solution's flow rate be slowly tapered over 2 to 3 days as enteral nutrition is being advanced. During this tapering process, blood glucose should be carefully monitored to guard against hypoglycemia. Close monitoring of oral or enteral nutrition with calorie counts should be done during the transition from parenteral nutrition to enteral or oral diet, and should be continued until adequate intake is achieved. If abrupt discontinuation of the TPN solution is needed, it is often recommended that a 5% or 10% glucose infusion be started in a peripheral vein and maintained for 24 hours.

Although it has been traditional to reduce the infusion rate of TPN solutions progressively over a period of several days, there are reports that acute discontinuation (tapering for 2 hours, then off) may be well tolerated by patients with no evidence of pancreatic abnormalities.[14]

PREVENTION OF INFECTIOUS COMPLICATIONS

Infectious complications can be minimized in malnourished patients receiving parenteral nutrition by careful

TABLE 12–7.
Care of Central Venous Catheters Used for Parenteral Nutrition

NURSING ACTION	RATIONALE
Clamp extension tubing when adding or changing parenteral nutrition or fat emulsion container.	Avoids blood backing into the catheter with promotion of internal fibrin sheath
	Decreases catheter occlusion
Blood transfusions are not given through catheters used for parenteral nutrition.	Catheters generally placed for long-term use
	Platelets may adhere to catheter and form fibrin sheath
Blood should not be drawn through catheter.	Possible formation of internal fibrin sheath
	Increased potential for catheter clotting
	Risk of air embolism
Catheter is not used for monitoring central venous pressure.	Possibility of formation of internal fibrin sheath increased
	Interferes with delivery of TPN solution and can lead to glucose problems (risk of hypoglycemia)
Transducers should not be used with parenteral nutrition catheter.	May increase possibility of bacterial contamination
Tape all connections securely (luer-lock connections may be helpful if standardized and attached appropriately).	To avoid accidental disconnection of catheter and connecting tubing
	Decreases risk of air embolism
Apply occlusive dressing to catheter site (dressing must be occlusive on all sides). Change as frequently as needed to keep dressing clean and dry. Use particular care for patients with tracheostomy, nasotracheal tubes, and neck wounds.	To prevent catheter contamination

TPN, total parenteral nutrition.

attention to general aseptic principles and rigid protocols for management of the central venous catheter. Relatively healthy patients may require dressing changes only every other day whereas critically ill patients may need daily changes. Handwashing remains the most important preventive measure; this is especially true when the patient has wounds, a tracheostomy, or Foley catheter.

General principles of central venous catheter management are provided in Chapter 10. Table 12-7 outlines the nursing measures that should be considered when a central venous catheter is used to deliver TPN solutions. Every effort should be made to maintain the integrity of the catheter for the delivery of TPN solutions and fat emulsions.

MONITORING FOR METABOLIC DISTURBANCES

A major nursing function in the delivery of TPN solutions is that of monitoring for metabolic complications. A summary of selected metabolic complications of TPN and their management is given in Table 12-8.

In conclusion, parenteral nutrition can be a lifesaving modality for the malnourished patient. Effective, safe delivery of parenteral nutrition is assured by careful nursing assessment and interventions.

TABLE 12–8.
Summary of Selected Metabolic Complications of Total Parenteral Nutrition and Their Management

GLUCOSE DISORDERS

Hyperglycemia

1. Characterized by: Fatigue; thirst; polyuria; dry, hot, flushed skin; glucosuria; elevated blood glucose
2. Etiology: Excessive total dose or rate of dextrose infusion, inadequate endogenous insulin production, glucocorticoid administration, or presence of sepsis
3. Treatment: Slow TPN infusion, administer regular insulin as indicated
4. Monitoring: Blood glucose, state of hydration, serum sodium and potassium levels

Hyperosmolar Hyperglycemic Nonketotic Coma

1. Characterized by: Hyperglycemia, dehydration, glucosuria, increased serum osmolality, somnolence, and perhaps seizure and coma (see Chapter 21)
2. Etiology: Untreated hyperglycemia resulting in osmotic diuresis, dehydration, and central nervous system derangements
3. Treatment: Insulin administration to gradually correct hyperglycemia; administration of 5% dextrose and hypotonic saline (¼ strength) rather than TPN solution to correct free water deficit
4. Monitoring: Serum glucose, serum osmolality, and serum sodium and potassium levels

Hypoglycemia

1. Characterized by: Weakness, diaphoresis, hunger, nervousness, irritability, palpitations, headache, blurring or double vision, numbness of lips and tongue
2. Etiology: Abrupt interruption or slowing of high carbohydrate infusion, excessive administration of insulin or persistence of endogenous insulin production secondary to prolonged stimulation of islet cells by high-carbohydrate infusion
3. Treatment: Immediately begin 10% dextrose infusion; 50% dextrose may be required for severe reaction (ie, blood glucose less than 50 mg/dL or if the patient is unconscious)
4. Monitoring: Serum glucose and potassium levels

PROTEIN DISORDERS

Prerenal Azotemia

1. Characterized by: Symptoms of fluid volume deficit, elevated BUN, decreased urine output, and increased urinary specific gravity
2. Etiology: Fluid volume depletion (probably due to osmotic diuresis), excessive total delivery of protein or amino acid infusion
3. Treatment: Correct FVD; insulin administration necessary if hyperglycemia is cause of FVD; increase nonprotein calories to achieve calorie : nitrogen ratio of about 200 : 1
4. Monitoring: BUN, body weight, urine output, and urinary specific gravity

(continued)

TABLE 12–8.
(continued)

FAT DISORDERS

Essential Fatty Acid Deficiency

1. Characterized by: Scaly dermatitis, poor wound healing, elevated SGOT, elevated triene:tetraene ratio
2. Etiology: Inadequate infusion of linoleic acid, arachidonic acid, or both
3. Treatment: Provide 4% of total calories as linoleic acid
4. Monitoring: Platelet count, serum triglycerides, liver function tests

Essential Fatty Acid Excess

1. Characterized by: Tachycardia, tachypnea, nausea, vomiting, headache, back pain, dyspnea, cyanosis, histamine-like reaction, fever, and chills
2. Etiology: Excessive delivery rate of fat emulsion, liver inability to metabolize fat emulsion
3. Treatment: Decrease infusion rate of fat emulsion
4. Monitoring: Platelet count, liver function tests, serum triglycerides

---

ELECTROLYTE ABNORMALITIES

Hypokalemia

1. Characterized by: Anorexia, nausea, vomiting, abdominal distention, paralytic ileus, muscle weakness, cardiac arrhythmias
2. Etiology: Inadequate potassium intake relative to increased requirements for protein anabolism, excessive urinary or gastrointestinal losses of potassium, metabolic alkalosis, insulin administration
3. Treatment: Potassium supplements, oral or intravenous route, as dictated by the patient's serum potassium level
4. Monitoring: Serum and urine potassium levels, degree of muscle strength, cardiac regularity, gastrointestinal motility

Hypophosphatemia

1. Characterized by: Paresthesias, mental confusion, coma, decreased erythrocyte 2, 3-diphosphoglycerate
2. Etiology: Anabolism, intracellular shift of phosphorus in response to concentrated glucose solution, inadequate phosphorus in TPN solution
3. Treatment: Phosphorus supplements, oral or intravenous route, as dictated by serum phosphorus level
4. Monitoring: Serum calcium carefully (rapid correction of hypophosphatemia may cause hypocalcemic tetany); monitor serum phosphorus, calcium, and glucose levels

Hypomagnesemia

1. Characterized by: Mental changes, paresthesias, tremor, ataxia, muscle cramps, tetany, tachycardia, hypotension, positive Chvostek sign
2. Etiology: Insufficient magnesium in parenteral solution relative to requirements for protein anabolism and glucose metabolism, excessive urinary and gastrointestinal losses, elevated aldosterone levels
3. Treatment: Addition of sufficient magnesium to TPN solution, emergency administration of magnesium sulfate
4. Monitoring: Serum magnesium levels

Hypocalcemia

1. Characterized by: Numbness and tingling of nose, ears, fingertips, or toes, carpopedal spasm, muscle twitching, convulsions, positive Trousseau's sign, positive Chvostek's sign, nausea, vomiting, diarrhea, cardiac arrhythmias
2. Etiology: Rapid correction of hypophosphatemia, vitamin D deficiency, increased urinary calcium excretion, decreased parathyroid hormone, acute pancreatitis, administration of large amounts of citrated products; if total calcium is measured, evaluate calcium level in relation to serum albumin level (see Chapter 6)
3. Treatment: Calcium supplementation, slow correction of hypophosphatemia
4. Monitoring: Serum calcium and phosphorus levels, monitor vitamin D level with home TPN patients

---

(continued)

TABLE 12–8.
(continued)

Hypozincemia

1. Characterized by: Ecxemoid skin rash, alopecia, poor wound healing, impaired cellular immunity, depression, anorexia, diarrhea, altered taste, insulin hypersensitivity
2. Etiology: Inadequate zinc intake, diminished zinc stores, and reticuloendothelial system uptake of zinc
3. Treatment: Zinc replacement
4. Monitoring: Serum zinc and urine levels in long-term patients; assess for signs and symptoms of zinc deficiency

TPN, total parenteral nutrition; BUN, blood urea nitrogen; FVD, fluid volume deficit; SGOT, serum glutonic oxaloacetic transaminase.

REFERENCES

1. Griggs B: Indications for nutritional support in the adult patient. In: Grant J, Kennedy-Caldwell C (eds): Nutritional Support in Nursing, p 75. Philadelphia, Grune & Stratton, 1988
2. Long C, Schaffel N, Geiger J: Metabolic response to injury and illness: Estimation of energy and protein needs for indirect calorimetry and nitrogen balance. JPEN 3:452, 1979
3. Caldwell M, Kennedy-Caldwell C: Normal nutrient requirements. Surg Clin North Am 61:497, 1981
4. Keusch G, Farthing M: Nutrition and infection. *Annu Rev Nutr* 134, 1986
5. Crocker K: Metabolic monitoring during nutritional support therapy. In: Grant J, Kennedy-Caldwell C (eds): Nutritional Support in Nursing, p 197, Philadelphia, Grune & Stratton, 1988
6. Alpers D, Clouse R, Stenson W: Manual of Nutritional Therapeutics, 2nd ed, p 238. Boston, Little, Brown, 1988
7. Silberman H: Parenteral and Enteral Nutrition, 2nd ed, p 306. Norwalk, CT, Appleton & Lange, 1989
8. Thomas Jefferson University Hospital: Formulary and Regulations Governing Drugs, 28th ed. Philadelphia, 1987
9. Weinsier R, Bacon J, Butterworth C: Central venous alimentation: a prospective study of the frequency of metabolic abnormalities among medical and surgical patients. JPEN 6:421, 1982
10. England B, Mitch W: Acid–base, fluid, and electrolyte aspects of parenteral nutrition. In: Kokko J, Tannen R (eds): Fluids & Electrolytes, 2nd ed, p 1024. Philadelphia, WB Saunders, 1990
11. Silberman, page 311
12. Weinsier et al
13. England, Mitch, p 1029
14. Wagman et al: The effect of acute discontinuation of TPN. Ann Surg 204:524, 1986

CLINICAL SITUATIONS ASSOCIATED WITH FLUID AND ELECTROLYTE PROBLEMS

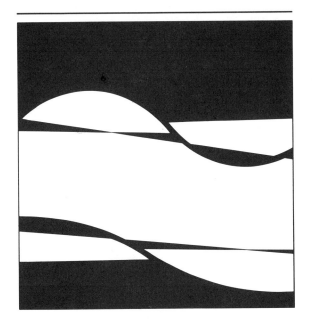

13

Tube Feedings

Enteral feedings are commonly used to provide nutritional support for patients who, for some reason, cannot consume adequate nutrients although they have functional gastrointestinal (GI) tracts. Indeed, enteral feedings are believed to be more beneficial physiologically and more cost-effective than total parenteral nutrition (TPN). However, there are problems associated with enteral feedings just as there are with most therapies. Those related to fluid and electrolyte balance are discussed in this chapter.

CHARACTERISTICS OF FORMULAS

Before discussing specific problems, it is helpful to review briefly some characteristics of tube feeding solutions. Formulas have evolved from the blenderized whole foods used several decades ago to a multitude of commercially available ones that can provide total nutrient needs. Whereas commercially available standardized formulas have many advantages, they must be selected carefully to meet patients' individual needs. Formulas differ in osmolality, protein and carbohydrate sources, fat content, caloric density, and electrolyte content.

OSMOLALITY

An important characteristic of a tube feeding formula is its osmolality (concentration). Osmolality is primarily a function of the number and size of molecular and ionic particles in a given volume. Commercially prepared feedings usually have this value printed on the product label; if not, this information, as well as the renal solute load, is usually available in product brochures. Major determinants of a formula's osmolality include protein, carbohydrate, and electrolyte con-

TABLE 13–1.
Selected Characteristics of Some Commercially Available Enteral Formulas

FORMULA	OSMOLALITY (mOsm/kg)	CALORIC DENSITY (cal/mL)	WATER CONTENT (mL/L)	SODIUM CONTENT (mEq/L)	POTASSIUM CONTENT (mEq/L)
Enrich	480	1.10	829	33.5	40.0
Ensure	470	1.06	845	32.0	32.5
Ensure HN	470	1.06	841	49.5	53.8
Ensure Plus	690	1.50	769	46.0	49.0
Jevity	310	1.06	833	39.8	39.5
Osmolite	300	1.06	841	23.5	27.0
Osmolite HN	300	1.06	841	40.0	46.0
Pulmocare	490	1.50	786	57.0	48.7
TwoCal HN	690	2.0	712	45.7	59.2
PediaSure	325	1.0	845	16.3	33.2
Replena	615	2.0	712	34.0	28.5

(Information from *Enteral Nutrition Handbook*, pp 1215–1217. Ross Laboratories, March 1989. With permission of Ross Laboratories, Columbus, OH 43216)

centrations as well as the protein form (intact versus partially hydrolyzed). The more predigested a formula is, the higher its osmolality.[1] Table 13-1 shows the wide variance in osmolalities of some commercially available tube feeding formulas. Whereas some formulas approximate the osmolality of plasma (and are thus deemed isotonic), others have considerably higher osmolalities (hypertonic). (Recall that plasma osmolality is approximately 300 mOsm/kg.) Of course, when feedings are diluted with water, they may become hypotonic.

A formula's osmolality affects tolerance to the feeding in several ways. First, it often affects the renal solute load and water requirements. (The primary determinants of renal solute load are protein, sodium, potassium, and chloride.)[2] A high renal solute load (formed during nutrient use) requires a large water volume for excretion. Another way in which osmolality affects tolerance to feedings is in its effect on gastric function. If given too quickly, hypertonic solutions slow gastric emptying and can lead to gastric retention, nausea, and vomiting. This effect is believed to be regulated by osmoreceptors in the duodenum.[3] Hypertonic solutions may also cause diarrhea if given too rapidly, especially into the small intestine (due to large shifts of fluid into the small bowel to dilute the hypertonic bowel contents).

ELECTROLYTES

Standard enteral formulas have fixed electrolyte contents, based on usual requirements. This can be a source of fluid and electrolyte problems in tube-fed patients as some require additional electrolytes whereas others cannot tolerate the preestablished amounts.

As with TPN, either deficiencies or excesses of electrolytes can occur, varying with the patient's underlying disease condition, general clinical status, and the electrolyte content of the formula being used. For example, starving patients beginning vigorous refeeding may suffer extracellular deficits of potassium, phosphorus, and magnesium as these electrolytes are pulled into the cells during anabolism. Such patients need relatively more of these electrolytes than those who are not undergoing this process. Conversely, patients with renal failure often need limitations on potassium, phosphorus, and magnesium intake. (The sodium and potassium contents of some commonly used enteral formulas are listed in Table 13-1.)

Commercial sources supply special products for patients with specific problems, such as trauma, renal failure, hepatic failure, and respiratory failure. For example, high fat, low carbohydrate formulas are available to reduce the respiratory quotient of pulmonary patients by lowering the production of carbon dioxide and thereby the $PaCO_2$.[4] (An example of such a formula is Pulmocare.) Because numerous products are available, it is important to study the literature supplied by the manufacturer. In summary, to avoid complicating existing metabolic derangements, nutritional prescriptions must be tailored in the direction of restoring homeostasis.

FLUID AND ELECTROLYTE DISTURBANCES ASSOCIATED WITH TUBE FEEDINGS

Tube-fed patients tend to have the fluid and electrolyte disturbances associated with their underlying disease and treatment conditions. Theoretically, therefore, it is possible to observe all types of electrolyte disturbances in tube-fed patients. Understandably, fluid and electrolyte disturbances are more common in patients with severe illness than in relatively healthy persons requiring tube feedings for only short periods. The discussion of imbalances in this chapter will be limited to the more commonly encountered disturbances.

HYPERNATREMIA

Hypernatremia has been described as a possible electrolyte abnormality in tube-fed patients.[5] However, it is less common today than in the past when very high osmolality formulas (approximately 1000 mOsm/kg) and protein content were often used.[6] Although formulas in use today tend to have lower osmolalities, hypernatremia can still develop in patients given inadequate water supplements. This problem is most prevalent in patients unable to make their thirst known (such as those who are unconscious, very young, aphasic, elderly, or debilitated). Elderly patients are more prone to develop hypernatremia with hyperosmolar feedings because of their decreased renal ability to conserve needed water.[7] The very young may also have difficulty in concentrating urine because of immature renal function. With decreased ability to concentrate urine, patients need more fluid to eliminate body wastes. If not provided via the feeding tube or the IV route, it is taken from internal fluid reserves.

Clinical studies have reported variable rates of hypernatremia in tube-fed patients. In one study it occurred in 10% of the tube-fed patients (primarily in neurosurgical patients who were unable to conserve free water because of transient diabetes insipidus).[8] In another study, a higher incidence (18%) was reported in an acutely ill tube-fed population, being greatest in patients over 60 years of age who were receiving feedings with osmolalities greater than 400 mOsm/kg.[9]

HYPONATREMIA

In two recent studies of tube-fed patients, the incidence of hyponatremia was higher than that of hypernatremia (24%–31% versus 10%–18%).[10,11] In both studies, the condition was often associated with the concomitant use of IV dextrose and water solutions for parenteral drug administration.

Factors contributing to hyponatremia in tube-fed patients include water-retaining states, including excessive antidiuretic hormone (ADH) secretion (such as occurs with syndrome of inappropriate ADH [SIADH]) and abnormal routes of sodium loss, such as diarrhea or diuretic use. Note in Table 4-2 that a number of conditions predispose to this condition. In the presence of excessive ADH activity, large water supplements (by any route) can cause dilution of the serum sodium level, particularly when hypotonic or isotonic feedings are used. Although water added to the formula is usually charted, it is often difficult to determine the amount of fluid used as flushes to maintain tube patency and to administer medications by the tube.[12] The latter can be a significant source of fluid intake, which is particularly important in patients with a water-retaining state (such as SIADH).

A summary of sodium imbalance causes in tube-fed patients is given in Table 13-2. Clinical indicators of hypernatremia and hyponatremia are described in Chapter 4.

FLUID VOLUME OVERLOAD

It is possible to cause fluid volume overload when attempting to provide sufficient calories to a patient with renal, cardiac, or hepatic disease. For such patients, a formula supplying 2 kcal/mL is often selected (as opposed to one supplying only 1 cal/mL). In addition, special low-sodium formulas are available for such patients. As noted in Table 13-1, some formulas have considerably more sodium than others. However, in most situations, the volume of formula needed to provide 2000 kcal will deliver 40 to 80 mEq of sodium.[13] Edema can also occur when a high-carbohydrate formula is fed to a previously fasting patient. Weight gains of 20 pounds in a single week have been reported, accompanied by massive pedal edema.[14] The mechanism for the antidiuretic effect of carbohydrate is not fully understood. Contributing to edema in tube-fed patients may be the presence of hypoalbuminemia, which favors shifting of fluid from the vascular to the interstitial space. One study of tube-fed patients found the incidence of edema to be 20% to 25%.[15]

POTASSIUM, PHOSPHORUS, AND MAGNESIUM IMBALANCES

Recall that potassium, phosphorus, and magnesium are major cellular electrolytes. When starving (catabolic) patients are started on vigorous enteral feedings, there is a shift of potassium, phosphorus, and magnesium from the extracellular space into the cells. This shift occurs as protein synthesis (anabolism) is initiated. Insulin administration further favors intracellular shifting of these electrolytes. Failure to detect early hy-

TABLE 13–2.
Possible Causes of or Factors Contributing to Sodium
Imbalances in Tube-Fed Patients

IMBALANCE	POSSIBLE CAUSES/CONTRIBUTING FACTORS
Hypernatremia with fluid volume deficit	Formula that produces a large renal solute load
	Inadequate free-water intake
	Inadequate thirst perception
	Impaired ability to concentrate urine (as occurs in old age)
	Increased insensible water loss, as occurs in hyperventilation and fever
	Diabetes insipidus (increased urinary water loss due to inadequate ADH activity)
	Watery diarrhea
Hyponatremia	Conditions predisposing to abnormal water retention, such as inappropriate ADH production in head-injured patients or in those with oat-cell lung tumors
	Excessive free-water supplements:
	▶ Can occur by routinely diluting isotonic formulas to half strength without consideration of other free-water intake or clinical status
	▶ Failure to consider glucose/water solutions given by IV route when calculating supplemental water needs
	▶ Failure to consider "flush" fluids (used to maintain tube patency and deliver medications) when calculating supplemental water needs
	Abnormal routes of sodium loss, as in diarrhea
	Vigorous use of diuretics

ADH, antidiuretic hormone.

pokalemia, hypophosphatemia, and hypomagnesemia, and to furnish replacements as needed, can result in serious consequences as these electrolytes have vital functions.

Hypokalemia is a common metabolic complication of enteral feeding that reportedly occurs in up to 50% of tube-fed patients.[16] Therefore, close attention should be paid to the potassium content of the formula as well as to other conditions predisposing to hypokalemia (such as diarrhea or use of potassium-losing diuretics). Note in Table 13-1 that there is variability in the potassium content in tube feeding formulas. Clinical indicators of hypokalemia are described in Chapter 5.

There is danger of hypophosphatemia during enteral feeding, since refeeding causes phosphates to shift into the cells where they are used for glucose phosphorylation and protein synthesis.[17] When this happens, the plasma phosphate level may drop precipitously. Some formulas contain considerably more phosphates than others.

In one study of tube-fed patients, a 30% incidence of hypophosphatemia was observed, even when phosphate-containing solutions were used.[18] This occurred primarily in patients who received insulin for treatment of hyperglycemia; thus, the hypophosphatemia was probably secondary to a shift of phosphorus into the cells. Others reported hypophosphatemia in malnourished patients receiving glucose infusions (again, related to a cellular shift).[19] Clinical indicators of hypophosphatemia are described in Chapter 8.

During anabolism, magnesium requirements increase as the intracellular mass expands. As with the other primary cellular electrolytes (potassium and phosphorus), extracellular deficiency may result if inadequate amounts are present in the formula or added as supplements (either enterally or parenterally). In a study by Holcombe and Adams,[20] 46% of the subjects had lower than normal serum magnesium levels (11 had the problem before the initiation of tube feedings and nine became hypomagnesemic during the course of tube feedings). Clinical indicators of hypomagnesemia are described in Chapter 7.

*Hyper*kalemia also may occur in the tube-fed patient. Note in Table 13-1 the potassium content of some common formulas. If excessive supplements are given in addition to the formula, hyperkalemia could result, particularly in high-risk patients. As explained in Chapter 5, several factors predispose to hyperkalemia (such as metabolic acidosis and advanced renal failure). Holcombe and Adams[21] observed hyperkalemia in 16% of their tube-fed population; it usually developed secondary to potassium supplementation after tube feedings were initiated. In a study of 13 patients receiving tube feedings, Primrose et al[22] reported a rise in serum potassium from a mean of 4.2 ± 0.5 mmol/L before feeding to 5.1 ± 0.5 mmol/L after 1 week.[22] Two subjects had elevations that were considered hazardous, necessitating discontinuance of the feedings. The researchers concluded that careful attention should be paid to monitoring serum potassium levels in patients receiving tube feedings.

Hyperphosphatemia has also been observed in tube-fed patients. In one study, a 14% incidence of hyperphosphatemia was reported; the elevated phosphate levels correlated with renal failure (a common cause of this imbalance).[23] This report reflects the close parallel between electrolyte abnormalities and underlying disease states in tube-fed patients.

FLUID VOLUME DEFICIT ASSOCIATED WITH HYPERGLYCEMIA

Tube-fed patients are at risk for hyperglycemia because of the high carbohydrate content of some formulas and because of the relative insulin resistance commonly present in acute illness.[24] Patients with mild to moderate hyperglycemia need extra fluid to replace increased urinary fluid losses until the disorder can be controlled by hypoglycemic agents. (When insulin is administered, it is important to remember its contributory effect on the shifting of potassium, phosphorus, and magnesium from the extracellular fluid into the cells.) Occasionally, tube feedings will cause severe hyperglycemia that may progress to a hyperosmolar reaction. In this situation, vigorous hydration is warranted (see Chapter 21).

ZINC DEFICIENCY

Although several trace element deficiencies may occur in patients receiving long-term enteral feedings as their only nutrient source, zinc deficiency has probably received the most attention. In one report, zinc deficiency was described in two patients who had received tube feedings for 4 and 7 months.[25] Both patients developed skin rashes around the groin and under the breasts and axilla; after supplementation with zinc sulfate, the rashes disappeared and the serum zinc levels returned to normal.

Below normal serum zinc levels occurred in 11% of the tube-fed patients in the study by Vanlandingham et al.[26]

ASSESSMENT FOR FLUID AND ELECTROLYTE DISTURBANCES IN TUBE-FED PATIENTS

ROUTINE LABORATORY AND CLINICAL MONITORING

Although recommendations vary regarding the frequency of metabolic monitoring in tube-fed patients, it seems reasonable to measure serum Na, K, glucose, blood urea nitrogen (BUN), and creatinine daily for the 1st week and once a week thereafter; and serum P, Mg, and Ca twice weekly during the 1st week and once a week subsequently. As stabilization evidence is gathered, the testing frequency can be gradually decreased. In many situations, the severity of illness dictates how frequently laboratory values are obtained.

Fluid intake and output (I&O) should be monitored and recorded every 8 hours (or hourly in acute situations such as hyperosmolar reaction). Body weight should be measured and recorded daily. Vital signs should be monitored at least once per shift. Urine glucose and acetone should be checked every 6 hours for the first 48 hours and then once daily if normal. If the renal threshold is in question (as it frequently is in elderly and very ill patients), capillary blood glucose should be monitored.

RISK FACTORS FROM UNDERLYING DISEASE AND TREATMENT CONDITIONS

Because various electrolyte disturbances can occur with tube feedings, each patient should be evaluated individually, with consideration of which factors are present that predispose to disturbances.

1. Consider disease conditions that may predispose to hyponatremia, such as:
   ▶ Excessive ADH secretion, as occurs with oat-cell carcinoma of the lung, subarachnoid hemorrhage, head injury, brain tumor, pneumonia, and acquired immunodeficiency syndrome.
   (For a more extensive listing, see Table 4-2.)
   If any of these are present, use of a hypotonic solution (isotonic solution further diluted with water) or excessive water flushes to keep the tube patent place the patient at increased risk.

2. Consider whether the patient is receiving medications that favor water gain and thus hyponatremia, such as:
   ▶ Intravenous cyclophosphamide (Cytoxan), vincristine (Oncovin), chlorpropamide (Diabenese), tolbutamine (Orinase), carbamazepine (Tegretol), amitriptyline (Elavil), haloperidol (Haldol), thioridazine (Mellaril), or nonsteroidal antiinflammatory drugs. See Chapter 4 for additional causes of increased ADH production.
   If so, use of a hypotonic solution (isotonic solution further diluted with water) or excessive water flushes to keep the tube patent put the patient at increased risk.

3. Consider whether the patient is at increased risk for hyponatremia because of use of relatively large volumes of D_5W as a vehicle for IV medications or to "keep the vein open." If so, the risk is compounded if the patient also has a disease condition favoring increased ADH activity or is receiving a medication favoring water retention.

4. Consider the presence of disease conditions predisposing to hypernatremia, such as:
   ▶ A neurological condition associated with decreased level of consciousness, inability to recognize thirst, or both
   ▶ Excessive water excretion in urine due to diabetes insipidus (ADH deficiency)

▶ Hyperventilation (causing increased insensible water loss from lungs)

▶ Fever (causing increased water loss)

If so, the risk is compounded if the patient is receiving hyperosmolar feedings with inadequate water supplements.

5. Consider whether the patient is at increased risk for fluid volume overload, such as occurs with renal, hepatic, or cardiac insufficiency. If so, use of a standard formula with a relatively high sodium content and low caloric density puts the patient at increased risk.

6. Consider whether the patient is at increased risk for sodium, potassium, and magnesium loss through diarrhea. Are other body fluids being lost abnormally?

7. Consider whether the patient is at increased risk for potassium imbalances, either hypokalemia because of use of potassium-losing diuretics, or hyperkalemia due to use of potassium-conserving diuretics.

8. Consider whether the patient is at risk for the "refeeding syndrome" because of an aggressive feeding regimen after sustaining a prolonged period of fasting or inadequate caloric intake. If so, observe for hypokalemia, hypomagnesemia, and hypophosphatemia as these electrolytes shift into the cells during the anabolic process. These electrolyte disturbances are aggravated by the administration of insulin.

9. Consider whether the patient is at increased risk for fluid volume deficit (FVD) because of osmotic diuresis associated with a carbohydrate intolerance. Although overt diabetes is direct evidence of carbohydrate intolerance, remember that nondiabetics who are highly stressed by illness may also have a temporary glucose intolerance.

RISK FACTORS RELATED TO TYPE OF FORMULA

1. What is the formula's osmolality, protein, and electrolyte content? Remember, generally speaking, the higher these are, the greater the need for water supplementation.

2. What is the formula's caloric density? (How many calories per milliliter?) Anticipate giving solutions with high caloric density to patients requiring fluid restriction.

3. What is the formula's electrolyte content? Recall that this content may need adjusting to the individual patient's electrolyte needs. When high-osmolality electrolyte supplements are added to the formula, they may greatly increase the formula's osmolality. When GI intolerance to the electrolytes is a problem, it may be necessary to use the parenteral route to achieve electrolyte replacement.

4. Is the formula being diluted unnecessarily? Needless

dilution of isotonic formulas with water not only decreases the caloric intake but can predispose to hyponatremia in susceptible patients. Most often, isotonic formulas can be administered at full strength.

HYDRATIONAL STATUS

Because tube-fed patients may develop either FVD or fluid volume excess (FVE), with or without sodium imbalances, monitor the hydrational status closely.

1. Monitor fluid I&O on all patients receiving tube feedings. In most instances, unless abnormal fluid losses are occurring from other routes, the urinary output should roughly equal the total fluid intake. Recorded intake should include all fluids given by mouth, tube, and the IV route. In addition to recording the amount of formula, chart the amount of free water given by the tube. This includes water used to flush the tube to maintain patency and to dilute medications given by the tube. Recorded output should include the volume of urine, liquid feces, vomitus, or drainage from fistulas or wounds, if present. Because diarrhea is a possible complication of tube feedings, monitor the character, frequency, and volume of stools closely. Also consider fluid losses associated with elevated body temperature, excessive perspiration, hyperventilation, and dry environmental conditions.

2. Monitor urine concentration. In FVD, the healthy kidney will conserve fluid and produce a visibly concentrated, low-volume urine. In neurologically impaired patients at risk for diabetes insipidus or syndrome of inappropriate antidiuretic hormone secretion (SIADH), it may be necessary to measure urinary specific gravity (SG). (See Chapters 4 and 20 for a discussion of these conditions.)

3. Monitor for glucosuria at least three times daily throughout the initial feeding period, particularly in middle-aged and elderly patients. If present, check blood glucose; hyperglycemia predisposes to FVD and deficits of potassium, phosphorus, and magnesium, especially when insulin is used to correct the elevated blood glucose. If the renal threshold is in question, check capillary blood sugars instead of urine sugars.

4. Monitor daily body weights. A slight daily increase in weight is anticipated in the anabolic patient. This gain should not exceed 0.7 kg (roughly 1.5 lb) per day[27]; a gain greater than this amount probably indicates fluid volume overload.

5. Monitor skin and tongue turgor. See assessment of skin turgor and tongue turgor in Chapter 2.

6. Monitor rate of vein filling. Rate of vein filling is a useful indicator of fluid volume status. See the discussion of this topic in Chapters 2 and 26.

7. Monitor for abnormal breath sounds and dependent edema, especially in elderly patients and those with underlying renal or cardiac disease.
8. Monitor the level of sensorium. Severe sodium derangements, high or low, can seriously affect the sensorium. Of course, if the patient has a decreased level of consciousness at the time feedings are initiated, a worsening of the condition would be anticipated. Also, a patient with a decreased level of consciousness is at greater risk for hypernatremia because of inability to perceive or respond to thirst.
9. Monitor serial determinations of blood chemistries (sodium, BUN, serum creatinine, and glucose). An elevated BUN:creatinine ratio indicates FVD. A greater than normal serum sodium level indicates excessive free water loss, whereas a decreased serum sodium level signals a water gain, sodium loss, or both. A markedly elevated serum glucose level will produce an osmotic diuresis and cause FVD if fluid replacement is inadequate.

NURSING DIAGNOSES

After completing the above assessment, it should be possible to formulate nursing diagnoses. See Table 13-3 for examples of nursing diagnoses related to potential fluid and electrolyte disorders in tube-fed patients. Also, see discussion of fluid and electrolyte disturbances associated with tube feedings earlier in this chapter. Chapters 3 through 9 provide in-depth discussions of specific imbalances.

TABLE 13–3.
Examples of Nursing Diagnoses Related to Fluid and Electrolyte Disorders in Tub-Fed Patients

NURSING DIAGNOSIS	ETIOLOGIES	DEFINING CHARACTERISTICS
FVD with hypernatremia ("hypertonic dehydration") related to hypertonic tube feedings and inadequate water supplements	Hyperosmolar feedings with inadequate water supplements, particularly in elderly or very young patients, or in those patients unable to respond to thirst	Polyuria initially, followed by oliguria; fluid intake totaled over several days much less than output; sticky mucous membranes, serum Na > 145 mEq/L, altered sensorium, slow-filling hand veins
FVE related to standard tube feedings in patients with cardiac or renal abnormalities	Use of a feeding formula with standard sodium content, at a rate exceeding the patient's tolerance	Intake totaled over several days much greater than output; moist crackles, dependent edema (see Chapter 3)
Alteration in sodium balance (hyponatremia) related to excessive water gain or loss of sodium	Isotonic or hypotonic tube feeding associated with high water intake (tube or IV), particularly in patient with excessive ADH activity or abnormal route of sodium loss	Serum Na < 135 mEq/L; lethargy, personality change, headache, decreased level of consciousness; if due to water excess, weight gain and greater fluid intake than output (see Chapter 4)
Alteration in phosphorus balance (hypophosphatemia) related to refeeding syndrome	Aggressive tube feeding in previously malnourished patient, results in shift of phosphorus into cells as patient becomes anabolic, particularly when PO_4 replacement is inadequate, or insulin is used to treat hyperglycemia	Progressive muscle weakness which may involve respiratory and cardiac function, decreased serum P level (see Chapter 8)
Alteration in potassium balance (hypokalemia) and magnesium balance (hypomagnesemia) related to refeeding syndrome or diarrhea	Same mechanism as for phosphorus imbalance since all three (PO_4, K, and Mg) are primarily cellular electrolytes Inadequate replacement Increased loss in diarrheal fluid	Symptoms of hypokalemia: fatigue, muscle weakness, arrhythmias, ECG changes, plasma K < 3.5 mEq/L (see Chapter 5) Symptoms of hypomagnesemia (arrhythmias, increased neuromuscular irritability serum Mg < 1.5 mEq/L [see Chapter 7])
Alteration in bowel elimination, diarrhea, related to rapid administration of hyperosmolar feedings into small intestine	Large fluid shifts into small bowel are induced by hyperosmolar feedings; diarrhea results from bowel distention	Loose, liquid stools, increased frequency, cramping, abdominal pain, increased frequency of bowel sounds

INTERVENTIONS

WATER SUPPLEMENTATION

A perplexing problem for the nurse is determining how much free water is needed for each tube-fed patient. The above discussion identified several variables affecting this decision. To reiterate, clinical assessment helps to determine whether a patient has normal volume status, is fluid volume deficient, or is overloaded. Review of the underlying disease condition(s) is imperative. For example, is there need for fluid restriction due to SIADH or renal or cardiac disease? Is extra fluid required due to delivery of high osmolality, high-protein feedings without sufficient water, or increased loss from other routes, such as diarrhea, fistula or wound drainage, hyperventilation, or fever? Is the patient receiving sizable amounts of fluid via the IV route? How does the I&O record look? All of these factors must be considered individually.

Given the above qualifiers, a few rough guidelines may be considered. Some suggest that adults need 1.0 mL of fluid per calorie delivered, whereas children require 1.5 mL per calorie.[28] Another method suggest that adults require from 25 to 35 mL of water per kilogram of body weight per day.[29] See Table 13-4 for a sample problem to calculate water needs of a hypothetical tube-fed patient. (Water requirements for children of various ages are presented in Chapter 25.)

TABLE 13–4.
Sample Calculation for Estimating Daily Fluid Requirements

A 56-year-old patient weighing 70 kg is being fed Osmolite HN, 75 mL/hr/day (75 × 24 = 1800 mL/day)

Step 1. Estimated daily fluid requirement = Estimated water need (mL) times body weight (kg)
For a person this age, 30 mL per kg of water is generally accepted as adequate. For this patient, therefore, estimated daily fluid requirement equals 30 mL times 70 kg = 2100 mL.

Step 2. Fluid provided by enteral formula = mL water/L times volume of formula/day (L). Fluid provided by enteral formula = 841 mL/L times 1.8 L. (See Table 13-1 for water content of formula.) Fluid provided by enteral formula = 1514 mL.

Step 3. Additional fluid required = Result 1 − Result 2
Additional fluid required = 2100 mL − 1514 mL.
Additional fluid required = 586 mL/day.

(Adapted from Enteral Nutrition Handbook, p 14. Ross Laboratories, March 1989. With permission of Ross Laboratories, Columbus, OH 43216)

PREVENTING DIARRHEA

Unfortunately, diarrhea is a common complication of tube feedings. Several possible causes have been identified and studied to varying degrees. Among these are osmolality of the formula, volume of formula, rate of delivery, site of delivery (gastric versus intestinal), formula contamination, severity of illness, and various treatments (such as medications and mechanical ventilation). Reported incidences of diarrhea vary widely, depending on the patient's clinical status and the individual researcher's definition of diarrhea.

When GI function is normal, the incidence of diarrhea in tube-fed patients is reported to be 12% to 25%.[30,31] In contrast, about half of the patients in intensive care units develop diarrhea.[32] Several factors may account for this higher incidence, such as increased rates of malnutrition (causing decreased ability of the intestinal mucosa to absorb nutrients), multiple-system organ disease, multiple medications, and infectious processes. Apparently, critically ill patients who are mechanically ventilated are at even greater risk for diarrhea. A study of 73 critically ill mechanically ventilated patients discovered a diarrhea incidence of 63%.[33] Another study of tube-fed patients found 26% had documented diarrhea (defined as stools greater than 500 mL/day for at least two consecutive days).[34] A single cause was specified in 29 of the 32 episodes of diarrhea. Medications were directly responsible in 61%, whereas tube feeding formulas were responsible in only 21%, and *Clostridium difficile* in 17%.

Because diarrhea places the patient at great risk for fluid and electrolyte problems, measures must be used to prevent its occurrence.

FORMULA AND MEDICATION DILUTION

As a rule, hyperosmolar solutions should be diluted to isotonic strength and started at a low flow rate. The concentration and flow rate can then be increased (one at a time) until nutritional needs are met. Hyperosmolar solutions are less well tolerated in the small intestine than in the stomach.

There is seldom need to dilute isotonic formulas. Two instances in which it may be recommended that isotonic (300 mOsm/kg) formulas be diluted to half strength (150 mOsm/kg) are (1) when the serum albumin is less than 2.5 g/dL or (2) when loose stools initially occur.[35] However, to dilute isotonic formulas routinely when initiating tube feedings can seriously interfere with the patient's caloric intake and perhaps predispose to hyponatremia in susceptible patients.

Several medications are hyperosmolar and can cause osmotic diarrhea if given undiluted, especially into the small intestine. Examples of osmolalities of such medications include 10% potassium chloride solution (Adria), 3000 mOsm/kg; acetaminophen elixir, 65 mg/mL [Roxanne] 5400 mOsm/kg; and sodium phosphate liquid, 0.5 g/mL (Fleet), 7250 mOsm/kg (Fleet).[36] Dilute hyperosmolar medications before administration and irrigate the tube with water before and after delivery.[37] This not only dilutes the medication but enhances its absorption. (This should be done with the patient's fluid requirements in mind.) At times, the parenteral route may be necessary for electrolyte supplements when they are not tolerated well by the GI tract.

OTHER FACTORS

In addition to hyperosmolar agents given through the tube, other medications the patient is receiving should be considered as possible causative agents of diarrhea. For example, diarrhea is a common side effect of penicillin-like antibiotics. Use of magnesium-containing antacids may also cause diarrhea.

Formulas with little or no lactose content are indicated for very ill patients with small-bowel conditions that predispose to lactose intolerance (such as intestinal resection, radiation enteritis, and malnutrition). The presence of mucosal damage reduces the total intestinal surface area available for absorption and produces secondary lactose deficiency.[38] Most commercially available feedings are lactose free. Of course, any feeding prepared with milk contains lactose.

Recently refrigerated formulas should be started at a slow rate to permit them time to warm to room temperature. (Research findings by Kagawa-Busby et al[39] suggest that cold feedings can predispose to cramping and diarrhea in some patients).

The complete delivery set (except the feeding tube itself) should be changed every 24 hours for patients in a hospital setting to reduce the incidence of contamination.[40] All equipment used in formula preparation should be handled aseptically. Some authors recommend the use of sterile water (versus tap water) when it is necessary to reconstitute or dilute enteral nutrition solutions.[41] Recent studies indicated that enteral nutrition solutions may be an important source of nosocomial infection.[42]

REFERENCES

1. MacBurney M, Russell C, Young L: Formulas, p 167. In: Rombeau J, Caldwell M (eds): Clinical Nutrition: Enteral and Tube Feeding, 2nd ed. Philadelphia, WB Saunders, 1990
2. Ibid
3. Ibid
4. Al-Saady N, Blackmore C, Bennett E: High fat, low carbohydrate, enteral feeding lowers PaCO$_2$ and reduces the period of ventilation in artificially ventilated patients. Intensive Care Med 15:290, 1989
5. Gault et al: Hypernatremia, azotemia, and dehydration due to high-protein feeding. Ann Intern Med 68:778, 1968
6. Silk D, Payne-James J: Complications of enteral nutrition, p 525. In: Rombeau J, Caldwell M (eds). Clinical Nutrition: Enteral and Tube Feeding, 2nd ed. Philadelphia, WB Saunders, 1990
7. Walike J: Tube feeding syndrome in head and neck surgery. Arch Otolaryngol 89:117, 1969
8. Vanlandingham et al: Metabolic abnormalities in patients supported with enteral tube feeding. JPEN 5:322, 1981
9. Bowman M: Sodium Imbalances in Tube-Fed Patients. Master's Thesis. St. Louis University, 1986
10. Vanlandingham et al, p 323
11. Bowman et al: Sodium imbalances in tube-fed patients. Critical Care Nurse 9(1):22, 1989
12. Bowman
13. Alpers D, Clouse R, Stenson W: Manual of Nutritional Therapeutics, 2nd ed, p 226. Boston, Little, Brown, 1988
14. Havala T, Shronts E: Managing the complications associated with refeeding. Nutrition in Clinical Practice 5(1):27, 1990
15. Heymsfield et al: Enteral hyperalimentation: An alternative to central venous hyperalimentation. Ann Intern Med 90:63, 1979
16. Silk, Payne-James, p 525
17. Ibid, p 526
18. Vanlandingham et al, p 324
19. Hayek M, Covey T, Eisenberg P: Hypophosphatemia in enteral tube feedings (abstr). Missouri Surgical Convention, St. Louis, MO, 1984
20. Holcombe B, Adams M: Metabolic complications associated with enteral nutritional support. Nutritional Support Services 5(3):26, 1985
21. Ibid
22. Primrose et al: Hyperkalemia in patients on enteral feedings. JPEN 5:130, 1981
23. Vanlandingham et al, p 324
24. Silk, Payne-James, p 525
25. Jhangiana et al: Clinical zinc deficiency during long-term total enteral nutrition. J Am Geriatr Soc 34:385, 1986
26. Vanlandingham et al, p 324
27. Heymsfield et al, p 69
28. Anonymous: Enteral Nutrition Handbook, p 13. Columbus, OH, Ross Laboratories, 1989
29. Ibid
30. Cataldi-Betcher et al: Complications occurring during enteral nutrition support: A prospective study. JPEN 7:546, 1983
31. Jones et al: Comparison of an elemental and poly-

meric enteral diet in patients with normal gastrointestinal function. Gut 24:78, 1983

32. Brinson R, Anderson W, Singh M: Hypoalbuminemia-associated diarrhea in critically ill patients. Journal of Critical Illness 2(9):72, 1987

33. Smith et al: Diarrhea associated with tube-feeding in mechanically ventilated critically ill patients. Nurs Res 39(3):148, 1990

34. Edes T, Walk B, Austin J: Diarrhea in tube-fed patients: Feeding formula not necessarily the cause. Am J Med 88:91, 1990

35. Guenter et al: Administration and delivery of enteral nutrition. In: Rombeau J, Caldwell M (eds): Clinical Nutrition: Enteral and Tube Feeding, 2nd ed, p 199. Philadelphia, WB Saunders, 1990

36. Melnik G: Pharmacologic aspects of enteral nutrition. In: Rombeau J, Caldwell M (eds): Clinical Nutrition: Enteral and Tube Feeding, 2nd ed, p 493. Philadelphia, WB Saunders, 1990

37. Edes et al, p 91

38. Eisenberg P: Enteral nutrition: Indications, formulas, and delivery techniques. Nurs Clin North Am 24(2):324, 1989

39. Kagawa-Busby K, Heitkemper M, Hansen B: Effects of diet temperature on tolerance of enteral feedings. Nurs Res 29:276, 1980

40. Perez S, Brandt K: Enteral feeding contamination: Comparison of diluents and feeding bag usage. JPEN 13(3):306, 1989

41. Fagerman K: Microbiological monitoring of enteral nutrition solutions needed. (Letter to the Editor) JPEN 13(6):670, 1989

42. Thurn et al: Enteral hyperalimentation as a source of nosocomial infection. J Hosp Infect 15:203, 1990

14

Fluid Balance in the Surgical Patient

Although surgical patients are at great risk for fluid and electrolyte imbalances, these disturbances can often be prevented or minimized by appropriate intervention. Assessment and management of the patient's fluid and electrolyte status begins in the preoperative period and continues in the postoperative recovery period.

PREOPERATIVE PERIOD

Before surgery, potential perioperative problems should be identified by review of the patient's history and assessment for specific indicators of problems.

FLUID AND ELECTROLYTE DISTURBANCES

Laboratory data should be reviewed carefully to detect fluid and electrolyte problems. (See Tables 2-3 and 2-4 for blood and urine tests useful in determining fluid balance status.) In patients without a contributing chronic illness, serum electrolytes are usually normal. If not, abnormalities should be called to the attention of the medical staff for early correction. (Specific fluid and electrolyte imbalances are discussed in Chapters 3–9.) Preoperative identification of hypokalemia is particularly important because this imbalance predisposes to cardiac arrhythmias during the intraoperative period. Correction of potassium deficit should be started only after an adequate urine output is established. Calcium and magnesium replacement may be needed for patients with massive subcutaneous infections, acute pancreatitis, or chronic starvation.[1] Anemia correction is important. A hematocrit increase of approximately 3% should follow the infusion of a unit of packed red blood cells in an average-sized adult.[2] In a patient with a contracted intravascular volume, a significantly greater rise may occur, indicating the need for concurrent fluid volume replacement.

Surgical patients are frequently subjected to oral fluid restriction for test preparation, and to prevent aspiration of gastric contents during anesthesia. Many have undergone fluid and electrolyte losses due to illness, use of cathartics and enemas for bowel preparation, or use of contrast agents for diagnostic radiograph procedures (causing osmotic diuresis). Fluid volume deficit (FVD) should be detected and corrected before induction of anesthesia as it is more difficult to correct intraoperatively. Before surgery, sufficient fluid must be given to stabilize blood pressure and pulse and increase hourly urine volume to an acceptable range (preferably 50 mL/hr in an adult). The rate of fluid administration varies considerably, depending on severity and type of fluid disturbances, presence of continuing losses, and cardiac status. Hemodynamic monitoring is indicated in the cardiac patient requiring aggressive fluid therapy.

CHRONIC CONDITIONS

Certain chronic illnesses predispose to fluid, electrolyte, and acid–base disturbances during the stressful perioperative period. For example, patients with renal failure are at risk for hyperkalemia, metabolic acidosis, hypermagnesemia, and hyponatremia; those with chronic obstructive pulmonary disease are predisposed to respiratory acidosis and hypoxemia. Patients with chronic illnesses should be in the best metabolic control possible before surgery.

MEDICATIONS

As discussed in Chapters 3 through 9, several medications can cause fluid and electrolyte disturbances. Some of the more problematic are potassium-losing diuretics. Examples of others include antibiotics predisposing to renal potassium wasting (such as carbenicillin and amphotericin B) and renal magnesium wasting (such as gentamicin).

Altered Adrenal Response

Factors that can interfere with the expected adrenal response to the stress of surgery must be identified preoperatively; one such factor is altered adrenal function related to use of therapeutic doses of corticosteroids. To review, the usual daily secretion of cortisol ranges from 15 to 30 mg/day.[3] However, increased secretion is needed to withstand the stress of surgery. (Estimates of endogenous cortisol production in patients undergoing major surgery vary from 75–150 mg/day.[4]) The adrenal glands of patients who have used corticosteroids for prolonged periods may not be able to respond during periods of high stress. Thus, patients maintained on chronic corticosteroid therapy require steroid replacement in the perioperative period to prevent acute adrenocortical insufficiency (adrenal crisis).[5] Symptoms of this relatively rare but dangerous complication may include lethargy, disorientation, confusion, hypotension, hyponatremia, and hyperkalemia. These signs, with or without cardiovascular collapse, in any intraoperative or postoperative patient should raise the suspicion of adrenocortical insufficiency.[6]

Controversy exists as to the steroid dosage needed in at-risk patients to prevent acute adrenocortical insufficiency in the postoperative period without producing other complications (such as impaired wound healing, increased catabolism, electrolyte disturbances, and more frequent infectious complications.) In general, however, it is well to remember that short-term excess of glucocorticoids is relatively harmless, but short-term deficiency during stress may be fatal.[7]

NUTRITIONAL STATUS

The reasonably well nourished and otherwise healthy individual undergoing an uncomplicated major surgical procedure has sufficient body fuel reserves to withstand catabolic insult and partial starvation for at least 1 week. However, the nutritionally depleted patient undergoes surgery with a serious handicap. It has been shown that operative morbidity and mortality are increased enormously in malnourished patients.[8] Increased susceptibility to infection results from a diminished ability to form antibodies and the superficial atrophy in the mucous membrane linings of the respiratory and gastrointestinal (GI) tracts that often accompanies malnutrition. Hypoproteinemia follows prolonged negative nitrogen balance and increases susceptibility to shock. Diminished supplies of protein and vitamin C retard wound healing. Because malnutrition greatly increases perioperative risk, the malnourished patient should be identified early so that appropriate intervention can be undertaken. The patient's nutritional history must be reviewed. For example, consider whether the weight is 20% above or below normal, 10% of usual body weight has been recently lost or gained, physical problems are present that interfere with eating, and the patient has been maintained for more than a week on "routine" intravenous (IV) fluids. (Recall that a liter of fluid with 5% dextrose contains only 170 calories, all from carbohydrates, and that electrolyte solutions without dextrose have essentially no calories.)

INTRAOPERATIVE PERIOD

INTRAOPERATIVE FLUID MANAGEMENT

Hypotension may develop promptly with the induction of anesthesia if preoperative correction of extracellular FVD has been inadequate. Further predisposing to hypotension in the operative period is fluid loss due to bleeding, shifting of intravascular fluid into the surgical site (third-space edema), evaporation of fluid from the exposed peritoneum during abdominal surgery, and inhalation of dry gases. Most patients tolerate a 500-mL blood loss without difficulty, as albumin synthesis and erythropoiesis will usually compensate for such minor losses. However, when this volume is exceeded, blood replacement must be considered.

Third-space fluid shift (which cannot be directly measured) can be substantial after extensive dissection of tissue; fluid can also sequester into the lumen and wall of the small bowel and accumulate in the peritoneal cavity. Judicious intraoperative correction of third-space fluid losses with an electrolyte solution (such as lactated Ringer's solution) markedly reduces postoperative oliguria. Although no accurate formula for intraoperative fluid administration is known, balanced salt solution needed during surgery is approximately 0.5 to 1 L/h (but only to a maximum of 2–3 L during a 4-hour major abdominal procedure unless there are other measurable losses).[9]

EFFECT OF CARDIOPULMONARY BYPASS ON FLUID AND ELECTROLYTE BALANCE

Cardiopulmonary bypass, used for patients undergoing cardiac surgery, has unique effects on body fluids and electrolytes. Since massive extracellular fluid (ECF) volume expansion is required for patients undergoing cardiopulmonary bypass, a 5- to 15-lb weight gain is expected.[10] Indeed, it has been shown that patients undergoing cardiopulmonary bypass without weight gain during the procedure develop significant postoperative problems (such as hypovolemia and poor cardiac function).[11] The expanded ECF can persist for up to 10 days postoperatively.[12] Management of this problem in the postoperative period includes use of diuretics and colloids (such as albumin or hetastarch) to help mobilize the accumulated fluid. (See Chapter 11 for a discussion of colloid solutions.)

There is a tendency to hyponatremia because plasma antidiuretic hormone (ADH) levels during cardiopulmonary bypass are higher than in other types of surgery (causing excessive water retention with sodium dilution).[13] During the postoperative period, free-water intake is minimized to avoid hyponatremia. In patients with preoperative congestive heart failure, both fluid and sodium restriction may be indicated.

Hypokalemia commonly occurs during bypass and requires treatment, usually over and beyond the hyperkalemic cardioplegia solutions used at the termination of bypass.[14] This is especially important in patients who were taking digoxin before surgery. (Recall that hypokalemia intensifies the action of digoxin on the myocardium.) Conditions aggravating the drop in serum potassium during cardiopulmonary bypass include the preoperative use of potassium-losing diuretics, urinary potassium losses, and shifting of potassium into the intracellular space. The obvious danger of hypokalemia is increased risk of arrhythmia.

Hypomagnesemia is also common during and after cardiopulmonary bypass (due to dilution of plasma magnesium by ECF volume expansion, and binding of magnesium by chelating agents in administered stored blood products).[15] Indicators of hypomagnesemia in the postoperative period can include hyperreflexia, enhanced digoxin toxicity, and cardiac arrhythmias.

POSTOPERATIVE PERIOD

NEUROENDOCRINE RESPONSE

The neuroendocrine response stimulated by many anesthetic agents is further heightened by surgical stress. Secretion of adrenocorticotrophic hormone (ACTH) and cortisol is increased according to the magnitude of surgery or trauma. Cortisol and ACTH levels generally remain elevated for 2 to 4 days after surgery; with extensive trauma or the complications of sepsis or shock, however, levels may remain elevated for weeks.[16]

Circulatory instability related to fluid losses during surgery and trauma produces decreased renal perfusion, which in turn stimulates production of substances (renin, angiotensin, and aldosterone) that support the blood pressure through vasoconstriction and sodium and water conservation.[17] Isotonic fluid volume reduction (as occurs in simple blood loss) is one of the most potent stimuli to aldosterone and ADH secretion in humans. Surgery and trauma also cause increased release of ADH through vasoconstriction of the renal artery and stimulation of the hypothalamus; these effects may persist 12 to 24 hours into the postoperative period. Reduced volumes of concentrated urine can be expected in the early postoperative period due to these hormonal changes. Unfortunately, increased aldosterone secretion results in greater urinary loss of potassium, predisposing to hypokalemia if potassium replacement is inadequate. Cerebrovascular surgical patients may have either prolonged inappropriate secretion of ADH (resulting in dilutional hyponatremia) or, possibly, suppression of ADH secretion (resulting in diabetes insipidus with hypernatremia). Therefore, careful monitoring of plasma osmolality and sodium levels is required (see Chapter 20).

METABOLIC CHANGES

During the first hours after surgical trauma, secretion of growth hormone and glucagon is stimulated whereas insulin secretion is suppressed, resulting in hyperglycemia. The second phase may last from days to weeks and occurs after tissue perfusion has been restored; it is characterized by catabolism, negative nitrogen balance, and hyperglycemia. The extent of negative nitrogen balance varies considerably and is largely related to the magnitude of the injury.[18] Normally, the patient should lose ¼ to ½ lb/day during the acute injury phase. The third phase of altered metabolism is associated with a slow but progressive reaccumulation of protein followed by a reaccumulation of body fat.

HEMODYNAMIC ALTERATIONS

With the increased circulating catecholamines, an increase in heart rate and cardiac output occurs, as does vasoconstriction. In persons with heart disease who cannot increase cardiac output (or in older individuals with chronic coronary insufficiency), four types of undesirable changes can result from this physiological challenge. These include (1) acute congestive heart failure, (2) acute cardiac arrhythmias, (3) peripheral tissue anoxia and lactic acidosis, and (4) outright visceral failure (brain or kidneys).[19] As circulating volume changes, the right and left atria and great veins of the mediastinum alter the production of aldosterone and ADH secretion.[20] If alkalosis occurs, a left shift in the oxyhemoglobin curve results; reduced oxygen delivery may reduce cerebral function, causing disorientation, hallucinations, extreme restlessness, or coma.

FLUID AND ELECTROLYTE IMBALANCES

Fluid Volume Deficit

By far the most common fluid disorder in the postoperative patient is extracellular FVD.[21] Contributing factors to postoperative FVD include loss of GI fluids, continued third-space fluid shifts, fever, overzealous blood sampling for repeated chemical determinations, hyperventilation of greater than 35 respirations per minute, injudicious administration of diuretics, and an unhumidified tracheostomy with hyperventilation.

Among the indicators of FVD are decreased urine output, postural hypotension and tachycardia, diminished skin turgor, decreased capillary refill time, and blood urea nitrogen (BUN) elevated out of proportion to the serum creatinine (see Chapter 3). If body fluids are directly lost from the body (as from vomiting or diuresis), body weight will decrease acutely. However, if FVD is due to third-spacing, decreased body weight does not occur because the fluid "lost" from the vascular space pools in another part of the body (such as the surgical site or bowel due to adynamic ileus). Actually, as parenteral fluids are administered to correct the vascular volume deficit, the patient will *gain* weight. Intake and output (I & O) measurements are mandatory when FVD is suspected; generally, an acceptable hourly urine volume is 30 to 50 mL in the adult. If the urine volume is decreased and is accompanied by tachycardia and depressed blood pressure, one should suspect a deficit of at least 2 to 3 L.

Of course, fluid replacement must be guided by the intravascular volume status (estimated by vital signs and urine output). Remember that third-spacing from surgical trauma is not limited to the operative period; indeed, it may continue slowly for a few hours or more during the 1st day of injury.[22] Unrecognized deficits of ECF volume during the early postoperative period may be manifested as circulatory instability. Later, as the third-spacing resolves and fluid shifts back into the intravascular space, diuresis and weight loss will occur. In patients with cardiac or renal dysfunction, the shift of fluid back into the vascular bed may result in congestive heart failure or pulmonary edema.

Treatment of FVD depends on the composition of lost fluids. Generally, it can be accomplished with either lactated Ringer's solution (LRS) or isotonic saline (0.9% NaCl). Use of a large volume of isotonic saline can produce hyperchloremic acidosis because it contains considerably more chloride than is normally present in plasma. In some situations, normal volume can be accomplished with albumin or other blood products. (See Chapter 11 for a discussion of IV replacement fluids and their recommended use.) Because fluid losses are only roughly estimated, careful monitoring of physiological indices must be done to warn of overhydration when large volumes of fluid are given rapidly. For example, central venous pressure values over 15 cm of water and wedge pressures over 18 mmHg are indications that fluids are being administered faster than they can be tolerated.[23]

Urine Output

Preferably, urinary output should be at least 30 to 50 mL/hr; an hourly urinary output lower than 25 mL should be investigated. The decreased urinary output of stress reaction (healthy physiological response to surgery) must be differentiated from pathological developments. Factors contributing to decreased urinary volume in the postoperative patient may include the following:

▶ Inadequate preoperative fluid replacement
▶ Hypovolemia resulting from fluid loss incurred during surgery (either direct loss or subtle third-space accumulation at the surgical site or intestinal ileus)
▶ Disturbance in myocardial function, causing decreased blood flow to the kidneys and thus decreased urine formation
▶ Renal failure (a serious cause of postoperative oliguria)

Although oliguric renal failure may occur postoperatively in the patient who has suffered poor renal perfusion during surgery, high-output renal failure is actually more frequent. The latter is characterized by uremia occurring with a daily urine volume greater than 1000 to 1500 mL. It probably represents the renal response to a less severe episode of renal injury than is required to cause the classic oliguric renal failure. Although it is generally easier to manage than oliguric renal failure, high-output failure is more difficult to recognize. Typically, the urine volume is normal or greater than normal (often reaching 3–5 L/day) whereas the BUN is increasing. A real danger for hyperkalemia exists when potassium is administered to a patient with unrecognized high-output failure.

Fluid Volume Excess

In trauma and postoperative patients, there may be seepage of large volumes of fluid from the vascular space into a third space (such as the surgical site, or generalized interstitial space due to decreased plasma oncotic pressure after albumin loss). As fluids are administered to correct these vascular losses, the body takes on an added fluid load. Technically, this positive salt and water retention is not considered fluid volume overload. Instead, fluid volume overload is defined as overexpansion of the *intravascular* volume.[24]

In the surgical patient without renal failure, the most common causes of volume overload are iatrogenic (overcorrection of a previous volume deficit, a poorly guarded "keep-open" IV line, or a positive gain of water in patients receiving constant humidified ventilatory support). Drugs such as morphine sulfate, and most of its substitutes, are markedly antidiuretic and thus can predispose to fluid retention.[25] Among the earliest signs is weight gain during the catabolic period when the patient is expected to lose ¼ to ½ lb/day. In addition to peripheral edema, overadministration of isotonic electrolyte solutions may cause pulmonary edema and increased local edema at the surgical site. The increased edema may be sufficient to cause partial or complete obstruction in intestinal surgery.

Although volume overload can occur at any time in the postoperative period, it is more common soon after surgery. Daily weight measurement is necessary to detect excessive weight gain due to retained fluid. If pulmonary edema is present, diuretics may be indicated. Observation for pulmonary edema is crucial since eventually the retained third-space fluid will shift back into the vascular space.

Hyponatremia

A frequent imbalance in the postoperative period is hyponatremia, related to excessive ADH secretion. Conditions favoring increased ADH secretion include the trauma of major surgery itself, premedication, anesthesia, decreased blood volume, and pain. Although it is not important to aggressively treat patients who have serum sodium levels between 130 to 135 mEq/L, this important clue to the risk of future serious hyponatremia should be heeded.[26] That is, the simple measure of restricting free water should be taken to avoid the full-blown syndrome of water intoxication (severe dilutional hyponatremia). Cases of permanent brain damage related to profound hyponatremia have been reported in postoperative patients receiving excessive free water.

Potassium Imbalances

Hypokalemia is the most common potassium imbalance in surgical patients. However, it is unnecessary and probably unwise to administer potassium during the first 24 hours postoperatively unless a definite potassium deficit exists.[27] This is because trauma causes release of potassium from cells in the surgical site into the extracellular space in the early postoperative period. For patients at risk for renal failure due to hypotensive episodes during the surgical procedure, even small potassium supplements can be detrimental. After the first 24 hours, potassium is administered daily as necessary to replace urinary and GI potassium losses.[28] Generally, a daily supplementation of 60 to 100 mEq is required postoperatively.[29] The needed potassium should be distributed evenly in the total daily maintenance fluids. For example, if 2 L of fluid are prescribed over 24 hours, and 80 mEq of potassium chloride is the required daily potassium supplement, 40 mEq/L should be added. This makes far more sense than routinely administering "K-runs" to meet maintenance potassium needs. (See the discussion of IV potassium replacement in Chapter 5.) Special considerations for patients undergoing cardiopulmonary bypass are discussed earlier in this chapter.

Hyperkalemia is rare in the postoperative patient, except when acute renal failure, rhabdomyolysis, massive hemolysis, or tissue necrosis is present. If hyperkalemia occurs at any time in the postoperative period, the possibility of impaired renal function (manifested by a rising serum creatinine in the presence of low, normal, or high urine output) should be explored. Release of cellular potassium by crush injuries and electrical injuries, plus acute renal failure, can lead to lethal hyperkalemia within hours.

Acid—Base Disorders

Surgical patients may have normal pH, or develop virtually any acid—base abnormality (depending on indi-

TABLE 14–1.
Examples of Nursing Diagnoses For a New Postoperative Patient After Abdominal Surgery

NURSING DIAGNOSIS	ETIOLOGICAL FACTORS	DEFINING CHARACTERISTICS
FVD related to actual fluid loss and third-space fluid shift during surgical procedure	Vomiting after reaction to anesthesia GI suction Third-space fluid shift at surgical site	Postural tachycardia Postural hypotension initially; later, low BP in all positions Decreased skin turgor Decreased capillary refill time Oliguria (<30 mL/hr in adult) Weight change depends on cause (decreased if actual fluid loss, as in GI suction; usually increased if fluid loss is due to third-space shift, provided parenteral fluids are given in an attempt to correct hypovolemia)
Altered tissue perfusion (renal) related to hypotension during surgical procedure	Hypotensive effects of anesthesia Hypovolemia due to direct or indirect loss of fluid Hypovolemia due to inadequate parenteral fluid replacement	Oliguria or polyuria in presence of elevated serum creatinine (see discussion of low-output and high-output renal failure in text.)
Alteration in sodium balance (hyponatremia) related to excessive ADH activity	Major surgery with its premedication, anesthesia, decreased blood volume, and postoperative pain results in increased ADH release (causing water retention with sodium dilution)	Serum sodium < 135 mEq/L May be asymptomatic if Na > 120 mEq/L Lethargy, confusion, nausea, vomiting, anorexia, abdominal cramps, muscular twitching (see Chapter 5).
Alteration in acid—base balance (metabolic alkalosis) related to vomiting or gastric suction	Vomiting after reaction to anesthesia Gastric suction, particularly if patient is allowed to ingest ice chips freely	Tingling of fingers, toes, and circumoral region, due to decreased calcium ionization pH > 7.45, bicarbonate above normal, chloride below normal
Altered nutrition (less than body requirements) related to negative nitrogen balance after surgical stress, and inadequate caloric intake	Catabolic response to stress of surgery Inability to tolerate oral feedings during first few postoperative days due to decreased GI motility, anorexia, nausea, and general discomfort Failure of health-care providers to administer sufficient calories via the parenteral route	Weight loss of approximately ¼ to ½ lb/day in adult (provided fluids are not abnormally retained) Perhaps a decrease in serum albumin, transferrin, and retinol binding protein levels (although delivery of a large volume of blood products or the long half-life of certain secretory proteins can interfere with correct interpretation)[32]

BP, blood pressure; FVD, fluid volume deficit; GI, gastrointestinal.

vidual circumstances). Respiratory acidosis may result from shallow respirations related to anesthesia, narcotics, abdominal distention, pain, or large cumbersome dressings. On assessment, decreased respirations and decreased breath sounds in the bases may be noted. Measures to increase gas exchange, such as frequent coughing and deep breathing, frequent suctioning of tracheobronchial secretions, avoidance of oversedation, and turning and ambulating the patient, will decrease the likelihood of respiratory acidosis. Subclinical respiratory alkalosis is common in surgical patients.[30] Common causes include hyperventilation due to pain, hypoxia, central nervous system injury, and assisted ventilation. In fact, most patients who require ventilatory support in the postoperative period will develop varying degrees of respiratory alkalosis. Therefore, frequent measurement of arterial blood gases is necessary to allow proper corrections of the ventilatory pattern when indicated. To prevent serious complications, the pCO_2 should not be allowed to drop below 30 mmHg.[31] This is particularly important in the presence of a complicating metabolic alkalosis (for which hypoventilation with subsequent carbon dioxide retention is needed for compensatory purposes).

The most common causes of metabolic acidosis in surgical patients include loss of alkali from biliary and pancreatic drainage, ketoacidosis, renal failure, and lactic acidosis associated with shock. Metabolic alkalosis generally results from loss of acid due to nasogastric drainage or vomiting, and therapy with potassium-losing diuretics.

Nursing Diagnoses

Table 14-1 lists some possible nursing diagnoses related to fluid and electrolyte balance for a patient who has undergone abdominal surgery.

FLUID RESUSCITATION

Chapter 11 discusses commonly prescribed water and electrolyte parenteral fluids and colloid solutions (hetastarch, albumin, and other blood products).

REFERENCES

1. Schwartz S, Shires G, Spencer F: Principles of Surgery, 5th ed, p 85. New York, McGraw-Hill, 1989
2. Ibid
3. Condon R, Nyhus L: Manual of Surgical Therapeutics, 7th ed, p 265. Boston, Little, Brown, 1988
4. Schwartz et al, p 1577
5. Ibid
6. Ibid, p 1575
7. Condon, Nyhus, p 265
8. Pestana C: Fluids and Electrolytes in the Surgical Patient, 4th ed, p 174. Baltimore, Williams & Wilkins, 1989
9. Schwartz et al, p 86
10. Kokko J, Tannen R: Fluids and Electrolytes, 2nd ed, p 1016. Philadelphia, WB Saunders, 1990
11. Ibid
12. Ibid
13. Ibid, p 1017
14. Ibid
15. Ibid
16. Ibid, p 993
17. Ibid
18. Schwartz et al, p 92
19. Moore F: Homeostasis: Bodily changes in trauma and surgery. In Sabaston D (ed): Textbook of Surgery, 12th ed, vol 1, p 39. Philadelphia, WB Saunders, 1981
20. Ibid, p 42
21. Schwartz et al, p 73
22. Ibid, p 87
23. Shoemaker et al: Textbook of Critical Care, 2nd ed, p 1139. Philadelphia, WB Saunders, 1989
24. Kokko, Tannen, p 1007
25. Moore, p 50
26. Kokko, Tannen, p 1008
27. Schwartz et al, p 87
28. Ibid, p 88
29. Kokko, Tannen, p 1010
30. Shires G: Fluids, Electrolytes and Acid–Bases, p 8. New York, Churchill Livingstone, 1988
31. Ibid, p 9
32. Rombeau J, Caldwell M: Clinical Nutrition: Enteral and Tube Feeding, 2nd ed, p 318. Philadelphia, WB Saunders, 1990

15

Cirrhosis with Ascites

PATHOPHYSIOLOGY

Cirrhosis is characterized by an extensive increase of fibrous tissue within the liver structure. As blood, lymph, and biliary channels become compressed by fibrotic changes, intrahepatic pressure increases, reducing the liver's capacity to fulfill its functions. At first the liver is enlarged with fatty tissue; later, it becomes small, hard, and nodular.

ASCITES FORMATION

A common complication of cirrhosis is ascites, a collection of serum-like fluid in the peritoneal cavity. This fluid accumulates as venous outflow is impeded through the fibrotic liver, and then seeps from the surface of the liver into the peritoneal cavity to produce ascites. Because of the fluid's high protein content, it pulls additional fluid from the surfaces of the gut and mesentery by osmosis.

Exact mechanisms in the development of ascites remain unclear; however, several theories have been proposed, including "overfilling" and "underfilling." Both are probably plausible, depending on the stage of hepatic disease. Early, intrahepatic hypertension activates a hepatic baroreceptor reflex that enhances renal sodium retention and increased plasma volume. As the cirrhotic disease progresses, this overflow spills into the peritoneal cavity as ascites. The fluid shift from the vascular system to the peritoneal space causes underfilling, which eventually dominates the clinical picture. Stimulation of the renin–angiotensin system increases renal sodium retention and thus plasma volume.

Decreased Effective Arterial Volume

Decreased effective arterial volume refers to a state in which the total extracellular fluid (ECF) volume is normal or even expanded, although the kidneys respond as if they were underperfused.[1] They do so by retaining sodium and producing a concentrated urine. This, presumably, is what occurs in the patient with cirrhosis and ascites formation.

Hypoalbuminemia

Severe *hypoalbuminemia* may also contribute to ascites formation. Causes of low serum albumin levels in cirrhotic patients include decreased synthesis of protein by the diseased liver, dilutional effect (due to salt and water retention), and a shift of protein from the vascular space to the peritoneal cavity. The protein content of ascitic fluid may be as high as half that of serum.[2] Because the serum albumin level is below normal, plasma oncotic pressure is reduced, an effect that favors shifting of fluid from the vascular space into the peritoneal cavity.

However, hypoalbuminemia is not nearly as important in ascites formation as is the increased pressure generated by hepatic postsinusoidal obstruction.[3] Relief from ascites has been reported when portal hypertension is corrected by surgical shunting procedures.

EDEMA

Edema formation in cirrhotic patients has several causes. Increased pressure in the vena cava (secondary to ascitic fluid and enlarged liver size) interferes with venous drainage of the lower extremities. Contributing to edema formation is the hypoalbuminemia that is frequently present in patients with advanced liver disease. By lowering the plasma oncotic pressure, hypoalbuminemia promotes shifting of fluid from the intravascular to the interstitial space.

At first edema appears in dependent areas; later it spreads to nondependent areas, varying in severity with the degree of sodium intake.[4] The edema associated with liver disease is of the "pitting" variety (see Fig. 2-6).

FLUID AND ELECTROLYTE DISTURBANCES

Fluid Volume Excess

The patient with advanced cirrhotic disease has a complex fluid balance problem. Although there is an excess of total body fluid with an accumulation in the peritoneal cavity (ascites) and in the interstitial space (edema), there is also a problem of decreased effective arterial blood volume. Because of this, the kidneys strive to build up the intravascular volume by retaining sodium and water (although the blood volume may actually be normal or even above normal). Plasma aldosterone levels are often above normal due to increased adrenal secretion and inability of the liver to deactivate this hormone. Aldosterone, of course, causes sodium and water retention. Nonsteroidal antiinflammatory drugs (NSAID) should be avoided because they may cause deterioration in renal function (with further fluid retention) if given in sufficient doses to patients with ascites due to liver disease.[5]

Hyponatremia

Hyponatremia is common in patients with advanced hepatic cirrhosis and is usually due to impaired ability to excrete water. Experimental and clinical evidence suggests that the impaired water excretion is related to persistent release of antidiuretic hormone (ADH).[6] A derangement in renal hemodynamics may also contribute to this effect. This hyponatremia occurs in addition to fluid volume excess. That is, although there is abnormal retention of both sodium and water, a relatively greater degree of water retention occurs. As such, the serum sodium level is diluted below normal although the total body sodium is excessive (see Fig. 4-2A). Other factors that can contribute to hyponatremia are sodium loss through frequent paracentesis or excessive diuretic use, or too stringent sodium restriction.

Additional possible fluid and electrolyte disturbances related to cirrhosis of the liver are listed in Table 15-1, along with probable etiological associations.

EFFECTS ON BODY SYSTEMS

Cirrhosis of the liver has an insidious onset and affects most body systems. Brief discussions of the effects on various body systems follow.

Gastrointestinal System

Development of esophageal varices is the most serious complication associated with hepatic failure and portal hypertension. Severity of bleeding from varices is intensified by coagulopathies associated with liver failure. Enlarged abdominal veins and internal hemorrhoids may also be caused by portal hypertension. Malnutrition is common in patients with hepatic failure because the frequently associated anorexia, nausea, and vomiting preclude the recommended dietary intake. Many gastrointestinal (GI) symptoms are related to venous engorgement of the GI organs. Muscle wast-

TABLE 15–1.
Possible Water and Electrolyte Disturbances in Patients With Advanced Cirrhosis and Ascites

DISTURBANCE	ETIOLOGY
Increased total ECF volume, but decreased effective arterial volume	Enhanced renal tubular reabsorption of sodium
	Increased plasma aldosterone level due to increased adrenal secretion (in response to decreased effective arterial volume) and decreased degradation of this hormone by the diseased liver
Increased water retention, causing dilutional hyponatremia	Impaired renal water excretion related to excess ADH secretion (in response to decreased effective arterial volume)
Hypokalemia	Direct loss in vomiting or diarrhea
	Decreased intake due to anorexia
	Excessive use of potassium-losing diuretics (Note that hypokalemia is especially harmful to patients with hepatic failure because it increases ammonia formation and can induce hepatic coma.)
Hyperkalemia	Excessive use of potassium-sparing diuretics, especially when renal insufficiency is present or potassium-containing salt substitutes are used to make the low-sodium diet more palatable
Elevated serum ammonia level	Under normal circumstances, the large amounts of ammonia formed in the intestines by bacterial action are absorbed into the bloodstream and carried to the liver to be converted to urea for renal excretion. However, in cirrhosis, the liver cannot convert the ammonia to urea; thus, the blood ammonia level increases.
Hypomagnesemia	Loss of magnesium in vomiting and diarrhea, poor dietary intake, and renal wasting of magnesium in patients with cirrhosis due to alcoholism
Hypocalcemia	Possibly a result of inadequate storage of vitamin D by diseased liver
Hyperventilation with respiratory alkalosis	May be related to hyperammonemia (high ammonia level acts as a respiratory stimulant)
Respiratory acidosis	May occur if ascites is severe enough to compromise diaphragmatic movement
Metabolic alkalosis	Common in patients treated with potassium-losing diuretics such as furosemide, thiazides, and ethacrynic acid
Mild metabolic acidosis	May occur in patients treated with spironolactone (Aldactone) alone (due to interference by spironolactone with sodium/hydrogen ion exchange in the distal tubules)

ECF, extracellular fluid; ADH, antidiuretic hormone.

ing and weight loss may be masked by fluid retention. Fetor hepaticus is often noted.

Cardiovascular System

Right ventricular heart failure often occurs in patients with hepatic failure secondary to high pressure in the portal system. Contributing to cardiac problems is the hypokalemia commonly found in cirrhotic patients due to use of potassium-losing diuretics. Potassium deficiency predisposes to ventricular arrhythmias. Of course, arrhythmias may also result from hyperkalemia, which can occur in patients treated with potassium-sparing diuretics, particularly if renal disease is present.

Renal System

Hepatorenal syndrome (HRS) encompasses a poorly explained type of renal failure in patients with liver disease. It is an ominous occurrence with an unclear pathophysiology, associated with a high mortality rate. Although HRS is usually fatal, cause of death in most patients is due to hepatic, rather than renal, insufficiency. Death usually occurs before uremia develops.[7] Hepatorenal syndrome is manifested by oliguria, increased serum creatinine (although usually <10 mg/dL), increased blood urea nitrogen (BUN), low urinary sodium output, and maintained ability of the kidneys to concentrate urine until the last stages of the syndrome. Evidently the abnormality is functional rather than structural because few or no histological changes are demonstrated. The latter statement is substantiated by reports that the kidney from a patient with HRS may be successfully transplanted into a patient with normal liver function.[8] Also, when liver transplants are performed on patients with HRS, renal function may normalize.[9]

Neurological System

Portal systemic encephalopathy (PSE) refers to the syndrome of disordered consciousness and altered neuromuscular activity seen in patients with hepatic failure. In the presence of hepatic failure, a variety of toxins bypass the liver (where they would normally be destroyed) and enter the systemic circulation in abnormal concentrations. Although the exact toxins are not defined, ammonia is one of the implicated substances. Recall that the normal liver converts ammonia into urea for renal excretion. When this process is altered by a diseased liver, the serum ammonia level may rise sharply. However, the degree of serum ammonia elevation is not always predictive of the severity of PSE. Whatever the precise biochemical trigger of PSE, interference with cerebral metabolism and neurotransmission appears to be the basic underlying mechanism. Symptoms may range from mild (sleep-wake disturbances and ataxia) to severe (coma and seizures).

Precipitating causes of PSE episodes include fluid volume depletion from overzealous use of diuretics, high protein diet, digestion of blood from GI bleeding, constipation, infection, progressive liver dysfunction, and hypokalemia with alkalosis. Inability of the liver to convert the end products of protein metabolism to urea results in an elevated serum ammonia level. Constipation increases the systemic absorption of toxins from the colon. Hypokalemia increases ammonia production and alkalosis promotes movement of ammonia and other toxins into the brain.

Not all neurological symptoms of hepatic failure patients are due to PSE. They may be related to sodium derangements, especially hyponatremia. For this reason, even mild hyponatremia may be treated aggressively. Another cause of neurological symptoms may be severe malnutrition, which often accompanies hepatic failure. For example, deficiencies of B vitamins can lead to paresthesias, sensory disturbances, peripheral nerve degeneration, palsy of the sixth cranial nerve, and ptosis.

Respiratory System

The primary respiratory complication associated with hepatic failure is decreased lung expansion secondary to upward pressure on the diaphragm from ascites. Lung capacity may also be reduced due to hydrothorax when ascitic fluid leaks through the diaphragm into the pleural cavity. Last, pulmonary hypertension is sometimes associated with uncontrolled portal hypertension. Hypoxemia and hypercarbia may result in all of the above circumstances. However, if a high serum ammonia level is present, hyperventilation with respiratory alkalosis may occur due to stimulation of the respiratory center.

Immune System

The patient with chronic hepatic failure has an increased risk for infection because the liver is no longer able to filter bacteria effectively from the blood. In addition, associated hypersplenism causes a decreased white blood cell count. Infection, particularly full-blown sepsis, places the patient at increased risk for fluid and electrolyte disturbances.

Dermatological System

There are dermatological signs of liver failure, including varying degrees of jaundice, palmar erythema, hair changes, and spider angiomas. Spider angiomas are small dilated superficial vessels resembling bluish-red spiders that may appear in the skin of the face, forearms, and hands. They may represent a large shunting of blood and can bleed profusely.

Hematological System

Anemia may occur in hepatic failure because the hypersplenism caused by portal hypertension increases the rate of red blood cell destruction. Also, the malnutrition that commonly accompanies hepatic failure decreases the rate of red blood cell formation.

Increased bleeding tendencies due to vitamin K deficiency and decreased prothrombin formation leave the patient at risk for excessive bleeding from menses, nosebleeds, gingivitis, GI mucosal changes, and even bruising. Recall that as bleeding in the GI tract is increased, buildup of ammonia secondary to digestion of blood (a protein-containing substance) is increased. Blood transfusions increase the hepatic failure patient's chance for developing hyperammoniemia if aged whole blood is used (see Chap. 11).

TREATMENT

Treatment of advanced cirrhotic patients is in part directed at controlling the excess fluid in the peritoneal cavity (ascites) and interstitial space (edema). Among the therapies for these problems are sodium restriction, bedrest, diuretics, water restriction (when hyponatremia is a problem), paracentesis, albumin administration, and peritoneovenous shunts. Other therapeutic interventions for patients with advanced hepatic disease are directed at preventing hepatic coma. Among these are dietary protein restriction and administration of lactulose, bowel-sterilizing antibiotics, and laxatives or enemas.

SODIUM RESTRICTION

Patients with ascites are first treated with sodium-restricted diets. Dietary sodium restriction varies according to need, but daily limitations of 500 mg are usually necessary initially.[10] A more liberal sodium intake (750–1000 mg/day) may be allowed when a diuresis is effected.[11] Low sodium diets are discussed in Chapter 3.

BEDREST

Approximately 5% to 15% of cirrhotic patients can be managed with bedrest and moderate sodium restriction.[12] Unless life-threatening complications of ascites are present, patients should be given a trial of 3 to 4 days of bedrest and sodium restriction.[13] After diuresis has been initiated, a gradual increase in activity can be allowed.[14]

DIURETICS

Diuretics should be considered for patients who do not respond to salt restriction and bedrest. The amount of ascites that can be mobilized via the peritoneal capillaries is limited to approximately 500 to 750 mL/day in most patients; therefore, diuretic dosage should be determined cautiously.[15] Overvigorous use of diuretics may result in severe contraction of the intravascular fluid volume, causing azotemia and worsening of hepatic encephalopathy. Of course, in edematous patients, diuretics promote fluid loss from the tissue space as well as from the pool of ascites. It is generally accepted that the goal of diuretic therapy is a daily weight loss of 0.5 to 1.0 kg in edematous patients with ascites and approximately 0.25 kg in those having ascites but no edema.[16] These figures are consistent with findings from the classic study reported by Shear and associates in 1970.[17] A more recent study reported that cirrhotic patients without peripheral edema could safely undergo diuresis of 0.75 kg/day as compared with more than 2 kg/day for those with peripheral edema.[18]

Spironolactone (an aldosterone-blocking agent) is usually the first diuretic prescribed when conservative measures (sodium restriction and bedrest) fail to induce an adequate diuresis. Loop diuretics (furosemide, bumetanide, or ethacrynic acid) may be added to spironolactone in patients who fail to respond to spironolactone alone. Because loop diuretics are potassium-losing agents, hypokalemia must be avoided because this imbalance can contribute to the development of hepatic encephalopathy. A frequently advocated method to avoid hypokalemia is the concomitant administration of a potassium-sparing agent, such as spironolactone, with a potassium-losing agent. This not only helps avoid hypokalemia but provides two agents to eliminate excess body sodium.

WATER RESTRICTION

Water restriction is not indicated for all patients. However, if dilutional hyponatremia occurs, a fluid restriction to 1000 to 1500 mL/day will usually suffice.[19] For severe hyponatremia, fluid restriction to the amount necessary to replace insensible loss plus urine output may be needed.

PARACENTESIS

Eventually, patients with ascites may become refractory to diuretics and require paracentesis to relieve respiratory distress and symptoms of marked intraabdominal pressure. Several studies suggested that paracentesis in patients with massive ascites results in a shorter hospital stay and a decreased incidence of fluid and electrolyte disturbances when compared with treatment with diuretics alone.[20,21] In a related study, it was reported that the intravenous (IV) administration of 40 g of albumin after each large-volume paracentesis appeared to minimize the risk of intravascular volume depletion due to rapid reaccumulation of ascites.[22]

The desired rate for removing ascites is somewhat unclear. Removing more than 1.5 to 2.0 L/day from patients with ascites but no peripheral edema may lead to a reduction in cardiac output, particularly if albumin infusions are withheld.[23] In contrast, a recent study suggested that patients with ascites who also have peripheral edema may be treated with daily 4- to 6-L paracenteses.[24] Another source indicated that up to 5 L of ascitic fluid can be safely removed if the patient has edema, the fluid is removed slowly (over 30–90 min), and a fluid restriction is initiated to avoid hyponatremia.[25] Excessive fluid removal by paracentesis may lead to circulatory collapse, encephalopathy, or renal failure in some patients. When paracenteses are performed regularly, the state of tissue perfusion must be monitored. This can be simply estimated by monitoring the BUN and plasma creatinine concentration; stable levels indicate that renal perfusion and, presumably, that of other organs is well maintained and paracentesis can be safely continued.[26]

ALBUMIN ADMINISTRATION

Although 25% albumin is sometimes administered IV to ascitic patients to help correct intravascular volume depletion, it is expensive and appears to offer little advantage over crystalloid solutions for volume expansion.[27] A study conducted in 1949 reported that albumin administered IV passed into the ascites pool in significant quantities, causing the researchers to conclude that albumin was not markedly beneficial in the management of the underlying liver disorder.[28] However, recent studies indicated that albumin infusion is helpful in preventing fluid volume complications when repeated large-volume paracenteses are performed on patients with massive ascites.[29]

PERITONEOVENOUS SHUNTS

Peritoneovenous shunts (such as the LeVeen or Denver shunt) are sometimes used for the 5% to 10% of patients with ascites who do not respond to sodium restriction, diuretics, or other types of medical therapy.[30] The *LaVeen shunt* consists of a long tube (with openings along the sides) inserted into the abdominal cavity, running under subcutaneous tissue into the jugular vein. With the shunt, reinfusion of ascitic fluid into the venous system is allowed (a one-way valve prevents backflow of blood). Pressure changes of respiration permit the shunt to operate. An average weight loss of 10 kg during the first week after shunt placement is not unusual.[31] To achieve adequate post-shunt diuresis, diuretics are essential; the response to diuretics is markedly improved after shunt placement.[32] Although the shunt may be effective in controlling ascites, its use is associated with a number of serious complications, which include episodes of disseminated intravascular coagulation (due to entry into the bloodstream of endotoxin or other procoagulant material in the ascitic fluid), frequent shunt thrombosis, sepsis, and hemodilution. Shunts should not be used in patients with recent variceal hemorrhage because the risk for further bleeding is increased by the volume expansion as the ascitic fluid is drained into the venous system. Other contraindications are coagulopathies or bacteria in the ascitic fluid. Shunt failure reportedly occurs in 10% of cases.[33] Mortality may approach 25% in the first month.[34]

Dietary Protein Restriction

Impending hepatic coma is an indication to eliminate protein temporarily from the diet. A reduced protein intake decreases ammonia formation, and thus the likelihood for hepatic encephalopathy. Adequate nonprotein calories (25–30 cal/kg) must be supplied by the enteral or parenteral route.[35] It appears that vegetable proteins are tolerated better by patients with portal-systemic encephalopathy than diets containing meat proteins.[36] As the patient improves, more protein can be added in small increments every few days as tolerated. Specialized enteral and parenteral formulas are commercially available for malnourished patients with hepatic failure and concomitant hepatic encephalopathy; these formulas are designed to correct the abnormal amino acid profile associated with hepatic encephalopathy. They contain low quantities of aromatic amino acids and methionine and high quantities of branched chain amino acids.[37]

Bowel-Sterilizing Antibiotics

Bowel-sterilizing antibiotics, such as neomycin, can reduce ammonia formation caused by excessive bacterial growth in the bowel. Recall that neomycin (given orally, by nasogastric tube, or by enema) kills urease-producing bacteria, causing less urease to be produced and, hence, less urea to be broken down into ammonia. There is a risk of nephrotoxicity and ototoxicity when neomycin is used, particularly in patients with renal impairment. Metronidazole is an agent that is useful for short-term therapy when neomycin is unavailable or poorly tolerated.[38]

Lactulose as Laxative

Constipation should be prevented because the systemic absorption of toxic nitrogenous substances from the intestinal lumen is more likely when constipation is allowed to occur. Lactulose is a poorly absorbed substance used to promote more frequent stools and thus prevent or treat PSE. About 97% of the lactulose taken orally reaches the colon unabsorbed. The mechanisms by which it reduces PSE are unclear, but three actions have been suggested. First, through the conversion of lactulose to organic acids (such as lactic acid) the *p*H of colonic contents decreases, inhibiting the diffusion of ammonia (NH_3) from the colon into the blood. Second, because the *p*H of the bowel vasculature is relatively higher than the contents of the colon under treatment with lactulose, ammonia is converted into ammonium (NH_4), preventing its absorption. Due to this same *p*H gradient, absorption of amines (also implicated in PSE) from the colon to the bloodstream is reduced. Third, lactulose has a cathartic effect caused by an osmotic effect, which increases the water contents of stool.

By monitoring the *p*H of stool (with regular *p*H paper) and adjusting lactulose accordingly, it is possible to reach more precisely a desired *p*H level of 5.[39] Oral dosage begins at 20 to 30 g three or four times a day for 1 or 2 days; the dosage is then adjusted so that two or three soft stools are produced daily.[40]

Lactulose can be administered rectally when it is not tolerated orally or when pulmonary aspiration is a great risk. (Two hundred grams can be diluted in 700 mL of water or saline, depending on risk of sodium absorption and current serum levels).[41] The solution is given through a rectal balloon catheter and retained for 30 to 60 minutes. If not retained, it can be repeated immediately. The process should be repeated every 4 to 6 hours until symptoms of PSE begin to reverse and oral administration can be started. Soapsuds or other enemas with alkalinizing agents are to be avoided because their use can reverse the effects of lactulose.

ASSESSMENT

Nursing assessment of cirrhotic patients with ascites focuses largely on fluid balance parameters, such as fluid gains and losses (as measured by I&O records, body weights, and abdominal girth). More specifically, the nurse is responsible for monitoring responses to therapy and for changes indicating metabolic abnormalities. Listed below are some of the more important nursing assessments with a brief discussion of rationales.

1. Monitor response to diuretics and sodium restriction by the following assessments:
   A. Determine abdominal girth on a serial basis, measuring the abdomen at the same place each time. To ensure accurate placement of the measuring tape, it is helpful to draw lines above and below the tape on each side of the abdomen. Be sure the tape is not kinked under the patient's body. Measurements should be made with the patient in the same position each time (Fig. 15-1).
   B. Measure I&O; expect to see output exceed intake during effective diuresis. Be aware of the danger of excessive diuresis (see Rationale below).
   C. Monitor vital signs at least twice daily. Be alert for hypotension and tachycardia, indications of

excessive diuresis and decreased circulating blood volume.
   D. Monitor for dependent pitting edema. This is helpful in assessing the degree of sodium and water retention.
   E. Measure body weight daily. Weights are most accurate when measured in the early morning before breakfast and after voiding, using the same scale each time. Compare the expected therapeutic weight loss with the actual weight loss (see Rationale below).

Rationale: With adequate sodium restriction and diuretic use, a decrease in abdominal girth, a urinary output relatively greater than the intake during period of diuresis, a decrease in peripheral edema, and a decrease in body weight should be anticipated. The desired weight loss with treatment varies with the patient's clinical status. However, as discussed in the section on treatment, an ascitic patient without peripheral edema might be expected to lose approximately 0.25 kg (½ lb) per day, whereas an ascitic patient with peripheral edema might be expected to lose 0.5 to 1.0 kg (approximately 1–2 lb) per day.[42] Also, as mentioned in the treatment section, one study suggested that weight loss might safely occur more rapidly (eg, 0.75 kg/day in ascitic patients without peripheral edema and >2 kg/day in those with peripheral edema).[43] Because of differences among patients and treatment plans to induce fluid diuresis, the need for careful clinical observations (such as vital sign variations) is evident. The treatment of ascites and edema must be undertaken cautiously. Although the fluid retained as ascites and edema is uncomfortable and cosmetically unpleasing, it is seldom life threatening. However, overly aggressive therapy can lead to hepatic encephalopathy and compromised renal function.

2. Monitor patients undergoing paracentesis carefully for the following adverse effects:

   ▶ Circulatory collapse (eg, pallor; weak, rapid pulse; hypotension; fall in central venous pressure)
   ▶ Decline in renal function (oliguria, rise in BUN, serum creatinine)
   ▶ Worsening of neurological function (lethargy, confusion, slurred speech)

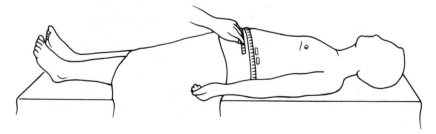

FIGURE 15–1.
Measurement of abdominal girth.

Rationale: Hypovolemia is most likely to result when too much fluid is removed at one time. The mechanism involves a rapid reaccumulation of ascitic fluid, resulting from flow of sodium and water from the intravascular compartment causing a diminished plasma volume. As indicated in the treatment section, the removal of as little as 1500 mL may precipitate hypotension in some patients, particularly in those without peripheral edema. However, some sources state that as much as 5 L may be safely removed in edematous patients, provided the fluid is removed slowly (over 30–90 min) and a fluid restriction is initiated to avoid hyponatremia.[44] Excessive fluid removal via paracentesis or diuresis can precipitate the hepatorenal syndrome (manifested by oliguria or rise in serum creatinine and BUN) or portal-systemic encephalopathy (manifested by, for example, lethargy, confusion, and slurred speech). As discussed earlier, some authors report that the administration of albumin helps prevent fluid balance problems after massive paracentesis.[45]

3. Monitor patients receiving diuretics for disturbances in potassium balance.

Rationale: Patients receiving potassium-losing diuretics (such as furosemide and thiazides) are at risk for hypokalemia. Symptoms include fatigue, muscle weakness, leg cramps, decreased bowel motility, paresthesias, ECG changes (flat T waves and depressed ST segments), arrhythmias, and increased sensitivity to digitalis. On the other hand, patients taking potassium-conserving diuretics (such as spironolactone, Dyrenium, and amiloride) are at risk for hyperkalemia. Symptoms include weakness, paresthesias, ECG changes (tented T waves), and arrhythmias. See Chapter 5 for a review of nursing responsibilities related to potassium imbalances.

4. Monitor patients receiving neomycin for hearing difficulty.

Rationale: Large doses of neomycin can damage both the kidneys and the ears; deafness may occur, particularly when neomycin is administered with furosemide (Lasix) or ethacrynic acid (Edecrin).

5. Monitor patients for symptoms of PSE.

Rationale: This disturbance is particularly likely to occur in individuals who are bleeding into the intestinal tract. Symptoms include lethargy, loss of memory, slurred speech, personality change, and disorientation. Convulsive seizures and coma may follow untreated or refractory PSE.

6. Monitor patients for hyponatremia.

Rationale: This imbalance must be detected early so that fluid restriction can be initiated before the im-

balance becomes severe. Symptoms are primarily those of cerebral swelling (lethargy and somnolence), making this imbalance difficult to distinguish from other disturbances affecting the neurological status.

NURSING DIAGNOSES

Examples of nursing diagnoses related to fluid and electrolyte balance in patients with cirrhosis are listed in Table 15-2, along with etiologies and defining characteristics. Nursing interventions and rationales are discussed below.

NURSING INTERVENTIONS

Nursing interventions are directed at promoting adaptation and minimizing ill effects of the disease process.

1. Continue ongoing assessment of fluid balance status as the basis for collaborative interaction with the physician in regulation of therapy. See section on assessment.
2. Prevent constipation by administering lactulose as prescribed and indicated (goal is to produce 2 or 3 soft stools per day).

   ▶ Attempt to minimize the unpleasant sweet taste of lactulose by diluting it with fruit juice, water, or milk or administering it in foods (such as desserts).
   ▶ If lactulose is given through a GI tube, it should be well diluted to prevent vomiting and the risk of pulmonary aspiration.
   ▶ If aspiration is likely, it may be necessary to administer the lactulose by retention enema.
   ▶ Monitor for excessive loose stools because severe fluid and electrolyte depletion could occur.

Rationale: Constipation should be prevented because it contributes to the accumulation of ammonia. Bleeding in the GI tract increases ammonia formation (due to digestion of blood proteins) and may precipitate hepatic coma. Bowel evacuation removes blood from the intestine and thus decreases a source of urea and other false neurotransmitters. Use of lactulose (orally and by enema) is described further in the section on treatment.

3. Encourage rest periods in which the patient lies down.

Rationale: Assumption of the supine position is often associated with a spontaneous diuresis, resulting in significant weight loss with mobilization of peripheral edema fluid and ascitic fluid. The diuresis induced by bedrest results from improvement in cardiac output

TABLE 15–2.

Examples of Nursing Diagnoses Related to Fluid and Electrolyte Problems in Patients with Cirrhosis

NURSING DIAGNOSIS	ETIOLOGICAL FACTORS	DEFINING CHARACTERISTICS
ECF volume excess (total body sodium and water increased), but decreased effective arterial volume, related to pathophysiological changes of cirrhosis	Despite increased total ECF content due to renal retention of sodium and water, body responds as if arterial volume is diminished (decreased effective arterial volume)	Ascites Peripheral edema first noted in lower extremities and later becoming generalized (dependent on sodium intake)
Risk for hypovolemia related to rapid reaccumulation of ascitic fluid after large volume paracentesis	Ascites may reaccumulate rapidly (particularly when albumin is not administered after paracentesis) following the removal of large volumes of ascites	Reduced cardiac output Decreased blood pressure Increased pulse rate
Alterations in thought processes related to increased toxins (such as ammonia)	Elevated serum ammonia level (results when liver is unable to convert ammonia formed in intestines to urea) Bleeding into GI tract increases protein metabolism Excessive diuresis contracts plasma volume and increases concentration of toxins	Slowed response, memory loss, sleep disturbances, confusion, disorientation, personality change, stupor, coma, seizures
Alteration in thought processes related to dilutional hyponatremia	Increased ADH secretion due to decrease in ineffective arterial volume	Lethargy, somnolence, personality change, serum sodium < 135 mEq/L (see Chapter 4)
Alteration in potassium balance (hypokalemia) related to use of potassium-losing diuretics	Potassium-losing diuretics (such as furosemide or bumetanide)	Fatigue, muscle weakness, leg cramps, decreased bowel motility, arrhythmias, ECG changes (see Chapter 5)
Risk for impaired gas exchange related to decreased lung expansion	Large accumulation of ascites causes diaphragm to press upward on lungs, causing decreased respirations. Condition is aggravated by generalized weakness, lethargy, and immobility	Decreased respiratory depth Increased $PaCO_2$

ECF, extracellular fluid; ADH, antidiuretic hormone.

and effective circulating blood volume. The patient with severe ascites is usually better able to tolerate the lateral recumbent position.

4. Maintain a safe environment for the patient with the potential for, or actual presence of, PSE.

   ▶ When deemed necessary, remove potential sources of harm (such as matches or sharp objects) from the immediate environment.
   ▶ Caution significant others that the patient's ability to drive or perform usual activities (such as cooking) should be closely monitored. Driver's licenses are often restricted or revoked for this group of patients, making it necessary for significant others to assume many additional responsibilities for home-bound patients (eg, cooking and transportation to treatment facilities).

Rationale: Because episodes of encephalopathy may interfere with thought and reasoning processes, physical safety of the patient and others must be considered.

5. Initiate patient instruction in self-care.

   A. Teach home-bound patients how to monitor their fluid I&O and body weights, and when to seek intervention from the health care provider.
   B. Instruct patient or significant other in how to manage a sodium-restricted diet at home; written information that can be taken home is advantageous, as is accessibility of a dietary consultant when questions arise.
   C. Promote the patient's understanding of his or her diuretic therapy. For example, the patient should be able to name the diuretic as well as its purpose and common side effects. The desirability of taking the diuretic in the morning

to avoid disturbing sleep at night should be emphasized.

D. Promote the patient's understanding or that of significant others of potassium supplements when they are required. The patient or caregiver should be able to name the agent, its dosage, the reason for taking it, and possible side effects. Because some potassium supplements can be unpleasant, the reason for taking the substance should be emphasized (recall that hypokalemia associated with metabolic alkalosis can lead to the development of portal systemic encephalopathy).

E. Promote the patient's understanding of salt substitutes, if used. For example, the patient should be able to name acceptable agents. Instruct patients receiving a combination potassium-conserving, potassium-losing diuretic (such as Aldactazide or Dyazide) that salt substitutes should be used sparingly (if at all). When only a potassium-conserving diuretic is used, the danger of hyperkalemia is present; for such patients, salt substitutes are generally not recommended. Recall that most salt substitutes contain sizable amounts of potassium (see Table 5-4).

Rationale: Understanding dietary and pharmacological regimens will promote adherence to these treatment modalities and promote optimal wellness.

REFERENCES

1. Kokko J, Tannen R: Fluids and Electrolytes, 2nd ed, p 672. Philadelphia, WB Saunders, 1990
2. Ibid, p 675
3. Rose B: Clinical Physiology of Acid–Base and Electrolyte Disorders, 3rd ed, p 442. New York, McGraw-Hill, 1989
4. Kokko, Tannen, p 675
5. Rose, p 582
6. Schrier R: Renal and Electrolyte Disorders, 3rd ed, p 109. Boston, Little, Brown, 1986
7. Kokko, Tannen, p 682
8. Koppel et al: Transplantation of cadaveric kidneys from patients with hepatorenal syndrome: Evidence for the functional nature of renal failure in advanced liver disease. N Engl J Med 280:1367, 1969
9. Iwatsuki et al: Recovery from hepatorenal syndrome after orthotopic liver transplantation. N Engl J Med 289:1155, 1973
10. Dunagan W, Ridner M: Manual of Medical Therapeutics, 26th ed, p 321. Boston, Little, Brown, 1989
11. Ibid
12. Rocco V, Ware A: Cirrhotic ascites: Pathophysiology, diagnosis, and management. Ann Intern Med 105:573, 1986
13. Ibid
14. Dunagan, Ridner, p 321
15. Rose, p 432
16. Dunagan, Ridner, p 321
17. Shear L, Ching S, Gabuzda G: Compartmentalization of ascites and edema in patients with hepatic cirrhosis. N Engl J Med 282:1391, 1970
18. Pockros P, Reynolds T: Rapid diuresis in patients with ascites from chronic liver disease: The importance of peripheral edema. Gastroenterology 90:1827, 1986
19. Dunagan, Ridner, p 322
20. Gines et al: Comparison of paracentesis and diuretics in the treatment of cirrhotics with tense ascites: Results of a randomized study. Gastroenterology 93:234, 1987
21. Kao et al: The effect of large volume paracentesis on plasma volume—a cause of hypovolemia? Hepatology 5:403, 1985
22. Gines et al: Randomized comparative study of therapeutic paracentesis with and without intravenous albumin in cirrhosis. Gastroenterology 94:1493, 1988
23. Ibid
24. Ibid
25. Kao et al, p 403
26. Rose, p 448
27. Dunagan, Ridner, p 322
28. Faloon et al: An evaluation of human serum albumin in the treatment of cirrhosis of the liver. J Clin Invest 28:583, 1949
29. Gines et al, p 234
30. Epstein M: Peritoneovenous shunt in the management of ascites and the hepatorenal syndrome. Gastroenterology 82:790, 1982
31. Wapnick S: Randomized prospective matched pair study comparing peritoneovenous shunt and conventional therapy in massive ascites. Br J Surg 66:667, 1979
32. Kokko, Tannen, p 676
33. LeVeen H: Peritoneovenous shunt for ascites. In: Schiff L, Schiff E (eds). Diseases of the Liver, 5th ed, p 1632. Philadelphia, JB Lippincott, 1982
34. Greig et al: Complications after peritoneovenous shunting for ascites. Am J Surg 139:125, 1980
35. Dunagan, Ridner, p 320
36. Uribe et al: Treatment of chronic portal-systemic encephalopathy with vegetable and animal protein diets. Dig Dis Sci 27(12):1109, 1982
37. Rombeau J, Caldwell M: Clinical Nutrition: Enteral and Tube Feeding, 2nd ed, p 300. Philadelphia, WB Saunders, 1990
38. Dunagan, Ridner, p 321
39. McEvoy G (ed): Lactulose. AHFS Drug Information, p 1412–1413. Bethesda, MD American Society of Hospital Pharmacists, 1990
40. Ibid
41. Ibid
42. Dunagan, Ridner, p 321
43. Pockros, Reynolds, p 1827
44. Kao et al, p 403
45. Gines et al, p 1492

16

Gastrointestinal Problems

Gastrointestinal (GI) fluid loss is the most common cause of water and electrolyte disturbances. This becomes evident when the large fluid volumes in the GI tract and the many ways in which these fluids can be lost, such as vomiting, diarrhea, suction drainage, fistulas, and sequestration into an obstructed bowel are considered. Along with the possibility of fluid volume deficit (FVD), there is the potential for various electrolyte imbalances. Nursing considerations related to these GI fluid and electrolyte losses are discussed in this chapter.

CHARACTER OF GASTROINTESTINAL FLUIDS

In normal individuals, approximately 3 to 6 L of gastric, pancreatic, biliary, and intestinal secretions are secreted into the GI lumen each day.[1] Counting normal fluid intake and endogenous GI secretions, approximately 9 L/day enter the upper intestinal tract. Most of these fluids are then reabsorbed in the ileum and proximal colon, resulting in daily loss of only 100 to 200 mL of water in feces.

TABLE 16–1.
Approximate Electrolyte Composition of Gastrointestinal Secretions

SECRETION	USUAL MAXIMUM VOLUME/DAY	SODIUM (mEq/L IN ADULTS)	CHLORIDE (mEq/L IN ADULTS)	POTASSIUM (mEq/L IN ADULTS)
Normal				
Saliva	1000	100	75	5
Gastric juice (pH < 4.0)	2500*	60	100	10
Gastric juice (pH > 4.0)	2000*	100	100	10
Bile	1500	140	100	10
Pancreatic juice	1000	140	75	10
Succus entericus (mixed small-bowel fluid)	3500	100	100	20
Abnormal				
New ileostomy	500–2000	130	110	20
Adapted ileostomy	400	50	60	10
New cecostomy	400	80	50	20
Colostomy (transverse loop)	300	50	40	10
Diarrhea	1000–4000	60	45	30

* Nasogastric suction volume is usually much less than this unless pyloric obstruction exists.
(Condon R, Nyhus L: Manual of Surgical Therapeutics, 9th ed, p 177. Boston, Little, Brown, 1988; with permission.)

With the exception of saliva, the GI secretions are isotonic with the extracellular fluid (ECF). In addition, material entering the GI tract tends to become isotonic during the course of its absorption. Because many liters of ECF pass into the GI tract and back again, as part of the normal digestive process, this movement is sometimes referred to as the "gastrointestinal circulation." The electrolyte content of GI secretions is summarized in Table 16-1. The usual pH of GI secretions is listed in Table 16-2.

TABLE 16–2.
Gastrointestinal Secretions and Their Usual pH

SECRETION	pH
Saliva	6.0–7.0
Gastric juice	1.0–3.5*
Pancreatic juice	8.0–8.3
Bile	7.8
Small intestine	7.5–8.0
Large intestine	7.5–8.0

* Gastric pH will probably be higher than 3.5 in patients receiving H₂-receptor antagonists and perhaps in a segment of the elderly population due to decreased acid secretion.

VOMITING AND GASTRIC SUCTION

FLUID AND ELECTROLYTE DISTURBANCES

Major electrolytes in gastric juice are hydrogen (H^+), chloride (Cl^-), potassium (K^+), and, to a lesser extent, sodium (Na^+). Gastric juice is the most acidic of the GI secretions with a pH of 1.0 to 3.5 in the fasting state in most individuals not receiving H_2 receptor antagonists. Imbalances most often associated with the loss of gastric juice include the following:

- Fluid volume deficit
- Metabolic alkalosis
- Hypokalemia
- Sodium imbalances
- Hypomagnesemia

Fluid Volume Deficit

If vomiting is prolonged and fluid replacement therapy is inadequate, severe FVD may result, manifested by decreased urinary output, postural hypotension, tachycardia, elevated hematocrit, and elevated blood urea nitrogen (BUN):creatinine ratio. It is not uncommon to see a 10-point drop in the hematocrit level during the first 12 to 24 hours after fluid replacement.[2] Also, because many liters can be removed daily by gastric suction (depending on the underlying disease process), FVD can easily occur in this situation if fluids are not replaced parenterally.

Metabolic Alkalosis

Excessive loss of gastric juice by vomiting or suction causes metabolic alkalosis (base bicarbonate excess) for several reasons. First, secretions from the stomach contains high concentrations of H^+ and Cl^-. With loss of Cl^-, there is a compensatory increase in bicarbonate ions. (Each mEq of HCl lost from the stomach represents 1 mEq of bicarbonate added to the ECF.[3]) The kidneys add to the metabolic alkalosis by failing to excrete all the excess circulating bicarbonate (HCO_3^-).[4] Symptoms are generally those of decreased calcium ionization related to the alkaline plasma. (Recall that calcium ionization is decreased in alkalosis.) Because it is the ionized fraction of calcium that controls neuromuscular excitability, symptoms of tetany can occur.

Hypokalemia

As noted in Table 16-1, gastric fluid contains approximately 10 mEq/L of potassium. With the loss of several liters of gastric fluid, it is clear that hypokalemia could easily develop. In addition to the direct loss of potassium with vomiting and gastric suction, there is a transient renal wasting of potassium early in the period of gastric fluid loss. The metabolic alkalosis described above accompanies hypokalemia.

Recall that the usual adult, not eating, requires the daily addition of approximately 40 to 60 mEq of potassium to intravenous (IV) fluids. A patient with large gastric fluid losses may require substantially more.

Sodium Imbalances

The plasma sodium level in patients losing gastric fluid by vomiting and gastric suction varies. Recall that gastric fluid is usually isotonic or mildly hypotonic; therefore, the plasma sodium level will usually remain essentially normal unless other factors are present. For example, in the hospital setting, if excessive amounts of free water (such as 5% dextrose in water) are given, the plasma sodium concentration may drop below normal. This is particularly likely to occur because vomiting is a potent stimulus for the release of antidiuretic hormone (ADH), thus causing water retention. Hyponatremia is less likely to occur in the home-bound patient because vomiting usually precludes oral fluid intake until the problem is resolved. Of course, in the presence of other factors that increase free water loss

(eg, fever and hyperventilation), it is possible that the plasma sodium level could be elevated.

Hypomagnesemia

Prolonged vomiting or gastric suction can result in magnesium deficit, an imbalance not as likely as those listed above because the magnesium concentration in gastric juice is relatively low (1.4 mEq/L). However, it is likely to occur if losses are prolonged (lasting several weeks) and no magnesium is supplied in the IV fluids. Unfortunately, most routine electrolyte-replacement solutions do not contain magnesium (eg, lactated Ringer's and isotonic saline have none).

NURSING MANAGEMENT OF GASTRIC FLUID LOSS

The reader is referred to Table 16-3 for a list of potential nursing diagnoses related to fluid and electrolyte problems associated with gastric fluid loss. Nursing interventions for patients with vomiting are listed in Table 16-4 and interventions for patients with gastric suction are listed in Table 16-5.

DIARRHEA

FLUID AND ELECTROLYTE DISTURBANCES

Diarrhea is characterized by increased frequency of stools with excessive water content. It can have many causes, such as infectious agents (viral, bacterial, and parasitic), toxins, and certain drugs. Viral enteritis and infections with noninvasive bacteria are the most frequent causes of diarrhea in the United States.[5] Common causes in hospitalized patients who develop diarrhea are antibiotics, lactose intolerance (unmasked by hospital diets), and fecal impactions.[6] Diarrhea is classified into several categories, including osmotic, secretory, structural, and primary motility disorders. Examples of osmotic diarrhea causes are ingestion of poorly absorbable solutes (eg, lactulose, sorbitol, mannitol, magnesium sulfate, magnesium hydroxide, and sodium phosphate), generalized malabsorption or maldigestion, and certain infections. Secretory diarrhea is caused by abnormal secretion of water and electrolytes into the bowel lumen. Examples of secretory diarrhea include enterotoxigenic bacteria (eg, *Escherichia coli* and *Vibrio cholerae*), elevated venous and lymphatic pressure (eg, diarrhea associated with severe hypoalbuminemia and portal hypertension), intestinal obstruction, and villous adenoma.[7] Diarrhea secondary to structural changes occur in inflammatory bowel disease,

TABLE 16–3.
Possible Nursing Diagnoses Related to Loss of Gastric Juice

NURSING DIAGNOSIS	ETIOLOGICAL FACTORS	DEFINING CHARACTERISTICS
Fluid volume deficit related to vomiting or gastric suction	Prolonged loss of isotonic-gastric fluid, particularly if replacement fluid therapy is inadequate	Decreased skin turgor, dry mucous membranes, furrowed tongue, oliguria, and acute weight loss (see Chapter 3)
Alteration in acid–base balance (metabolic alkalosis) related to vomiting or gastric suction	Loss of hydrogen and chloride ions causes a compensatory increase in bicarbonate ions (base bicarbonate excess)	Tingling of fingers and toes (due to decreased calcium ionization), compensatory depressed respirations (usually not evident in an alert patient) Lab values: increased HCO_3; pH > 7.45; Cl < 100 mEq/L (see Chapter 9)
Alteration in potassium balance (hypokalemia) related to vomiting or gastric suction	Potassium loss in gastric fluid; also, potassium loss is associated with metabolic alkalosis; inadequate IV potassium replacement	Muscular weakness, irregular pulse, gaseous intestinal distention, muscle cramps Lab values: serum K < 3.5; HCO_3 usually elevated; pH often > 7.45 (see Chapter 5)
Alteration in sodium balance (hyponatremia) related to vomiting or gastric suction	Prolonged loss of sodium in gastric fluid, particularly if water is ingested orally in liquid or ice-chip form, or if nasogastric tube is irrigated with plain water	Anorexia, weakness, abdominal cramping, lethargy, confusion Lab values: serum Na < 135 mEq/L (see Chapter 4)
Alteration in magnesium balance (hypomagnesemia) related to vomiting or gastric suction	Prolonged loss of magnesium in gastric fluid, particularly if IV fluids contain no magnesium (as is commonly the case)	Tachycardia, arrhythmias, increased neuromuscular irritability, paresthesias Lab values: serum Mg < 1.5 mEq/L (see Chapter 7)

TABLE 16–4.
Nursing Interventions for Patients with Vomiting

1. Discourage the intake of plain water if vomiting is prolonged. Instead, encourage the frequent intake of small volumes of fluids containing electrolytes. (See Tables 3-1 and 25-4 for a summary of the electrolyte content of commonly available oral fluids.)
2. Report vomiting early so that appropriate treatment can be started before fluid and electrolyte disturbances become severe. The physician will likely prescribe a medication to relieve nausea. If vomiting is prolonged and oral fluids are not retained, parenteral fluids are indicated.
3. Alter physical environment as much as possible to lessen stimuli for nausea (eg, remove sources of unpleasant odors).
4. Promote bedrest when vomiting is severe; avoid quick movements because they often make nausea more severe.
5. Measure, or estimate as accurately as possible, the amount of vomitus so that lost water and electrolytes can be replaced by the parenteral route. In fact, all fluids lost and gained from the body should be measured.
6. Measure body weight daily to detect significant changes in fluid balance. Daily weights are helpful in detecting FVD, particularly if vomitus has not been measured. A patient on a starvation diet should lose about ½ lb/day; a loss in excess of this amount probably implies FVD. A weight gain in this situation implies FVE. Routine IV fluids are low in calories; for example, a liter of 5% dextrose solutions contains only 170 calories.
7. Monitor for imbalances associated with loss of gastric fluid (see preceding discussion).
8. Be familiar with parenteral fluids commonly used to replace gastric fluid. Solutions that may be prescribed include routine solutions (such as isotonic or half-strength saline) with added potassium and magnesium, or special gastric replacement solutions (see Chapter 11).

FVD, fluid volume deficit; FVE, fluid volume excess.

TABLE 16–5.
Nursing Interventions for Patients with Gastric Suction

1. Irrigate suction tube with isotonic NaCl solution (or other electrolyte solution as prescribed by physician). Realize that plain water is not recommended as an irrigating solution because it can wash out electrolytes.

   When plain water is instilled through the tube, gastric secretions are increased in an attempt to make the water "isotonic" to allow absorption. However, before the fluid can be absorbed, the gastric suction apparatus triggers on and pulls both the water and electrolytes out through the tube. This phenomenon is sometimes referred to as *electrolyte washout*.
2. Prohibit the intake of large quantities of water or ice chips by mouth because water washes electrolytes from the stomach. Profound states of metabolic alkalosis and sodium deficit have been caused by the unwise practice of giving large quantities of plain water to a patient undergoing gastric suction.

   Be aware that some physicians prefer that patients with gastric suction receive nothing by mouth; others allow small quantities of ice chips (such as 1 oz/hr). Be particularly careful when orders are written to give ice chips "sparingly"; this term is open to interpretation by the staff, and more ice may be given than was intended, especially if the patient asks frequently. Occasionally physicians will prescribe ice chips made from electrolyte solutions for patients experiencing great discomfort (dry mouth or thirst). Remember that true thirst should not be present if the patient is adequately hydrated via the parenteral route. The patient's desire for ice chips may be lessened by supplying a wet washcloth to apply to the lips and mouth.
3. Measure and record the amount of fluid lost by suction, as well as by all other fluid losses and gains.
4. Measure daily weight variations to help detect early fluid volume deficit (or excess related to excessive fluid replacement).
5. Monitor for imbalances associated with loss of gastric fluid (see previous discussion in this chapter).

---

collagen vascular disease, and sprue. Imbalances likely to be associated with diarrhea include the following:

▶ Fluid volume deficit
▶ Metabolic acidosis
▶ Hypokalemia
▶ Hypomagnesemia
▶ Sodium imbalances

Fluid Volume Deficit

Volume depletion is secondary to sodium and water loss in the diarrhea fluid. Severe diarrhea can lead to a daily loss of 2 to 10 L of fluid, together with large quantities of electrolytes.[8] Obviously, prolonged diarrhea is a serious threat to water and electrolyte balance.

Metabolic Acidosis

The incidence of acid–base disorders in patients with severe diarrhea is about 70%, and the entire spectrum of disturbances may be seen.[9] However, metabolic acidosis is by far the most common disorder and is especially likely to occur in pediatric patients, and in those with secretory or infectious diarrhea.[10] Recall that intestinal fluids are relatively alkaline because of their bicarbonate content. As a result, loss of intestinal fluid is likely to lead to metabolic (hyperchloremic) acidosis. (The plasma chloride level elevates as the bicarbonate decreases.)

Hypokalemia

Relatively large amounts of potassium (approximately 20–30 mEq/L) are contained in the intestinal fluid; therefore, hypokalemia usually occurs with diarrhea, particularly when many liters of fluid are lost. The typical electrolyte disorder in patients with diarrhea is hypokalemia with hyperchloremic metabolic acidosis, due to the loss of bicarbonate ions (see section above on metabolic acidosis).

Hypomagnesemia

Relatively large amounts of magnesium (approximately 10–15 mEq/L) are contained in intestinal fluid; therefore, magnesium deficit will likely occur with prolonged diarrhea. This is particularly likely if IV replacement fluids are deficient in magnesium. Unfortunately, this is often the case. Recall that most routine electrolyte solutions do not contain magnesium (eg, lactated Ringer's solution and isotonic saline have none). Thus, if losses are prolonged and there is no IV replacement, magnesium deficit should be anticipated.

Sodium Imbalances

The plasma sodium concentration varies in patients with diarrhea, depending on the cause of the problem and related clinical events. As discussed below, the diarrheal fluid may have a sodium content that is similar to, higher than, or lower than that of plasma. Extraneous factors also affect the plasma sodium concentration; among these are the amount of water intake (orally or IV), and the degree of water loss due to fever or hyperventilation. (Recall that hyperventilation is a compensatory reaction to metabolic acidosis.)

When the diarrheal fluid's sodium content is similar to that of plasma, its loss causes an isotonic FVD (with no change in the plasma sodium level). This is often the case with diarrheal conditions classified as secretory diarrhea. In contrast, diarrheas caused by osmotic conditions tend to be associated with relatively greater losses of water than sodium, resulting in a tendency for an elevated plasma sodium concentration.[11] In some types of diarrhea, sodium is lost in excess of water, causing a tendency toward hyponatremia. See Chapter 25 for a discussion of diarrhea in children.

MANAGEMENT OF DIARRHEAL FLUID LOSS

Most acute diarrheal episodes of viral or bacterial origin are self-limited and do not require specific therapy. A clear liquid diet is usually recommended while fluid status is carefully observed.[12] If FVD or electrolyte con-

centration imbalances occur, parenteral fluids are indicated. If diarrhea is due to the accumulation of poorly absorbed solutes in the intestine (osmotic diarrhea), it usually subsides with fasting. However, the diarrhea will usually persist despite fasting if it is a form of secretory diarrhea.[13]

Oral rehydration with glucose and electrolytes in infantile diarrhea is described in Chapter 25. It has been found that glucose in the solution promotes small intestinal sodium reabsorption while providing extra calories.

Table 16-6 lists possible nursing diagnoses related to water and electrolytes in the patient with diarrhea; selected nursing interventions are listed in Table 16-7.

TABLE 16–6.
Possible Nursing Diagnoses Related to Diarrhea

NURSING DIAGNOSIS	ETIOLOGICAL FACTORS	DEFINING CHARACTERISTICS
FVD, related to diarrhea	Large loss of isotonic diarrheal fluid resulting in decreased bowel absorption	Decreased skin turgor, dry mucous membranes, furrowed tongue, oliguria, acute weight loss, tachycardia, postural hypotension (see Chapter 3)
Alteration in acid–base balance (metabolic acidosis) related to diarrhea	Loss of bicarbonate-rich diarrheal fluid causes HCO_3 deficit (recall that intestinal secretions are alkaline)	Compensatory increase in respirations, headache, confusion, warm flushed skin Lab values: decreased HCO_3; pH < 7.35 (see Chapter 9)
Alteration in potassium balance (hypokalemia) related to diarrhea	Loss of potassium-rich diarrheal fluid (contains approximately 20 mEq/L) Particularly likely in patients with villous adenomas (type of colonic tumor with high potassium content, such as 80 mEq/L)	Muscular weakness, irregular pulse, muscle cramps Lab values: serum K < 3.5 mEq/L (see Chapter 5)
Alteration in magnesium balance (hypomagnesemia) related to diarrhea	Loss of magnesium-rich diarrheal fluid (contains as much as 10–15 mEq/L), particularly in association with inadequate magnesium in IV fluids	Tachycardia, arrhythmias, increased neuromuscular irritability, parenthesias Lab values: serum Mg < 1.5 mEq/L (see Chapter 7)
Alteration in sodium balance (hyponatremia) related to diarrhea and high water intake	Loss of sodium, particularly in association with excessive water intake (orally or IV as D_5W)	Anorexia, nausea and vomiting, confusion, lethargy Lab values: serum Na < 135 mEq/L (see Chapter 4)
Alteration in sodium balance (hypernatremia) related to diarrhea and low water intake	Relatively greater loss of water than sodium, related to fever (if infection is present) or hyperpnea (if metabolic acidosis is present); particularly likely when water intake is poor	Thirst, dry sticky mucous membranes, irritability, restlessness Lab values: serum Na > 145 mEq/L (see Chapter 4)

FVD, fluid volume deficit.

TABLE 16–7.
Nursing Interventions for Patients with Diarrhea

1. Measure, or estimate as accurately as possible, the amount of liquid feces so that lost water and electrolytes can be replaced (either by oral electrolyte solutions or via the parenteral route). All fluids gained and lost from the body should be measured and recorded on the I & O record. (See discussion of I & O measurement in Chapter 2.)
2. Measure body weight daily to detect significant changes in fluid balance. Daily weights are helpful in detecting fluid volume deficit, particularly if liquid stools have not been measured.
3. Monitor for clinical and laboratory indicators of imbalances commonly associated with the loss of intestinal fluid (see text). Specific imbalances are described in Chapters 3–9.
4. Offer oral electrolyte-containing liquids if allowed by the type of diarrhea present. (Some types of diarrhea respond better to temporary fasting and parenteral fluid replacement.)
5. Monitor response to parenteral fluids (if they are indicated) to replace fluid losses. Commonly used fluids for this purpose are lactated Ringer's solution and half strength saline (0.45% NaCl) with added potassium. Other electrolytes (such as magnesium) are replaced as indicated. Nursing responsibilities in fluid replacement therapy are described in Chapter 11.

I&O, intake and output.

IMBALANCES ASSOCIATED WITH BOWEL PREPARATION FOR DIAGNOSTIC STUDIES AND SURGERY

STANDARD BOWEL PREPARATIONS VERSUS POLYETHYLENE GLYCOL LAVAGE

Two commonly used regimens to cleanse the colon before colonoscopy or colon surgery consist of (1) a clear liquid or low-residue diet for 1 to 3 days, plus laxatives and enemas, and (2) the rapid ingestion (either orally or by nasogastric tube) of a balanced electrolyte–polyethylene glycol (PEG) solution. Polyethylene glycol is a nonabsorbed osmotic agent. Commercially available PEG lavage solutions include GoLytely (Braintree Laboratories, Inc.) and Colyte (Reed and Carnrick). When reconstituted with water, Colyte contains 125 mEq/L sodium, 10 mEq/L potassium, 20 mEq/L bicarbonate, 80 mEq/L sulfate, 35 mEq/L chloride, and 18 mEq/L PEG 3350.[14] Approximately 1.5 L/hour of a PEG lavage solution are ingested in adults until the rectal effluent is clear or up to 4 L are consumed. According to the manufacturers, large volumes may be administered without significant changes in fluid and electrolyte balance because the osmotic activity of the PEG lavage results in virtually no net absorption or excretion of ions or water.

A recent survey of 206 physicians regarding preferences for a primary mechanical bowel cleansing method indicated that 51% preferred cathartics and enemas, 43% the PEG lavage method, 4% an oral mannitol solution, and less than 1% a saline lavage method.[15] A major disadvantage of the saline lavage method is the large volume of fluid that must be administered (7–10 L) over 2 to 3 hours. Also, several clinical studies have indicated that there is significant absorption of the saline solution, causing rapid intravascular expansion; thus, this method is contraindicated in patients with impaired cardiovascular or renal status.[16–18]

The same group of physicians described above estimated the incidence of fluid and electrolyte complications at 10% for patients receiving cathartics and enemas and 5% for patients receiving the PEG lavage method. The authors noted that complications are usually underreported in survey research. Several studies indicated that neither of the two commonly used methods (traditional bowel preparation and PEG lavage) results in clinically significant changes in body weight, blood chemistries, and hematological values. In the studies, changes associated with PEG lavage were less pronounced than those associated with the traditional mechanical method.[19–21] For example, Beck et al described an average weight loss of 2.2 lb with a standard bowel preparation as opposed to 0.1 lb loss with PEG lavage (GoLytely). Ambrose et al[22] found that the serum sodium increased an average of 0.35 mEq/L with the PEG lavage method and decreased an average of 1.2 mEq/L with a cathartic and rectal washout method.

Compared with the traditional method, the major advantage of PEG lavage is the considerably shorter time needed for preparation. Because the food restriction period is shortened by as much as 2 or 3 days, hunger and associated weakness are less problematic. A disadvantage is nausea, abdominal fullness, and bloating (occurring in up to 50% of patients) associated with rapid ingestion of the PEG lavage.[23] Some patients complain that the PEG lavage solution has a disagreeable mildly salty taste and refuse to drink it. Chilling the solution makes it more palatable. The manufacturers recommend that patients fast for approximately 3 or 4 hours before ingesting the solution. They emphasize that solid food should not be allowed for at least 2 hours before the solution is given. Only clear liquids are allowed during the interval between PEG lavage solution ingestion and examination.

A major disadvantage of the traditional method is the 1- to 3-day period of reduced food intake, resulting in hunger and weakness. Adding to the discomfort is the use of laxatives and enemas. Rigorous use of cathartics and numerous cleansing enemas after several days of dietary restrictions can present problems for elderly patients, particularly those with cardiovascular disease. Thus, the elderly patient undergoing rigorous bowel preparation should be observed closely for adverse reactions. Care should be taken to perform the procedure correctly the first time to avoid the need for repeated roentgenograms (requiring more cathartics, more enemas, and more fluid restriction). The elderly patient cannot afford to undergo one test after another without a rest period in between; it is frequently the nurse's responsibility to intervene in this area on the patient's behalf. The already-reduced glomerular filtration rate (GFR) in the elderly potentiates the hazards of any further decrease in ECF volume (as occurs in vigorous catharsis). The aged patient having GI roentgenograms should probably receive IV fluids during the preparation period of reduced oral intake and increased fluid loss by catharsis and enema. Note also that use of radiocontrast agents in diagnostic radiology (particularly in large doses) has been incriminated as predisposing to acute renal failure, especially when the patient has a severe FVD. See Chapter 26 for further discussion of the effect of standard bowel preparations on elderly patients.

In a clinical study, serum magnesium levels were found to be increased in patients receiving the standard preparation when compared with those in patients receiving a PEG lavage solution.[24] Presumably the higher magnesium levels resulted from use of magnesium citrate as a laxative. Although the serum magnesium concentrations remained within a normal range, the potential for hypermagnesemia could be an important consideration in patients with renal insufficiency because they lack the ability to excrete magnesium normally.

ENEMAS AS BOWEL PREPARATIONS

Enema administration as bowel preparation for diagnostic studies or surgery can also present problems. For example, repeated tap water enemas can result in excessive water absorption and dilutional hyponatremia. Even more problematic are sodium phosphate (Fleet, C. B. Fleet Co., Lynchburg, VA) enemas in at-risk patients (eg, infants, small children, patients with GI abnormalities interfering with elimination of the solution, patients with severe renal impairment, and patients with preexisting electrolyte abnormalities).

Several recent case studies involving sodium phosphate (Fleet) enemas as bowel preparation for surgery or radiology pointed out the dangers to small children.

A tragic occurrence involved the administration of four adult-sized sodium phosphate (Fleet) enemas to an 11-month-old male infant admitted for surgical correction of an imperforate anus.[25] The child had a sigmoid colostomy constructed shortly after birth. Two enemas were given in each barrel of the colostomy. Before the enemas, the child received 800 mL of a GI lavage solution (Golytely). Approximately 2½ hours after the enemas were administered, cardiac arrest occurred. Despite extensive resuscitative efforts with IV calcium, phosphate-binding resins per ostomy, and peritoneal dialysis, the child died. The marked hypernatremia, acidemia, hyperphosphatemia, and hypocalcemia observed before the child's death were replicated in an animal model in which the same enemas were administered before anal obstruction with balloon catheters. In the pig model, the retained enema solution was lethal at a dose of 20 to 30 mL/kg. Another situation involved the administration of two sodium phosphate pediatric enemas to a girl aged 2 years, 6 months in preparation for a radiographic procedure.[26] Subsequently she developed coma, tetany, dehydration, hypotension, tachycardia, and hyperpyrexia. Laboratory results indicated severe hyperphosphatemia, hypocalcemia, hypernatremia, and acidosis. Apparently about one third of the administered enema solution was absorbed systemically.

The manufacturer of Fleet enemas warns that adult-sized (4.5 oz) enemas should not be administered to children younger than 12 years and that the children's size (2.25 oz) enema should not be administered to children younger than 2 years.[27] The authors of one of the case studies described above recommended that sodium phosphate enemas not be used in small children and infants, indicating that it is incorrect to assume that sodium phosphate solutions are not absorbed by the colon.[28] Many clinicians favor the use of isotonic saline (0.9% NaCl) as an enema solution for patients of all ages to minimize fluid and electrolyte changes associated with absorption of the enema solution.

IMBALANCES RELATED TO LAXATIVES AND ENEMAS FOR CONSTIPATION

Constipation is defined as a decrease in the frequency of bowel movements combined with a prolonged and difficult evacuation of stool. Among the causes of constipation are several medications, psychological conditions, mechanical disorders, and a variety of metabolic conditions (eg, dehydration, hypercalcemia, and hypokalemia). Whenever possible, constipation should be treated by nonpharmacological measures (Table 16-8). When these measures are not feasible or are ineffective,

TABLE 16–8.
Nursing Interventions Related to Laxative and Enema Abuse

1. Encourage patients to avoid the repeated use of cathartics and enemas and rely on other methods to achieve bowel evacuation regularity.
2. Encourage maximum level of tolerated physical activity. Regular exercise stimulates gut motility and is an important part of a bowel management program. Walking 20 to 30 minutes a day is a good form of exercise. For immobilized patients, even small increases in activity may be helpful. For example, modest activities such as sitting up in bed or turning and twisting in a chair cause changes in colonic motility.[29]
3. Encourage ingestion of a glass of warm fluid first thing in the morning to stimulate the evacuation reflex.
4. Encourage regular fluid intake to act as a stool softener. For example, a glass or two of water on rising, between meals, and before bedtime should be consumed if tolerated.[30]
5. Encourage adequate bulk in the diet. Wheat bran is an excellent source that is available in many cereals and breads; approximately 3 tbl supplies roughly 10 grams of dietary fiber.[31] Most fruits and vegetables are good sources of fiber. Dietary fiber holds water, causing stools to be softer, bulkier, and heavier. The increased bowel bulk causes quicker movement of stool through the colon.
6. Encourage patients to attempt to develop a regular bowel routine. The best time to attempt a bowel elimination is probably after breakfast because this is the time when the strongest propulsive contractions occur.

occasional use of laxatives or enemas may be indicated. However, the fluid and electrolyte problems that may accompany the injudicious use of laxatives and enemas must be considered.

LAXATIVES

Laxatives can lead to sodium and water depletion (usually with no change in serum sodium) and hypokalemia.[32] Patients with impaired renal function are at risk for hypermagnesemia and hyperphosphatemia when magnesium salts (such as magnesium citrate, magnesium sulfate, and milk of magnesia) or sodium phosphate solutions are administered because they are unable to excrete these substances adequately.[33] Magnesium-containing laxatives are frequently administered in quantities sufficient to cause toxic serum levels of magnesium when renal function is impaired.[34] Magnesium cathartics are further contraindicated in patients with poor bowel motility, as occurs in adynamic ileus, and in those ingesting drugs with anticholinergic activity. This is because slowed motility increases the likelihood of magnesium absorption. Of interest, several instances

have been described in which hypermagnesemia developed in patients with normal renal function who received large doses of magnesium sulfate to facilitate poison removal from the GI tract.[35] Osmotic laxatives can cause large fluid losses, increasing the need for fluid replacement.

ENEMAS

As indicated earlier, repeated tap water enemas can predispose to dilutional hyponatremia after absorption of water from the colon, particularly in children with megacolon or chronic constipation. Also, as discussed earlier, hypertonic sodium phosphate enema solutions (available over the counter) may produce a series of fluid and electrolyte problems in some patients. Among these are hyperphosphatemia, hypocalcemia, and hypernatremia. These disturbances occur primarily in patients unable to eliminate the enema solution adequately before significant absorption occurs. Hyperphosphatemia and hypernatremia are the direct result of absorption of these electrolytes from the enema solution. Hypocalcemia is a reciprocal response to hyperphosphatemia. There have been reports of profound electrolyte disturbances (primarily hyperphosphatemia, hypocalcemia, and hypernatremia) after the use of sodium phosphate enemas in patients with GI disorders that interfere with prompt elimination.[36,37]

The manufacturer warns that sodium phosphate (Fleet) enemas should not be used in patients with conditions predisposing to retention of the enema solution (eg, congenital megacolon, imperforate anus, or colostomy) or congestive heart failure because hypernatremic dehydration may occur. Also, the manufacturer advises caution in the use of these enemas in patients with impaired renal function, heart disease, or preexisting electrolyte disturbances, or in patients on calcium channel blockers, diuretics, or other medications that can affect electrolyte levels because hyperphosphatemia, hypocalcemia, hypernatremia and acidosis may occur.[38]

Use of adult-sized sodium phosphate enemas for constipation in children can produce disastrous results. A case of hypocalcemia and severe hyperphosphatemia was reported in a four-year-old boy who received adult sodium phosphate enemas for the treatment of constipation.[39] Due to tetany from the hypocalcemia, the child's extremities were stiff and could not be actively or passively moved. After treatment with IV calcium gluconate and oral calcium supplements to reduce the phosphate load, and hydration to promote diuresis, the child's condition improved. A similar case was described in which a previously healthy 5-month-old child suffered severe hyperphosphatemia, hypocalcemia, acidosis, and shock after administration of an adult-sized sodium phosphate enema for the treatment of constipation.[40]

Although more likely in high-risk patients, electrolyte disturbances from sodium phosphate enemas have also been reported in patients with no obvious underlying disease process.[41-43] Because most reports of these enemas' adverse effects involve small children, some authors recommend against the use of sodium phosphate enemas entirely in small children and infants.[44] Others recommend that parents be made aware that such enemas can be dangerous to infants, and that the enema's manufacturers have more prominent labeling indicating the dangers of such enemas to infants.[45] Nurses should take an active part in educating at-risk patients (or their parents) about the dangers of injudicious use of enemas. As indicated earlier, many clinicians favor the use of isotonic saline (0.9% NaCl) when enemas are needed for patients of any age.

LOSS OF FLUID THROUGH FISTULAS

Fistulas are abnormal communications between the intestine and the skin (external fistula) or another hollow viscus (internal fistula). They can result from trauma or occur spontaneously as a complication of pancreatitis, inflammatory bowel disease, neoplasia, or other GI disorders. Surgical procedures have been implicated as etiological factors in 67% to 80% of cases.[46] Fistulas may develop at any level in the GI tract. Loss of fluid from these abnormal openings can produce serious fluid and electrolyte disturbances. Intestinal fluids, including pancreatic and biliary secretions, are relatively alkaline because of their bicarbonate content. Thus, loss of these fluids would likely lead to metabolic acidosis. In contrast, loss of gastric fluid would likely lead to metabolic alkalosis. In addition to pH changes, high-output fistulas can cause a serious contraction of the ECF volume. For example, a duodenal fistula may drain 1 to 4 L of fluid daily.

Obviously, the amount and kind of fluid lost through a fistula depend on its location. An educated guess regarding imbalances likely to accompany a specific fluid's loss can be made by reviewing the usual electrolyte content of fluid in the region of the fistula (see Table 16-1). When doubt about the fistula's origin exists, measurement of the drainage's pH and electrolyte content can be done in the laboratory.

Although fluid and electrolyte problems are possible with any fistula, they are most likely to be substantial in patients with pancreatic, duodenal stump, and gastrojejunal anastomotic fistulas.[47] Biliary and pancreatic fistulous drainage contains sizable amounts of sodium and bicarbonate, predisposing to FVD and metabolic acidosis. Hyponatremia can easily occur if fluid replacement contains more free water than needed. High chloride content of drainage from gastric fistulas predisposes to metabolic alkalosis.

Large amounts of drainage can most often be collected with a well-fixed stoma appliance. The amount of the loss should be recorded, along with all other fluid losses. If the drainage cannot be directly measured, an estimate should be made of the volume. Statements regarding how much of a dressing is saturated, as well as the extent of gown and linen saturation, help in planning fluid replacement therapy. Skin care is essential to guard against the effects of autodigestion by GI enzymes. A variety of skin barrier sheets and powders are available for this purpose. Encouraging adequate nutritional intake will promote spontaneous closure of enterocutaneous fistulas. Most fistulas that close spontaneously do so within 6 weeks.[48] Often total parenteral nutrition (TPN) is needed to achieve the level of calories needed. Healing is retarded when the fistula has a high fluid output. Preliminary findings from a clinical study indicated that the continuous infusion of somatostatin facilitates considerable decrease in fistula output (thereby facilitating acceleration of healing).[49]

IMBALANCES ASSOCIATED WITH BULIMIA

Bulimia nervosa is an eating disorder characterized by eating binges coupled with measures designed to promote weight loss (eg, self-induced vomiting, laxative abuse, abuse of diuretics, use of diet pills, and prolonged periods of fasting). This syndrome is most common in women during late adolescence or early adulthood.[50] Serious fluid and electrolyte abnormalities can accompany bulimia. One study of 168 patients with bulimia or related eating disorders found about 50% had some sort of electrolyte abnormality.[51] Most common among the electrolyte abnormalities are hypochloremic metabolic alkalosis, hypokalemia, and hyponatremia. These imbalances are understandable given the loss of gastric fluid. Also, FVD is expected with loss of vomitus, diarrheal stools, and diuretic abuse. Hypokalemia is common in patients taking potassium-losing diuretics and in those with large diarrheal fluid losses. If metabolic acidosis is present, the likely cause is laxative-induced diarrhea.

Bulimic patients must be monitored for fluid and electrolyte disturbances. Individuals who abruptly stop using laxatives or diuretics for weight control often develop reflex fluid retention. If this happens, the individual needs reassurance that this is only temporary and that salt restriction may be helpful during this transient period. With withdrawal of cathartics, measures to assist with bowel function are indicated, such as bulk-type laxatives or bran, exercise, and adequate hydration.

IMBALANCES ASSOCIATED WITH INTESTINAL OBSTRUCTION

Intestinal obstruction causes interference with the normal progression of intestinal contents; it may be complete or incomplete. A mechanical obstruction is defined as an actual physical barrier (eg, adhesions, hernia, tumor, or diverticula) blocking normal passage of intestinal contents. A mechanical obstruction is termed *simple* when there is no compromise in vascular supply; it is termed *strangulated* when the vascular supply is inhibited. A functional obstruction is sometimes referred to as *paralytic ileus,* or an *adynamic* or *neurogenic ileus.* As the name implies, the obstruction is caused by ineffective or nonpropulsive peristalsis. Although motor activity is slowed, it is not completely absent. Causes of paralytic ileus can include intraabdominal conditions such as peritonitis, appendicitis, cholecystitis, and pancreatitis. Other causes involve trauma and systemic conditions such as hypokalemia, uremia, and septicemia.

Mechanical small-bowel obstruction is manifested by distention of the bowel lumen with gas and fluid proximal to the obstruction. Most of the gas is due to swallowed air, although some results from bacterial fermentation within the gut. Because of distention, large quantities of water and electrolytes are secreted into the bowel lumen, even in the absence of oral intake. The edematous bowel wall is not able to absorb the large volume of intestinal secretions; thus, distention becomes progressively greater, leading to isotonic contraction of the ECF compartment as fluid is sequestered in the bowel (third-space effect). Ten liters or more of fluid can collect in this third space, and lead to hypovolemic shock. (Nursing assessment for third-space fluid shift is described in Chap. 3, and an example of the nursing process applied to the most frequent fluid balance-related diagnosis in bowel obstruction is given in Table 16-9.)

In adynamic ileus, decreased propulsive motility can affect the small intestine and colon, separately or together. As in mechanical obstruction, gas accumulates in the involved intestine, producing marked distention. Fluid also accumulates in the intestine because of decreased absorption. Although third-space fluid loss may be significant, it is not as great as in mechanical obstruction.

Plasma concentrations of electrolytes are initially preserved because the fluid lost is primarily isotonic; however, the patient usually becomes thirsty and drinks

TABLE 16-9.
Example of Nursing Process in Care of 68-Year-Old Man with Acute Intestinal Obstruction and Nursing Diagnosis of Fluid Volume Deficit Related to Third-Space Fluid Shift

ASSESSMENT	INTERVENTIONS	EXPECTED OUTCOMES
Postural hypotension: BP, 136/86 supine BP, 118/78 sitting up Pulse rate 118/min Urinary output 20 mL/hr; SG, 1.025 Hand veins take 7 seconds to fill in dependent position Decreased capillary refill time CVP, 1 cm H$_2$O BUN, 70 mg/dL; creatinine 2.1 mg/dL Hematocrit 55% Lethargy; patient responds appropriately when aroused	Monitor response to fluid replacement at hourly or more frequent intervals In collaboration with physician, administer fluids at rate needed to return vital signs, hourly urine output, and other parameters to within normal limits (without overloading circulatory system)	BP within normal limits (determined by patient's baseline) Pulse rate < 100/min Urine volume > 40 mL/hr Normal or improved skin and tongue turgor Hand veins fill in 3 to 5 seconds Normal capillary refill time CVP between 4 and 11 cm water BUN: creatinine ratio close to 10:1 (return to baseline levels) Hematocrit within normal limits Improved sensorium Normal breath sounds

SG, specific gravity; CVP, central venous pressure.

water, thereby developing hyponatremia. Contributing to hyponatremia is the endogenous release of water produced by oxidation. Sodium and other electrolytes (such as potassium and magnesium) are also lost by vomiting or as a result of GI suction after treatment is initiated. If the lost electrolytes are not replaced, deficits will eventually result.

Metabolic alkalosis is common with pyloric or high jejunal obstruction in which copious vomiting produces loss of acidic gastric juice. Sometimes in upper small-intestinal obstruction, the patient will vomit approximately equal volumes of gastric and intestinal juice, thus preventing serious disturbances in pH levels. If the obstruction is in a distal segment of the small intestine, the patient may vomit larger quantities of alkaline fluids than of acid fluids. (Recall that secretions below the pylorus are mainly alkaline.) Thus, metabolic acidosis can result from a low intestinal obstruction. If the obstruction is below the proximal colon, most of the GI fluids will be absorbed before reaching the point of obstruction, and thus acid–base balance may remain intact. In this situation, solid fecal matter accumulates until symptoms of discomfort develop. Respiratory acidosis can develop in patients with abdominal distention because respirations are compromised by upward pressure on the diaphragm, resulting in carbon dioxide retention.

REFERENCES

1. Rose B: Clinical Physiology of Acid–Base and Electrolyte Disorders, 3rd ed, p 721. New York, McGraw-Hill, 1989
2. Kokko J, Tannen R: Fluids and Electrolytes, 2nd ed, p 924. Philadelphia, WB Saunders, 1990
3. Maxwell M, Kleeman C, Narins R: Clinical Disorders of Fluid and Electrolyte Metabolism, 4th ed, p 704. New York, McGraw-Hill, 1987
4. Kokko, Tannen, p 924
5. Dunagan W, Ridner M: Manual of Medical Therapeutics, 26th ed, p 305. Boston, Little, Brown, 1989
6. Ibid
7. Maxwell et al, p 870
8. Ibid, p 871
9. Ibid
10. Kokko, Tannen, p 931
11. Rose, p 374
12. Dunagan, Ridner, p 306
13. Ibid
14. Physician's Desk Reference, 44th ed, p 1722. Oradell, NY, Medical Economics Company, 1990
15. Beck D, Fazio V: Current preoperative bowel cleansing methods. Dis Colon Rectum 33:12, 1990
16. Crapp et al: Preparation of the bowel by whole-gut irrigation. Lancet ii:1239, 1975
17. Rhodes et al: Oral electrolyte overload to cleanse the colon for colonoscopy. Gastrointest Endosc 24:24, 1977
18. Skucas et al: Whole-gut irrigation as a means of cleansing the colon. Radiology 121:303, 1976
19. Fleites et al: The efficacy of polyethylene glycol-electrolyte lavage solution versus traditional mechanical bowel preparation for elective colonic surgery: A randomized prospective, blinded clinical trial. Surgery 98(4):708, 1985
20. Beck D, Fazio V, Jagelman D: Comparison of oral lavage methods for preoperative colonic cleansing. Dis Colon Rectum 29:699, 1986
21. Beck et al: Comparison of cleansing methods in preparation for colonic surgery. Dis Colon Rectum 28:491, 1985
22. Ambrose et al: A physiological appraisal of polyethylene glycol and a balanced electrolyte solution as bowel preparation. Br J Surg 70:428, 1983
23. PDR, p 717
24. DiPalma et al: Comparison of colon cleansing methods in preparation for colonoscopy. Gastroenterology 86:856, 1984
25. Martin et al: Fatal poisoning from sodium phosphate enema: Case report and experimental study. JAMA 257(16):2190, 1987
26. Sotos et al: Hypocalcemic coma following two pediatric phosphate enemas. Pediatrics 60(3):305, 1977
27. PDR, p 950–951
28. Martin et al
29. Ellickson E: Bowel management plan for the homebound elderly. Journal of Gerontological Nursing 14(1):16, 1988
30. Yakabowich M: Prescribe with care: The role of laxatives in the treatment of constipation. Journal of Gerontological Nursing 16(7):4, 1990
31. Preece C, Judd C: Constipation in the elderly: Are drugs the only alternative to irregularity? Canadian Pharmaceutical Journal 115(4):136, 1982
32. Alpers D, Clouse R, Stenson W: Manual of Nutritional Therapeutics, 2nd ed, p 122. Boston, Little, Brown, 1988
33. Yakabowich
34. Shires GT: Fluids, Electrolytes, and Acid Bases, p 16. New York: Churchill Livingstone, 1988
35. Jones et al: Cathartic-induced magnesium toxicity during overdose management. Ann Emerg Med 15:1214, 1986
36. Martin et al
37. Mosley P, Segar W: Fluid and serum electrolyte disturbances as a complication of enemas in Hirschsprung's disease. Am J Dis Child 115:714, 1968
38. PDR, 950
39. Edmondson S, Almquist T: Iatrogenic hypocalcemic tetany. Ann Emerg Med 19:938, 1990
40. Wason S, Tiller T, Cunha C: Severe hyperphosphatemia, hypocalcemia, acidosis, and shock in a 5-month-old child following the administration of an adult Fleet[R] enema. Ann Emerg Med 18:696, 1989

41. Swerdlow D, Labow S, D'Anna F: Tetany and enemas: Report of a case. Dis Colon Rectum 17:786, 1974
42. Davis et al: Hypocalcemia, hyperphosphatemia, and dehydration following a single hypertonic phosphate enema. J Pediatr 90:484, 1977
43. Levitt M, Gessert C, Finberg L: Inorganic phosphate (laxative) poisoning resulting in tetany in an infant. J Pediatr 82:479, 1973
44. Martin, p 2192
45. Wason et al
46. Schwartz S, Shires G, Spencer F: Principles of Surgery, 5th ed, p 493. New York, McGraw-Hill, 1989
47. Kokko, Tannen, p 937
48. Schwartz et al, p 493
49. Geersden J, Pedersen V, Kjaergard H: Small bowel fistulas treated with somatostatin: Preliminary results. Surgery 100(5):811, 1986
50. Mitchell et al: Medical complications and medical management of bulimia. Ann Intern Med 107:71, 1987
51. Mitchell et al: Electrolyte and other physiological abnormalities in patients with bulimia. Psychol Med 13:273, 1983

17

Acute Pancreatitis

PATHOPHYSIOLOGY

Acute pancreatitis is a severe abdominal condition produced by inflammation in the pancreas. Damage to the pancreas and surrounding tissue stems from release of digestive enzymes. The pancreas becomes edematous and may pull enough fluid into itself to produce hypovolemia; swelling may be severe enough to compress the vascular bed and cause ischemia and necrosis. In addition, severe pancreatitis can produce irritation of the peritoneal surface (measuring 1.0–1.5 sq. m^2) and cause the transudation of substantial volumes of protein-rich fluid.[1]

ETIOLOGICAL ASSOCIATIONS

About 60% of nonalcoholic patients with acute pancreatitis have gallstones.[2] The mechanism by which gallstones cause pancreatitis is unclear; on occasion, a calculus impacted on the ampulla of Vater may produce the problem.[3]

Another major cause of acute pancreatitis is alcoholism. Apparently, alcoholism causes pancreatitis by a combination of mechanical and nutritional factors. Among other possible causes of pancreatitis are trauma and operation, certain drugs (such as steroids and thiazide diuretics), mumps, and the coxsackie virus. Sometimes the cause is unknown and is labeled idiopathic.

FLUID AND ELECTROLYTE DERANGEMENTS

Hypovolemia

In acute pancreatitis, pancreatic inflammation and autodigestion lead to peripancreatic edema and loss of fluid into the retroperitoneal tissue. Release of digestive enzymes from the inflamed pancreas can cause a peritoneal burn that, when severe, equals a burn covering up to a third of the body's surface.[4] The resulting fluid shifts from the vascular space may produce profound hypovolemia. This hypovolemia's severity depends on

(1) the extent of fluid and blood lost in the retroperitoneum and peritoneal cavity (as much as 10 L of plasma and blood may be sequestered into these areas),[5] (2) the volume of fluid sequestered in the bowel during adynamic ileus, and (3) the volume of vomitus. A myocardial depressant factor (MDF), demonstrated to be released from the pancreas during pancreatitis, may also contribute to the shock.[6]

The decrease in plasma volume may be as much as 30% to 40% over a 6-hour period, causing hypotension, tachycardia, oliguria, and hemoconcentration.[7] Acute renal failure may follow untreated severe intravascular volume depletion.

Hypocalcemia

Hypocalcemia has been reported to occur in 10% to 80% of patients with acute pancreatitis.[8] In part, drop in the total serum calcium (sum of the ionized and bound fractions) is related to the concurrent hypoalbuminemia predictably associated with acute pancreatitis. (Recall that when hypoalbuminemia is present, the total serum calcium appears lower than it actually is.) However, there is also, apparently, a true decrease in ionized calcium.[9]

Several hypotheses have been proposed to explain the hypocalcemia of acute pancreatitis. For example, discovery of calcium ions deposited in areas of fat necrosis in the pancreas led to the proposal that calcium soap formation was the main cause of hypocalcemia in pancreatitis. However, if this were the only cause, it would be difficult to explain why parathyroid hormone (PTH) does not quickly stimulate the release of calcium stored in the bones. It has more recently become clear that decreased secretion of PTH contributes to the hypocalcemia. There are also suggestions that increased glucagon secretion and hypercalcitonemia may contribute to the development of hypocalcemia in some patients, as may hypomagnesemia and hypoalbuminemia.

The extent of hypocalcemia is often used as a predictive measure for quantifying the severity of acute pancreatitis. See Table 17-1 for additional indicators validated by Ranson and Pasternak[10] in a clinical study. When fewer than three criteria are present, the mortality is predicted to be 1%; when three or four are present, 15%; when 5 or 6 are present, 40%; and when 7 or more are present, 100%. Awareness of prognostic indicators is helpful in planning the degree of aggressiveness required in therapy for acute pancreatitis.

Hypomagnesemia

Mild hypomagnesemia may occur during acute pancreatitis. As is the case with hypocalcemia, hypomagnesemia has been attributed to precipitation of magnesium ions in the inflamed tissues in and around the pancreas as insoluble magnesium soaps.[11] Also, like hypocalcemia, hypomagnesemia is often at least partially related to hypoalbuminemia (meaning that much of the change may be in bound rather than in ionized magnesium). Of course, contributing to the hypomagnesemia may be direct loss by means of vomiting, gastric suction, and diarrhea. If the pancreatitis is due to alcoholism, the hypomagnesemia is likely to be more severe (because of the multiple magnesium-lowering effects of alcohol). A recent study concluded that patients with acute pancreatitis and hypocalcemia commonly have intracellular magnesium deficiency despite normal serum magnesium concentrations, and that magnesium deficiency may play a significant role in the pathogenesis of hypocalcemia.[12]

Acid—Base/Oxygenation Disturbances

Acid—base disturbances may vary widely, depending on clinical circumstances. For example, metabolic alkalosis may result from the frequent vomiting associated with acute pancreatitis, as well as from the gastric suction used during treatment to put the pancreas "at rest" and to alleviate adynamic ileus. On the other hand, metabolic acidosis is likely if acute renal failure occurs secondary to severe hypovolemia.

Respiratory acid—base problems are possible due to a variety of conditions. For example, severe pain may stimulate ventilation and cause respiratory alkalosis. Also, the pulmonary complications (such as pneumonia, pleural effusions, pulmonary edema, pulmo-

---

TABLE 17—1.
Signs Used to Classify Severity of Acute Pancreatitis

At admission

1. Age > 55
2. WBC > 16,000/mm^2
3. Glucose > 200 mg/dL
4. LDH > 350 IU/L
5. SGOT > 250 Frankel units (%)

During initial 48 hours

1. Hematocrit fall > 10%
2. BUN rise > 5% per mg/dL
3. Ca < 8 mg/dL
4. Arterial PaO$_2$ < 60 mmHg
5. Base deficit > 4 mEq/L
6. Fluid sequestration > 6 L

(Adapted from Schwartz S, Shires G, Spencer F [eds]: Principles of Surgery, 5th ed, p 1422. New York, McGraw-Hill, 1989, with permission.) BUN, blood urea nitrogen; LDH, lactic dehydrogenase; SGOT, serum glutamic oxaloacetic transaminase; WBC, white blood count.

nary emboli, and atelectasis) to which patients with pancreatitis are predisposed may cause respiratory acid–base problems. Factors contributing to respiratory complications may include the following:

▶ Immobility and retained secretions
▶ Release of pancreatic enzymes into the systemic circulation, which may cause damage to pulmonary tissues[13]
▶ Pleural effusions, more prominent on the left (a result of inflammation from pancreatic enzymes and extravasation of fluids)
▶ Ascites (which interferes with respiratory excursions)[14]
▶ Overzealous fluid replacement therapy

Respiratory complications are among the more frequent life-threatening features of patients with acute pancreatitis.[15] Respiratory difficulty of sufficient magnitude to require ventilator support is an ominous prognostic sign.[16]

TREATMENT

FLUID REPLACEMENT

Maintenance of an adequate circulating blood volume is of paramount importance in the patient with acute pancreatitis. The importance of restoring volume cannot be overemphasized because the death rate from this disease in the acute stage is directly correlated with the adequacy of fluid resuscitation.[17] Fluid losses through fluid pooling in the abdomen and retroperitoneal area, as well as from nasogastric suction, vomiting, and diaphoresis, must be considered and replaced. As a rule, crystalloid solutions (such as lactated Ringer's) will suffice because the fluid lost into the retroperitoneum has the composition of the extracellular fluid (ECF).[18] However, in severe cases of hemorrhagic pancreatitis, blood products and colloid solutions may be needed (sometimes in a volume as great as 7 L over a 24-hour period).[19]

Close monitoring of vital signs and urine output is mandatory in guiding fluid replacement therapy (see section on assessment). In seriously ill patients with underlying cardiovascular disease, a Swan-Ganz catheter may be necessary to make decisions regarding fluid administration.

ELECTROLYTE REPLACEMENT

Because hypocalcemia and hypomagnesemia are frequently present in acute pancreatitis, it may be necessary to administer these electrolytes by the parenteral route. Ionized fractions (Ca^{++} and Mg^{++}) should be measured when possible because they are significant in physiological functioning. When evaluating total calcium or magnesium, the effect of hypoalbuminemia should be considered. Hypokalemia is frequently a problem that must be dealt with by potassium replacement.[20]

PAIN MANAGEMENT

The pain of pancreatitis is caused by edema and distention of the pancreatic capsule, obstruction of the biliary tree, and peritoneal irritation caused by pancreatic products.[21] Management of the severe pain is important. Meperidine is the drug of choice for this purpose as it has less effect on the sphincter of Oddi than does morphine or other opiates.[22,23] Patients should be given no oral feedings until several days after pain ceases. Premature introduction of food can exacerbate a severe recurrence. Striking relief from pain may follow insertion of a nasogastric (NG) tube.

NASOGASTRIC SUCTION

Most clinicians favor the use of NG suction in patients with acute pancreatitis until nausea, vomiting, and pain subside. The major objective of this therapy is to "put the pancreas at rest" by stopping the secretin-pancreozymin stimulus to pancreatic secretion. Another benefit of NG suction is relief from the intestinal ileus so frequently present in acute pancreatitis. Several clinical studies have failed to prove the effectiveness of NG suction in patients with pancreatitis, unless vomiting is a problem.[24,25]

RESPIRATORY CARE

Supportive respiratory care should be given during the course of acute pancreatitis. As stated earlier, a number of respiratory complications have been described in patients with acute pancreatitis (including diaphragmatic elevation, fleeting infiltrates, pleural effusions, atelectasis, and arterial hypoxemia).[26] For this reason, blood gases should be monitored in acutely ill patients and respiratory support provided when indicated (such as humidified oxygen, intratracheal intubation, and assisted ventilation). Nursing management is discussed in the section on interventions.

NUTRITIONAL SUPPORT

As described above, it is important to "put the pancreas at rest" during an attack of acute pancreatitis. Thus, oral intake must be stopped during the acute phase.

Still, patients are often hypercatabolic because of the severity of their illness. The problem becomes one of deciding how to supply nutrients in adequate amounts. The choice is essentially between total parenteral nutrition (TPN) or enteral delivery of an elemental formula into the jejunum. The decision as to which is indicated must be made on an individual basis. Patients with mild disease can often be managed with enteral feeding of an elemental formula via a nasojejunal tube.[27] However, it may be difficult to achieve adequate levels of calories and protein because the feeding must be introduced slowly and the rate reduced if intolerance develops. For more seriously ill patients, enteral feeding may be precluded by ileus or other gastrointestinal (GI) malfunction. It may be necessary to start out with TPN and then gradually convert to enteral feeding as tolerance allows.

Although it seems logical that patients nourished with TPN during the course of their pancreatitis would fare better than those not receiving this treatment, clinical trials failed to indicate a significant difference in outcomes between the two groups. Also of note is that a high incidence of unexplained catheter-related sepsis occurs in patients with acute pancreatitis receiving TPN.[28]

INSULIN ADMINISTRATION

Small doses of regular insulin may be needed to treat the transient hyperglycemia that may occur in 25% to 50% of patients with acute pancreatitis. Apparently this is due to damage to the beta cells (thus decreasing insulin secretion) and increased glucagon release from the alpha cells (elevating the blood sugar).[29] In some patients, permanent diabetes may follow.

NURSING ASSESSMENT

Nursing care of the patient with acute pancreatitis is complex and requires sophisticated monitoring for complications and response to medical therapy. The monitoring role requires a firm understanding of physiological processes and expected responses to treatment. The following steps are necessary to detect changes in the patient's often rapidly fluctuating status:

1. Carefully measure and record fluid intake and output (I & O) from all routes. Fluid replacement is partially based on fluid losses that are directly measurable (for example, vomiting and gastric suction). Because of third-space fluid shifts into the retroperitoneum and abdomen, not all of the fluid loss can be measured directly. Therefore, in the early phase of the third-space fluid shift, it is often necessary to give more fluid than would be indicated by measured losses. Fluid replacement is primarily guided by hourly urine outputs and vital signs.

2. Monitor for the following signs of hypovolemia due to excessive fluid loss:
   ► Decreased skin turgor
   ► Dry mucous membranes
   ► Postural hypotension initially; later, systolic pressure less than 80 mmHg in all positions
   ► Pulse rate greater than 100/min
   ► Urinary output less than 30 mL/hr in adult
   Low urine volume may be a function of insufficient fluid replacement or may indicate renal failure (acute tubular necrosis).
   ► BUN elevated out of proportion to serum creatinine
   ► Central venous pressure (CVP) less than 4 cm water
   ► Pulmonary artery capillary pressure less than 6 mmHg
   ► Cardiac output less than 4 L/min
   ► Hematocrit may be elevated (red cells are suspended in less plasma as intravascular fluid is shifted into third space)
   Because of sequestering of fluid in abdominal and retroperitoneal areas, plus vomiting and NG suction, fluid loss may be severe enough to induce serious hypovolemia. This situation must be detected before perfusion to vital organs is compromised, leading to permanent renal or cerebral damage. As stated above, monitoring I & O alone is not sufficient to guide fluid replacement therapy.

   With adequate fluid replacement, the above parameters will remain within or return to normal limits.

3. Monitor for the following signs of hemorrhagic shock if patient has necrotizing hemorrhagic pancreatitis:
   ► Hypotension
   ► Tachycardia
   ► Anxiety
   ► Oliguria
   ► Cool, clammy skin
   ► Falling hematocrit
   ► CVP less than 4 cm water
   ► Pulmonary artery capillary pressure less than 6 mmHg
   Blood loss can be significant in necrotizing hemorrhagic pancreatitis and must be detected before serious perfusion problems develop. While this condition looks very much like simple fluid volume

deficit, it tends to occur more rapidly and is associated with a falling rather than an elevated hematocrit.

4. Monitor response to fluid replacement therapy. Fluid replacement therapy should be aggressive enough to keep the vital signs and hourly urine volume within normal limits. If the patient has underlying cardiovascular problems, it may be necessary to monitor the CVP and pulmonary capillary wedge pressure (PCWP). A close working relationship between the nurse and physician is necessary if the correct volume of fluid replacement is to be achieved. With adequate replacement therapy, expect to see:
   ▸ Normal BP and pulse rate (appropriate for age group)

5. Monitor for the following signs of respiratory distress or infection:
   ▸ Hypoxemia (as evidenced by low PaO_2)
   ▸ Breath sounds indicating the presence of infiltrates
   ▸ Tachypnea and labored respirations
   ▸ Cyanosis
   ▸ Temperature elevation

   Patients with pancreatitis are predisposed to pulmonary complications, such as adult respiratory distress syndrome (ARDS), fleeting infiltrates, pleural effusions, and atelectasis.

6. Monitor for the following signs of hypocalcemia:
   ▸ Complaints of numbness or tingling in the extremities or circumoral region
   ▸ Latent tetany as indicated by Trousseau's and Chvostek's signs (see Chapter 2, Figs. 2-13, 2-14)
   ▸ Laryngospasm and convulsions (signs of severe hypocalcemia). Monitor serum calcium levels (consider albumin level and pH). Look for a prolonged Q–T interval on electrocardiogram. See Chapter 6 for further discussion of hypocalcemia.

7. Monitor for the following signs of hypomagnesemia:
   ▸ Tremors, confusion, hallucinations, tachycardia, and positive Chvostek's and Trousseau's signs
   ▸ Lowered serum magnesium levels

   See Chapter 7 for a more thorough discussion of magnesium.

   Magnesium deficiency is most likely to be present in patients who were previously malnourished or alcoholic. Note that this imbalance looks a lot like hypocalcemia. Unfortunately, magnesium is not an ingredient in commonly used intravenous (IV) fluids; nor, for that matter, is calcium (except for the small amount in lactated Ringer's solution). Magnesium salts are available for parenteral use and are discussed in Chapter 7.

8. Monitor for the following signs of hypokalemia:
   ▸ Arrhythmias, weakness, GI hypomotility, and paresthesias
   ▸ Lowered serum potassium levels

   See Chapter 5 for further discussion of hypokalemia

9. Assess for infection (such as pancreatic abscess) by monitoring pain and temperature. Consider the location, severity, and duration of pain. Be aware that subtle changes in the nature and frequency of pain may be indicative of pancreatic abscess. Also, be aware that a temperature above the usual low-grade fever may signal a complicating infection. Several potential sources of fever exist in patients with acute pancreatitis, including pancreatic necrosis, abscess, infected pseudocyst, and aspiration pneumonia.[30] Development of fever after 2 weeks or longer suggests pancreatic abscess formation.

10. Monitor serum glucose levels to detect hyperglycemia. Serum glucose levels (determined by capillary "sticks") are more valid than urinary glucose levels. Once the renal threshold for glucose has been determined to be normal, one can rely on urine glucose measurements.

11. Assess bowel sounds and abdominal girth at regular intervals to monitor degree of adynamic ileus.

NURSING DIAGNOSES

Alterations associated with acute pancreatitis involve rapidly changing derangements in fluid, electrolyte, and, perhaps, acid–base balance. Because of these changes, a number of physiological nursing diagnoses may be appropriate. When possible, the North American Nursing Diagnosis Association (NANDA) list of accepted diagnoses should be used; however, the list is not yet fully developed. For this reason, the nurse must formulate additional diagnoses based on results of the nursing assessment. Table 17-2 lists possible nursing diagnoses related to the care of patients with acute pancreatitis. The list is not all-inclusive; it focuses primarily on derangements in metabolism.

NURSING INTERVENTIONS

Nursing interventions must be executed in a timely fashion and tailored to the individual patient's rapidly fluctuating status. As such, much of what the nurse does in caring for the critically ill patient with acute pancreatitis revolves around monitoring the current clinical status and working collaboratively with the physician to provide supportive care. The following interventions are often needed:

TABLE 17–2.
Examples of Nursing Diagnoses Related to Acute Pancreatitis

NURSING DIAGNOSIS	ETIOLOGICAL FACTORS	DEFINING CHARACTERISTICS
FVD, related to third-spacing of fluid and gastric loss by vomiting and suction	Escape of secretions into abdomen and retroperitoneum, vomiting, and nasogastric suction (aggravated by fever and diaphoresis)	Tachycardia, hypotension, urine output < 30 mL/hr, concentrated urine, BUN elevated out of proportion to creatinine, poor skin turgor (see Chapter 3)
Alteration in tissue perfusion: renal, related to FVD	Severe FVD due to fluid shift into abdomen and retroperitoneum, vomiting, and nasogastric suction	Oliguria or anuria, symptoms of renal failure (see Chapter 18)
Ineffective breathing pattern related to immobility, pain, and pleural effusions	Immobility, retained secretions, and pleural effusions (result of inflammation from pancreatic enzymes and extravasation of fluid), aggravated by overzealous fluid administration	Dyspnea, shortness of breath, tachypnea, cyanosis, cough, nasal flaring, decreased arterial oxygenation
Alteration in nutrition: less than body requirements, related to being NPO for prolonged period	Being NPO and receiving nasogastric suction during acute phase of illness; if prolonged, serious caloric deficiency can result, particularly if hypercatabolism is present due to severe illness	Loss of lean body mass as evidenced by decreased arm circumference, decreased serum albumin, pale mucous membranes and conjunctiva
Pain related to pancreatic disease process	Edema of pancreatic capsule, obstruction of biliary tree, irritation of peritoneum	Verbalizing of severe pain in mid-epigastric region; about half of patients experience radiation to upper left lumbar area. Verbalizing of pain made worse by supine position, relieved somewhat by sitting and leaning forward
Alteration in calcium balance (hypocalcemia) related to calcium binding in inflamed tissues, and altered PTH secretion	Binding of calcium in areas of fat necrosis caused by action of pancreatic enzymes on peritoneal fat, alteration in PTH secretion	Tingling of fingers and circumoral region, positive Chvostek's and Trousseau's signs, seizures, and laryngeal stridor (see Chapter 6)
Alteration in magnesium balance (hypomagnesemia) related to binding in inflamed tissues and loss in vomiting and diarrhea	Binding of magnesium in areas of fat necrosis caused by action of pancreatic enzymes on peritoneal fat, direct loss of GI fluids (most pronounced in alcoholics)	Weakness, tremors, arrhythmias, confusion, disorientation (see Chapter 7)

FVD, fluid volume deficit; BUN, blood urea nitrogen; PTH, parathyroid hormone.

1. Collaborate with physician to safely administer fluids and electrolytes, based on physiological indices. (See section on assessment.)
2. Maintain correct position and patency of the NG tube to alleviate nausea and vomiting and relieve distention.
    ▶ The tip of the tube should be well into the stomach (near the pylorus); if the tip rests high in the stomach, hydrochloric acid (HCl) may escape through the duodenum and theoretically stimulate secretions.
    ▶ Once the tube has been correctly positioned, mark the exterior portion and make every effort to maintain the position.
    ▶ Maintain patency of the tube by irrigating with approximately 20 mL of isotonic saline every 2 hours. Viscous gastric secretions may necessitate more frequent irrigations.

► Check suction apparatus periodically to be sure it is working correctly.

3. Implement measures to relieve pain.

► Administer prescribed analgesics as frequently as indicated. Pain can be quite severe and should be treated with regular analgesic injections. Medical directives frequently call for meperidine. If pain persists despite analgesics, discuss problem with physician. In addition to promoting comfort, pain relief from analgesics decreases restlessness and anxiety, which probably also decreases pancreatic secretions.

► Assist the patient to achieve a position of comfort. Pain relief may sometimes be partially attained by sitting up or lying curled on the right or left side.[31] Patients with peritoneal irritation are likely to remain very still. (This may present a problem in terms of retained respiratory secretions.)

4. Attempt to prevent or minimize respiratory complications.

► Turn patient at regular intervals to foster drainage of secretions.

► Encourage deep breathing at regular intervals.

► Suction retained secretions if necessary to keep airway open.

► Monitor rate of fluid replacement to avoid overloading the circulatory system and predisposing to pulmonary edema.

The physician may prescribe humidified oxygen to help support the patient. In severe situations, intubation and mechanical ventilation will be indicated. It should be noted that impaired pulmonary function may occur in all patients with pancreatitis (regardless of severity of illness).

5. Administer insulin per medical directives as indicated, based on capillary blood sugars, to control hyperglycemia.

6. Provide patient with periods of rest between nursing activities and attempt to minimize anxiety-producing situations.

7. Consider the patient's need for nutrients.

► Administer TPN or jejunal feedings if prescribed. (See section on nutritional support under treatment.)

► Be aware that after NG suction is discontinued, the patient is usually maintained without oral feedings for at least 24 to 48 hours before a low-fat diet is gradually introduced. Great care must be taken to avoid feeding too quickly as this can exacerbate another episode of acute pancreatitis.

► When the acute phase subsides and clear liquids are allowed by mouth, monitor bowel sounds and watch for recurring pain and nausea.

► Keep a record of the patient's nutrient intake so that deficiencies can be brought to the attention of the physician and dietitian.

REFERENCES

1. Switz D: Pancreatitis. In: Shoemaker et al (eds): Textbook of Critical Care, 2nd ed, p 734. Philadelphia, WB Saunders, 1989
2. Ranson J: The role of surgery in the management of acute pancreatitis. Ann Surg Apr 21 1(4): 386, 1990
3. Silen W, Steer M: Pancreas. In: Schwartz S, Shires G, Spencer F (eds): Principles of Surgery, 5th ed, p 1418. New York: McGraw-Hill, 1989
4. Switz, p 734
5. Wyngaarden J, Smith L: Cecil's Textbook of Medicine, 17th ed, p 774. Philadelphia, WB Saunders, 1985
6. Silen, Steer, p 1420
7. Starker P, Gump F: Gastrointestinal disorders. In: Askanazi J, Starker P, Weissman C (eds): Fluid and Electrolyte Management in Critical Care, p 257, Boston, Butterworths, 1986
8. Ryzen E, Rude R: Low intracellular magnesium in patients with acute pancreatitis and hypocalcemia. West J Med 152:145, 1990
9. Weinberg J, Moseley R: Fluid and electrolyte disorders and gastrointestinal diseases. In: Kokko J, Tannen R: Fluids and Electrolytes, 2nd ed, p 938. Philadelphia, WB Saunders, 1990
10. Ranson J, Pasternack B: Statistical methods for quantifying the severity of clinical acute pancreatitis. J Surg Res 185:43, 1977
11. Vanatta J, Fogelman M: Moyer's Fluid Balance: A Clinical Manual, 4th ed, p 131. Chicago, Year Book Medical Publishers, 1988
12. Ryzer, Rude, p 146
13. Orr et al: Acute Pancreatic and Hepatic Dysfunction, p 81. Bethany, CT, Fleschner, 1981
14. Switz, p 735
15. Ranson J, Rifkind K, Turner J: Prognostic signs and nonoperative peritoneal lavage in acute pancreatitis. Surg Gynecol Obstet 143:209, 1976
16. Baker R, Duarte B: The current status and recognition of treatment of severe necrotizing pancreatitis. Surg Annu 18:129, 1986
17. Starker, Gump, p 257
18. Ibid
19. Ibid, p 258
20. Switz, p 735
21. Given B, Simmons S: Gastroenterology in Clinical Nursing, p 421. St. Louis, CV Mosby, 1984
22. Dunagan W, Ridner M (eds): Manual of Medical Therapeutics, 26th ed, p 308. Boston, Little, Brown, 1989
23. Silen, Steer, p 1421
24. Fuller R, Loveland J, Frankel M: An evaluation of the efficacy of nasogastric suction treatment in alcoholic pancreatitis. Am J Gastroenterol 75:349, 1981

25. Switz D: Acute alcoholic pancreatitis: Effect of clinical presentation and therapies on outcome at a VA hospital. Ann Intern Med 78:816, 1973

26. Toledo-Pereyra L: The Pancreas: Principles of Medical and Surgical Practice, p 184. New York, John Wiley & Sons, 1985

27. Howard L, Michalek A, Alger S: Enteral nutrition and gastrointestinal, pancreatic, and liver disease. In: Rombeau J, Caldwell M (eds): Clinical Nutrition: Enteral and Tube Feeding, 2nd ed. Philadelphia, WB Saunders, 1990

28. Maxwell M, Kleeman C, Narins R: Clinical Disorders of Fluid and Electrolyte Metabolism, 4th ed, p 774. New York, McGraw-Hill, 1987

29. Fain J, Amato-Vealey E: Acute pancreatitis: A gastrointestinal emergency. Crit Care Nurs 8(5):4, 1988

30. Dunagan, Ridner, p 308

31. Fain, p 56

18

Renal Failure

The renal system is the primary regulator of homeostasis of the body's internal environment. It performs its essential maintenance functions by participating in the following physiologic processes: (1) regulation of the volume, concentration, and pH of body fluids; (2) detoxification and elimination of waste products; (3) regulation of blood pressure; (4) regulation of erythropoiesis; (5) synthesis of prostaglandins; and (6) metabolism of Vitamin D. Thus, when the renal system becomes dysfunctional, the result is an altered internal environment that is not compatible with life. Individuals who experience this dysfunction must rely on a complex set of therapeutic interventions that includes dietary and fluid restrictions, pharmacological agents, and renal replacement therapies to sustain life. The biochemical and metabolic alterations that these individuals endure severely compromise their well-being and present a major challenge for clinicians. To assist the clinician in meeting this challenge, this chapter discusses the following: definitions of renal failure; differentiation between acute and chronic renal failure, particularly with regard to etiologies and clinical courses; overview of the systemic manifestations of renal failure; specific effects of renal failure on fluid, electrolyte, and acid–base balance; assessment of the patient experiencing renal failure; overview of the nursing diagnoses appropriate for delivering care to a patient experiencing renal dysfunction and the appropriate management therapies specific for those nursing diagnoses related to the fluid, electrolyte, and acid–base imbalances.

DEFINITION

Renal failure is the cessation of renal function, resulting in biochemical, metabolic, fluid, electrolyte, and acid–base derangements in the individual's internal environment that seriously threaten life. There are two types of renal failure, acute and chronic, that can be differentiated by their definitions, etiologies, and clinical courses, or disease progression.

ACUTE RENAL FAILURE

Acute renal failure is the abrupt, reversible cessation of renal function, rapidly accompanied by azotemia and uremia. Various etiologies can produce acute renal failure. However, they can be categorized into three major types: prerenal, postrenal, and parenchymal. Prerenal etiologies are perfusion related, whereas postrenal etiologies are associated with obstruction. The parenchymal, or intrinsic, renal etiologies reflect damage to functioning kidney tissue as a result of a prolonged or major cellular insult. In general, the prerenal and postrenal etiologies are reversible if corrective interventions are implemented rapidly enough. Table 18-1 summarizes the three classifications of etiologies and delineates specific examples of frequently occurring clinical conditions that illustrate each category.

The clinical course of acute renal failure is relatively short, lasting approximately 10 to 25 days, during which time the individual progresses through four phases of the pathophysiological process. The four phases are onset; oliguria or anuria; diuresis, both early and late, or recovery stages; and convalescence. Technically, however, convalescence constitutes a separate phase because it actually occurs beyond the 10- to 25-day clinical course. A definition of each of these phases presents the clinician with an overview of the progression of the disease process.

THE ONSET PHASE

The onset phase extends from 0 to 2 days and is the period that elapses from occurrence of the precipitating event until the beginning of the oliguria or anuria. During this phase, the patient's renal blood flow and oxygen consumption decrease to 25% of normal, urine volume decreases to about 20% of normal, and filtration clearance decreases to 10% of normal.

THE OLIGURIC–ANURIC PHASE

This phase is approximately 8 to 14 days in length and constitutes the period during which the patient's urine volume remains less than 400 mL/day. Four hundred mL/day is the classic definition of an oliguric state. It should be noted that, although this phase is labeled oliguric-anuric, anuria rarely occurs in these patients. Indeed, the presence of anuria should lead the clinician to assess the patient further for indications of a urinary tract obstruction.

During this phase, the patient's renal blood flow and oxygen consumption remain at about 25% of normal, urine volume decreases further to an obligatory 5% of normal, and filtration clearance remains decreased at 10% of normal level. The longer the patient remains in this phase, the poorer the prognosis due to the additional opportunities for serious complications to occur as a result of excesses in fluids, electrolytes, and metabolic waste products.

THE DIURETIC PHASE

The diuretic phase lasts about 10 days and is comprised of two distinct segments, early and late diuresis. The early diuretic stage is the period from when the urine output becomes greater than 400 mL/day until the serum laboratory values stop rising. The laboratory values do not begin to fall during this stage but merely cease rising. During this stage of diuresis, the patient's renal blood flow and oxygen consumption increase slightly to about 30% of normal, urine volume soars to 150% of normal, and filtration clearance remains at 10% of normal. The increase in urine volume during this stage usually reflects more the change in renal perfusion and the existing serum's hyperosmolality than it does a change in actual renal function. This is evident in the continuing low percentage of filtration clearance.

Late-stage diuresis occurs from the time when the serum laboratory values begin to decrease until they stabilize at new, lower values. The new, lower values usually will not fall within the normal range for the patient but will remain somewhat elevated. The decrease and stabilization of the laboratory values at a higher

TABLE 18–1.
Common Causes of Acute Renal Failure

CLASSIFICATION	EXAMPLES OF CLINICAL CONDITIONS
Prerenal	
Hypovolemia	Vascular loss: hemorrhage Gastrointestinal loss: vomiting, diarrhea Renal loss: diuretic abuse, osmotic diuresis associated with diabetes Integumentary loss: burns, diaphoresis
Cardiovascular failure	Myocardial infarction Tamponade Vascular pooling: sepsis Vascular occlusion: thrombosis, embolism
Postrenal	
Obstruction	Ureteral: fibrosis, calculi, crystals, clots, accidental ligation Bladder: neoplasms Urethral: stricture, prostatic hypertrophy
Parenchymal	
Glomerulonephritis	Acute poststreptococcal, systemic lupus erythematosus, Goodpasture's syndrome, bacterial endocarditis
Vasculitis	Periarteritis, hypersensitivity angiitis
Interstitial nephritis	Acute pyelonephritis, allergic nephritis, hypercalcemia, uric acid nephropathy, myeloma of the kidney
Renal vascular disease	Renal artery occlusion, renal vein thrombosis
Acute tubular necrosis	
Postischemia	Hypovolemia, cardiogenic shock, endotoxic shock
Nephrotoxins	Heavy metals, organic solvents, glycols, antibiotics, anesthetics, radiographic contrast media
Pigments	
Hemoglobin	Intravascular hemolysis: transfusion reactions, toxic hemolysis
Myoglobin	Rhabdomyolysis: trauma, muscle disease, seizures, severe exercise, prolonged coma

(Schoengrund L, Balzer P: *Renal Problems in Critical Care*, p 27. New York, Delmar, 1985, with permission.)

than normal level is a reflection of the continuing improvement of renal blood flow and filtration clearance during this stage. Renal blood flow and oxygen consumption increase to about 50% of normal, urine volume peaks at about 200% of normal and then declines, and filtration clearance increases to 50% of normal. During this stage of the diuretic phase, the individual is vulnerable to developing fluid and electrolyte imbalances; at this time, however, they are likely to be deficits rather than excesses. These imbalances are easier to manage, and, although they still constitute a threat to the patient's well-being, they present much less of a hazard than the excesses that can occur during the oliguric–anuric phase. That they are less critical is related to the increased number of therapeutic options available because of the return of some real function.

THE CONVALESCENT PHASE

The convalescent phase lasts from 4 to 6 months and is the period from the stabilization of the serum laboratory values until the patient attains either totally normal or optimal renal function. In some patients, particularly the elderly and those with a preexisting renal disease, the renal dysfunction will result in a 1% to 2% degree of residual impairment. Those patients, therefore, may not regain 100% of their previous renal function. In most cases, however, the degree of residual impairment is clinically insignificant.

CHRONIC RENAL FAILURE

Chronic renal failure involves the slowly progressive, and often insidious, irreversible cessation of renal function accompanied by the sequential intensification of biochemical, metabolic, fluid, electrolyte, and acid–base imbalances. Many etiologies can result in chronic renal failure. Most can be classified as belonging to one of the following nine categories: glomerular diseases, tubular diseases, vascular diseases, infectious diseases, obstructive diseases, collagen diseases, metabolic renal diseases, congenital diseases, and neoplastic diseases. Table 18-2 summarizes these categories and gives some examples of clinical conditions that are illustrative of each category. The clinical conditions that occur most frequently appear to be chronic glomerulonephritis,

TABLE 18–2.
The Categories of Etiologies of Chronic Renal Failure

CATEGORY	EXAMPLES OF CLINICAL CONDITIONS
Glomerular diseases	Chronic glomerulonephritis Nephrotic syndrome Rapidly progressive glomerulonephritis
Tubular diseases	Renal tubular acidosis Chronic electrolyte imbalances ▶ Hypercalcemic nephropathy ▶ Hypokalemic nephropathy
Vascular diseases	Hypertension Arteriosclerosis Nodular glomerulosclerosis ▶ Kimmelsteil-Wilson's syndrome
Infectious diseases	Pyelonephritis Tuberculosis
Obstructive diseases	Obstructive uropathy ▶ Urethral strictures ▶ Congenital deformities
Collagen diseases	Scleroderma Lupus nephritis Necrotizing vasculitis ▶ Polyarteritis nodosa ▶ Hypersensitivity angiitis
Metabolic renal diseases	Amyloidosis Hyperoxaluria
Congenital diseases	Polycystic kidney disease Medullary cystic disease Hypoplastic kidneys Hereditary nephritis ▶ Alport's syndrome
Neoplastic diseases	Multiple myeloma Lymphoma

hypertension, nodular glomerulosclerosis due to diabetes mellitus, and obstructive uropathy. In addition, many etiological categories can produce a broad pathological process called chronic interstitial nephritis, which also occurs frequently.

The clinical course of chronic renal failure progresses gradually, and the patient often is not aware that there is a problem until very late in the process. During the disease progression, the patient progresses through four phases of functional deterioration, including diminished renal reserve, renal insufficiency, renal failure, and the uremic syndrome. During the third phase, renal failure, the patient usually recognizes that there is a problem. The time from the onset of the renal dysfunction through the progressive deterioration phases is very specific to each patient and the pathological processes associated with the etiology. Thus it is difficult to identify any precise time frames for each phase.

DIMINISHED RENAL RESERVE

The first phase of functional deterioration involves only a mild reduction in renal function. In this phase, the patient's creatinine clearance will decrease from an average normal level of 120 mL/min to approximately 50 mL/min, accompanied by an increase in the serum creatinine level from a normal range of 0.7 to 1.5 mg per 100 mL to a range of 1.6 to 2.0 mg per 100 mL. During this phase the patient still has about 50% of normal renal function and the kidney's primary regulatory, excretory, and metabolic functions remain intact. Consequently, there is little change in the individual's internal environment and no warning of what is to come.

RENAL INSUFFICIENCY

As the functional deterioration continues, the patient experiences renal insufficiency. During this phase, creatinine clearance continues to decrease to about 10 mL/min and is accompanied by an increase in the serum creatinine level to a range of about 2.1 to 5.0 mg/100 mL. The patient experiences mild alterations in the internal environment that are usually not significant enough to seek health care interventions. If, however, the patient experiences additional physiological stress such as an infection or dehydration, during this phase, the alterations in the internal environment will intensify and usually require therapeutic intervention.

RENAL FAILURE

During this phase of functional deterioration the patient usually realizes that a problem exists. There is now sufficient deterioration in renal function, usually a loss of more than 75% of normal function, to produce significant, constant alterations in the internal environment that threaten the patient's well-being. The patient now experiences clinical signs and symptoms that require management so that the activities of daily living can continue. During this phase, the individual's creatinine clearance has decreased to about 5 mL/min, and the serum creatinine level is greater than 8.0 mg per 100 mL.

THE UREMIC SYNDROME

The final phase of chronic renal failure is the onset of the uremic syndrome. At this point, the functional deterioration of the renal system is almost complete, and the individual experiences clinical manifestations in every body system. The patient's creatinine clearance level is less than 5 mL/min, and the serum creatinine level is greater than 12 mg per 100 mL and continues to rise.

THE SYSTEMIC MANIFESTATIONS OF RENAL FAILURE

The clinical signs and symptoms that manifest the presence of renal failure are collectively labeled the uremic syndrome. The uremic syndrome accompanies both acute and chronic renal failure. However, due to the relatively rapid resolution of acute renal failure, the syndrome may be less severe and may not evidence all components. For example, it is not likely that reproductive or chronic skeletal system alterations will be observed in a patient with acute renal failure, primarily due to the short duration of the renal dysfunction. Table 18-3 summarizes the clinical manifestations and their associated pathophysiological mechanisms according to body system. The fluid, electrolyte, and acid–base imbalances are so critical to caring for these patients that they require additional discussion.

FLUID VOLUME IMBALANCES

Fluid volume excess is usually evident in patients during either the oliguric–anuric phase of acute renal failure or in chronic renal failure. In both pathophysiological processes, the primary factor is the inability of the kidneys to excrete the appropriate amounts of fluid to maintain a homeostatic internal environment. The fluid volume excess may be a more serious problem in the oliguric–anuric phase of acute renal failure due to the rapidity of the onset of cessation in renal function. The rapid cessation of renal function does not allow time for the development of the adaptive mechanisms that patients with chronic renal failure experience. Thus the patient in the oliguric–anuric phase of acute

renal failure is much more vulnerable to the fluid imbalance.

The fluid volume excess that accompanies the oliguric–anuric phase of acute renal failure results from several etiologies. Certainly the decreased excretion of fluids due to a decreased glomerular filtration rate and tubular dysfunction is a major factor. The following may also contribute: (1) excessive ingestion or administration of oral or intravenous (IV) fluids; (2) accumulation of water resulting from the metabolism of nutrients; and (3) accumulation of water that is released from injured or catabolized tissues.

As the patient progresses through the acute renal failure episode and enters the diuretic phase, the fluid imbalance is likely to shift to a deficit. During this phase the glomerular filtration rate and tubular functional capacities have improved sufficiently so that a marked increase in the volume of urine excreted is noted. The volume of urine that is excreted depends not only on the degree of functional improvement that has occurred but on the amount of excess water and solute that was retained by the individual since the onset of the disease process. Fortunately, because of more aggressive dialysis therapy and other therapeutic interventions employed recently, the degree of excess water and solute retention has been somewhat minimized. Thus, these individuals do not seem to experience the massive fluid volume shifts and depletion characteristic of the diuretic phase in the past.

The patient with chronic renal failure usually experiences a fluid volume excess. In general, this fluid volume imbalance results primarily from the decreased glomerular filtration rate and decreased excretion of free water. In addition, it is enhanced by a dysfunctional concentrating and diluting mechanism and an increased solute load. The deficit in the concentrating mechanism probably occurs due to several pathophysiological alterations, including the following: (1) decreased medullary blood flow; (2) decreased response or resistance of the collecting tubules to the presence of vasopressin or antidiuretic hormone (ADH); (3) impaired sodium and chloride transport in the ascending limb of Henle's loop; (4) diminished urea gradient in the medullary interstitium due to dilution; (5) decreased physiological functioning of Henle's loop, distal convoluted tubules, and collecting tubules due to pathology and cellular injury; and (6) increased secretion or synthesis of vasoconstrictor substances, such as renin or prostaglandins to support glomerular blood flow, which further suppresses the response to ADH. The ultimate outcome of the decrease in concentrating ability is an increased solute load for the patient.

Patients with chronic renal failure also cannot dilute urine. The defect in the diluting mechanism probably

(text continues on page 250)

TABLE 18–3.
The Systemic Manifestations of Renal Failure

SYSTEM	MANIFESTATION	PATHOPHYSIOLOGICAL MECHANISMS
Vascular	Fluid overload	Decreased excretion
	Electrolyte imbalances	Decreased excretion
	Metabolic acidosis	Decreased hydrogen ion secretion
		Decreased sodium ion reabsorption
		Decreased bicarbonate ion reabsorption and generation
		Decreased excretion of phosphate salts or titratable acids
		Decreased ammonia synthesis and ammonium excretion
	Hypertension	Fluid overload
		Increased sodium retention
		Inappropriate activation of the renin–angiotensin system
Cardiac	Congestive heart failure	Fluid overload
		Hypertension
	Dysrhythmias	Electrolyte imbalances, especially hyperkalemia, hypocalcemia and variations in sodium
	Pericarditis (more frequently seen in chronic renal failure patients)	Uremic toxins
		Increased pericardial membrane permeability
	Peripheral or systemic edema	Fluid overload and increased hydrostatic pressure (associated decrease in osmotic pressure would increase the degree of edema)
		Right ventricular dysfunction
Hematopoietic	Anemia	Decreased erythropoietin secretion
		Loss of red blood cells through the GI tract, mucous membranes, or dialysis
		Decreased red blood cell survival time due to uremic toxins
		Burr cells are produced by a hypertonic serum due to uremic toxins
		Uremic toxins interfere with folic acid action
	Alterations in coagulation	Platelet dysfunction due to uremic toxins
		Hypocalcemia could contribute but rarely does because of the metabolic acidosis
	Increased susceptibility to infection	Decreased neutrophil phagocytosis and chemotaxis due to uremic toxins
Respiratory	Pulmonary edema	Fluid overload
		Increased pulmonary capillary permeability
		Left ventricular dysfunction
	Pneumonia or pneumonitis	Thick, tenacious oral secretions due to decreased fluid intake
		Weak, lethargic patient with depressed cough reflex due to uremia
		Decreased pulmonary macrophage activity
		Fluid overload
	Kussmaul respirations	Increase in rate and depth of respirations to decrease the carbon dioxide in the body to compensate for metabolic acidosis

(continued)

TABLE 18–3.
(continued)

SYSTEM	MANIFESTATION	PATHOPHYSIOLOGICAL MECHANISMS
Gastrointestinal	Anorexia, nausea, and emesis	Uremic toxins Decomposition of urea in the GI tract releasing ammonia that irritates mucosa
	Stomatitis and uremic halitosis	Uremic toxins Decomposition of urea in the oral cavity releasing ammonia
	Gastritis and bleeding	Uremic toxins Decomposition of urea in the GI tract releasing ammonia that irritates GI mucosa producing small ulcerations Increased capillary fragility
	Bowel problems Diarrhea	Uremic toxins Hypermotility due to electrolyte imbalances, especially hyperkalemia
	Constipation	Hypomotility due to electrolyte imbalances, decreased fluid intake, decreased activity, and decreased bulk in diet
Neuromuscular	Drowsiness, confusion, coma, and irritability	Uremic toxins produce uremic encephalopathy Metabolic acidosis
	Tremors, twitching, and convulsions	Electrolyte imbalances Uremic toxins produce uremic encephalopathy

	Peripheral neuropathy
	  Stage 1: restless leg syndrome and paresthesias
	  Stage 2: motor involvement leading to footdrop
	  Stage 3: paraplegia
	(Stages 2 and 3 are rare in acute renal failure patients.)
		Decreased nerve conduction, both motor and sensory, due to uremic toxins

Psychosocial	Decreased mentation, decreased concentration, and altered perceptions (even to the point of frank psychoses)	Uremic toxins produce uremic encephalopathy Electrolyte imbalances Metabolic acidosis Tendency to develop cerebral edema
Integumentary	Pallor	Uremic anemia
	Yellow hue	Retained urochrome pigment is excreted through skin
	Dryness	Decreased secretions from oil and sweat glands due to uremic toxins
	Pruritis	Dry skin Calcium or phosphate deposits in the skin or both Uremic toxins effects on nerve endings
	Purpura and ecchymoses	Increased capillary fragility Platelet dysfunction
	Uremic frost (seen only in terminal or severely critically ill patients)	Urea or urate crystals are excreted through the skin
Endocrine	Glucose intolerance (usually not clinically significant)	Peripheral insensitivity to insulin due to uremia Prolonged insulin half-life due to decreased renal metabolism

(continued)

TABLE 18–3.
(continued)

SYSTEM	MANIFESTATION	PATHOPHYSIOLOGICAL MECHANISMS
Skeletal	Hypocalcemia	Hyperphosphatemia due to decreased renal excretion Decreased GI reabsorption due to decreased renal conversion of vitamin D
	Osteodystrophy	Increased osteoclastic activity in response to an increased secretion of parathormone
	Soft tissue calcification	Deposition of calcium phosphate crystals in soft tissue and other structures
Reproductive	Infertility	Decreased sperm production and decreased ovulation due to uremia
	Decreased libido	Combination of the pathophysiological and psychological effects of uremia

(Schoengrund L, Balzer P: Renal Problems in Critical Care, pp 29–31. New York, Delmar Publishers, 1985; with permission.)

results from the decreased glomerular filtration rate, the decreased number or functional nephrons due to pathology, and the increase in overall solute load. The result is the excretion of an isosthenuric urine with a fixed osmolality that is similar to the plasma. Thus, the individual cannot dilute the urine and is unable to excrete excess free water.

ELECTROLYTE IMBALANCES

The patient with renal failure experiences deviations in almost every electrolyte. In general, the patient is hypernatremic (or dilutionally hyponatremic), hyperkalemic, hyperchloremic, hypocalcemic, hyperphosphatemic, and normomagnesemic (unless exogenous sources of magnesium are ingested or administered). Understanding the specific pathophysiological mechanisms that produce these imbalances during renal failure will assist the clinician in planning and implementing appropriate therapeutic measures to assist the individual in coping with these alterations in the internal environment.

Sodium

Patients with either acute or chronic renal failure often present initially with hyponatremia. This state, however, usually changes to hypernatremia during the progression and management of the disease process. The patient with acute renal failure tends to retain sodium due to a decreased glomerular filtration rate and tubular dysfunction. The increased sodium retention results in increased water retention and, thus, an extracellular

fluid (ECF) volume expansion with a concomitant dilutional hyponatremia. Other factors that contribute to producing this almost "pseudo" hyponatremic state include increased ingestion or administration of free water; increased accumulation of water resulting from increased metabolic processes; increased ECF volume resulting from cellular catabolism or injury; and intracellular shifts of sodium that occur as a result of the extracellular–intracellular exchanges among sodium, hydrogen, and potassium due to metabolic acidosis and hyperkalemia. Thus the patient appears to have a dilutional hyponatremia when, in fact, a hypernatremic state exists. The hypernatremic state may gradually appear as the patient's water intake is restricted. In some patients, however, the hypernatremia may never be evident because of the early, aggressive initiation of renal replacement therapy, usually in the form of hemodialysis.

As the individual with acute renal failure progresses to, and through, the late stage of diuresis, the possibility of a true hyponatremic state occurring becomes more distinct. The solute-induced diuresis, as well as the cellular shifts of electrolytes, is likely to create at least a transient sodium deficit. The imbalance will, however, usually resolve without therapeutic intervention as the diuresis decreases and more normal renal function occurs.

The sodium imbalances that accompany chronic renal failure usually shift from hyponatremia to hypernatremia as the renal function deteriorates to an end-stage level. The concept that sodium excretion decreases as the functional renal mass decreases certainly is valid. However, during the progressive deterioration in function, numerous adaptive mechanisms are stimulated that serve to maintain a certain degree of sodium balance. Those adaptive mechanisms appear to include the following: (1) extracellular fluid volume expansion as a result of sodium retention, which may increase the glomerular filtration rate; (2) Na-K-ATPase inhibition resulting in natriuresis; (3) increased circulating amounts of atrial natriuretic factor; (4) increased prostaglandin synthesis; (5) hypertrophy and hyperfiltration of the remaining nephrons; (6) tubular adaptation due to altered Starling forces at the peritubular membrane and an increased solute load; and (7) altered proximal tubule sodium reabsorption due to metabolic acidosis. These adaptive mechanisms appear to remain operative throughout the renal dysfunction but decrease in effectiveness as the disease process progresses to an end-stage level. Thus, as their effectiveness decreases, the occurrence of hypernatremia increases.

Potassium

Hyperkalemia is a significant electrolyte imbalance for patients in either acute or chronic renal failure. However, it is a greater threat to the patient with acute renal failure due to the rapidity of its onset and the patient's overall decreased capacity to activate appropriate adaptive mechanisms in response to the abrupt alteration. In fact, for patients with acute renal failure, hyperkalemia-induced complications are second only to sepsis as the leading cause of death.

The primary mechanisms present in acute renal failure that enhance the development and maintenance of a hyperkalemic state include (1) decreased glomerular filtration rate, loss of distal tubular function, and oliguria; (2) intracellular release of potassium from lysed, necrotic, or injured cells; (3) presence of acute metabolic acidosis; (4) cellular catabolism; and (5) inhibition of ATPase and its resulting defect in potassium transport mechanisms. In addition, any new stresses that occur, such as infection, fever, or gastrointestinal (GI) bleeding, will further compromise the patient and serve to enhance the hyperkalemia.

The patient with chronic renal failure employs adaptive mechanisms for handling the increased potassium load resulting from the decrease in renal function. These adaptive mechanisms remain intact and operative throughout the progression of the chronic renal failure until the patient becomes oliguric. Once oliguria is present, the adaptive mechanisms cease to be effective. Included among those adaptive mechanisms are (1) increased potassium per nephron excretion rate by the remaining intact nephrons; (2) increased potassium excretion by the large intestine; (3) increased renal Na-K-ATPase activity level; (4) increased tubular intra-

luminal flow rate; (5) increased peritubular potassium reabsorption; (6) increased potassium secretion by the collecting ducts; (7) increased distal tubular potassium secretion due to an increased aldosterone production; and (8) presence of chronic metabolic acidosis. Certainly if the patient with chronic renal failure experiences additional stressors that would further compromise the adaptive mechanisms, the hyperkalemic state could be exacerbated and rapidly become life threatening. Such stressors might include volume depletion or catabolic events like infection, GI bleeding, trauma, or surgery.

Chloride

Overall, chloride imbalance does not seem to be a significant problem for patients with either acute or chronic renal failure. Any imbalance that does occur reflects either the alterations in sodium, water, bicarbonate, and hydrogen ions or the presence of uremic manifestations or complications. Patients with acute renal failure are likely to have an actual increase in chloride as a result of the decreased glomerular filtration rate, tubular dysfunction, sodium retention, and bicarbonate deficit. The increase, however, may be masked by the dilutional effect of the excessive water that is retained.

Patients with chronic renal failure tend to remain normochloremic due to the adaptive mechanisms that are activated. Such balance appears to be evident throughout the progression of the chronic renal failure process, including during the uremic state. Although little is known regarding the adaptive mechanisms that can facilitate chloride balance maintenance during chronic renal failure, one hypothesis suggests that a chloruretic factor may be a primary contributor.

Calcium

Hypocalcemia is an imbalance frequently occurring in both acute and chronic renal failure. In acute renal failure, the decline in serum calcium levels can be noted as early as 48 hours after the onset of oliguria. In most instances, the decrease will stabilize at approximately 6 mg per 100 mL. In acute renal failure due to rhabdomyolysis, however, the levels may be much lower due to an exacerbated deficit of calcium as it shifts into the injured and necrotic tissues. The hypocalcemia that accompanies acute renal failure results from the following mechanisms: (1) phosphate retention due to a decreased glomerular filtration rate and tubular dysfunction, (2) exaggerated hyperphosphatemia due to the release of phosphate ions from injured tissues, (3) decreased 1,25 dihydroxycholecalciferol production by the kidneys and its concomitant decrease in the GI absorption of calcium, and (4) increased secretion of parathyroid hormone (PTH) in response to the hyperphosphatemia and suppressed serum calcium level. PTH acts directly on the bone to cause resorption of calcium and phosphate. Since the additional phosphate added to the bloodstream cannot be disposed of through the usual renal route, the serum calcium concentration cannot increase and remains a stimulus for increased PTH secretion. The clinical significance of hypocalcemia in patients with acute renal failure lies not so much in its ability to produce tetany as a result of altering neuron permeability as in its potentiation of the effect of hyperkalemia on cardiac function. Indeed, the acute metabolic acidosis that is present in acute renal failure serves to modulate some of the effects of the hypocalcemia by increasing the proportional amount of ionized calcium that is available in the serum.

In chronic renal failure, the hypocalcemic imbalance has greater clinical significance. It often results in the following complications for the patient: renal osteodystrophy, soft tissue calcification, secondary hyperparathyroidism, and enhanced signs and symptoms of uremia. The mechanisms responsible for creating and maintaining the hypocalcemia include (1) excessive phosphate retention due to decreased renal parenchymal mass, (2) increased PTH production as a compensatory response, (3) impaired vitamin D metabolism by the kidneys, and (4) the physiologically depressive effects of the uremic toxins in the body. These mechanisms result in decreased GI calcium absorption, the formation of calcium-phosphate complexes, decreased bone mobilization of calcium due to a skeletal resistance to PTH, and suppression of the normal metabolic processes used to restore calcium to normal levels.

Initially in chronic renal failure an adaptive hypocalciuria occurs. Unfortunately, it is not sufficient to overcome the effects of the hyperphosphatemia and uremia producing the hypocalcemic state. Thus, the patient remains hypocalcemic, and the imbalance is accentuated as the chronic renal failure progresses to end-stage level.

Phosphorus

Patients with either acute or chronic renal failure experience hyperphosphatemia. In acute renal failure, the imbalance is created by (1) inadequate excretion due to a decreased glomerular filtration rate and tubular dysfunction; (2) intracellular shift of phosphate ions to the ECF due to catabolism, cellular injury, and tissue necrosis; and (3) acute metabolic acidosis that decreases glycolysis resulting in the hydrolysis of intracellular sugar phosphates that increase the concentration of diffusible inorganic phosphate ions. Thus, this imbalance may be exaggerated in patients who are very catabolic.

Individuals with chronic renal failure do not experience hyperphosphatemia until renal function has deteriorated to a creatinine clearance level of from 20 to 30 mL/min. At that point, not only are there reductions in the filtered load of phosphate due to a decreased glomerular filtration rate, but there is also impairment of the intrinsic tubular adaptive mechanisms that would normally decrease the reabsorption of phosphate in a hyperphosphatemic state. Increased PTH secretion is another adaptive mechanism that tends to blunt the severity of the hyperphosphatemic state. Unfortunately, the result of this compensatory response is secondary hyperparathyroidism that merely complicates the patient's clinical condition even more. Thus, the excess phosphate not only creates additional problems by secondary hyperparathyroidism but also appears to (1) decrease the calcium mobilizing ability of PTH; (2) decrease GI calcium absorption; (3) inhibit the hydroxylation of vitamin D to 1,25 dihydroxycholecalciferol in the kidney; (4) facilitate the deposition of calcium in soft tissues; and (5) have a direct nephrotoxic effect.

Magnesium

Patients with either acute or chronic renal failure usually retain magnesium as a result of a decreased glomerular filtration rate and tubular dysfunction. In most instances, however, the hypermagnesemic state does not become clinically significant unless the patient ingests or receives additional magnesium from exogenous sources. The usual exogenous sources of magnesium include magnesium-based antacids and cathartics, pharmacological agents, IV solutions, and hyperalimentation solutions.

During acute renal failure, the degree of magnesium retention in the oliguric–anuric phase is usually not sufficient to produce clinically significant alterations. Such clinical signs and symptoms are not frequently manifested until the serum magnesium level is in excess of 7 mEq/L. Fortunately, because acute renal failure is usually of short duration, the patient rarely experiences serum magnesium levels greater than 3 or 4 mEq/L unless an exogenous load of magnesium is provided. Thus, hypermagnesemia is present in patients with acute renal failure but usually is not clinically apparent.

In chronic renal failure, the serum magnesium level remains within the normal range until the glomerular filtration rate decreases to less than 30 mL/min. As the disease progresses to end-stage level, adaptive mechanisms are initiated that tend to lessen the clinical impact of the continuing accumulation of magnesium due to decreased excretion. Those adaptive mechanisms include (1) increased fractional magnesium excretion due to the increased filtered magnesium load; (2) increased total volume of magnesium excreted as a result of natriuresis and the overall increased osmotic load; (3) increased magnesium excretion due to acidosis, which decreases magnesium tubular reabsorption; (4) decreased tubular response to PTH; (5) decreased intestinal absorption of magnesium due to uremia and the decreased production of 1,25 dihydroxychyloecalciferol; and (6) increased deposition of magnesium in the bone and perhaps intracellularly. Eventually these adaptive mechanisms are unable to compensate for the excessive magnesium that is retained. As a result, the patient is more likely to accumulate magnesium, attain higher serum levels, and experience the clinical signs and symptoms associated with hypermagnesemia. Certainly the addition of any exogenous source of magnesium will exacerbate the imbalance and result in further clinical manifestations.

Acid–Base

Metabolic acidosis is the predominant acid–base imbalance that accompanies both acute and chronic renal failure. In both disease processes, there is a retention of hydrogen ions due to a decreased glomerular filtration rate, tubular dysfunction, and an overall decrease in the number of functioning nephrons. The primary physiological alterations that contribute to producing the acidosis seem to be deficits in bicarbonate reabsorption and ammoniagenesis. The result is that the usual daily load of nonvolatile acids produced by the metabolism of dietary protein and the catabolism of endogenous tissue cannot be excreted. Thus, those acids, normally averaging about 1 mEq/kg/day of body weight accumulate and result in metabolic acidosis.

Patients with acute renal failure usually experience more severe acid–base imbalances due to the rapid onset of the disease process and their catabolic state. The rapidity of the onset decreases the patient's ability to initiate complex adaptive mechanisms to modulate the effects of the imbalance. In addition, cellular catabolism releases anions (sulfate, phosphate, and organic ions) into the plasma that enhance the high anion gap metabolic acidosis (see Chapter 9). Because the patient rapidly uses the existing buffering substances and, due to renal dysfunction, cannot provide sufficient replacements, the acidosis persists. The respiratory compensatory mechanisms that are stimulated appear to ameliorate some of the negative effects of the acidosis, but the imbalance is usually too severe for those mechanisms to significantly affect the patient's overall situation.

In chronic renal failure, the metabolic acidosis appears to remain mild until renal function deteriorates below a creatinine clearance level of 25 mL/min. At that time, the acidosis intensifies and gradually becomes more severe. The imbalance is even more exaggerated because the usual renal adaptive mechanisms are insufficient to contribute significantly to modulating the adverse effects of the acidosis. Fortunately, however, there are other adaptive physiological mechanisms that are triggered by the acidosis that can substitute for the defective renal mechanisms. These mechanisms include (1) buffering by tissue alkali from the bone stores; (2) respiratory compensation, which seems to operate effectively until the bicarbonate level decreases below 18 mEq/L; and (3) intracellular shift of hydrogen ions. Unfortunately, these mechanisms are not sufficient to maintain any semblance of homeostasis in acid–base balance in the patient. Thus, patients with chronic renal failure almost always have some degree of metabolic acidosis. Even the combination of maintenance renal replacement therapies, pharmacological agents, and dietary restrictions does not seem to restore or maintain a normal acid–base balance. Instead, the therapeutic management tends to decrease the hazardous effects of the imbalance and create a more stable internal environment for the patient.

CLINICAL ASSESSMENT

The clinical assessment of a patient experiencing renal dysfunction incorporates the following components: (1) documenting the patient's history, (2) inspection, (3) evaluation of vital signs, (4) palpation and percussion, (5) assessment of laboratory data, (6) noninvasive monitoring of the system, and (7) invasive monitoring of the system.

HISTORY

The individual's history contains four aspects that are very relevant to the renal system: (1) renal-related symptoms, (2) systemic diseases, (3) family history, and (4) pharmacological history.

Renal-Related Symptoms

Exploring the symptoms a patient reports in relation to the renal system can provide essential information that will assist in structuring the assessment to obtain more relevant and specific data. For example, certain symptoms are more indicative of one or two specific pathological conditions than they are of others. Table 18-4 lists the most frequently reported renal-related symptoms and their correlated potential pathologies.

Systemic Diseases

Numerous systemic diseases can affect the renal system as part of their inherent pathological processes. These

TABLE 18–4.
Selected Renal-Related Symptoms and Their Correlated Potential Pathologies

SYMPTOM	POTENTIAL PATHOLOGY
Dysuria	Infection
Dribbling	Prostatic enlargement
	Strictures
Edema	Failure
	Nephrotic syndrome
Frequency	Infection
	Diabetes
Hematuria	Trauma
	Glomerular membrane diseases
	Neoplasms
Hesitancy	Prostatic enlargement
Incontinence	Infection
	Neoplasms
	Prolapsed uterus
Nocturia	Infection
	Insufficiency
Oliguria	Insufficiency
	Neoplasms
	Failure
Proteinuria	Glomerular membrane diseases
	Nephrotic syndrome
Pyuria	Infection
Renal colic	Calculi
Urgency	Infection
	Prostatic disease

(Hartshorn J, Lamborn M, Noll ML: *Introduction to Critical Care Nursing*. Philadelphia, WB Saunders [in press]; with permission.)

systemic diseases originate in another primary body system that has a direct effect on the renal system. Specific clinical examples of such diseases include cardiovascular diseases such as hypertension and chronic congestive heart failure, respiratory diseases such as Goodpasture's syndrome and tuberculosis, endocrine diseases such as diabetes mellitus and hepatic dysfunction, and reproductive diseases such as disseminated intravascular coagulation and hemolytic–uremic syndrome.

Family History

The family history data is important in the assessment process because it not only indicates those systemic diseases which the patient may be prone to develop but also delineates specific hereditary or metabolic renal diseases that may already be present, or be likely to develop in the future. Examples include hereditary pathologies such as hereditary glomerulonephritis, Al-

port's syndrome, polycystic disease, medullary cystic disease, and metabolic abnormalities such as calculi, amyloidosis and hyperoxaluria.

Pharmacologic History

A medication history is important in assessing the renal system because the clinician not only documents and evaluates the currently prescribed and unprescribed medications ingested or administered but also specifically assesses for any drug use or abuse that might result in nephrotoxicity. Analgesic and antibiotic medications are primary offenders in this respect.

INSPECTION

Inspection is useful because many of the systemic manifestations of renal failure, which are reflected in almost every body system, are easily discernable visually. Table 18-5 depicts the various aspects and specific pa-

TABLE 18–5.
Inspection Components for Clinically Assessing the Renal System

ASPECT	SPECIFIC PARAMETERS
General appearance	Posture
	General strength
	Motor functioning
	Affect and mental attitude
	General hygiene
Skin	Color
	Turgor and elasticity
	Odor
	Degree of intactness
	Texture
	Presence, severity, and location of edema
Mucous membranes	Color
	Characteristics of secretions
	Odor
	Intactness
	Hydration state
Eyes	Visual acuity
	Periorbital edema
Ears	Auditory acuity
Activity	Level or amount
	Gait
	Motor functioning
Muscle movement	Purposeful
Cognitive functioning	Orientation
	Level of consciousness
	Responses to various types of stimuli

rameters that should be included when a clinician inspects a patient with renal dysfunction.

VITAL SIGNS

When assessing a patient's vital signs in relation to renal dysfunction, it is important for the clinician to recall the following: (1) patients with renal dysfunction are usually hypertensive due to fluid and electrolyte imbalances and, possibly, hyperactivity of the renin–angiotensin system; (2) they usually exhibit a strong, irregular, and somewhat rapid pulse as a result of the fluid and electrolyte imbalances; (3) they often exhibit Kussmaul's respirations as a compensatory mechanism for their metabolic acidosis; and (4) they are usually hypothermic but may exhibit temperature elevations due to susceptibility to infection from decreased phagocytic and chemotoxic mechanisms caused by uremia, as well as to their debilitated state overall. Thus, a patient with renal dysfunction may exhibit vital signs comparable to the following: BP, 160/98; pulse, 104 and irregular; respiration, 30; and oral temperature, 99° F (37.2° C).

PALPATION AND PERCUSSION

The kidneys are palpated in the lower portions of the upper right and left quadrants of the abdomen. Normally, only the lower pole of the right kidney is palpable because other anatomical structures obscure the left kidney and the remaining portions of the right kidney. The primary purposes for palpating the kidneys are to determine size and to elicit pain if an infective process is present. The kidneys should be palpated both anteriorly and posteriorly, particularly in the flank area at the costovertebral angle.

Percussion of the kidneys is performed in the same areas that have been designated for palpation. The purposes of percussion are to determine size and to assess for the presence and degree of abnormally sequestered amounts of perinephric fluid.

LABORATORY DATA

Renal dysfunction is rapidly evident in the patient's serum laboratory values. Thus, these data should be assessed at least daily for patients with acute renal failure and at least weekly for those with chronic renal failure. Table 18-6 presents the substances that should be included in a laboratory data assessment and their variations associated with acute and chronic renal failure.

The urine laboratory values vary with the pathological processes and the progression of the acute or chronic renal failure. Therefore, they are less helpful overall but may be important for differentiating various aspects of the therapeutic interventions. For example, urine sodium is a significant parameter for differentiating between prerenal oliguria and the intrinsic oliguria of acute renal failure. In addition, urine values may assist in determining the dietary needs of patients with chronic renal failure. In general, however, the concept

TABLE 18–6.
Variations in Serum Laboratory Values Accompanying Acute and Chronic Renal Failure

SUBSTANCE	VARIATION IN ACUTE RENAL FAILURE	VARIATION IN CHRONIC RENAL FAILURE
Sodium	Increases or varies	Normal or varies
Potassium	Increases	Increases
Chloride	Increases or varies	Varies
Blood urea nitrogen	Increases	Increases
Creatinine	Increases	Increases
Calcium	Decreases	Decreases
Phosphorus	Increases	Increases
Uric acid	Increases	Increases
Carbon dioxide combining power	Decreases	Decreases
Magnesium	Increases or normal	Increases or normal
Osmolality	Increases or varies	Increases or varies
Hematocrit	Decreases	Decreases
Hemoglobin	Decreases	Decreases

in renal failure is that substances are being retained in the serum and not excreted in the urine.

The best measure of renal function is creatinine clearance. Unfortunately, in many clinical situations it is not pragmatic to measure creatinine clearance. Instead, serum creatinine and blood urea nitrogen (BUN) can be used to assess renal function. Significant increases in both of those serum values indicate renal dysfunction. Of the two values, however, BUN is the least reflective of renal function because it is easily influenced by other factors such as catabolism, internal bleeding, and dehydration. Also of note is that the volume of urine output is not a good measure of renal function. Urine volume is more reflective of perfusion levels than of function. Thus, a decrease in urine volume may reflect perfusion deficits or renal pathology.

NONINVASIVE MONITORING

Noninvasive monitoring techniques include obtaining intake and output (I & O) measurements, obtaining daily weights, and consulting with the physician regarding existing radiographs. Intake and output measurements and daily weights provide some data regarding the patient's hydration state, but, as mentioned previously, they are not a valid measure of renal function. Of course, for these techniques to be useful, they must be accurate. Chapter 2 describes some frequently occurring errors associated with these simple measurements that the clinician may want to review.

The radiograph is one of the most frequently used techniques for obtaining gross assessment data regarding the renal system. A plain film of the abdomen called a KUB (for kidneys, ureters, and bladder), is obtained for almost every patient before any other invasive techniques. This radiograph provides data regarding the size, shape, position, and possible areas of kidney calcification.

INVASIVE MONITORING

Invasive monitoring of the renal system includes several diagnostic procedures that provide essential information for the clinician. Any and all of the following procedures may be used with patients experiencing renal dysfunction: IV pyelography, computerized axial tomography, nephrosonography, nephrotomography, renal angiography, renal scan, and renal biopsy. Table 18-7 summarizes these diagnostic procedures including their purposes and potential problems.

NURSING DIAGNOSES

The patient with acute or chronic renal failure experiences systemic manifestations that require nursing support to maintain life. The care that is planned and delivered to these patients is based on a comprehensive assessment of all the ramifications of the renal failure for the patient. In general, the care that is provided is based on the nursing diagnoses summarized in Table 18-8. All the nursing diagnoses, except sexual dysfunction, apply equally to patients with acute or chronic renal failure.

MANAGEMENT THERAPIES

The primary therapeutic intervention for patients experiencing acute or chronic renal failure is renal replacement therapy. Aggressive renal replacement therapy is usually instituted early in the disease process for patients with acute renal failure in an attempt to keep the serum creatinine level lower than 10 mg per 100 mL and the BUN lower than 100 mg/dL. The maintenance of serum values at the lower levels provides an internal biochemical environment that is more conducive to preventing many of the complications that usually accompany uremia. In addition, initiating early dialysis also broadens the scope of other therapeutic interventions that can be used with patients with acute renal failure. In chronic renal failure, renal replacement therapies are not instituted until the disease progresses to end-stage level, usually characterized by a urinary creatinine clearance level of less than 5 mL/min.

In addition to renal replacement therapy, the patient will require dietary, pharmacological, and other types of therapeutic support. The specific management therapies that are included in this discussion relate to the alterations in fluid, electrolyte, and acid–base balance.

HYPERVOLEMIA

In the oliguric phase of acute renal failure or the end stage of chronic renal failure, fluids are restricted to an amount sufficient to replace the fluids lost through insensible mechanisms, as well as via the urine. In most instances, the amount is 600 to 1000 mL plus the volume of urine from the previous 24 hours. If the individual experiences unusual amounts of insensible losses due to hyperventilation or pyrexia, the fluid restriction is augmented by an additional amount, often based on changes in body weight.

Individuals in the progressive stages of chronic renal failure before end stage, however, will not have fluid restrictions imposed until their creatinine clearance values and urine volumes decrease to levels that can no longer support the homeostasis of the internal environment. Instead, these patients are encouraged to ingest 2 to 3 L/day of fluid to support the fluid volume necessary for excreting waste products as effectively as possible by the remaining intact nephrons.

TABLE 18–7.
Invasive Diagnostic Procedures for Assessing the Renal System

PROCEDURE	PURPOSE	POTENTIAL PROBLEMS
Intravenous pyelography	To visualize renal parenchyma, calyces, pelves, ureters, and bladder to obtain information regarding size, shape, position, and function of kidneys	Hypersensitivity reaction Acute renal failure Postinjection hematoma
Computerized axial tomography	To visualize renal parenchyma to obtain data regarding size, shape, and presence of lesions, cysts, masses, calculi, obstructions, congenital anomalies, and abnormal accumulations of fluid	Hypersensitivity reactions if a contrast medium is used Postinjection hematoma
Nephrosonography	To visualize renal parenchyma, calyces, pelves, ureters, and bladder to obtain data regarding size, shape, position, and internal structure of kidneys and perirenal tissue; to assess and localize urinary obstructions and abnormal accumulations of fluid	No potential problems currently identified
Nephrotomography	To visualize renal parenchyma, calyces, and pelves in layers to obtain information regarding tumors, cysts, lacerations, or areas of nonperfusion	Hypersensitivity reaction Postinjection hematoma
Renal angiography	To visualize arterial tree, capillaries, and venous drainage of kidneys to obtain data regarding presence of tumors, cysts, stenosis, infarction, aneurysms, hematomas, lacerations, and abscesses	Hypersensitivity reaction Hemorrhage at the catheter insertion site Acute renal failure
Renal scan	To determine renal function by visualizing appearance and disappearance of radioisotopes within kidney; also provides some anatomical information	Hypersensitivity reaction Postinjection hematoma
Renal biopsy	To obtain data for histological diagnosis to determine extent of pathology, appropriate therapy, and possible prognosis	Hemorrhage Postbiopsy hematoma Acute renal failure

HYPERNATREMIA

Patients in the oliguric phase of acute renal failure and in the end-stage level of chronic renal failure have difficulty maintaining sodium balance and require dietary restrictions. The usual restrictions are 500 mg/day in acute renal failure and 1000 to 2000 mg/day in chronic renal failure. In the diuretic phase of acute renal failure and all other phases of chronic renal failure, the sodium intake must be individualized for each patient, usually in accordance with the amount excreted in the urine.

HYPERKALEMIA

Management of hyperkalemia is a primary therapeutic goal for patients with either acute or chronic renal failure. In oliguric acute renal failure and end-stage chronic renal failure, dietary restrictions are necessary. The usual dietary restriction is 40 mEq/day. (In contrast, a healthy adult typically consumes 50–100 mEq of potassium in the diet.) If the patient is severely catabolic,

additional restrictions may be required. Table 18-9 summarizes the various therapeutic approaches, specific methods, and their efficacy in treating hyperkalemia. In general, the approaches that attempt to antagonize the membrane effect of hyperkalemia and shift the potassium intracellularly are used primarily as emergency measures.

When implementing measures to decrease both the total body and serum potassium levels, the clinician should (1) discourage the patient from using salt substitutes that are potassium based, (2) avoid administering pharmacological agents that contain potassium, and (3) avoid administering pharmacological agents that are likely to exacerbate the potassium imbalance. Such pharmacological agents include potassium-sparing diuretics, beta-adrenergic antagonists, and nonsteroidal antiinflammatory agents. In addition, recall the following facts regarding the use of the cation exchange resin, Kayexalate: (1) sodium ions are exchanged for potassium ions in the intestine; thus sodium is reabsorbed and potassium is excreted in the feces; (2) the exchange process is slow and requires

TABLE 18–8.
Summary of Nursing Diagnoses Appropriate for Providing Care for Patients with Renal Failure

NURSING DIAGNOSIS	RELATED TO
Alterations in fluid, electrolyte and acid–base balance	Decreased excretion
	Catabolism
Examples:	Accumulation due to retention
▶ Alteration in potassium balance (hyperkalemia) related to decreased excretion	Intracellular–extracellular shifts
	Extracellular–intracellular shifts
▶ Fluid volume excess related to inability to excrete fluid	Excessive ingestion or administration
▶ Alteration in acid–base balance (metabolic acidosis) related to retention of acid metabolites	Systemic effects of uremic toxins
Alterations in cardiac output	Fluid overload and hypertension
	Electrolyte imbalances
	Uremic toxins
Potential for infection	Uremic toxins
	Catabolism
Alterations in coagulation	Uremic toxins
Alterations in breathing patterns	Metabolic acidosis
	Fluid overload
Alterations in nutrition	Uremic toxins
	Decomposition of urea in the oral cavity and gastrointestinal tract
	Electrolyte imbalances
	Dietary restrictions
Alterations in bowel elimination	Electrolyte imbalances
	Decreased activity
	Fluid restrictions
	Decreased dietary bulk
Impaired physical mobility	Uremic toxins
	Anemia
	Electrolyte imbalances
Risk for injury	Uremic toxins
	Fluid, electrolyte, and acid–base imbalances
Sensory–perceptual alterations	Uremic toxins
	Uremic encephalopathy
	Fluid, electrolyte, and acid–base imbalances
Alterations in thought processes	Uremic toxins
	Uremic encephalopathy
	Fluid, electrolyte, and acid–base imbalances
Risk for impaired skin integrity	Uremic toxins
	Anemia
	Retained urochrome pigment
	Decreased sebaceous and sweat gland secretion
	Calcium–phosphate deposition
	Increased capillary fragility
	Urea or urate crystal deposition
Altered oral mucous membranes	Uremic toxins
	Decomposition of urea in oral cavity
	Hyperosmolality
	Increased capillary fragility
	Fluid restrictions
Sexual dysfunction	Uremic toxins
Knowledge deficit	All facets of renal failure and renal replacement therapies

TABLE 18–9.
Approaches to Treating Hyperkalemia

APPROACH	METHODS	EFFICACY
Reduce the body potassium content	1. Decrease potassium intake	May decrease plasma and total body potassium content over time
	2. Increase fecal excretion of potassium using cation exchange resins such as Kayexelate	Takes several hours to be effective but will eventually decrease both plasma and total body potassium content
	3. Increase renal excretion of potassium by using mineralocorticoid agents, increasing salt intake, or using diuretic agents	Any of these is effective in decreasing both plasma and total body potassium content if the individual has normal renal function
	4. Dialysis	Decreases both plasma and total body potassium content within 4–6 hours
Shift the potassium intracellularly	1. Administer glucose and insulin intravenously	Decreases plasma potassium for about 2 hours but has no effect on total body potassium content
	2. Administer an alkali such as sodium bicarbonate	Decreases plasma potassium for short time but has no effect on total body potassium content
Antagonize the membrane effect	1. Administer calcium salts	Has no effect on either plasma or total body potassium content
	2. Administer hypertonic sodium salts	Has no effect on either plasma or total body potassium content

(*Hartshorn J, Lamborn M, Noll ML: Introduction to Critical Care Nursing. Philadelphia, WB Saunders [in press]; with permission.*)

hours and several repeated administrations to be maximally effective; (3) the exchange resin was designed to be given orally to maximize its contact with the surface area of the GI tract, but because many patients cannot ingest it orally due to nausea and regurgitation, it may be given rectally as a retention enema; (4) when the resin is administered as a retention enema it must be retained at least 20 to 30 minutes to be effective; (5) approximately 1 mEq of potassium is exchanged per gram of resin; and (6) the resin is usually mixed with a sorbitol solution to promote an osmotic diarrhea to facilitate excretory processes and prevent constipation.

HYPERCHLOREMIA

In most patients with renal failure, the chloride imbalance is clinically insignificant. If it is a problem, however, it is usually managed by dietary salt restriction, avoiding the administration of chloride-containing pharmacological agents, and administering exogenous bicarbonate.

HYPOCALCEMIA

Therapeutic management of hypocalcemia that accompanies both acute and chronic renal failure requires a combined approach aimed at replacing the deficient calcium, controlling the excess phosphate, and slowly correcting the acid–base imbalance. The first component of this combined approach will be discussed here and the other components as the specific imbalances are addressed. Usually, pharmacological replacement of 1 to 2 g/day of elemental calcium orally is sufficient to replace the deficit, particularly if it is augmented by the administration of 1,25 dihydroxycholecalciferol. The calcium replacement can take many forms, ranging from calcium carbonate to calcium gluconate or calcium gluceptate.

HYPERPHOSPHATEMIA

Hyperphosphatemia is an imbalance that occurs in patients with either acute or chronic renal failure. It is usually managed by restricting dietary intake and administering pharmacological phosphate-binding agents. The dietary restriction is usually accomplished by limiting the daily phosphate intake to less than 700 mg and the daily protein intake to about 1 g/kg. Unfortunately, the dietary restrictions are often difficult to implement and thus the patient may not achieve the desired reduction in phosphate by using dietary restrictions alone. Consequently, phosphate-binding agents, such as aluminum hydroxide gels or calcium-based antacids, are administered concurrently. These agents, usually administered within 20 minutes of meals, supply cations to the intestinal lumen that bind with the phosphate that is present to form an insoluble complex that is excreted in the feces. Use of these agents frequently results in constipation for the patient, and the aluminum-based binders may produce sufficiently high serum aluminum levels to interfere with bone mineralization.

HYPERMAGNESEMIA

Clinically insignificant elevations of serum magnesium levels are the norm in both acute and chronic renal failure. In most patients, dietary restrictions and avoiding pharmacological agents that contain magnesium are adequate measures to prevent the retention of excessive amounts of magnesium. For patients who do experience clinically significant elevations of serum magnesium levels, dialysis is usually the therapeutic intervention of choice.

METABOLIC ACIDOSIS

The metabolic acidosis that accompanies oliguric acute renal failure usually develops rapidly, is severe, and necessitates early initiation of therapeutic measures. In fact, the daily acid production during catabolic oliguric acute renal failure may decrease the serum bicarbonate level by greater than 15 mEq/L. Thus, replacement therapy is frequently a high therapeutic priority and is usually accomplished by sodium bicarbonate administration. In addition, because the metabolism of ingested exogenous protein will produce approximately 1 mEq/g of nonvolatile acid, dietary protein is usually restricted. Table 18-10 summarizes the general daily dietary restrictions and requirements for patients experiencing renal failure. These amounts are always adjusted upward or downward in accordance with the patient's specific physiological needs.

Patients with end-stage chronic renal failure usually experience approximately a 2 mEq/L/day decrease in serum bicarbonate. Therefore, they also require replacement therapy, often in the form of either sodium bicarbonate or sodium citrate and dietary protein restrictions. In addition, the management of metabolic acidosis in either acute or chronic renal failure also encompasses the following: (1) minimizing all catabolic processes, including infections and GI bleeding; (2) rapidly correcting any diarrhea that occurs; and (3) avoiding catabolic pharmacological agents, such as corticosteroids.

The clinician should monitor the patient frequently for other fluid and electrolyte imbalances that might occur as a result of the therapeutic management of metabolic acidosis. The primary possibilities include hypervolemia, hypernatremia, more clinically significant hypocalcemia, an exaggerated hyperphosphatemia, and transient hypokalemia. With the exception of hypocalcemia, these imbalances are not usually clinically significant in most patients. The patient may, however, require additional IV or oral calcium supplement to manage the tetany and neuromuscular effects of the rapidly induced exaggerated hypocalcemia re-

TABLE 18–10.
Daily Dietary Requirements and Restrictions in Renal Failure

DIETARY COMPONENT*	DAILY AMOUNT IN ACUTE RENAL FAILURE	DAILY AMOUNT IN CHRONIC RENAL FAILURE
Water	400–600 mL plus the urine output	1000 mL or 600 mL plus the urine output
Calories	35–50 kcal/kg	35–50 kcal/kg
Protein	0.5–1.5 g/kg	1–1.2 g/kg
Sodium	500–1000 mg	2 g
Potassium	20–50 mEq	40–60 mEq
Phosphate	700 mg or less	700 mg or less
Calcium	800–1200 mg	1000–1200 mg
Carbohydrate	Unrestricted	Unrestricted
Fats	Variable	Variable

* *Daily water-soluble vitamin supplements are also required in both acute and chronic renal failure.*

sulting from the overcorrection of the metabolic acidosis to an alkalotic state.

Overall, it is clear that the patient who experiences either acute or chronic renal failure is in a very compromised state. Not only does the patient lack the ability to maintain a homeostatic internal environment compatible with life, but he or she also exhibits the clinical effects of the renal failure on all other body systems. Thus many of the normal adaptive mechanisms are also dysfunctional. The result is a patient in jeopardy who must rely on external management therapies to sustain life. Such patients challenge clinicians not only to provide these therapeutic interventions competently and effectively, but also to anticipate and prevent other potential threats. This challenge demands that clinicians use their vast stores of intellectual resources to provide the requisite quality nursing care. It is hoped that this discussion has expanded those intellectual resources and increased the clinician's ability to meet the challenge presented by patients experiencing either acute or chronic renal failure.

BIBLIOGRAPHY

Baer CL: Acute Renal Failure. In Hartshorn J, Lamborn M, and Noll ML: *Introduction to Critical Care.* Orlando, FL, WB Saunders (in press)

Baer CL: Acute renal failure. Nursing 90 20:6: 34–39, 1990

Baer CL: Regulation and assessment of fluid and electrolyte balance. In Kinney MR, Packa DR, Dunbar SB: *AACN's Clinical Reference for Critical Care Nursing,* 2nd ed, pp 193–236, New York: McGraw-Hill, 1988.

Baer, CL: Regulation and assessment of acid–base balance. Ibid, pp 237–248

Bergstrom J: Toxicity of uremia: physiopathology and clinical signs. Contrib Nephrol 71:1–9, 1989

Brenner BM, Coe FL, Rector FC: *Clinical Nephrology.* Philadelphia, WB Saunders, 1987

Brenner BM, Lazarus JM: *Acute Renal Failure.* Philadelphia, WB Saunders, 1983

Drukker W, Parsons FM, Maher JF: Replacement of Renal Function by Dialysis, 2nd ed. Martinus Nijhoff, 1983

Eknoyan G, Knochel JP: *The Systemic Consequences of Renal Failure.* Orlando, FL, Grune & Stratton, 1984

Finn WF: Diagnosis and management of acute tubular necrosis. Med Clin North Am 74:4: 873–891, 1990

Goldstein MS: Acute renal failure. Med Clin North Am 67: 1325–1341, 1983

Harper J: Rhabdomyolysis and myoglobinuric renal failure. Crit Care Nurse 10:3: 32–34, 36, 1990

Lancaster LE: The Patient with End Stage Renal Disease, 2nd ed. New York, John Wiley & Sons, 1985

Lancaster LE, Baer CL: The pathophysiology of acute renal dysfunction. In Schoengrund L, Balzer P (eds): Renal Problems in Critical Care. New York, John Wiley & Sons, pp 21–46, 1985

Maxwell MH, Kleeman CR: Clinical disorders of fluid and electrolyte metabolism, 3rd ed. New York, McGraw-Hill, 1980

Mitch WE, Klahr S: *Nutrition and the Kidney.* Boston, Little, Brown, 1988

Norris MKG: Acute tubular necrosis: preventing complications. Dimens Crit Care Nursing 8:1: 16–26, 1989

Porush JG: New concepts in acute renal failure. Am Fam Physician 33:3: 109–118, 1986

Schoengrund L: Nursing management of the patient with acute renal failure. In Schoengrund L, Balzer P (eds): Renal Problems in Critical Care. New York, John Wiley & Sons, pp 47–67, 1985

Schrier RW: Renal and Electrolyte Disorders, 3rd ed. Boston, Little, Brown, 1986

Stein J: Nephrology. New York, Grune & Stratton, 1980

Strupp TW: Post shock resuscitation of the trauma victim: preventing and managing acute renal failure. Crit Care Nurs Quart 11:2: 1–9, 1988

Swartz RD: Fluid, electrolyte, and acid–base changes during renal failure. In Kokko J, Tannen R: Fluids and Electrolytes, 2nd ed. Philadelphia, WB Saunders, 1990

Whittaker AA: Acute renal dysfunction: assessment of patient at risk. Focus Crit Care 12:3: 12–17, 1985

Wilkins RG, Faragher EB: Acute renal failure in an intensive care unit: incidence, prediction, and outcome. Anaesthesia 7: 628–624, 1983

Wills MR: Effects of renal failure. Clin Biochem 23: 55–60, 1990

Wolfson M: Nutritional support in acute renal failure. Dial Transplant 16: 493, 496, 1987

19

Heart Failure

DEFINITION

Heart failure refers to an inability of the heart to pump enough blood to meet the metabolic needs of tissues throughout the body. Common causes of heart failure (often referred to as congestive heart failure) include hypertension, myocardial infarction, cardiomyopathies, and valvular disease.

Left-ventricular failure, as seen in hypertensive heart disease or mitral stenosis, typically presents with pulmonary but not peripheral edema. In contrast, pure right-ventricular failure initially seen in patients with cor pulmonale typically presents with edema in the lower extremities and perhaps ascites. Failure of one ventricle often leads to failure of the other, so that both types of failure are present. Patients with cardiomyopathies tend to have simultaneous failure of both ventricles, presenting with both pulmonary and peripheral edema. Heart failure can be chronic or become acutely manifested in the form of pulmonary edema or cardiogenic shock.

PATHOPHYSIOLOGICAL MECHANISMS AFFECTING FLUID BALANCE

The patient with heart failure presents with the classic picture of an expanded extracellular fluid volume (ECF), that is, swollen legs, engorged neck veins, congested liver, and pulmonary crackles. Although the ECF is increased, the kidneys respond as if a reduced blood volume were present. This paradoxical renal response is postulated to be due to a decreased "effective" blood volume.[1] It has been suggested that the fluid retentive responses are initiated by a reduced "fullness" of the arterial vascular system.[2] Theoretically, decreased cardiac output reduces the effective blood volume. Another factor affecting the fullness of this compartment is peripheral vascular resistance.[3]

Responses to circulatory failure include stimulation of the sympathetic nervous system, activation of the renin–angiotensin–aldosterone mechanism, and stimulation of hormones such as arginine vasopressin (antidiuretic hormone [ADH]) and atrial natriuretic peptide. Although these responses are initially adaptive, some may later become the source of additional problems.

STIMULATION OF SYMPATHETIC NERVOUS SYSTEM

Stimulation of the sympathetic nervous system increases heart rate and contractility, which in turn increases cardiac output (Fig. 19-1). Blood is preferentially shunted to the brain and heart (away from the skin, skeletal muscles, abdominal organs, and kidneys). This shunting increases arteriovenous oxygen extraction, which can become so severe that the cells shift to anaerobic metabolism (leading to metabolic [lactic] acidosis).

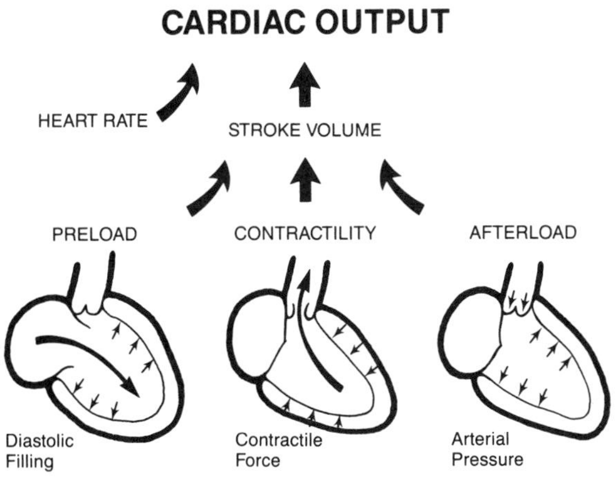

CARDIAC OUTPUT

FIGURE 19–1.
Factors determining cardiac output.

RENIN–ANGIOTENSIN–ALDOSTERONE MECHANISM

A second powerful mechanism active in heart failure is the renin–angiotensin–aldosterone mechanism. Shunting of blood away from the kidneys stimulates secretion of renin, which acts on angiotensinogen to produce angiotensin I which is subsequently converted to angiotensin II. Angiotensin II is a strong arterial vasoconstrictor that helps to support arterial blood pressure when cardiac output falls. This arterial vasoconstriction increases the work of the left ventricle as it pumps against the increased pressure (increased afterload). Angiotensin II also stimulates the secretion of aldosterone, which strongly promotes the reabsorption of sodium in the distal tubules and collecting ducts of the kidney. Another effect is venous vasoconstriction, which tends to increase venous return to the heart (increased preload).

OTHER HORMONES

In heart failure there is an increased secretion of ADH, also known as arginine vasopressin. Antidiuretic hormone acts on the distal tubules to cause water retention, which can lead to an increased preload as well as hyponatremia. Remember that, although there is a total excess of sodium and water (due to aldosterone effect), the added water retention produced by ADH can cause dilutional hyponatremia. Thus, the patient has a fluid volume excess with a relatively greater retention of water than sodium (see Fig. 4-2A). Another harmful effect of ADH is its vasoconstrictive property, which can increase the left ventricle's workload and oxygen need. Atrial natriuretic peptide is a hormone stimulated by atrial distention. It produces the positive effects of increased renal sodium excretion and inhibition of aldosterone, renin, and ADH production.

ASSESSMENT

Knowledge of the pathophysiological mechanisms associated with the usual signs and symptoms of heart failure, especially those affecting fluid and electrolyte balance, contributes to effective management of this complex situation (Tables 19-1 and 19-2). The following discussion of assessment of patients with heart failure includes both noninvasive and invasive measures.

NONINVASIVE MONITORING

Left ventricular failure is associated with decreased cardiac output, which leads to symptoms of weakness

TABLE 19–1.
Fluid and Electrolyte Disturbances Associated with Congestive Heart Failure

FLUID AND ELECTROLYTE DISTURBANCE	ETIOLOGY
Fluid volume excess	Secondary hyperaldosteronism (result of decreased renal blood flow associated with decreased cardiac output)
	Excessive aldosterone causes sodium and water retention
Low serum sodium level (hyponatremia)	Although total body sodium content is above normal, excessive secretion of ADH causes relatively greater retention of water, diluting the serum level (see Fig. 4-2A)
	Contributing to hyponatremia can be the movement of extracellular sodium into the cells to replace the potassium so frequently lost in treatment of heart failure
	Contributing to hyponatremia is loss of sodium in, for example, vomiting, diarrhea, and paracentesis; most hazardous if patient is on severely restricted sodium diet and large doses of diuretics
Potassium deficit	Excessive aldosterone levels predispose to potassium excretion
	Excessive use of potassium-losing diuretics and prolonged loss of potassium by vomiting or diarrhea represent typical causes of potassium deficit
Metabolic alkalosis if potassium-losing diuretics are used	Potassium-losing diuretics (particularly the thiazides) cause a greater excretion of chloride than of sodium ions; loss of chloride causes a compensatory increase in bicarbonate ions, hence alkalosis
Metabolic (lactic) acidosis	Slowing of circulation interferes with the excretion of metabolic acids
	Increased liberation of lactic acid from anoxic tissues and failure of body to metabolize it rapidly
Respiratory acidosis	Pulmonary congestion interferes with elimination of CO_2 from lungs
Shift of intravascular fluid into interstitium (edema)	Hydrostatic pressure is increased by excessive venous blood volume

ADH, antidiuretic hormone.

and fatigue as tissue oxygenation is impaired. Dyspnea is also commonly present, at first experienced only with exercise. As heart failure worsens, dyspnea shows up with progressively less exercise and finally even on rest. Other pulmonary symptoms associated with left ventricular failure include orthopnea, paroxysmal nocturnal dyspnea, dry cough, and fine moist crackles in the lungs. Patients may also demonstrate expiratory wheezing and Cheyne-Stokes respirations. Severe left ventricular failure results in acute pulmonary edema, a potentially life-threatening condition characterized by severe dyspnea and profound anxiety.

Physical signs associated with left ventricular failure may include third and fourth heart sounds, sinus tachycardia, or any dysrhythmia. The point of maximal impulse is shifted to the left when cardiomegaly occurs. Patients may also demonstrate pulsus alternans.

Right-sided heart failure is associated with jugular vein distention and hepatojugular reflux, which reflect increased venous pressure. The degree of jugular vein distention provides important data regarding fluid volume status and cardiac function; of importance, it can be performed noninvasively (see Fig. 2-8).

Dependent pitting edema (see Fig. 2-6) reflects excessive fluid in the interstitial space and is a major indication in right-sided heart failure. As such, the degree of peripheral edema should be assessed at regular intervals. This can be accomplished by measuring the extremities with a millimeter tape (Fig. 2-7). The patient should be taught to monitor for fluid retention by noting, for example, tight shoes or tight clothing as the day progresses.

Weight gain usually occurs with heart failure because of abnormal retention of sodium and water. Early in the therapeutic period, a baseline body weight should be obtained to compare with subsequent weight measurements to monitor response to treatment. For accuracy, it is best to use the same scale and perform the procedure at the same time each day. Any change in daily weight of more than 0.25 kg (0.5 lb) can be

TABLE 19–2.
Signs and Symptoms of Congestive Heart Failure and Their Causes

SYMPTOM OR SIGN	CAUSE
Fatigue with little exertion or at rest, confusion, headache	Tissue anoxia due to decreased cardiac output
Dyspnea on exertion, later at rest	Cardiac output inadequate to provide for increased oxygen required by exertion (results in increased breathing effort)
PND in left-sided heart failure	When recumbent, edema fluid from the dependent parts returns to the bloodstream, increasing preload and causing decompensation
Cough; sputum may at times be brownish or blood-tinged	Pulmonary capillary pressure greater than 30 mmHg causes transudation of serum with hemosiderin-filled macrophages into the alveoli, which causes
Adventitious lung sounds	pulmonary congestion and diminished oxygen–carbon dioxide exchange
Tachycardia, various dysrhythmias	Effort to compensate for decreased cardiac output; arrthythmias may be stimulated by hypoxia, digitalis toxicity, hypokalemia, or hypomagnesemia
Presence of third/fourth heart sounds	Associated with rapid ventricular/atrial filling in noncompliant ventricles/atria
Cardiomegaly	Hypertrophy of myocardium helps to maintain stroke volume
Decreased urinary output	Decreased cardiac output and renal blood flow
	Sodium and water retention caused by excess aldosterone level
	Increased water retention caused by excess antidiuretic hormone (ADH) secretion
Nocturia	While resting at night, deficit in cardiac output in relation to oxygen demands is reduced, leading to decreased renal vasoconstriction and increased glomerular filtration rate (GFR)
Elevated pulmonary capillary wedge pressure or left ventricular end-diastolic pressure	Left ventricle cannot maintain stroke volume in face of increased venous return
Edema (initially in dependent parts, later generalized)	Hydrostatic pressure is greatest in dependent parts of body
	Progressive cardiac failure causes substantial increase in hydrostatic pressure in all parts of body
Distention of peripheral veins, most noticeable on face, neck, and hands	Elevated venous pressure secondary to cardiac failure
Elevated CVP (greater than 11 cm H_2O in vena cava)	
Palpable liver, positive hepatojugular reflux	Decreased cardiac output causes damming of venous blood
	Increase in total blood volume and interstitial fluid volume
Nausea and vomiting	Edema of liver and intestines
	Impulses arising from the dilated myocardium in acute heart failure
	Digitalis toxicity
Anorexia	Potassium deficit
	Digitalis toxicity
Constipation	Poor nourishment and inadequate bulk in diet
	Lack of activity
	Depression of motor activity by hypoxia
Orthopnea	Increased interstitial edema decreasing lung compliance and increasing work of breathing; upright position fosters air exchange in upper lungs
Cyanosis, particularly of lips and nail beds	Inadequate oxygenation of blood
Pulmonary edema with severe dyspnea, profound anxiety, coughing of pink frothy fluid, cyanosis, shock, and death	Increased pulmonary venous pressure, which cause serum and blood cells to transudate into the alveoli

PND, paroxysmal nocturnal dyspnea; CVP, central venous pressure.

assumed to have resulted from alterations in total body fluid and can be used to monitor therapy with diuretics and other medications to improve cardiac performance. The patient can be taught to monitor daily weight changes at home.

An important measurement during hospitalization is daily fluid intake and output (I&O). With diuretic administration, urinary output is expected to increase significantly. This increase should parallel the decrease in body weight. Discrepancies in these findings are an indication to check for errors in measurement.

INVASIVE HEMODYNAMIC MONITORING

Hemodynamic monitoring by means of multilumen flow-directed catheters has made it possible to assess pressures directly within the heart chambers and great vessels and to monitor cardiac output. Measurements can be made of arterial pressure, central venous pressure (CVP), right atrial pressure (RAP), pulmonary artery pressure (PAP), pulmonary capillary wedge pressure (PCWP), and cardiac output (CO). The obtained pressure measurements provide information concerning the fluid volume status of both sides of the heart. Several other hemodynamic indices can be derived from these measurements (eg, stroke volume index, right and left ventricular stroke work, and systemic and pulmonary vascular resistance). All these findings are used to monitor the patient's initial status and response to therapy.

In the patient experiencing heart failure, CVP and RAP are used to monitor the intravascular volume status. These measurements will decrease during periods of hypovolemia (which may occur with overdiuresis) and will increase with hypervolemia, increased venous return, and when right-sided failure worsens.

As indicators of the left ventricle's status in the absence of mitral valve disease, chronic obstructive pulmonary disease, or pulmonary hypertension, PAP and PCWP are more sensitive than the CVP or RAP. The pulmonary artery end-diastolic pressure (PAEDP) and the PCWP reflect the left ventricular end-diastolic pressure (LVEDP). Left ventricular end-diastolic pressure represents the left ventricular filling pressure (preload), which is one of the determinants of stroke volume. An increase in PAEDP or PCWP is due to the diminished ability of the left ventricle to empty its contents. Symptoms of pulmonary congestion occur when the PAEDP or PCWP exceeds 18 mmHg. This is the usual situation in pulmonary edema. Cardiac output is another hemodynamic measurement that can be obtained with flow-directed catheters. Decrease in cardiac output can indicate the degree of failure and help determine needed therapy to increase the heart's contractility.

NURSING DIAGNOSES

Table 19-3 presents three nursing diagnoses that occur with high frequency in patients experiencing acute or chronic heart failure. Also included is information needed for assessment, intervention, and evaluation.

INTERVENTIONS

Because the nurse works closely with physicians in the management of fluid balance problems in heart failure patients, the principles of treatment are presented with collaborative actions as a focus.

When possible, therapy is directed at eliminating the disease condition producing heart failure (eg, surgical correction of a valvular disorder). When this is not possible, therapy must focus on making the most efficient use of remaining cardiac function. Unfortunately, most persons with congestive heart failure have irreversible cardiac damage. There is some evidence, however, that relief of pressure or volume overload (preload and afterload) may lessen or even reverse the decline in contractility; thus, this is an important therapeutic objective.[4]

DECREASING MYOCARDIAL WORKLOAD

Rest causes a reduction in oxygen need and thus decreases cardiac workload. It also produces a physiological diuresis. Sometimes rest alone is sufficient to alleviate the symptoms of congestive heart failure because it diminishes the discrepancy between the heart's ability to pump blood and the tissue oxygenation needs. The amount of rest required varies with the person and may range from complete bedrest to only slight restriction of activity.

The patient should be helped to identify an appropriate level of activity that is as nondisruptive to the usual lifestyle as possible. Even somewhat strenuous activities may be tolerated if they are done slowly and are accompanied with frequent rest periods.

Another important nursing responsibility involves monitoring the patient's response to exercise, including changes in pulse and respiratory rate. An increase in heart rate greater than 10% over the baseline indicates that an activity may exceed the capacity of the failing heart to respond. Careful reporting of these observations helps to determine the desired amount of activity and aids in evaluation of the therapeutic regime.

Other interventions to ensure decreased myocardial workload include relief of pain and reduction of fever, if present. Also, patients with heart failure often receive oxygen therapy to maintain a PaO_2 of at least 80 mmHg.

This reduces hypoxia and the work of breathing. Positioning the patient in a semi-Fowler's position facilitates ventilation by allowing full chest expansion and diaphragmatic excursion. The upright position may also decrease venous return by sequestering blood in the dependent areas.

DECREASING VENOUS RETURN

Venous return is one of the most important determinants of ventricular preload. As preload is increased, so is peripheral edema and pulmonary congestion.

Dietary Sodium Restriction

Restriction of dietary sodium is a valuable aid in the management of heart failure (see Chapter 3). In general, the fewer sodium ions are in the body, the less water is retained. The degree of sodium restriction necessary to control edema varies with the severity of heart failure. The dietary sodium intake often can be cut in half by avoiding added salt at the table and in cooking and foods with a high salt content (see Chapter 3). Often, limitation of sodium intake to 2 g daily, in conjunction with diuretic therapy, is sufficient to control congestive symptoms while maintaining a reasonably palatable diet.[5] A stricter diet limited to only 0.5 to 1 g of sodium may be required; if so, the patient will need help to achieve the knowledge and motivation necessary to adhere to the recommended diet.

The degree of sodium restriction necessary to control edema also varies with the degree of rest, dosage, and type of diuretic. For example, an ambulatory patient requires a more severe sodium restriction than a patient at bedrest because rest in itself encourages diuresis. A patient receiving potent diuretics has less need for severe sodium restriction than one not receiving diuretics. Indeed, drastic restriction of sodium intake can be dangerous in the patient receiving a potent diuretic, particularly during bouts of abnormal sodium loss, such as occurs with vomiting or diarrhea.

Diuretics

Diuretics are a valuable aid in the symptomatic treatment of heart failure. Their primary purpose is to promote the excretion of sodium and water from the body, thus lowering intravascular volume. If hemodynamic monitoring is being used, it may be noted that diuretics produce a decrease in LVEDP (preload) and move the heart's function to a more favorable portion of the Starling curve (Fig. 19-2). This effect decreases pulmonary and systemic congestion and also decreases the degree of backward failure. These effects, in turn, will tend to decrease myocardial need for oxygen. Another advantage of certain diuretics, eg, furosemide, is an increase in venous capacitance with decreased venous return. At times, it is necessary to administer diuretics by the intravenous (IV) route to achieve a posi-

(text continues on page 270)

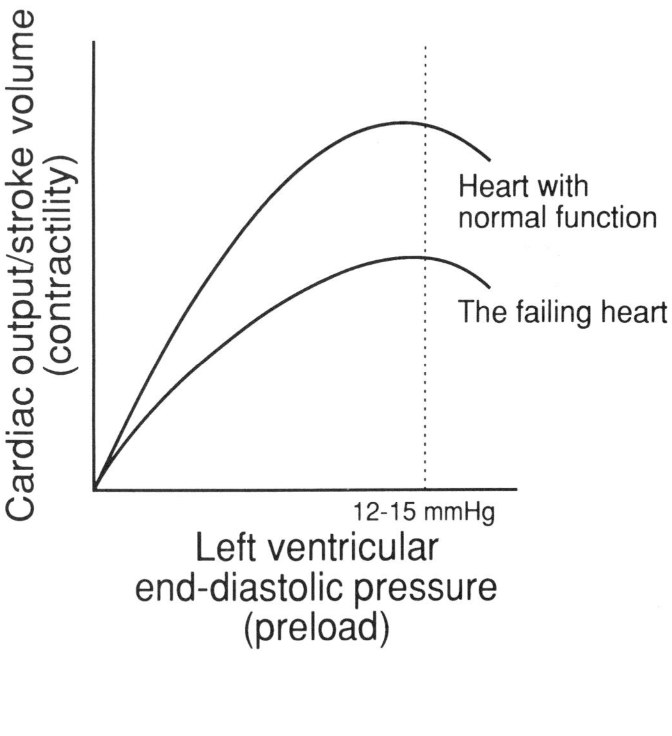

FIGURE 19–2.
The Starling mechanism in normal heart function and heart failure.

TABLE 19–3.
Examples of Nursing Process in Care of Patients with Heart Failure

NURSING DIAGNOSIS	ASSESSMENT	INTERVENTIONS	EXPECTED OUTCOMES
Fluid volume excess related to compromised regulatory mechanisms (cardiac failure) *Pathophysiology:* Decreased GFR; kidneys respond by retaining sodium and water (under the influence of aldosterone and ADH)	Weight gain Peripheral edema Intake greater than output Decreased urinary volume, increased urinary specific gravity Peripheral venous distention Paroxysmal nocturnal dyspnea Increased CVP, PCWP, LVEDP Abnormal breath sounds (crackles) Orthopnea and dyspnea Tachypnea Frothy sputum Hepatomegaly	Assess for fluid volume excess: ▲ Measure I & O; look for I > O ▲ Weigh daily (same scale, same amount of clothing, and same time each day) ▲ Assess lung fields for crackles (compare to baseline) ▲ Monitor changes in vital signs (compare to baseline) Instruct in dietary restrictions (sodium restriction favors diuresis) Restrict fluids as prescribed (may be necessary in patients with severe heart disease to decrease ECF volume) Monitor response to diuretics: ▲ Weight should decline no faster than 1 kg/day (2.2 lb) with diuretic administration ▲ Look for inadequate response to diuretics ▲ Look for excessive response to diuretics (such as weight loss exceeding 2.2 lb/day and BUN elevated out of proportion to serum creatinine) Instruct patient to weigh self daily and report significant weight variations to health care provider Encourage rest periods in which patient lies down (rest, particularly in supine position, favors diuresis) Promote calm environment to decrease sympathetic nervous system stimulation (again, rest favors diuresis) Place in Fowler's position (reduced upward pressure on diaphragm, facilitating ease of breathing) Measures for management of acute pulmonary edema are described in text	Urine output will increase Weight will decrease to baseline as diuresis occurs Peripheral edema will lessen Peripheral venous distention will lessen Crackles will be absent or diminished Sputum production will diminish Dyspnea and tachypnea will diminish Liver size will diminish Patient and significant other will verbalize understanding of sodium-restricted diet Patient will demonstrate ability to weigh self and will verbalize significant variations requiring reporting to health care provider

Nursing Diagnosis	Assessment Data	Nursing Interventions	Expected Outcomes
Activity intolerance related to decreased cardiac reserve *Pathophysiology:* Decreased contractility and increased preload leads to decreased cardiac output and tissue hypoxia	Heart rate increased greater than 10% over baseline with activity Heart rate remains increased 2 minutes after exercise Increased LVEDP	Provide bedrest during acute phase of failure (reduces metabolic requirements and, thus, myocardial workload) Encourage patient to sit in chair when tolerated (pooling of blood in legs decreases venous return and thus preload) Encourage rest 1 hour after meals (since digestion increases metabolic requirements, tolerance to activity is diminished at this time) Monitor response to increases in activity; encourage rest when heart rate increases significantly over baseline and when heart rate remains elevated for longer than 2 minutes after exercise Promote emotional rest (decreases workload of heart by decreasing sympathetic nervous system stimulation) Instruct patient and significant other in prescribed activity regimen Institute measures to maintain normal body temperature, such as avoiding extremes in environmental temperature and prevention of fever (decrease tissue metabolic needs and thus the myocardial workload)	Heart rate will not increase greater than 10% above baseline with allowed activity Heart rate will return to baseline within 2 minutes after allowed activity Patient or significant other will verbalize understanding of balance between rest and activity
Impaired gas exchange related to pulmonary congestion *Pathophysiology:* Decreased cardiac output, increased preload, transudation of fluid into alveoli	Dyspnea, orthopnea, PND Crackles Cough Cyanosis $PaO_2 < 80$ mmHg $PaCO_2 > 45$ mmHg pH < 7.35 ↑ LVEDP ↑ PCWP Alveolar congestion (radiograph)	Elevate head of bed (facilitates ventilation by allowing full chest expansion, draining uppermost alveoli) Tracheal suctioning (removes secretions and thus increases alveolar surface area for gas exchange) Lower feet (decreases venous return and thus preload) Implement medical regimen as appropriate: ▲ Bronchodilators (increases airway diameter) ▲ Oxygen (maintains PaO_2 at greater than 80 mmHg to reduce hypoxia and work of breathing)	Absence or diminishing of dyspnea, crackles $PaO_2 > 80$ mmHg $PaCO_2 < 45$ mmHg pH $\geq$ 7.35 (important to correct acidemia since it predisposes to decreased myocardial contractility) Hemodynamic parameters within normal limits

ADH, antidiuretic hormone; CVP, central venous pressure; BUN, blood urea nitrogen; ECF, extracellular fluid; GFR, glomerular filtration rate; LVEDP, left ventricular end diastolic pressure; I & O, intake and output; PCWP, pulmonary capillary wedge pressure; PND, paroxysmal nocturnal dyspnea.

tive therapeutic result. Remember that gastrointestinal (GI) absorption may be impaired when right-sided heart failure is accompanied by congestion of the abdominal organs.

Because thiazides (eg, hydrochlorothiazide) and loop diuretics (furosemide, bumetanide, and ethacrynic acid) predispose to hypokalemia, potassium supplementation is often needed. A potassium-sparing diuretic (eg, spironolactone) may also be indicated, particularly since secondary hyperaldosteronism often plays a significant role in advanced heart failure. (Recall that spironolactone is an aldosterone-blocking agent.) It should be remembered that angiotensin-converting enzyme inhibitors (such as captopril) cause potassium retention and should not be given simultaneously with potassium-retaining diuretics nor with potassium supplements.

As discussed above, possible side effects of diuretics are disturbances in potassium balance. For example, thiazides and loop diuretics promote renal potassium loss whereas spironolactone, amiloride, and dyrenium promote potassium retention. Acid–base disturbances usually accompany disruptions in potassium balance (metabolic alkalosis with hypokalemia, and metabolic acidosis with hyperkalemia.) Excessive reduction in the intravascular volume caused by too vigorous diuresis may actually worsen heart failure by diminishing the preload stimulus to cardiac contractility. As cardiac output decreases, so does renal blood flow and glomerular filtration rate (GFR), resulting in prerenal azotemia and increased blood urea nitrogen (BUN).

In intractible heart failure, the kidney is unable to respond to the usual diuretics. Treatment may then consist of a combination involving more severe sodium restriction, more potent diuretics in higher dosage, and fluid restriction to 1000 mL/day.

Priority nursing responsibilities in the care of patients with heart failure include keeping an accurate account of fluid I&O and daily weight measurements. Data obtained from these measurements, in addition to revealing changes in edema accumulation, are invaluable in regulating diuretic dosage and dietary sodium restriction.

Fluid Restriction

Fluid restriction may be indicated in patients with intractible heart failure to minimize fluid volume overload. It may also be necessary to alleviate the hyponatremia that is common in patients with heart failure due to excessive ADH secretion. Consequences of severe hyponatremia are primarily neurological in nature (see Chapter 4). Contributing to hyponatremia in some patients is the tendency of sodium to shift from the ECF

into the cells to replace the potassium loss associated with hyperaldosteronism and use of potassium-losing diuretics. Water intake is usually not restricted in the long-term management of heart failure unless there is dilution of the serum sodium (<130 mEq/L) by excessive water retention.

Although fluid restriction may be indicated at times, the patient should not be allowed to become volume depleted. As described above, volume depletion further impairs cardiac output by decreasing the preload's stimulus on cardiac contractility. It is desirable to use hemodynamic monitoring to guide fluid replacement therapy in seriously ill heart failure patients. Frequent checks of venous pressure and pulmonary wedge pressure during fluid administration can give early warning of circulatory overload or underload and guide the safe administration of needed water and electrolytes. Fluid should be given until the LVEDP rises no higher than 15 mmHg. This level assures maximum cardiac output while preventing pulmonary edema caused by increased preload. The patient at home must understand the precise fluid regimen best suited for his or her condition, and situations that can complicate this regimen (such as increased fluid loss in vomiting and diarrhea).

Monitoring volume, speed, and composition of IV fluids given to congestive heart failure patients is important. Oral fluids should also be carefully monitored in those requiring fluid restriction; the patient's cooperation in this endeavor should be sought. As is the case with most patients, an ongoing assessment of response to fluid intake must occur, and alterations made as indicated in the treatment plan.

Venous Vasodilators

Two of the major venous vasodilator drugs used in congestive heart failure are nitroglycerin and isosorbide dinitrate. These medications reduce venous tone and thereby increase venous pooling. This effect reduces venous return and preload, which places the heart on a more favorable point on the Frank Starling curve because less blood is left in the ventricle after contraction. As a result, there is decreased pulmonary congestion and dyspnea. Vasodilators are now considered one of the first-line medications to treat congestive heart failure because of their positive effect on exercise tolerance and their ability to prolong life.

INCREASING MYOCARDIAL CONTRACTILITY

Administration of positive inotropic agents (medications that increase the strength of cardiac contractility) affects one factor contributing to stroke volume and, therefore, to cardiac output.

Digitalis

The most commonly used inotropic agent is digitalis. This medication increases the force and velocity of myocardial contraction. As the heart contracts more forcefully, tissue perfusion increases and the compensatory responses caused by hypoxia decrease, allowing a corresponding improvement in renal function with diuresis. Digitalis increases the intracellular calcium concentration by inhibiting the Na-K-ATPase pump, resulting in increased intracellular sodium, which then exchanges with calcium.

The role of digitalis in heart failure has been evaluated.[6] It was found that digitalis is effective in treating patients with heart failure complicated by atrial fibrillation with a rapid ventricular response. It is now recommended that therapy, in the absence of atrial fibrillation, not begin until the patient is experiencing a dilated heart, reduced ejection fraction, and a third heart sound. Administration of digitalis preparations before this time is not associated with increased survival potential.

When digitalis preparations are used, be alert for toxic symptoms, such as aversion to food, nausea and vomiting, blurred or distorted vision, confusion, and dysrhythmias. Increased myocardial automaticity may reflect alterations in transmembrane concentrations of sodium, potassium, and calcium. Conduction disturbances can occur secondary to changes in the refractory period.

Remember that symptoms of digitalis toxicity may be induced by hypokalemia, hypomagnesemia, hyponatremia, or hypercalcemia because these imbalances sensitize the heart to digitalis. Hypokalemia occurs frequently in patients with heart failure because of the simultaneous administration of potassium-losing diuretics. Often, a potassium supplement (see Chapter 5) or potassium-sparing diuretics will be used to prevent hypokalemia in a digitalized patient. Potassium replacement is often the initial therapy of choice for ectopic rhythms associated with digitalis toxicity. The serum potassium level should be maintained in the high normal range.[7] If potassium administration does not correct the arrhythmia, hypomagnesemia should be suspected.

Other Positive Inotropic Agents

Dopamine, a precursor of norepinephrine, as well as norepinephrine itself, may be used to increase myocardial contractility. Their usefulness is limited by the other natural effect of catecholamines, which is peripheral arteriolar constriction. This constriction increases afterload and thereby increases the workload of the heart.

Dobutamine is a synthetic catecholamine that increases myocardial contractility while limiting the side effects of tachycardia and elevation of arterial blood pressure. There is also a reduced left ventricular filling pressure and decrease in heart size. Dopamine may be given simultaneously with dobutamine to cause renal artery vasodilation and increased renal blood flow, and to promote sodium and water excretion.

Amrinone is one of a new class of positive inotropic agents that work through a mechanism different from that of digitalis or the catecholamines. These medications inhibit phosphodiesterase type III, which increases the level of cyclic AMP. In turn, this enhances calcium entry into the myocardium and peripheral smooth muscle cells. The effect is an increase in cardiac output and reduced left ventricular filling pressure without tachycardia or increased arterial pressure. There is also an arteriolar vasodilation that decreases afterload and, therefore, the workload of the heart.

DECREASING AFTERLOAD

Afterload refers to the pressure against which the ventricle must work to achieve blood flow during systole. In heart failure, even in the presence of normal arterial blood pressure, there is a relative worsening of the relationship between contractility and afterload that causes an even greater workload and oxygen need. To reduce the resistance against which the heart must work and to increase cardiac output, arterial vasodilators are one of the first-line medications used in the treatment of heart failure.

Hydralazine is one of the most effective arterial vasodilators. It works by increasing cardiac output while reducing systemic vascular resistance (afterload). Minoxidil is another potent arterial vasodilator. Hydralazine and isosorbide dinitrate can be given simultaneously to affect both preload and afterload; this combination results in better exercise tolerance and prolonged survival. If hydralazine or minoxidil cause fluid retention, the diuretic dose may be increased.

The angiotensin-converting enzyme (ACE) inhibitors are also arterial vasodilators. Three medications belonging to this class are captopril, enalapril, and lisinopril. These agents achieve their positive effects by inhibiting the converting enzyme responsible for the formation of angiotensin II. This illustrates the principle that one of the most powerful mechanisms associated with heart failure is the inappropriate response of the renin–angiotensin–aldosterone system. Administration of ACE inhibitors results in reduced blood pressure, systemic vascular resistance, and left and right atrial pressures. Because of their pressure-lowering effects, these agents may reduce irreversible myocardial hypertrophy (if given early in the treatment of heart failure).[8] Among these agents' other benefits are increase in cardiac output, a gradually occurring, improved exercise tolerance, and prolonged survival. Because aldosterone is inhibited, there is retention of potassium and magnesium (supplements of these electrolytes, therefore, should not be given). Blood pressure must be monitored when therapy is initiated because the patient may experience hypotension due to the effect of the drug. This hypotensive effect is heightened by the concurrent presence of a low intravascular volume (as occurs with too vigorous use of diuretics).

The calcium channel blockers (nifedipine, verapamil, and diltiazem) are not indicated for the routine treatment of systolic heart failure but may be helpful in the less frequent diastolic failure, eg, dilated cardiomyopathy. These agents inhibit the influx of extracellular calcium during muscular contraction, producing arterial vasodilation and decreased afterload. They may also improve myocardial relaxation during diastole, thus allowing more complete filling when diastolic compliance is impaired.[9]

TREATMENT OF PULMONARY EDEMA

Pumonary edema is an emergency situation. To deal with it, the patient should be quickly placed in a high-Fowler's position to reduce venous pressure and preload. This position facilitates fluid gravitation to the pleural bases so that less dependent areas of the lung are better ventilated and the work of breathing is decreased. Humidified oxygen is best delivered by a face mask. In extreme cases, endotracheal intubation and mechanical ventilation may be needed. Positive end-expiratory pressure (PEEP) may be used but should be done with caution because excessive increase in intrathoracic pressure compromises cardiac output.

Intravenous administration of morphine sulfate may be used to achieve multiple effects:

1. Reducing preload through peripheral venous dilation, and thereby decreasing venous return to the heart
2. Reducing afterload by decreasing arterial blood pressure
3. Reducing anxiety (and thereby decreasing sympathetic nervous system stimulation)

Diuretics may be given by intravenous push (IVP) to promote a rapid diuresis and, thus, decreased preload and pulmonary congestion. A vasodilator such as nitroglycerin may be given IV or sublingually to decrease preload. However, remember that an excessive drop in preload may abolish the stimulus for contrac-

tility caused by myocardial stretching. To monitor the patient's response and allow early detection of complications, measure arterial pressure, cardiac output, and LVEDP at regular intervals. An inotropic agent such as digitalis may be given IV. Digitalis is most effective if the patient is experiencing a supraventricular tachycardia.

Patients with acute pulmonary edema may develop severe acid–base problems (respiratory acidosis and metabolic [lactic] acidosis). Reversal of the pulmonary edema is usually effective in restoring acid–base balance by improving gas exchange and allowing metabolism of excess lactate into bicarbonate. Alkali therapy should be used only for refractory and severe metabolic acidosis ($pH < 7.00-7.10$).[10]

TREATMENT OF CARDIOGENIC SHOCK

Cardiogenic shock develops when the cardiac output is insufficient to meet the metabolic demands of the body due to either an absolute decrease in cardiac output or a severe increase in metabolic demands. Acute myocardial infarction is the most common cause.

Cardiogenic shock is characterized by left ventricular failure, low cardiac output, arterial hypotension, and peripheral vasoconstriction. Most often the patient will have a systolic blood pressure less than 90 mmHg. When the mean arterial pressure falls below 75 to 85 mmHg, there is danger that coronary blood flow will be inadequate, leading to further damage to the myocardium. A urinary output less than 20 mL/hr is also common, reflecting decreased glomerular filtration rate. Mental status is impaired due to cerebral hypoxia. Poor skin perfusion secondary to peripheral vasoconstriction can cause cold, clammy skin.

Treatment of cardiogenic shock depends on the underlying cause. One basic problem that many patients will encounter is cellular hypoxia related to decreased cardiac output. Oxygen may be given by a high-flow system such as a Venturi mask or endotracheal intubation. Atelectasis and retention of carbon dioxide must be prevented by initiating measures to mobilize secretions and then suctioning the patient as often as necessary. The goal of these interventions is to prevent or minimize acidosis, and to maintain a PaO_2 greater than 80 mmHg. When acidosis is pronounced ($pH < 7.2$), myocardial contractility is reduced.

Inotropic agents such as dopamine, dobutamine, norepinephrine, or amrinone may be given to strengthen contractility, maintain adequate blood pressure, and redistribute blood flow to the vital organs. Arterial vasodilators, such as nitroprusside, may be given to decrease afterload in the presence of severe, persistent vasoconstriction.

Intravenous fluids should be given to correct hypovolemia, if present. However, fluids must be given cautiously to prevent overload and pulmonary congestion. Maintaining PCWP at 15 mmHg ensures adequate left ventricular filling.

An intraaortic balloon pump (IABP) may be used in the presence of severe cardiac injury when recovery is still possible. In this procedure, a catheter with a balloon is placed in the aorta. The pump is set so that the balloon inflates during ventricular diastole and deflates during systole. This cycle provides better coronary artery and systemic perfusion with no increase in peripheral resistance to left ventricular output.

ELECTROLYTES IN CARDIAC RESUSCITATION

Sodium Bicarbonate

Recommendations and practice concerning pharmacological management of cardiopulmonary resuscitation (CPR) suggest a cautious use of sodium bicarbonate to manage acidosis. Sodium bicarbonate can cause hyperosmolarity, hypernatremia, or metabolic alkalosis with resultant hypokalemia and hypocalcemia. The oxyhemoglobin curve may be shifted to the left so that there is a decreased release of oxygen to already hypoxic tissues. Also, concomitant administration of catecholamines and bicarbonate may result in inactivation of the catecholamines.

Arterial *p*H is now believed to remain above 7.20 for 12 minutes with basic life support.[11] Venous *p*H, however, is markedly lower because anaerobic cellular metabolism produces carbon dioxide, which is not circulated to the lungs for excretion. Therefore, mixed venous blood most accurately reflects the acid–base state during CPR. Venous acidosis results in an intracellular hypercarbia and acidosis which is particularly deleterious to cardiac and cerebral function. Administration of sodium bicarbonate releases carbon dioxide, which can rapidly enter cells and aggravate the already existing hypercarbia.

Adequate ventilation and perfusion are now advocated as the best ways to prevent or treat acidosis early in cardiac arrest. If the arrest is prolonged, (ie, > 10 minutes) and definitive treatment has been initiated, or if severe acidosis existed before the arrest, sodium bicarbonate may be given to raise the arterial *p*H to 7.20. When used, 1 mEq/kg should be given initially, with no more than half this dose given every 10 minutes thereafter.[12]

Carbicarb is a mixture of sodium carbonate and sodium bicarbonate that has been shown to buffer excess hydrogen ions in laboratory animals without increasing the venous level of carbon dioxide.[13] However, any IV administered buffer may not reach the ischemic area because of marked reduction in coronary perfusion and contractility.[14]

Potassium

Extracellular potassium levels are often elevated during CPR. The energy-dependent sodium–potassium pump is impaired by cellular ischemia. This allows potassium to leak out of the cells, and extracellular levels to rise.[15] One result of this can be myocardial electromechanical dissociation (EMD). When hyperkalemia is the cause, calcium chloride may be used if the QRS complexes are greater than 0.12 seconds. Remember that calcium enhances the toxicity of digitalis and should not be given IV to the digitalized patient.

Magnesium

Magnesium infusions can be given to correct selected life-threatening arrhythmias, especially torsade de pointes or dysrhythmias refractory to other agents. It can also be given prophylactically to patients with a myocardial infarction and hypomagnesemia. Magnesium ions are involved in keeping intracellular potassium, calcium, and phosphorus levels constant (which may explain the effectiveness of magnesium in reversing dysrhythmias).

REFERENCES

1. Kokko J, Tannen R: Fluids and Electrolytes, 2nd ed, p 93. Philadelphia, WB Saunders, 1990
2. Schrier R: Pathogenesis of sodium and water retention in high-output and low-output cardiac failure, nephrotic syndrome, cirrhosis, and pregnancy. N Engl J Med 319:1065, 1988
3. Kokko, Tannen, p 93
4. Parmley W: Pathophysiology and current therapy of congestive heart failure. J Am Coll Cardio 13:771, 1989
5. Dunagan W, Ridner M: Manual of Medical Therapeutics, 26th ed, p 115. Boston, Little, Brown, 1989
6. Spann J, Hurst J: The recognition and management of heart failure. In: Hurst J (ed): The Heart, Arteries and Veins, 7th ed. New York, McGraw-Hill, 1990
7. Dunagan, Ridner, p. 119
8. Sonnenblick E, LeJemtel T: Pathophysiology of congestive heart failure: Role of angiotensin-converting enzyme inhibitors. Am J Med 87(suppl 6B):88S, 1989
9. Shub C: Heart failure and abnormal ventricular func-

tion: Pathophysiology and clinical correlation (Part 2). Chest 96:906, 1989

10. Rose B: Clinical Physiology of Acid–Base and Electrolyte Disorders, 3rd ed, p 438. New York, McGraw-Hill, 1989

11. Jaffe A: New and old paradoxes: Acidosis and cardiopulmonary resuscitation. Circulation 80:1079, 1989

12. Standards and guidelines for cardiopulmonary re-suscitation (CPR) and emergency cardiac care. JAMA 255:2942, 1986

13. Bersin R, Arieff A: Improved hemodynamic function during hypoxia with carbicarb, a new agent for the management of acidosis. Circulation 77:277, 1988

14. Jaffe, p 1081

15. Martin et al: Hyperkalemia during human cardiopulmonary resuscitation: Incidence and ramifications. J Emerg Med 7:109, 1989

Fluid Balance in the Head-Injured Patient

Approximately 120,000 severe head injuries occur annually. About 50% of such patients reach the hospital alive; of this number, 25% have irreversible damage.[1] The remaining 75% have some degree of reversible damage and require sophisticated management, part of which involves fluid and electrolyte imbalances. This chapter discusses nursing management of these disorders, especially as they relate to increased intracranial pressure (ICP) and disruptions in antidiuretic hormone (ADH) release.

PATHOPHYSIOLOGY

CEREBRAL EDEMA

Brain swelling in the early posttraumatic period results primarily from vascular engorgement due to impaired autoregulation; brain swelling that occurs 24 to 48 hours after impact is due to cerebral edema.[2] By definition, cerebral edema is an increase in brain volume caused by an increase in brain water.[3] In addition to being associated with trauma, cerebral edema is commonly associated with a wide variety of cerebral disorders such as tumor growths, infections, and toxic, anoxic, and metabolic conditions. In turn, cerebral edema commonly coexists with elevated ICP. Most head-injured patients suffer from increased ICP; failure to prevent this problem is the most frequent cause of death in hospitalized head-injured victims.[4]

Classification

Cerebral edema can be classified into three different forms: (1) vasogenic, (2) cytotoxic (or cellular), and (3) interstitial.[5] It is helpful to briefly review the features of these types of brain edema because therapeutic interventions for them can vary.

Vasogenic Edema

The most common form of brain edema is vasogenic edema; it is associated with conditions such as brain tumor growths, abscess, hemorrhage, infarction, and contusion.[6] In this type of edema, the extracellular fluid (ECF) volume is increased with an elevation in plasma protein.[7] There is increased capillary permeability and a predilection for white matter. It is believed that white matter offers less resistance to the bulk flow than does gray matter.[8]

Cytotoxic (Cellular) Edema

In this type of edema, all the cellular elements of the brain (neurons, glia, and endothelial cells) may swell, with a consequent reduction in the brain's ECF space.[9] Most commonly associated with this form of edema are acute hypoosmolality (hyponatremia) and cerebral hypoxia (such as occurs after cardiac arrest or asphyxia). Cellular swelling is related to failure of the ATP-dependent sodium pump within the cells, which causes sodium to accumulate rapidly within the cell and water to follow to maintain osmotic equilibrium.[10]

Current in vitro research suggests that free radicals (polyunsaturated fatty acids and excitatory amino acids) may induce brain cellular edema associated with ischemia and hyperosmolar states by inhibiting (Na^+ + K^+) − ATPase activity.[11] The role played by biochemical substances is under investigation.

Patients with chronic hyponatremia do not suffer cerebral swelling (because the brain cells have had time to adapt by losing intracellular osmoles, chiefly potassium). In this form of edema, both gray and white matter are affected.[12]

Interstitial Edema

As the name implies, interstitial edema is characterized by an increase in the portion of the ECF surrounding the cells. It is related to blockage of cerebro-spinal fluid absorption, most commonly by obstructive hydrocephalus.

Disruption in Pressure and Volume Equilibrium

Cerebral edema represents a disruption in the pressure and volume equilibrium within the intracranial compartments. These compartments, encased in the rigid cranial vault, contain brain, blood, and cerebrospinal fluid (CSF). The pressure is maintained by approximately 85% brain volume, 5% to 6% blood volume, and 9% to 10% CSF volume. When one compartment increases in volume, there must be a reciprocal compensatory change in one or both of the other components to maintain a constant total pressure. The brain can accommodate minimal changes by a compensatory shunting of CSF into the spinal dural sac, an increased CSF absorption, or a decreased cerebral blood volume. When the total volume of brain mass, blood, or spinal fluid exceeds the compensatory capacity, intracranial pressure rises. Once ICP is raised in a particular region of the brain as a result of a pathological process, brain displacement with the threat of herniation occurs.

CENTRAL DIABETES INSIPIDUS

As discussed in Chapter 4, diabetes insipidus is a disorder of water metabolism characterized by polyuria and polydipsia due to either insufficient production of ADH (central diabetes insipidus [CDI]), or renal unresponsiveness to ADH (nephrogenic diabetes insipidus).

Head trauma is a very frequent cause of CDI, and is usually related to a transient swelling of the brain (including the hypothalamus). This, in turn, temporarily prevents the release of ADH, thereby causing CDI. As the cerebral edema subsides, there is usually complete restoration of neurohypophyseal function. However, at times the diabetes insipidus may be permanent.

SYNDROME OF INAPPROPRIATE ANTIDIURETIC HORMONE SECRETION

As discussed in Chapter 4, a variety of central nervous system disorders may produce Syndrome of Inappropriate Antidiuretic Hormone Secretion (SIADH). Among these are head injury, subarachnoid hemorrhage, encephalitis, meningitis, and brain tumors. The exact mechanisms by which SIADH is produced are unknown; presumably, relatively excessive vasopressin (ADH) is released from the neurohypophysis.[13] In any event, when hyponatremia occurs in a patient with head injury, despite adequate salt administration, it is believed to be due to excessive ADH secretion with resultant water retention.[14] By itself, SIADH can cause cerebral edema due to cellular swelling (cytotoxic edema). This, with the cerebral edema produced by trauma, compounds the patient's problems. For the most part, SIADH is self-limiting and subsides as the brain tissue heals; however, it can last for weeks or even months.

ASSESSMENT

ELEVATED INTRACRANIAL PRESSURE

The most reliable data for assessing ICP are obtained through continuous ICP monitoring. Normal ICP is a mean pressure up to 12 mmHg. Readings between 12 and 19 mmHg are suspicious, and those of 20 mmHg or higher are definitely elevated.[15]

Several techniques exist for ICP monitoring. These include intraventricular catheters, subarachnoid screws, subdural catheters, and the newer fiberoptic transducers. Most neurosurgical centers use continuous ICP monitoring in all severely head-injured patients to detect deterioration and guide therapy. Direct monitoring is most valuable when used in conjunction with clinical assessment.

The classical signs and symptoms of elevated ICP include papilledema, headache, and vomiting. Unfortunately, these symptoms do not become evident until relatively late. Therefore, monitor for earlier changes by assessing the neurological status and vital signs. Without direct monitoring, clinical assessment becomes the primary method by which changes in ICP are determined. Baseline assessment should be performed and compared with data obtained from subsequent assessments for early recognition of significant changes. These include changes in the level of consciousness, motor and sensory function, pupil size and reactivity, vital signs, and other signs.

Deterioration in the Level of Consciousness

This is often the first sign of deterioration in the patient's condition because an increase in the ICP results in decreased cerebral oxygenation. The cells most sensitive to a reduction in oxygen supply are those of the cerebral cortex involved with higher intellectual functions, including thinking processes such as memory and orientation. Changes in wakefulness should also be noted.[16]

Loss of Motor and Sensory Function

As the ICP rises, motor and sensory functions are compromised. Motor loss progresses from hemiparesis to hemiplegia on the side of the body that is opposite the cerebral lesion. As the increase in ICP continues, the patient becomes progressively less responsive to light

and deep touch and painful sensations. As the condition further deteriorates, decortication or decerebration may be observed either spontaneously or in response to painful stimuli.

Pupillary changes

Change in pupil size usually occurs on the same side as the lesion (or pressure increase) and progresses from constriction to dilatation. The response to direct light in this pupil progresses from sluggish to nonreactive. With continued deterioration, the patient reaches the terminal stage of pupils bilaterally nonreactive to light stimuli. The pupillary changes are all related to compression of the third (oculomotor) cranial nerve.

Alterations in Vital Signs

During the compensatory phase of increased ICP there is an increase in systemic blood pressure with a widening pulse pressure. These alterations result from ischemia of the vasomotor center of the brain. As the patient's condition continues to deteriorate and the decompensatory phase begins, the blood pressure drops.

During the compensatory phase, the pulse drops to less than 60. On palpation, the pulse is full and bounding. This change in rate and quality is related to an attempt by the heart to pump blood into vessels with increased resistance as a result of the increased ICP. During the decompensatory phase, the pulse rate becomes rapid and irregular, and the quality becomes thready.

Abnormalities in respiratory patterns vary according to the level of brain dysfunction. Cheyne–Stokes respiration is often the first irregular breathing pattern observed, although as brain dysfunction progresses, other abnormal breathing patterns become apparent.[17] Increased ICP can also result in acute neurogenic pulmonary edema, which further contributes to alterations in the respiratory pattern.[18]

During the compensatory phase of increased ICP, the temperature usually remains within normal limits. In the decompensatory phase, however, it rises very high as a result of hypothalamic dysfunction.

Papilledema

Usually by the time papilledema occurs, the ICP has reached markedly elevated levels. The aforementioned signs and symptoms, therefore, are more reliable indicators of the beginning stages of increased ICP.

Headache

Although not always present with increased ICP, headache represents pressure against those intracranial structures that are sensitive to pain. These structures include the middle meningeal arteries and branches, the large arteries at the base of the brain, the venous sinuses, and the dura at the base of the skull. When headache is present in the patient with increased ICP, it typically is worse on arising in the morning.

Vomiting

Vomiting is not always present with increased ICP. When it occurs, it is characteristically projectile in nature and indicates pressure against the vomiting center in the medulla.

CENTRAL DIABETES INSIPIDUS

As described in Chapter 4, CDI is manifested by abrupt onset of polyuria and polydipsia. The usual urine volume is 8 to 10 L/day.[19] Conscious patients usually exhibit extreme thirst and will drink large volumes of fluid if able. For unknown reasons, there may be a preference for iced drinks. Because of the sustained polyuria, sleep deprivation can be a problem. Failure to consume fluid adequate to match the large urine volume will produce profound volume depletion. Because the unconscious patient cannot experience thirst, or respond to it, there is great need to replace fluids by the parenteral route, titrated according to urine output and laboratory results. Classic laboratory findings include hypernatremia and slight serum hyperosmolality. Urine specific gravity is usually less than 1.005 and urine osmolality less than 200 mOsm/kg.

It should be noted that CDI may be triphasic in critically ill patients. That is, it may occur transiently for a few days after surgery or trauma and then resolve for a few days, only to recur.[20] Therefore, one should closely monitor urine output and laboratory values, such as serum sodium and osmolality, and urine specific gravity or osmolality.

The reader is referred to Table 4-10 for a summary of clinical manifestations of diabetes insipidus and to Table 4-11 for a summary of assessments for this condition.

SYNDROME OF INAPPROPRIATE ANTIDIURETIC HORMONE SECRETION

The reader is referred to Table 4-4 for a summary of clinical manifestations and laboratory findings in SIADH, and to Table 4-6 for a summary of nursing assessment for this condition.

NURSING DIAGNOSES RELATED TO FLUID BALANCE

See Table 20-1 for a list of possible nursing diagnoses related to fluid and electrolyte problems in patients with head injuries. Interventions related to these nursing diagnoses are discussed below.

INTERVENTIONS

ELEVATED INTRACRANIAL PRESSURE

Management of the patient with elevated ICP is complex, evolving, and to some extent controversial. Nursing and medicine are both modifying protocols based on new research findings. However, basic to all interventions is on-going neurological assessment. Depending on the patient's condition, the neurological and vital signs must be assessed every 15 minutes to every 4 hours. The assessment should include mental status, level of consciousness, motor and sensory function, pupillary size, reaction to light, and eye movements. Results of each examination should be compared with those of previous assessments; significant changes should be promptly reported. Early subtle signs must be identified and acted on immediately because these signs can herald a change from a compensatory neurological status to one of irreversible decompensation.

In addition to continuing assessments, nursing interventions must be performed to meet the patient's basic needs. Nursing interventions for patients with elevated ICP have been the subject of much nursing research and have, in some cases, produced conflicting results. Some interventions have been shown to increase ICP (Table 20-2). Activities that increase ICP should not be clustered together due to their cumulative effects.[21] In addition, efforts should be directed toward nursing interventions that prevent or minimize increased ICP (Table 20-3).

Standard therapeutic interventions that continue to be used in the management of increased ICP include hyperventilation, osmotic diuretics, fluid restriction, temperature control, and ventricular drainage.

Maintenance of Adequate Ventilation

If respiratory insufficiency is present as a result of cerebral trauma, elevated levels of carbon dioxide (hypercapnia) and decreased levels of oxygen (hypoxemia) would be expected. Both hypercapnia and hypoxemia are potent vasodilating factors and thus contribute to increased ICP. Although hypercapnia and hypoxemia often occur together, hypercapnia alone will stimulate vasodilation.

TABLE 20–1.
Examples of Nursing Diagnoses Related to Fluid Balance in the Head-Injured Patient

NURSING DIAGNOSIS	ETIOLOGICAL FACTORS	DEFINING CHARACTERISTICS
Alteration in cerebral perfusion related to cerebral edema	Interruption of cerebral venous and arterial blood flow	Decreased cognitive functioning, decreased level of consciousness
Hypervolemia related to early use of osmotic diuretic	Osmotic diuretic pulls fluid from cellular and interstitial spaces into bloodstream	Moist crackles
	Decreased renal function (interferes with ability to excrete excess fluid)	Urine volume below level designated by physician (usually should be at least 30–50 mL/hr)
Alteration in sodium balance (hyponatremia) related to early use of mannitol, SIADH, or abnormal water gain or sodium loss	Diffusion of water into bloodstream caused by early use of mannitol dilutes the serum Na^+ level	Serum $Na^+ < 135$ mEq/L
	Excessive secretion of ADH	Serum osmolality < 280 mOsm/kg
	Excessive administration of freewater in tube feedings or parenterally as D_5W	ICP may increase because acute hyponatremia favors cellular swelling
		Neurological symptoms may worsen
Alteration in sodium balance (hypernatremia) with FVD related to prolonged use of osmotic diuretics or to diabetes insipidus	Osmotic diuretics (most often mannitol) cause a relatively greater loss of water than sodium (prolonged use can lead to an excess of sodium in the bloodstream)	Serum $Na^+ > 145$ mEq/L
		Serum osmolality > 300 mOsm/kg
	Deficiency of ADH leads to large renal water losses, causing serum Na^+ concentration to elevate	Signs of FVD
Alteration in potassium balance (hypokalemia) related to use of osmotic and loop diuretics	Both osmotic and loop diuretics increase urinary K^+ losses	Serum $K^+ < 3.5$ mEq/L
		Weakness, fatigue, decreased bowel motility, arrhythmias
Potential for greater increase in ICP related to ineffective breathing	Respiratory insufficiency (due to cerebral edema)	$PaO_2 < 70$ mmHg
	Obstruction of airway with mucus	$PaCO_2 > 30$ mmHg
		Decreased rate and depth of respirations
		Signs of increased ICP
Sensory–perceptual alteration (visual, auditory, gustatory, kinesthetic, tactile, olfactory) related to cerebral edema	Altered sensory perception, transmission, or integration	Disorientation, altered conceptualization, reported or measured changes in sensory acuity, changes in behavior pattern

ADH, antidiuretic hormone; FVD, fluid volume deficit; ICP, intracranial pressure; SIADH, syndrome of inappropriate antidiuretic hormone secretion.

TABLE 20–2.
Nursing Activities That May Increase Intracranial Pressure [23–25]

- ▶ Suctioning the patient frequently (particularly when rotating the head to reach the mainstem bronchi)
- ▶ Turning the patient frequently
- ▶ Discussing the patient's condition or prognosis at the bedside*
- ▶ Placing the patient on the bedpan
- ▶ Rotating the patient's head
- ▶ Rapidly shifting the patient's position
- ▶ Range of motion exercises
- ▶ Applying noxious stimuli during nursing assessment

* A recent study by Johnson et al[26] indicated that neither an emotionally referenced conversation about the patient's condition nor any type of conversation significantly increased intracranial pressure over baseline.

TABLE 20–3.
Interventions to Minimize Increased Intracranial Pressure

- Elevate the head of the bed to a 30° angle.
- Keep the patient's head in a neutral position; avoid neck flexion and extension.
- Use a turn sheet to move the patient.
- Encourage the patient to exhale while turning or pushing self up in bed.
- Minimize noxious stimuli; use medications as indicated.
- Prevent constipation (straining for stools elevates ICP).
- Maintain a patent airway.
- Use intermittent brief suctioning if necessary (remember, hypoxemia predisposes to vasodilation and increased ICP). Mild manual hyperventilation before respiratory care helps mitigate the harmful effects of endotracheal suctioning, as does sedation.
- Maintain a quiet environment (noise can precipitate elevated ICP in the patient with an unstable ICP).
- Administer fluids cautiously to avoid accidental fluid overload.
- Monitor blood gases. Be alert for changes in PaO_2 and $PaCO_2$; be aware that the PaO_2 should be maintained at a suitable level (such as > 70 mmHg) and the $PaCO_2$ should not be allowed to elevate above normal. (Indeed, the prescribed regimen frequently calls for decreasing it to below normal levels, such as 25–30 mmHg when ICP is elevated.)
- Monitor ICP readings and neurological signs. Implement prescribed medical regimen as appropriate.
- Monitor serum electrolytes and osmolality. Be particularly alert for hyponatremia since this condition tends to favor cerebral edema by promoting cellular swelling.
- Monitor temperature; administer antipyretics when appropriate.
- Use gentle tactile stimulation.[27]
- Use gentle auditory stimulation, calling the patient by name.[28]

ICP, intracranial pressure.

Because of the harmful effect of inadequate ventilation on ICP, it is important to maintain ventilation. Rate and quality of respirations should be assessed, and breath sounds should be auscultated at regular intervals. Interference with breathing related to complete or partial obstruction of the airway by mucus can be alleviated by periodic suctioning. The drainage of secretions pooled in the mouth can be facilitated by turning the patient from side to side at least every 2 hours. Regardless of clinical assessment, one must ultimately rely on arterial blood gas analyses to adequately assess ventilation. Findings from blood gas studies are crucial in planning measures to minimize increases in ICP. Some authorities recommend that the PaO_2 be maintained at least at 70 mmHg (by intubation if necessary).[22] The $PaCO_2$ is often purposely lowered below

normal as both a short- and long-term therapeutic measure for increased ICP.

Hyperventilation

Lowering the arterial carbon dioxide level by inducing hyperventilation results in cerebral vasoconstriction and, therefore, prompt lowering of ICP. Clinical studies indicate an acute reduction in arterial $PaCO_2$ of 5 to 10 torr lowers ICP 25% to 50% in most patients.[29] The inability to lower ICP by hyperventilation is a grave prognostic indicator identifying a patient with a massive area of damaged brain.[30]

Usually the $PaCO_2$ is maintained at a level of 25 to 30 mmHg.[31] This level is adequate to maintain cerebral blood flow. The net result is a reduction of intracranial volume with a subsequent decrease in ICP. Care should be taken to avoid dropping the $PaCO_2$ below 20 mmHg because, at that low level, severe vasoconstriction and decreased cerebral blood flow occur. Secondary brain ischemia due to severe vasoconstriction has been observed.[32] It is believed ischemia causes vasodilatation, which, in turn, offsets the effects of further hyperventilation.[33]

Before administering high concentrations of oxygen during the hyperventilation process, the respiratory system should be assessed for lung pathology, and, if present, specific guidelines for oxygen therapy must be provided by the physician.

Osmotic Agents and Other Diuretics

If elevating the head of the bed and hyperventilating the patient are ineffective, it may be necessary to administer osmotic diuretics (such as mannitol) or loop diuretics (such as furosemide). In patients with vasogenic cerebral edema, osmotic diuretics reduce cerebral volume by pulling fluid out of normal brain tissue into the bloodstream for subsequent excretion by the kidneys. Osmotherapy also reduces brain volume in patients with hypoosmolality but is rarely useful in interstitial edema.[34] Furosemide has a diuretic effect on the renal tubules and possibly reduces CSF formation.[35] Used in combination, mannitol and furosemide seem to have a synergistic effect in controlling elevated ICP.[36]

The primary osmotic diuretic is mannitol (Osmitrol). Mannitol has been shown to reduce ICP consistently and increase cerebral perfusion pressure within 10 to 20 minutes or less in head-injured patients with increased ICP.[37] Dosage varies and is calculated according to body weight. Before administering the drug, check the vital signs, urinary output, and body weight, and review the chart for serum electrolytes and renal-function studies. Cardiac status should also be evaluated.

Hemodynamic Monitoring

Soon after administration of mannitol, the intravascular volume is expanded as fluid is pulled into the bloodstream from the tissues. Because of the potential for pulmonary edema, some authorities favor monitoring CVP, and even pulmonary wedge pressures, in patients with questionable cardiovascular function.

Assessment of Hydration

The status of hydration should be monitored closely. Measurement of fluid intake and output (I&O) is mandatory; frequency should be designated by the physician (such as every 15–30 minutes, or hourly). To facilitate accurate measurements, an indwelling urinary catheter is usually used for adults, and a pediatric collection device for children. At times it may be helpful to measure the urinary specific gravity to assess renal function and hydrational status. Vital signs should be monitored every 30 minutes or as ordered. The rate of infusion is usually adjusted to maintain a urine flow of at least 30 to 50 mL/hr.[38] A volume less than this amount (or an amount designated by the physician) should prompt discontinuance of mannitol to prevent fluid overload and fulminant congestive heart failure. (Recall that the kidneys must be able to excrete the fluid being pulled into the bloodstream.) Serum creatinine and blood urea nitrogen (BUN) levels should be monitored to evaluate renal function and hydration status. (Osmotic diuretics are contraindicated in patients with significant renal disease because these individuals cannot effectively eliminate the excess fluid volume.) Variations in body weight should be monitored to detect excessive fluid retention or loss; an accurate in-bed scale is most useful. The serum osmolality should be measured at regular intervals. It should not exceed 320 mOsm/kg because higher levels cause intracellular dehydration with resultant renal failure and systemic acidosis.[39]

Assessment of Electrolyte Levels

Measurement of electrolytes, primarily sodium and potassium, is of vital importance in monitoring response to mannitol therapy. Be alert for imbalances in sodium and potassium and report their occurrence immediately. With mannitol use, there is initially an expansion of the plasma volume caused by diffusion of water into the bloodstream; therefore, hyponatremia is a possible complication. Later, as the fluid is excreted through the kidneys, hypernatremia may be observed (since relatively more water is excreted than sodium).[40] Because the serum sodium level can be either decreased or increased in mannitol therapy, measured serum levels should be observed closely and abnormalities reported at once. Similarly, serum potassium levels may be variable. Hyperkalemia can occur when potassium levels build up in the bloodstream during presence of oliguria; conversely, hypokalemia can result when potassium is eliminated during the osmotic diuresis. See Chapters 4 and 5 for descriptions of sodium and potassium imbalances.

A potential problem associated with mannitol use (and other osmotic diuretics) is a rebound increase in ICP.[41] The rebound may result from retention of mannitol in the brain tissue as the blood mannitol level is dropping; this situation reverses the pressure gradient and allows water to diffuse back into the brain tissue, increasing ICP.

Corticosteroids

Steroids are used frequently to manage elevated ICP. They are believed to be beneficial in vasogenic edema (as seen in brain tumor and abscess) but are not effective in cytotoxic edema (as in acute hyponatremia or hypoxia) and are of uncertain effectiveness in interstitial edema.[42] The most common corticosteroid given for control of increased ICP is dexamethasone (Decadron). When dexamethasone is administered, be alert for complications such as hyperglycemia, gastrointestinal (GI) bleeding, and increased incidence of infection. It is customary to monitor blood glucose levels during massive steroid therapy. Antacids are usually administered to patients receiving large doses of steroids, and H_2-receptor antagonists may be used to decrease gastric acidity.

High-Dosage Barbiturate Therapy

In recent years, barbiturates (most commonly pentobarbitol) have been used to manage elevated ICP, primarily in patients who have not responded to more conventional methods. Barbiturates induce significant decrease in cerebral blood flow and cerebral metabolism.[43] The subsequent effect is a lowering of cerebral blood volume and ICP. It is not known if the effects are sustained and if the eventual outcome is altered. With barbiturate therapy, continuous monitoring of ICP, arterial and preferably pulmonary capillary wedge pressures, and cardiac output is indicated.[44]

A major risk of barbiturate therapy is acute hypotension. This can profoundly affect the patient with a compromised myocardium. Hypothermia may also develop; however, core body temperature should not be allowed to drop below 34° C (93.2° F) because of the risk of cardiac instability.[45]

Certain components of neurological assessment (such as level of consciousness and ability to follow commands) are, of course, negated by barbiturate therapy. However, pupillary dilatation as a result of brain stem compression will still occur at serum barbiturate levels of up to 3 or 4 mg%.[46] After achievement of a satisfactory ICP (<20 mmHg for 24–48 hours), gradual reduction of the barbiturate can begin.[47]

Fluid Restriction

In some patients, restriction of fluids from a half to two thirds of maintenance needs is all that is required to control ICP. Fluid type, as well as fluid volume, selected is important. Most clinicians avoid the administration of free water (such as D_5W) in patients at risk for cerebral edema because a lowered serum sodium predisposes to this condition. Instead, half-strength normal saline (0.45% sodium chloride) is considered a suitable fluid.[48] For patients who are hyponatremic, or likely to become that way, the physician may consider the use of 5% dextrose in normal saline (or its equivalent).[49] In those patients who require osmotic or other diuretic therapy, liberalization of isoosmotic fluid intake to prevent dehydration is appropriate,[50] based on the following clinical parameters. These factors must be considered in determining fluid needs of patients at risk for cerebral edema:

▶ It is generally agreed that the desired amount of fluid to be administered should be based on the patient's serum osmolality, BUN, and electrolyte levels. Remember that the neurological patient is at risk for sodium imbalances in either direction.
▶ Of course, in the traumatized patient, fluid therapy must also provide for abnormal losses (such as occur from gastric suction or are due to other injuries, such as abdominal bleeding or third-space fluid shifts related to major fractures). Always remember that the head-injured patient frequently has marked extremity fractures and thoracoabdominal injuries; such injuries predispose to severe hypovolemia.
▶ Failure to maintain an adequate vascular volume interferes with cerebral perfusion pressure (CPP). Recall that CPP equals mean arterial pressure (MAP) minus intracranial pressure (ICP). [CPP = MAP − ICP]. Thus, a low MAP associated with hypovolemia has serious implications for the cerebral perfusion pressure. Ideally, CPP should be maintained within a range of 60 to 70 mmHg.[51]
▶ Care must be taken not to restrict fluids excessively in patients receiving dehydrating agents (such as osmotic or loop diuretics).

Obviously, the amount of fluid to be administered to patients at risk for cerebral edema and elevated ICP requires careful consideration. Physician's orders should be specific and the patient's response to the fluids carefully monitored. Significant findings should be quickly communicated to the physician for necessary modifications in the fluid directives.

Temperature Control

Any elevation in body temperature must be controlled because this will increase the brain's need for oxygen, thereby increasing cerebral blood flow (and, in turn, ICP). Elevated temperature can be treated with antipyretic medications used alone or in conjunction with a cooling blanket.

Ventricular Drainage

In an attempt to control erratic increases in the ICP, a ventriculostomy may be performed in some patients. This involves the insertion of a drainage catheter into a cerebral ventricle for the purpose of draining off excess cerebrospinal fluid. Because of the continual threat of infection, ventriculostomy patients are frequently given prophylactic antibiotics. Nursing responsibilities in caring for a patient with ventricular drainage include

▶ Promoting absolute sterility of the equipment
▶ Maintaining a sterile dry dressing at the catheter and incision site
▶ Keeping the collection container adjusted to a level indicated by the physician
▶ Observing the drainage system for kinks to assure patency of the tube
▶ Observing and recording the amount of drainage in the collection container

CENTRAL DIABETES INSIPIDUS

Patients with large urinary losses from CDI need water replacement. It may be given by mouth if the patient is conscious. If not, it may be given by the parenteral route in the form of 5% dextrose in water or half-normal saline, depending on the patient's volume status and degree of water deficit.[52] To avoid producing cerebral edema, only half of the water deficit plus insensible water loss should be replaced in the first 24 hours; the rest of the deficit can be replaced over the next 24 to 48 hours.[53] Frequent assessment of neurological status is indicated to look for cerebral edema, a complication that can result from accumulation of intracellular solute during dehydration.[54] In addition to water, magnesium and potassium may be needed to replace losses of these electrolytes in the urine.

Acute diabetes insipidus after surgery or trauma may be treated with short-acting aqueous Pitressin. After a period, the treatment may be temporarily discontinued to determine if the diabetes insipidus is transient or permanent.

With administration of ADH substances, it is conceivable that the patient may become fluid overloaded if fluid intake (intravenous and oral) exceeds fluid output. Fluid overload may also result if third-space fluid from other injuries shifts back into the vascular space at the time ADH is being administered. Excessive water retention may cause the serum sodium level to drop below normal. Close assessment of neurological signs and laboratory data are required to maintain the delicate balance required with ADH replacement therapy in the patient with CDI.

SYNDROME OF INAPPROPRIATE ANTIDIURETIC HORMONE SECRETION

As is the case with all causes of SIADH, restriction of electrolyte-free water intake is indicated.[55] Adequate free-water restriction will eventually increase the serum sodium concentration. In nonedematous patients in some situations, extra salt may be given in the diet or in the form of salt tablets in combination with mild fluid restriction.[56] However, if severe symptoms are present, it may be necessary to cautiously infuse a hypertonic saline solution (such as 3% of 5% NaCl). As discussed in Chapter 4, these solutions are extremely dangerous and should be handled with care. Hypertonic saline should be administered only in intensive care units under close observation. They are best administered in 100-mL containers to avoid an inadvertent excessive dosage. The reader is referred to Table 4-5 for additional information regarding nursing considerations in administering hypertonic saline, and to Table 4-7 for a list of nursing interventions related to SIADH therapy.

REFERENCES

1. Shoemaker et al: Textbook of Critical Care, 2nd ed, p 1238. Philadelphia, WB Saunders, 1989
2. Ibid
3. Marshall et al: Neuroscience Critical Care: Pathophysiology and Patient Management, p 152. Philadelphia, WB Saunders, 1990
4. Shoemaker et al, p 1238
5. Schmidley S: Cerebrospinal fluid, blood brain barrier and brain edema. In: Pearlman A, Collins R (eds): Neurological Pathophysiology, 3rd ed, p 337. New York, Oxford Press, 1984
6. Ibid, p 340
7. Ibid
8. Ibid, p 341
9. Ibid, p 337–338
10. Ibid, p 340
11. Ibid
12. Ibid, p 338
13. Kokko J, Tannen R: Fluids and Electrolytes, 2nd ed, p 169. Philadelphia, WB Saunders, 1990
14. Maxwell M, Kleeman C, Narins R: Clinical Disorders of Fluid and Electrolyte Metabolism, 4th ed, p 922. New York, McGraw-Hill, 1987
15. Shoemaker et al, p 292
16. Rudy E: Advanced Neurological and Neurosurgical Nursing, p 129. St. Louis, CV Mosby, 1984
17. Ibid, p 127–129
18. Marshall et al, p 400
19. Kokko, Tannen, p 833
20. Shoemaker et al, p 748
21. Parsons C, Smith A, Page M: The effects of hygiene interventions on the cerebrovascular status of severe closed head injured patients. Res Nurs Health 8:178, 1985
22. Marshall et al, p 193
23. Mitchell P, Mauss N: Relationship of patient–nurse activity to intracranial pressure variations. Nurs Res 27:4, 1978
24. Boortz-Marx R: Factors affecting intracranial pressure: A descriptive study. J Neurosci Nurs 4:89, 1985
25. Mitchell P, Ozuma J, Lipe H: Moving the patient in bed: Effects on intracranial pressure. Nurs Res 30:216, 1980
26. Johnson S, Omery A, Nikas D: Effects of conversation on intracranial pressure in comatose patients. Heart & Lung 18:56, 1988
27. Walleck C: Controversies in the management of head-injured patients, Crit Care Nurs Clin North Am 1(1):72, 1989
28. Pollack L, Goldsteen G: Lowering of intracranial pressure in Reye's syndrome by sensory stimulation. N Engl J Med 304:732, 1981
29. Ropper A, Rockoff M: In: Ropper A, Kennedy S (eds): Neurological and Neurosurgical Intensive Care, p 24. Rockville, MD, Aspen Publishing, 1988
30. Ibid, p 24
31. Shoemaker et al, p 294
32. Ropper, Rockoff, p 25
33. Ibid
34. Schmidley, p 338
35. Shoemaker et al, p 294
36. Ibid
37. Ropper, Rockoff, p 26
38. Marshall et al, p 195
39. Shoemaker et al, p 297
40. Rose B: Clinical Physiology of Acid–Base and Electrolyte Disorders, 3rd ed, p 304. New York, McGraw-Hill, 1989
41. Ropper, Rockoff, p 27
42. Schmidley, p 338
43. Ropper, Rockoff, p 34

44. Shoemaker et al, p 294
45. Ibid
46. Marshall et al, p 200
47. Ibid
48. Walleck, p 69
49. Ropper, Rockoff, p 26
50. Ibid, p 123
51. Marshall et al, p 200
52. Kokko, Tannen, p 835
53. Ibid
54. Ibid
55. Ibid, p 172
56. Ibid

21

Diabetic Ketoacidosis and Hyperosmolar Coma

A relative or absolute insulin deficiency can result in severe hyperglycemia, which in turn leads either to diabetic ketoacidosis (DKA) or hyperosmolar hyperglycemic nonketotic coma (HHNC), depending on which type of diabetes mellitus is present.

Type I, insulin dependent diabetes mellitus (IDDM), can develop at any age although most cases are generally diagnosed before age 30.[1] Persons with type I diabetes mellitus are insulinopenic and require exogenous insulin to prevent ketoacidosis and sustain life. An absolute deficiency of insulin, resulting from destruction of pancreatic beta cells, predisposes type I diabetics to ketosis. In some cases, DKA may be the first manifestation of diabetes. Diabetic ketoacidosis is life threaten-

ing and, despite treatment advances, mortality rates remain between 6% and 10%.[2]

Type II, noninsulin dependent diabetes mellitus (NIDDM), usually begins in middle or later adulthood, is typically diagnosed after age 40 and accounts for 80% to 90% of the diabetic cases in the United States.[3] Persons with type II diabetes mellitus may have decreased, normal, or even increased serum insulin levels. The metabolic problems associated with type II diabetes mellitus are believed to result from peripheral insulin resistance, with decreased tissue sensitivity or responsiveness to exogenous or endogenous insulin.[4] Approximately 80% of type II diabetics are obese,[5] and many can be managed by dietary and weight control

TABLE 21–1.
Oral Hypoglycemia Agents Used in Management of Type II Diabetes

GENERIC NAME	BRAND NAME
Tolbutamide	Orinase
Chlorpropamide	Diabinese
Acetohexamide	Dymelor
Tolazamide	Tolinase
Glyburide	DiaBeta
	Micronase
Glipizide	Glucotrol

measures. In some cases, oral hypoglycemic agents (OHA) are required. Table 21-1 lists the OHA currently used in the management of type II diabetes mellitus.

A percentage of type II diabetics may require some exogenous insulin for good blood glucose control, at least initially or during times of stress (such as illness or surgery).[6] Persons with NIDDM are not as prone to ketosis; instead, they are at risk for hyperosmolar hyperglycemic nonketotic coma (HHNC) when their hyperglycemia is severe. It is not fully understood why these individuals are ketosis resistant. Although HHNC occurs less frequently than DKA, it is on the increase because of the rising population of elderly adults who have type II diabetes mellitus. Indeed, it is a serious complication of many types of medical and surgical therapies in the elderly diabetic.

Use of the term "coma" for these conditions is somewhat misleading because only a small percentage of patients are actually comatose when treatment is initiated.[7] However, both DKA and HHNC cause severe derangements of fluid and electrolyte balances, affecting almost all systems of the body; these emergency situations require expert and prompt intervention.

DIABETIC KETOACIDOSIS

HYPERGLYCEMIA AND HYPEROSMOLALITY

Diabetic ketoacidosis results from insulin deficiency and the effects of the counter-regulatory hormones, glucagon, catecholamines, cortisol, and growth hormone. Underuse of glucose (most cells are relatively impermeable to glucose in the absence of insulin), excessive production of glucose from fats and amino acids by the liver (gluconeogenesis), and excessive production of glucose from glycogen (glycogenolysis) all lead to hyperglycemia.[8] Because of these processes, the blood glucose concentration rises markedly and increases plasma osmolality.

The following formula is used to calculate plasma osmolality, the normal range of which is 280 to 300 mOsm/L:

$$pOsm = 2(Na^+ + K^+) + \frac{G}{18} + \frac{BUN}{2.8}$$
$$= 280–300 \text{ mOsm/kg}$$

In the following example it is possible to see how hyperglycemia elevates plasma osmolality:

Example: Patient with hyperglycemia

$$Na^+ = 139 \text{ mEq/L}$$
$$K^+ = 4 \text{ mEq/L}$$
$$\text{Serum glucose} = 1800 \text{ mg/dL}$$
$$BUN = 30 \text{ mg/dL}$$
$$pOsm = 2(139 + 4) + \frac{1800}{18} + \frac{30}{2.8}$$
$$= 397 \text{ mOsm/kg}$$

This elevated osmolality of extracellular fluid (ECF) produces cellular dehydration as water shifts from the cells to the ECF.

Other authors use the following formula (omitting the urea component) to calculate the effective osmolality, because urea diffuses freely across cell membranes and does not create an osmotic gradient between the intracellular and extracellular spaces:

$$\text{Effective } pOsm = 2(Na^+ + K^+) + \frac{G}{18}$$

These authors reason that this equation can calculate a more clinically relevant value.[9, 10]

OSMOTIC DIURESIS AND FLUID VOLUME DEFICIT

When the blood glucose level exceeds the renal threshold (normally 180 mg/dL), glucose spills into the urine, taking water and electrolytes with it and increasing urine volume. Specific gravity (SG) of the urine is elevated due to the high glucose content. The polyuria eventually leads to fluid volume deficit (FVD). As the FVD worsens, glomerular filtration rate (GFR) decreases, as does renal blood flow, causing the patient to become oliguric or even anuric in spite of marked hyperglycemia. This FVD presents a potential renal tubular damage danger with resultant acute renal failure.

ELECTROLYTES

Potassium

Probably the most important electrolyte disturbance that occurs in DKA is the marked deficit in total body potassium. Causes of potassium depletion include:

1. Starvation effect with lean tissue breakdown
2. Loss of intracellular potassium
3. Potassium-losing effect of aldosterone (aldosterone is stimulated by FVD)
4. Loss of potassium with osmotic diuresis
5. Severe anorexia (reducing intake) and vomiting (increasing loss of potassium)

Before treatment, the patient with DKA may have a normal or elevated serum potassium although there is a marked deficit of total body potassium. Factors that tend to elevate the serum potassium level in the untreated patient include:

▸ Plasma volume contraction with oliguria, which interferes with renal excretion of potassium
▸ Metabolic acidosis (potassium shifts out of the cells into the extracellular compartment as hydrogen is buffered intracellularly).

This hyperkalemia is quickly alleviated by fluid replacement therapy and reestablishment of urine output.

After treatment is begun, the serum potassium falls rapidly and usually reaches its lowest point within 1 to 4 hours. Reasons for the decreased serum potassium level at this time include:

▸ Dilution by the intravenous (IV) fluids
▸ Increased urinary potassium excretion due to plasma volume expansion
▸ Formation of glycogen within the cells using potassium, glucose, and water from the ECF (a shift of potassium into the cells)
▸ Correction of acidosis with reentry of potassium into the cells

It is believed that use of low-dose insulin therapy in the management of DKA is less likely to be associated with rapid falls in serum potassium than is the use of high-dose insulin therapy.

Phosphorus

Hypophosphatemia almost invariably occurs during treatment in the patient with DKA, and for many of the same reasons that hypokalemia occurs. (Recall that both involve primarily cellular electrolytes.) One potentially serious consequence of phosphorus deficiency is decreased erythrocyte 2,3-DPG (diphosphoglycerate); a low level of 2,3-DPG may result in decreased peripheral oxygen delivery. Decreased myocardial function has also been observed when the serum phosphate concentration is less than 2 mg/dL.[11] When the serum phosphate concentration goes below 0.5 mg/dL, serious disturbances in metabolism may result; seizures, respiratory failure, impaired leukocyte and platelet function, and gastrointestinal bleeding have been reported.[12]

Sodium

Plasma sodium concentration is usually below normal as a result of hyperosmolality, despite losses of water in excess of solute in DKA. Accumulation of glucose in the ECF creates an osmotic gradient, causing water to be pulled out of the cells into the ECF and resulting in lowering of the plasma sodium level. If vomiting is present, the hyponatremia becomes more severe. Sodium also moves into the cells as they become depleted of potassium, further lowering the plasma sodium level.

KETOSIS

Insulin deficiency allows greater release of free fatty acids (FFA) from peripheral fat stores and activates ketogenic pathways in the liver; the excess fatty acids are converted by the liver to ketones, resulting in ketosis. The insulin deficiency also interferes with uptake of the ketones by peripheral tissues, further increasing the buildup of ketones in the bloodstream. The ketones (ketoacids) present in DKA are B-hydroxybutyrate and acetoacetate. Because ketones are strong acids, with one hydrogen ion created with each ion of B-hydroxybutyrate and acetoacetate, this overproduction and impaired metabolism soon overload the body's buffers, resulting in metabolic acidosis.[13] The anionic charge of bicarbonate is replaced by the negatively charged ketones.

The type of metabolic acidosis that occurs in DKA is manifested by a fall in bicarbonate with a reciprocal rise in the anion gap (AG) as large amounts of unmeasured anions are produced. Calculate AG using the following formula:

$$AG = Na^+ - (HCO_3^- + Cl^-) = 12\text{--}15 \text{ mEq/L}$$

Example: Patient with ketoacidosis

$$Na^+ = 131 \text{ mEq/L}$$
$$Cl^- = 95 \text{ mEq/L}$$
$$HCO_3 = 5 \text{ mEq/L}$$
$$AG = 131 - (5 + 95) = 31 \text{ mEq/L}$$

Calculation of AG is important in the assessment of acid–base disturbances in DKA because other findings may be misleading. For example, the vomiting that frequently accompanies DKA can superimpose a metabolic alkalosis on the preexisting ketoacidosis, making the plasma pH appear nearly normal. Measurement of AG will reveal the abnormal levels of ketone ions that are disrupting metabolism.

The ketones (ketoacids) present in DKA are β-hydroxybutyrate and acetoacetate. Excessive ketosis leads to ketonuria and even excretion of volatile acetone from the lungs (resulting in the classic "fruity" odor of the breath associated with DKA). It is not unusual for the plasma pH to drop to 7.25 or below and for the bicarbonate level to drop to 12 mEq/L or less. Possibly the greatest risks of prolonged uncorrected acidosis are decreased cardiac function, arrhythmia, and impaired hepatic handling of lactate.[14]

The body attempts to compensate for the metabolic acidosis associated with DKA by means of the kidneys and lungs. The kidneys eliminate hydrogen ions and conserve bicarbonate ions, resulting in decreased urinary pH. The lungs attempt to lighten the acid load by blowing off extra carbon dioxide, resulting in the deep, rapid breathing known as Kussmaul respiration. The expected fall in $PaCO_2$ for compensation of metabolic acidosis can be calculated by the following formula:

$$Expected\ PaCO_2(mmHg) = 1.5\ (HCO_3) + 8 \pm 2$$

Example: The expected $PaCO_2$ in a patient with a bicarbonate level of 12 mEq/L would be between 24 and 28 mmHg:

$$PaCO_2 = 1.5\ (12) + 8 \pm 2 = 24–28\ mmHg$$

A fall below the calculated amount indicates a superimposed respiratory alkalosis; failure of the $PaCO_2$ to decrease to the expected level indicates a complicating respiration acidosis (a dangerous combination).

HYPEROSMOLAR HYPERGLYCEMIC NONKETOTIC COMA

Hyperosmolar hyperglycemic nonketotic coma is a syndrome that develops in the middle-aged or elderly type II diabetic (sometimes not yet diagnosed), often as a result of stress caused by physical impairment such as renal or cardiovascular disease, infections, or effects of pharmacological therapy with drugs such as steroids or diuretics. Too rapid introduction of total parenteral nutrition (TPN) may also precipitate HHNC (see Chapter 12). The condition develops more slowly than DKA; it is not uncommon for patients to experience polyuria, polydipsia, weight loss, and weakness for days and even weeks before seeking medical attention. Hyperglycemia may be extreme (400–4800 mg/dL), but without the ketosis of DKA.[16] The plasma pH is usually normal or only slightly low. The absence of ketoacidosis was formerly attributed to the higher residual insulin levels in these patients, but this explanation is no longer considered entirely adequate.[17-19]

Fluid volume deficit is profound in HHNC and may be life threatening. Some sources report mortality rates as high as 50%, depending on the severity of the hyperosmolality and the occurrence of sequelae such as thromboembolic and respiratory complications.[20] Although there is a deficit of total body sodium, the serum sodium may be normal or elevated because of a relatively greater loss of water. The plasma bicarbonate level is normal or slightly reduced. The BUN is usually more elevated than in DKA (60–90 mg/dL) and reflects the more severe FVD and the catabolic state. The serum creatinine is often elevated in HHNC, reflecting the common association of HHNC with underlying renal impairment. Potassium and phosphate depletion may occur, as they do in DKA.

RULING OUT HYPOGLYCEMIA AND OTHER CAUSES OF COMA

Before treatment of the comatose diabetic patient, hypoglycemia must be ruled out. Hypoglycemia is characterized by anxiety, sweating, hunger, headache, dizziness, visual disturbances, nausea, pale, moist skin, dilated pupils, twitching, convulsions, and normal breathing and blood pressure. When in doubt, it is best that glucose (50 mL of 50% dextrose in water) be administered IV. Without IV access, severe hypoglycemia is best treated by administering glucagon, 1 mg (for adults) subcutaneously or intramuscularly.[21] If hypoglycemia is the problem, the patient's condition will improve quickly; if DKA or HHNC is the problem, the small amount of dextrose or the mobilization of hepatic glycogen stores by glucagon will do no harm. Of course, a blood glucose determination should be made as quickly as possible.

Serum glucose measurement is an important first step in evaluation of the diabetic patient with altered consciousness. A finding of hypoglycemia or hyperglycemia, however, may not fully explain the cause of the altered consciousness or coma. A thorough evaluation is needed so that other pathology, such as stroke, uremia, or drug intoxication, does not go untreated. Conversely, the signs and symptoms of hypoglycemia or hyperglycemia may mimic other conditions; for example, abdominal pain in patients with DKA may simulate an abdominal emergency. For this reason, even when there is no history of diabetes, serum glucose should be measured promptly in acutely ill patients. Recall that DKA or HHNC may be the first manifestation of diabetes in some individuals. Patients with alcoholic ketoacidosis may also occasionally have some degree of hyperglycemia, making differential diagnosis problematic.[22]

TREATMENT OF DKA AND NKHC

FLUID REPLACEMENT

Adequate and prompt rehydration is vital and must consider the patient's cardiovascular and renal status. Fluid replacement is usually begun with the administration of 1 to 3 L of isotonic saline (0.9% NaCl) infused at the rate of approximately 1 L/hr. Isotonic (normal) saline will expand the ECF and will begin to correct the hyperosmolality. In some cases of HHNC, in which there is significant hypernatremia, hypertension, or risk for congestive heart failure, half-strength saline (0.45% NaCl) may be used. When there is a concern about the adequacy of the patient's cardiovascular status, central venous pressure or hemodynamic monitoring may be needed to help gauge the best rate of fluid replacement.

After the initial infusion of normal saline, the IV fluid may be changed to half-strength saline to dilute the hyperosmolar plasma and provide free water for renal excretion. As fluid replacement continues, the rate and volume will be determined by the status of the patient. Patients with HHNC may need larger amounts of fluids to correct the FVD. When the plasma glucose levels fall to the 250 to 300 mg/dL range, solutions containing dextrose should be used to prevent hypoglycemia and other complications that might occur as a result of a too rapid fall in blood glucose. As soon as oral intake is adequate, IV fluids can be discontinued.

INSULIN ADMINISTRATION

The aim of insulin therapy is to give enough rapid-acting (regular) insulin to correct the problem without subjecting the patient to the risk of hypoglycemia. Regular insulin, which is a clear preparation, is the only insulin that may be used IV. While it can also be given intramuscularly or subcutaneously, the continuous IV route is best for the very ill patient because absorption of insulin from poorly perfused muscle and fat depots may be erratic, especially if the patient is hypotensive.

Studies have demonstrated that large insulin doses are generally no more effective in correcting DKA than small doses. The low-dose regimen has been shown to lower blood sugar smoothly, improve ketosis, and repair acidosis at rates indistinguishable from those ob-

tained by higher-dose regimens. In addition, patients are less likely to develop hypoglycemia and hypokalemia than are patients receiving large doses.[23] Of course, when low doses do not achieve the desired effect, as in cases of insulin "resistance," larger doses must be given. Patients with HHNC will require somewhat less insulin than those with DKA.

The insulin dose for continuous IV infusion is usually 4 to 10 U/hr or 0.1 U/kg/hr. Sometimes an initial bolus of 5 to 10 units is given when therapy is initiated. The adsorption of insulin to IV containers and tubing has been documented, but there is disagreement about the extent to which it affects insulin delivery, particularly in low-dose therapy. Methods used to minimize the effect of adsorption include addition of human serum albumin to infusion solutions or flushing the infusion set with the insulin solution to saturate the binding sites before connecting it to the patient. According to Peterson et al,[24] the insulin binding effect will be minimal if the solution contains a concentration of at least 25 units of insulin to 500 mL of saline, and 50 mL of the solution are flushed through the entire apparatus before patient infusion.

Of primary importance is the individualization of the dosage of insulin to the response of each patient, and adjustment of that dosage on the basis of ongoing blood glucose determinations. A too rapid drop in blood glucose creates the risk of complications such as hypoglycemia and hypokalemia. There is also a risk that cerebral edema may occur from the osmotic gradient created between brain and serum osmolality by a too rapid decline in blood glucose.[25] A controlled-rate infusion pump should be used to ensure accurate administration of the insulin. If one is not available, the solutions should be administered through a volume-controlled administration set. When the patient's condition is sufficiently stabilized, the insulin can be administered subcutaneously.

ELECTROLYTE REPLACEMENT

Potassium

Potassium is not added to the IV fluids until the first 2 or 3 L have been administered and adequate urinary output has been established, unless serum potassium levels have already decreased to normal or below. Potassium replacement is usually accomplished by adding 20 to 40 mEq of potassium to a liter of half-normal saline (0.45% NaCl), infused at a rate appropriate to the status of the patient. Occasionally, larger amounts of potassium are needed if the hypokalemia is severe. Since the IV administration of potassium is always associated with risk of hyperkalemia, it is wise to monitor the serum potassium level at 1- or 2-hour intervals and to use serial ECG tracings. (Rules for safe potassium administration are discussed in Tables 5-6 and 5-7.) Oral potassium-containing fluids may be given when the patient is able to tolerate them. (See Table 3-1 for a summary of the electrolyte content of commonly available beverages.)

Phosphorus

Because phosphate is lost during the osmotic diuresis of DKA and HHNC, some authorities favor replacing at least a part of the lost potassium with potassium phosphate. This can also reduce the risk of hyperchloremia associated with sole use of potassium chloride salts.[26] It is imperative, however, that significant renal failure be ruled out before phosphate is administered IV; serum phosphate levels should be monitored to prevent possible hyperphosphatemia. Administering too much phosphate can induce hypocalcemia. Therefore, calcium levels should also be monitored if phosphate is administered. When oral intake is tolerated, skim milk is a good source of phosphorus. It is thought that phosphate replacement accelerates the recovery of reduced red blood cell 2,3-DPG levels, thereby decreasing hemoglobin–oxygen affinity and improving tissue oxygenation.

Bicarbonate

There has been controversy over the use of bicarbonate in the treatment of DKA. It is used for management of hyperkalemia,[27] and is generally considered to be necessary in cases of severe acidosis ($pH < 7.1$). When bicarbonate is used to correct pH, it is not corrected above a level of 7.1; to normalize the pH could result in paradoxical CNS acidosis.[28] Too rapid correction of acidosis can also induce hypokalemia (as potassium shifts into the cells). When bicarbonate is given, it should be infused with the IV fluids, not administered by bolus. Some authorities believe that bicarbonate replacement is unnecessary because insulin therapy reverses the biochemical abnormalities of DKA including the bicarbonate deficit.

Sodium

Isotonic saline that is administered initially supplies enough sodium to correct any sodium loss. Because the patient with DKA or HHNC has lost proportionately more water than sodium, a hypotonic solution (such as 0.45% NaCl) will be ordered after the 2 to 3 L of isotonic saline. Hypotonic solutions provide free water to correct cellular dehydration.

Other Electrolytes

Losses of calcium and magnesium may occur as a result of the osmotic diuresis. Often they are not con-

TABLE 21–2.
Factors Contributing to Development of DKA or HHNC in Susceptible Persons

DKA	HHNC
Infections, illness	Chronic renal disease
Physiological stresses (eg, trauma, surgery, myocardial infarction, dehydration, pregnancy)	Chronic cardiovascular disease
	Acute illness, infection
Psychological/emotional stress	Surgery, burns, trauma
	Hyperalimentation, tube feedings
Omission/reduction of insulin	Peritoneal dialysis
Failure of insulin delivery system (pump)	Mannitol therapy
Excess alcohol intake	Pharmacological agents:
	▶ Chlorpromazine
	▶ Cimetidine
	▶ Diazoxide
	▶ Diuretics (thiazide, thiazide-related and loop diuretics)
	▶ Glucocorticoids and immunosuppressive agents
	▶ L-asparaginase
	▶ Phenytoin
	▶ Propanolol

DKA, diabetic ketoacidosis; HHNC, hyperosmolar hyperglycemic nonketotic coma.

sidered of clinical consequence, but in some cases, magnesium is replaced if renal function is adequate.[29]

TREATMENT OF PRECIPITATING FACTORS

In addition to the above therapies, treatment will include identification and treatment of concurrent health problems, particularly those that might have been precipitating factors in the development of DKA or HHNC. Table 21-2 lists common precipitating factors for each condition.

USE OF THE NURSING PROCESS

NURSING ASSESSMENT

Nursing care of the patient with HHNC or DKA involves meticulous, ongoing assessment to detect significant changes. Tables 21-3 and 21-4 outline the clinical manifestations of HHNC and DKA. To achieve

TABLE 21–3.
Clinical Signs of DKA and Their Probable Causes

CLINICAL SIGNS	PROBABLE CAUSES
Hyperglycemia (Normal blood glucose is 80–120 mg/dL. Elevations associated with DKA may be as high as 4000 mg/dL.)	Faulty glucose metabolism causes glucose to accumulate in the bloodstream (lack of insulin decreases glucose uptake by most cells and also increases gluconeogenesis in the liver)
Glucosuria	Blood glucose level exceeds renal threshold (normally 180 mg/dL, higher in the elderly) causing glucose to spill into the urine
Polyuria (initially) with high specific gravity	Osmotic diuretic effect of hyperglycemia, high renal solute load
Polydipsia	Thirst due to cellular dehydration (cells become dehydrated when water is drawn from them by the hypertonic ECF)
Anorexia, nausea, vomiting	Follows onset of DKA; interferes with fluid intake (hastening the development of fluid volume deficit)
Poor skin turgor, dry mucous membranes, poor tongue turgor	Fluid volume deficit
Acute weight loss	Fluid volume deficit (parallels degree of this imbalance)
Ketonemia and ketonuria	Excessive accumulation of ketones in the bloodstream causes them to spill out into the urine
Cherry red skin and mucous membranes	Marked peripheral vasodilatation associated with ketosis
Deep "air hunger" respirations (Kussmaul)	Compensatory mechanism to increase plasma pH by the elimination of large amounts of carbon dioxide
Acetone odor to breath (similar to that of overripe apples)	Acetone, a volatile ketone, is vaporized in the expired air (may be obscured by the odor of vomitus)
Abdominal pain (can simulate acute appendicitis, pancreatitis, or other acute abdominal problems)	Apparently due to the DKA per se (*Note:* Anorexia, nausea, and vomiting precede the abdominal pain when it is due to DKA; this is in contrast to most surgical emergencies in which the pain usually occurs first.)
Postural hypotension	Fluid volume deficit (eventually may be hypotensive even when supine)
Fatigue, muscular weakness	Lack of carbohydrate use, hypokalemia
Hypothermia or normal temperature	Fever is present only when there is a concurrent illness causing it
Blurred vision	Osmotic changes in lenses of eyes
Oliguria, anuria (late)	Fluid volume deficit causes decreased renal blood flow and decreased GFR. (Before assuming that urine formation is scanty, check for a distended, atonic bladder.)
Depressed sensorium (ranging from somnolence to frank coma)	Level of consciousness correlates best with level of hyperglycemia and plasma osmolality
Laboratory Data:	
Hyperglycemia	Related to insulin lack (see above)
Elevated serum osmolality (normal is 280–295 mOsm/kg)	Related primarily to high glucose level; elevated BUN contributes to elevated level
Potassium variations	Serum potassium concentration may be elevated before treatment; later, however, may drop to seriously low levels (see explanation in text)

(continued)

TABLE 21–3.
(continued)

CLINICAL SIGNS	PROBABLE CAUSES
Laboratory Data:	
Hypophosphatemia	Osmotic diuresis
Increased BUN (often increased to 40 mg/dL; normal is 10–20 mg/dL)	Fluid volume deficit, decreased GFR, increased protein metabolism, increased hepatic production of urea (due to insulin lack)
Increased creatinine (normal is 0.7 to 1.5 mg/dL)	Prerenal azotemia due to FVD
Leukocytosis	Flukd volume deficit, acidosis, adrenocortical stimulation
Decreased serum bicarbonate (usually <15 mEq/L, may be extremely low; normal is 24 mEq/L)	Excessive ketonic anions in the bloodstream cause a compensatory drop in bicarbonate
Decreased arterial *pH* (usually <7.25 may be as low as 6.8 in severe cases; normal is 7.35–7.45)	Associated with the metabolic acidosis caused by ketosis
High anion gap (AG) acidosis (normal AG is <12–15 mEq/L)	Due to excessive ketones in the bloodstream
Increased hemoglobin, hematocrit, total protein	FVD (causes concentration of formed elements in blood)
Increased liver function tests	Does not necessarily reflect acute or chronic liver damage, as most often values return to normal in several weeks

BUN, blood urea nitrogen; DKA, diabetic ketoacidosis; ECF, extracellular fluid; GFR, glomerular filtration rate; FVD, fluid volume deficit.

TABLE 21–4.
Summary of Hyperosmolar Hyperglycemic
Nonketotic Coma

The typical patient at risk for HHNC has either undiagnosed diabetes or a form of the disease mild enough to be managed with oral hypoglycemic agents or diet alone; the typical patient at risk for DKA requires insulin for everyday management.

HHNC tends to occur in middle-aged or elderly type II diabetics, often those suffering from underlying renal and cardiovascular impairment. In at-risk patients, the condition is often precipitated by the stress of an acute illness, or by treatment with corticosteroids, diuretics, mannitol, phenytoin, and glucose solutions.

Onset of HHNC tends to be more gradual and insidious than that of DKA. (It is not uncommon for patients to experience polyuria, polydipsia, weight loss, and weakness for many days, and even weeks, before seeking medical attention).

Hyperglycemia and related symptoms of hyperosmolality are often more pronounced in HHNC than in DKA. Abnormal neurological signs may occur, such as focal or generalized seizures. If water loss leads to hypernatremia, fever may occur.

HHNC is *not* associated with ketoacidosis; it has been postulated that in HHNC there is sufficient insulin to prevent ketosis but not enough to prevent hyperglycemia.

HHNC, hyperosmolar hyperglycemic nonketotic coma; DKA, diabetic ketoacidosis.

ongoing assessment, it is best to use a diabetic flow sheet, often including the following data:

1. Vital signs (BP, temperature, pulse, and respirations)
2. Fluid therapy (type, amount, and flow rate)
3. Insulin therapy (number of units per hour IV, IM, and SQ)
4. Hourly urine volume
5. ECG tracings
6. Level of consciousness
7. Deep-tendon reflexes
8. Relevant lab data, which may include:
   ▶ Blood and urine glucose
   ▶ Blood and urine ketones
   ▶ *p*H (blood gases)
   ▶ K^+
   ▶ HCO_3
   ▶ Na^+/Cl^-
   ▶ Ca^+/PO_4
   ▶ BUN/creatinine
9. Calculations
   ▶ Anion gap
   ▶ Serum osmolality

Decisions as to which of the above parameters will be monitored, by whom, and at what intervals, will be made based on the patient's status and protocols related to the care setting (such as the emergency room, critical care unit, and nursing unit). Response to therapy must be observed and recorded carefully. This involves constant vigilance over the patient's clinical status so that critical judgments can be made to provide optimal therapy.

NURSING DIAGNOSES

The alterations associated with DKA and HHNC will lead to the formation of some nursing diagnoses that involve effects of, or responses to, these alterations. However, because patients with DKA and HHNC also have severe and rapidly changing derangements in fluid, electrolyte, and acid–base balances, nursing diagnoses will frequently coincide with the domain of other health professionals. This is a necessary and important characteristic because the nursing role in caring for the patient with DKA or HHNC includes monitoring and decision making related to the physiological status of the patient and the response to medical therapies.

Whenever possible, the nurse should use the North American Nursing Diagnoses Association (NANDA) nursing diagnosis labels, refining them to make them specific to each individual patient. It should be remembered, however, that the NANDA list is not yet comprehensive enough to meet all situations. For that reason, one must formulate additional diagnoses based on results of the nursing assessment.

Although there are many nursing diagnoses relevant to the diabetic patient, Table 21-5 deals with diagnoses that relate primarily to fluid, electrolyte, and acid–base balance aspects of nursing care of patients with, or at risk for, DKA or HHNC. The listed etiologies and defining characteristics are those most likely to be applicable. In some situations, there may be others. See Chapters 3–9 for detailed descriptions of specific imbalances.

NURSING INTERVENTIONS

Nursing care of the patient with DKA or HHNC is complex and involves many traditional nursing actions plus sophisticated monitoring of the responses to medical therapy. The care plan will include many interventions that relate to the fluid and electrolyte status of the patient. Some of those most frequently used are outlined below:

1. Monitor degree of FVD and response to fluid replacement therapy.
   A. Assess blood pressure (supine and sitting, if possible) and pulse. (A drop in systolic pressure by more than 10 mmHg on position change from lying to sitting is indicative of FVD. Remember that a severely volume-depleted patient will be hypotensive even in the supine position. The pulse will be rapid and of a weak volume as the heart pumps faster to compensate for the below-normal plasma volume.)
   B. Observe neck veins. (Collapse of the neck veins when the head is raised is a sign of FVD.)
   C. Check skin and tongue turgor and degree of moisture of mucous membranes. (Poor skin turgor is indicative of FVD, as is the presence of a smaller-than-normal tongue with extra longitudinal furrows, and dry mucous membranes. Review assessment of these parameters in Chapter 2.)
   D. Monitor urinary output.
      i. If patient is too stuporous to void, insert a retention catheter, using meticulous aseptic technique. (Recall that diabetic patients are very prone to urinary infections.) Remove the catheter as soon as the patient is able to empty the bladder by voiding.
      ii. Measure hourly urine volume in a device calibrated for accurate reading of small amounts (see Figure 2-2). (Output should be at least 30–50 mL/hr. Oliguria related to FVD can lead to renal tubular damage and must be prevented. The hourly urinary output should increase if parenteral fluid replacement is adequate. Report a urine volume less than 30 mL/hr as well as failure of output to increase with fluid replacement.)
      iii. Measure SG of urine. (Urinary SG is elevated in FVD; if low with a scanty volume, renal damage may be present and should be reported. Heavy glucosuria invalidates SG readings; see Table 2-4.)
      iv. Total and compare the 8-hour and 24-hour intake and output. (During treatment, intake must exceed output until the FVD is corrected.)
      v. Monitor the BUN and creatinine levels. (Recall that an elevated BUN reflects FVD when elevated out of proportion to the serum creatinine level. See Table 2-3 for further discussion of these tests.)
   E. Calculate approximate degree of FVD.
      i. Weigh patient on admission and ascertain, if possible, the pre-illness weight. (A rapid loss of 1 kg [2.2 lb] of body weight is roughly equivalent to a loss of 1 L of body fluid. Loss of weight from not eating may amount to 0.5 lb/day. Acute weight loss of 5% body weight constitutes a moderate FVD; 8% or greater is a severe FVD. Many cases have been reported in which as much as 10% to 20% of body weight has been lost acutely in patients with DKA and HHNC).
      ii. Weigh patient each morning before break-

TABLE 21–5.
Examples of Nursing Diagnoses Related to Patients with Diabetic Ketoacidosis or Hyperosmolar Hyperglycemic Nonketotic Coma

NURSING DIAGNOSIS	ETIOLOGICAL FACTORS	DEFINING CHARACTERISTICS
Fluid volume deficit related to hyperosmotic diuresis	Hyperglycemia Hyperosmolality	Initially: Polyuria Later: Oliguria or anuria Other symptoms of FVD (see Chapter 3)
Alteration in potassium balance (hypokalemia) related to increased potassium loss and insulin therapy (shift into cells)	Osmotic diuresis Dilution by IV fluids Increased excretion Reentry into cells	Drop in serum potassium for 1–4 hours after therapy (symptoms of hypokalemia in Chapter 5)
Alteration in tissue perfusion: Renal, related to FVD	Severe FVD Decreased GFR Decreased renal blood flow	Oliguria or anuria symptoms of renal failure (see Chapter 18)
Risk for alteration in phosphorus balance (hypophosphatemia) and magnesium balance (hypomagnesemia) related to osmotic diuresis and insulin therapy	Osmotic diuresis Rapid fall in levels (especially phosphate) once fluid therapy is begun Reentry into cells	Symptoms of hypophosphatemia (see Chapter 8) Symptoms of hypomagnesemia (see Chapter 7)
Alteration in acid–base balance (metabolic acidosis) related to increased production and decreased use of ketones in DKA	Insulin deficiency in type I diabetes Increased activity of counterregulatory hormones Release of FFA from peripheral fat stores	Ketonemia Decreased plasma pH Ketonuria Decreased plasma HCO_3 Elevated anion gap Kussmaul respirations "Fruity" breath odor Clinical signs of acidosis (see Chapter 9)
Alteration in nutrition: less than body requirements, related to insulin deficiency	Decreased glucose uptake and storage Decreased protein synthesis and fat assimilation Gastric retention Anorexia, nausea, and vomiting	Early: Weight loss and hunger in spite of adequate food intake; abdominal pain Later: Reduction in muscle mass and fat stores
Sensory-perceptual alteration related to effects of DKA and HHNC	Elevated serum osmolality FVD Severe elevated BUN Acidemia in DKA	Changes in level of consciousness Change in usual response to sensory stimuli
Risk for hypoglycemia related to insulin therapy	Insufficient dextrose in IV fluids Erratic absorption of insulin from peripheral sites Excess insulin	Rapid drop in blood glucose <250 mg/dL Negative urine glucose
Risk for uncontrolled diabetes related to inadequate management or stress factors	Insulin supply or use not adequate for metabolic needs Food intake excessive for exogenous or endogenous insulin supply Physiological or psychological stressors such as illness, surgery, personal crisis	Lack of adjustment of regimen during illness, infection, or severe emotional stress Decreased insulin dosage when food intake decreases Manipulation of insulin dose related to fear of hypoglycemic reaction Inadequate health care during periods of illness or severe crisis
Potential for HHNC related to pharmacological or other medical therapy	Type II elderly diabetic receiving drugs or therapies that can precipitate HHNC (see Table 21-2)	Hyperglycemia Polyuria Water intake inadequate to compensate for osmotic diuresis
Lack of knowledge of diabetic sick day management related to development of DKA during period of illness	No previous history of attending diabetic education program Poor understanding of diabetic sick day management	Does not follow sick day diet; does not monitor blood glucose levels; does not manipulate insulin dosage during illness

FFA, free fatty acid; FVD, fluid volume deficit; DKA, diabetic ketoacidosis; HHNC, hyperosmolar hyperglycemic nonketotic coma; GFR, glomerular filtration rate.

fast. (Monitor for acute changes in body weight; anticipate that weight gain will parallel correction of the FVD.)

iii. If pre-illness weight cannot be determined, FVD may be calculated with a formula using the patient's plasma osmolality:

FVD (liters)

$$= \frac{\text{Patient's pOsm} - \text{Normal pOsm}}{\text{Normal pOsm}}$$
$$\times \text{ liters of body fluid}$$
$$(0.6 \times \text{body weight/kg})$$

Example: Assume an adult patient has a plasma osmolality of 340 mOsm/kg and weighs 70 kg. (Use 280 mOsm/kg as the normal value.)

$$\text{Liters of body fluid} = 0.6 \times 70 = 42$$

$$\text{FVD (liters)} = \frac{340 - 280}{280} \times 42 = 9 \text{ liters}$$

F. Monitor neurological status. Look for depressed sensorium and focal neurological signs. A depressed sensorium results most often from hyperosmolality of body fluids and occurs to some degree in most cases of DKA and HHNC. Because of this it is necessary to consider the following points:

i. Maintain an adequate airway (a comatose patient with airway obstruction will require intubation).

ii. Insert nasogastric tube when indicated (gastric retention with regurgitation of contents is not uncommon).

G. Regulate fluid replacement rate and volume according to protocol and patient status. Consider the following facts:

i. After the initial infusion of saline solutions to rehydrate the patient, dextrose solutions are indicated to keep the serum glucose from falling too rapidly.

ii. Central venous pressure or hemodynamic monitoring may be needed in elderly patients and those with compromised cardiovascular or renal status.

iii. The patient with HHNC may need larger amounts of fluid than the patient with DKA because the degree of FVD is often worse in HHNC.

2. Monitor electrolyte status and response to replacement therapy.

A. Monitor potassium levels at frequent (1–2 hour) intervals during the initial period of therapy. (Recall that the initial potassium level may be normal or elevated because of plasma volume contraction and shift from the intracellular fluid to the ECF, and that the potassium level drops rapidly with plasma dilution and reentry of potassium into the cells. Replacement therapy after the first 2 to 3 L of fluid should prevent a precipitous drop in serum potassium. Recall that potassium should not be administered to a patient with oliguria. Review Tables 5-6 and 5-7 for nursing considerations in the safe administration of potassium solutions.)

B. Use serial ECG tracings and other appropriate assessment parameters to detect effects of hypokalemia and to monitor responses to potassium infusion (see Chapter 5).

C. Promptly report abnormal laboratory levels of other electrolytes, such as a low phosphorus level. (Recall that decreased serum phosphorus levels often parallel those of low potassium. In fact, these electrolytes are often replaced together, in the form of potassium phosphate. See Chapter 8 for a description of hypophosphatemia.)

3. Monitor degree of hyperglycemia and response to insulin therapy.

A. Monitor blood sugar levels closely by use of capillary blood (finger stick) and a blood glucose meter plus regular laboratory determinations. Of course, a fall in the plasma glucose level is the earliest sign of effective therapy.[30] (Recall that blood sugar determinations are much more accurate than urine glucose tests. Renal threshold varies among individuals, increases with age, and may be affected by renal disease.)

B. Monitor administration of insulin-containing IV infusions to prevent too rapid decrease in blood sugar and serum osmalality. (*Cerebral edema* may occur with a too rapid drop in blood sugar. Blood glucose usually falls to a level of at least 300 mg/dL by 4–6 hours, somewhat longer in HHNC.[31] At this point, IV solutions containing dextrose in saline should be used for both fluid replacement and insulin infusion to prevent the development of hypoglycemia.[32] As stated earlier, some clinicians recommend maintaining the serum glucose level at approximately 250 mg/dL for at least 24 hours before allowing it to drop to normal.)

C. Observe the patient closely to prevent occurrence of hypoglycemia, and evaluate serum and urine glucose measurements. (*Hypoglycemia* can be a major complication of therapy. When severe, it may have serious CNS effects and is potentially fatal. Urine dipstick measurements are useful adjuncts to serum glucose monitoring when carefully done on fresh urine in patients with a normal renal threshold. These measurements will not be useful in patients who have neurogenic bladders with urinary retention and overflow. Of course, one should report a rapid drop in blood sugar.)

4. Monitor altered acid–base balance (acidemia) and response to therapy in type I diabetics with DKA.
   A. Monitor serum and urine ketones. (As a result of overproduction and decreased use, ketones build up in the blood and are excreted in the urine.)
   B. Observe rate and depth of respirations. (Extra carbon dioxide is blown off by Kussmaul respirations, which are stimulated by the acidemia and help to bring arterial pH back toward normal. Be alert for a change from deep, rapid respirations to rapid, shallow, gasping breaths. This may indicate a severe drop in blood pH [<7] or impaired flow to the respiratory center because of FVD and circulatory collapse. The patient loses the compensatory action of Kussmaul breathing when this occurs and the acidosis becomes more severe.)
   C. Check for "fruity" breath odor. (This occurs as acetone is excreted from the lungs but may be masked by the odor of vomitus.)
   D. Observe for cherry-red color of skin and mucous membranes. (This is characteristic of DKA due to marked peripheral vasodilation; improvement of skin color indicates response to therapy.)
   E. Observe for signs of decreased cardiac function and arrhythmias. (This constitutes the greatest risk of prolonged, uncontrolled acidosis.)
   F. Monitor blood and urine pH and serum bicarbonate levels. (Plasma pH may fall to 7.25 or below and urine pH falls as kidneys eliminate hydrogen ions in an attempt to correct the acidosis. The serum HCO_3 may fall to 12 mEq/L or lower. An increase in serum bicarbonate to 15–20 mEq/L may be expected within 8–12 hours.)[33]
   G. Assess for presence and characteristics of abdominal pain. (Recall that abdominal pain may occur in DKA and is preceded by nausea and vomiting. Other abdominal emergencies, eg, pancreatitis and surgical abdomen, may coexist with or may have triggered DKA. In these conditions, the pain usually precedes other symptoms.)

5. Use nursing measures to prevent and monitor for other complications that may occur with DKA or HHNC, such as:
   A. Respiratory or urinary tract infections, septic shock, adult respiratory distress syndrome (ARDS)
   B. Thromboembolic complications
   C. Central nervous system deterioration, prolonged coma
   D. Gastrointestinal bleeding
   (These complications have been responsible for deaths in some cases of DKA and HHNC.)

6. Use nursing measures to teach the recovering patient how to prevent recurrences of DKA and HHNC.
   A. Have the patient describe his or her daily routine and demonstrate methods used to carry out the diabetic regimen.[34] This enables one to assess the patient's understanding of the regimen and the degree of accuracy with which procedures such as glucose self-monitoring, meal planning, and insulin administration are being carried out. Some reteaching may be necessary and should be carefully evaluated for effectiveness.)
   B. Review with the patient factors that could disrupt control of diabetes, leading to hyperglycemia and DKA or HHNC. (Many persons with diabetes are not aware of the less obvious precipitating factors. See Table 21-2. The patient should be able to describe the factors and their effect on diabetes control.)
   C. Discuss early symptoms of hyperglycemia with the patient. (Polyuria, polydipsia, polyphagia, fatigue, weakness, blurred vision, and headache should be discussed with the patient as commonly occurring symptoms of poor control.)
   D. Assist the patient to learn a method of testing for elevated serum glucose and ketones. (Self-monitoring of serum glucose with a blood glucose meter is best, but even urine dipstick methods can reveal hyperglycemia greater than the renal threshold. Ketones can also be detected by the dipstick method. The patient should demonstrate testing methods in a simulated or real home setting and should interpret the results accurately.) Instruct the patient to monitor urine ketones anytime the blood glucose level is greater than 240 mg/dL or when illness occurs.
   E. Provide the patient with realistic "sick day instructions" and identify different health care resources for daily routines, in emergencies, and when away from home. (See example of "sick day instructions" in Table 21-6. Stress the importance of keeping regular appointments with the health care provider to prevent loss of control. An "after-hours" phone number to be used in serious or emergency situations should be provided when possible. Instruct the patient, when traveling, to seek help at emergency rooms of medical centers or community hospitals.)
   F. Employ careful and tactful assessment methods

TABLE 21-6.
Sick Day Instructions

1. Contact your physician immediately if you are vomiting and cannot hold down food or liquid or if you have persistent severe diarrhea, fever, or pain.
2. Always take your usual daily dose of insulin or oral hypoglycemic agents. Never omit your medication even if you are unable to eat.
3. Test your urine or blood glucose level every 4 hours (a minimum of four times a day, before each meal and at bedtime, is essential). It is usually preferable to test every 4 hours around the clock, setting an alarm during the night. If you use urine testing, use freshly made samples of urine. If you are feeling too sick to test, ask someone to do it for you.
4. If the urine glucose levels are 1% or higher, or the blood glucose levels are greater than 240 mg/dL, you should also test for urine ketones. Do this when ill from any cause. If ketones are present, along with high glucose levels, you will need extra insulin. Regular (short-acting) insulin should be used. Consult your physician immediately to obtain guidelines for how much regular insulin you should use and how often to take it.
5. Take liquids every hour and refer to the food suggestions for sick days. If you are unable to take liquids because of nausea or vomiting, contact your physician immediately. He or she may prescribe a medication to stop the nausea or vomiting.
6. If you are too ill to follow your usual meal plan, refer to the food suggestions for sick days.
7. Rest and keep warm. Do not exercise. Have someone take care of you.

Food Suggestions for Sick Days

Following are suggestions on how to eat if you do not feel like following your usual eating plan due to illness. Eat and drink whatever your body can tolerate, but you must consume at least 6 to 8 glasses of fluid a day. Take some each hour, alternating fluids with sugar one hour, without sugar the next. Fluids that may be used include

Water	Fruit juices
Tea	Regular (nondietetic) soft drinks
Consommé	Broth made from bouillon cubes

If you cannot drink liquids because of nausea and vomiting, call your physician.

Upon recovery from an illness, food sources of carbohydrate that may be more easily digested include (each portion provides 15 g of carbohydrate, or about one bread exchange)

Apple sauce (sweetened)	½ cup
Apple juice	½ cup
Baked custard	½ cup
Coke syrup	1½ tbl
Cooked cereal	½ cup
Cream soups	1 cup
Eggnog	½ cup
Fruit yogurt	⅓ cup
Frozen yogurt	
on a stick	1 bar
from container	⅓ cup
Grape juice	3 oz
Honey	3 tsp
Hershey's syrup	2 tbl
Life Savers	7
Popsicle (twin-pop)	1
Pudding (sweetened)	¼ cup
Regular ice cream	½ cup
Regular Jello	⅓
Regular soft drinks	¾ cup (6 oz)
Saltine crackers	6
Sherbet	¼ cup
Toast	1 slice

(Adapted from Krall L, Beaser R: Joslin Diabetes Manual, 12th ed, pp 262–264. Philadelphia, Lea & Febiger, 1989.)

to identify cultural and socioeconomic factors that may interfere with maintaining the diabetes regimen.[35]

i. Provide services of a social worker or counselor as indicated.

ii. Review the meal plan with the client and suggest low-cost substitutes when possible.

iii. Identify with the patient less expensive sources of food, equipment, and supplies. (Economic factors such as low income and unemployment, or pressing family needs, may prevent even the most committed patient from maintaining the proper regimen.)

iv. Make sure the meal plan and exercise and medication schedules have been adjusted to the patient's lifestyle and work schedule. (Shift workers and others who have unusual schedules may experience difficulty maintaining control with a "typical" regimen.)

v. Tailor instructional materials to the reading and learning level of the patient. (Functional illiteracy and perceptual learning disabilities are more widespread than is commonly recognized.)

vi. When indicated, include family members or significant others in the education process. (When a family member has diabetes, the whole family must cope with it. Family conflict can interfere with good control. Some patients may need family assistance with certain aspects of the regimen.)

EVALUATION

This important step of the nursing process measures the effectiveness of nursing care for the patient with DKA or HHNC. Evaluation is based on progress made toward short-term and long-term goals.

Short-term goal achievement is demonstrated by:

1. Return of blood sugar to desired levels without any episodes of hypoglycemia
2. Correction of FVD with optimal cardiovascular function and urinary output
3. Electrolyte levels approaching or within normal limits
4. Prevention or correction of complications
5. Prevention of immediate recurrence of DKA or HHNC

Long-term goal achievement is demonstrated by:

1. Control of blood glucose levels within a range appropriate for the individual
2. Prompt intervention when stressors are present that precipitate hyperglycemia

3. Maintenance of general health and activity levels appropriate to the individual

The importance of the nurse's role in the care of the diabetic patient cannot be overemphasized. Skillful use of the nursing process in the care of the patient with DKA or HHNC will contribute greatly to a successful outcome. Equally challenging is the nurse's role as a clinician and health care educator preparing the patient to maintain control of the diabetes in a way that will prevent recurrences of DKA or HHNC and will enable the best possible level of health.

REFERENCES

1. Sperling et al (eds): Diagnosis and classification/ Pathogenesis. Physician's Guide to Insulin-Dependent (Type I) Diabetes: Diagnosis and Treatment, p 3. Alexandria, VA, American Diabetes Association, 1988
2. Israel R: Diabetic ketoacidosis. Emerg Med Clin North Am 7:859, 1989
3. Rifkin et al (eds): Diagnosis and classification of diabetes mellitus. Physician's Guide to Type II Diabetes (NIDDM): Diagnosis and Treatment, p 5, American Diabetes Association, 1984
4. Ibid
5. Olefsky J: Diabetes mellitus. In: Wyngaarden J, Smith L (eds): Cecil's Textbook of Medicine, 18th ed, p 1362. Philadelphia, WB Saunders, 1988
6. Guthrie D, Guthrie R: The disease process of diabetes mellitus. Nurs Clin North Am 18:617, 1983
7. Carroll P, Matz R: Uncontrolled diabetes mellitus in adults: Experience in treating diabetic ketoacidosis and hyperosmolar nonketotic coma with low-dose insulin and a uniform treatment regimen. Diabetes Care 6:579, 1983
8. Grekin R, Tannen R: Ketoacidosis, hyperosmolar states, and lactic acidosis. In: Kokko J, Tannen R (eds): Fluids and Electrolytes, 2nd ed, p 873. Philadelphia, WB Saunders, 1990
9. Matz R: Hyperosmolar nonacidotic uncontrolled diabetes: Not a rare event. Clinical Diabetes 6:30, 1988
10. Pope D, Dansky D: Hyperosmolar hyperglycemic nonketotic coma. Emerg Med Clin North Am 7:854, 1989
11. Martin et al: Effect of hypophosphatemia on myocardial performance in man. New Engl J Med 297:901, 1977
12. Kyner J: Diabetic ketoacidosis. Crit Care Q 10:73, 1980
13. Grekin, Tannen, p 875
14. Park R, Arieff A: Lactic acidosis. Ann Intern Med 23:33, 1980
15. Sypniewski H, Mirtallo J, Schneider P: Hyperosmolar, hyperglycemic, nonketotic coma in a patient receiving home total parenteral nutrient therapy. Clinl Pharm 6:69, 1987

16. Boehm T: Hyperglycemia in critical care medicine. Crit Care Q 6(3):48, 1983
17. Olefsky, p 1377
18. Boehm, p 54
19. Grekin, Tannen, P 884
20. Olefsky, p 1377
21. Levandoski L: Hypoglycemia. In: Guthrie D, Hinnen D, DeShelter E (eds): Diabetes Education: A Core Curriculum for Health Professionals, p 140. Chicago, American Association of Diabetes Educators, 1988
22. Olefsky, p 1376
23. Kitabchi A, Matteri R, Murphy M: Optimal insulin delivery in diabetic ketoacidosis (DKA) and hyperglycemic, hyperosmolar nonketotic coma (HHNK). Diabetes Care 5(1) (Suppl):78, 1982
24. Peterson L, Caldwell J, Hoffman J: Insulin adsorbance to polyvinyl chloride surfaces with implications for constant infusion therapy. Diabetes 25:72, 1976

25. Grekin, Tannen, p 881
26. Carroll, Matz, p 580
27. Ibid
28. Bergenstal R: Diabetic ketoacidosis. Postgrad Med 77:152, 1985
29. Boehm, p 56
30. Olefsky, p 1376
31. Boehm, p 56
32. Moorman N: Acute complications of hyperglycemia and hypoglycemia. Nurs Clin North Am 18:707, 1983
33. Boehm, p 56
34. Macheca M: Educating the hospitalized diabetic: A nurse's responsibility. Current Concepts in Nursing 2(4):15, 1988
35. Resler M: Teaching strategies that promote adherence. Nurs Clin North Am 18:799, 1983

Major Thermal Injuries

Thermal injuries cause a series of major changes in the body's water and electrolyte balances. This chapter explores these changes and their implications for nursing care.

EVALUATION OF BURN SEVERITY

Multiple factors influence the severity of a burn. They include the extent, depth, and cause of the injury, the patient's age, and preexisting medical conditions. Two major factors are the percentage of body surface area involved and the depth of tissue damage. Various terms have been used to describe the depth of burn injury.

First-, second-, and third-degree classifications are commonly used to describe partial-thickness or full-thickness burns. Partial thickness indicates that only a portion of the skin layers (the epidermis and dermis) is damaged; burn depth may vary from superficial to deep. Full-thickness burns extend beyond the epidermis and dermis into the subcutaneous or muscle tissue, and possibly even to the bone.

First-degree burns are typically pink (or darker than the normal skin color), dry, slightly edematous, and painful. No blistering occurs because only the superficial layer of skin, the epidermis, is damaged. This injury depth is normally of little clinical importance because the epidermis, the skin's water vapor barrier, remains intact. First-degree burns are not considered in estimating percentage of body surface area burned or in planning fluid replacement needs.

Second-degree (partial-thickness) burns destroy the epidermis and injure a varying portion of the dermis. This burn depth is characterized by damaged capillaries and the appearance of blisters. The injury may be superficial or deep, depending on the length of exposure and degree of heat; symptoms therefore vary. Generally, second-degree burns are painful, blistered, and reddened with capillary blanching and refilling present. As partial-thickness burns approach destruction of the dermis, their appearance begins to resemble that of third-degree burns. Partial-thickness injuries have some viable skin elements remaining from which epithelial regeneration may occur if the wound is properly managed.

Third-degree (full-thickness) burns go beyond the dermis, destroying all the skin elements. Spontaneous regeneration of the epithelium is impossible, and skin grafting is necessary to close wounds larger than a few centimeters. Third-degree burns are dry, usually without blisters, inelastic (hard and leatherlike), and painless. The color varies from ivory to tan, charred black, or cherry red that will not blanch with pressure, indicating death of the capillary bed.

The rule of nines is commonly used by emergency personnel to estimate the percentage of body surface area (BSA) burned. This method divides the body's surface into areas equal to 9% or multiples of 9%. The portion of these areas that have sustained either second- or third-degree burns is determined. This calculation's total represents the percentage of total body surface area (TBSA) burned. The rule of nines is only a rough estimate and, unless used cautiously, a dangerously high calculation of the adult's TBSA burned can result. Because there is a significant change in the BSA of the head, thigh, and leg from infancy through adulthood, this method is extremely inaccurate for use with children. A detailed breakdown of the BSA will contribute to a more complete and accurate estimate of the TBSA burned, yielding a more accurate assessment of fluid needs. More specific charts focusing on the body areas affected by growth are widely available (such as the one shown in Fig. 22-1) and should be used to assess the percentage of BSA burned properly.

Factors other than depth and percentage of surface area must be considered when determining the burn severity. Burns become more serious in the presence of existing medical conditions such as renal, cardiac, or metabolic disorders; when there is associated trauma; when they occur in areas difficult to treat, such as the face, hands, feet or perineum; and when they occur in the very young and the elderly.

The American Burn Association has defined major burns as follows:

1. Second-degree burns covering more than 25% of the BSA in an adult, or more than 20% in a child
2. Third-degree burns covering more than 10% of the BSA in any age
3. Burns of "special areas" (the hands, face, eyes, ears, feet, or perineum)
4. Inhalation injuries
5. Electrical burns
6. Burn injuries complicated by fractures or other major trauma
7. All burns in poor-risk patients (children younger than 2 years and adults older than 60 years, as well as those individuals with preexisting medical conditions)

SUMMARY OF WATER AND ELECTROLYTE CHANGES AFTER BURN TRAUMA

The primary water and electrolyte changes occurring in patients with major burn trauma are given in Table 22-1. Most imbalances are time related, according to the burn phase. Other factors affecting fluid and electrolyte balance are directly related to treatment methods for the burns. The nurse should be aware of the potential water and electrolyte changes in burn patients so that significant clinical signs can be readily recognized and appropriate interventions promptly initiated.

NURSING MANAGEMENT

Care of the burned patient is complex and requires a high level of skill in both the physiological and psychosocial domains. Promoting independence, maintaining functional joints, and fostering a positive psychological outlook for both the patient and family are additional major challenges to the nurse. Much effort must be devoted to maximizing the quality of life after the acute phase of the burn injury. Obviously, a complete picture of what is required for burn care is far more complex than the scope of this chapter allows. That chapter's purpose is to explore the major fluid and electrolyte-related alterations in the major phases of burn injury from a nursing perspective.

It is helpful at this point to consider pertinent nursing diagnoses related to fluid and electrolyte balance. See Table 22-2 for examples of fluid balance-related nursing diagnoses for patients with major thermal

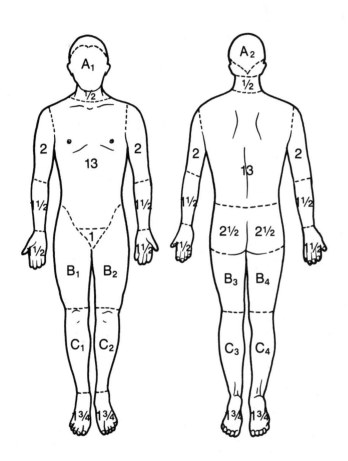

	ANTERIOR	POSTERIOR
HEAD	A_1 _____	A_2 _____
NECK	_____	_____
RT. ARM	_____	_____
RT. FOREARM	_____	_____
RT. HAND	_____	_____
LT. ARM	_____	_____
LT. FOREARM	_____	_____
LT. HAND	_____	_____
TRUNK	_____	_____
BUTTOCK	(L) _____	(R) _____
PERINEUM	_____	_____
RT. THIGH	B_1 _____	B_4 _____
RT. LEG	C_1 _____	C_4 _____
RT. FOOT	_____	_____
LT. THIGH	B_2 _____	B_3 _____
LT. LEG	C_2 _____	C_3 _____
LT. FOOT	_____	_____

▨ PARTIAL THICKNESS_____

■ FULL THICKNESS_____

TOTAL %_____

DATE OF BURN_____

DATE OF DIAGRAM_____

SIGNATURE_____

PERCENT OF AREAS AFFECTED BY GROWTH:			
AGE	A = ½ Head	B = ½ One Thigh	C = ½ One Leg
0	9½	2¾	2½
1	8½	3¼	2½
5	6½	4	2¾
10	5½	4¼	3
15	4½	4½	3¼
Adult	3½	4¾	3½

FIGURE 22–1.
Calculation of amount of skin surface involved in burns.

TABLE 22–1.
Some Possible Water and Electrolyte Changes in Burned Patients

IMBALANCE	COMMENTS

THIRD-SPACE FLUID SHIFTS

Phase I: fluid accumulation phase
(first 36–48 hours postburn)
- Plasma-to-interstitial fluid shift
  - Hypovolemia
  - Edema at burn site (maximal speed of edema formation is reached in first 6–8 hours)

Plasma leaks out through the damaged capillaries at the burn site; edema forms at expense of the circulating blood volume, causing hypovolemia

Decreased urinary output, secondary to decreased renal perfusion after hypovolemia; contributing factor is renal retention of sodium and water in response to stress hormones (aldosterone and ADH); more serious cause is oliguric renal failure due to ATN

Elevated hematocrit may be present and reflects the relatively greater loss of plasma than red blood cells at the site of injury

Phase II: fluid remobilization phase (diuresis stage)
(starts approximately 48 hours postburn)
- Interstitial-to-plasma fluid shift
  - Hypervolemia (if excessive IV fluids administered)
  - Edema at burn site begins to resolve

Fluid shifts back into the intravascular compartment as edema fluid is reabsorbed

Increased urine formation follows the shift of fluid back into the intravascular compartment

Potential for dangerous hypervolemia exists if IV fluid administration is not cutback appropriately

Hemodilution after shift of fluid from the burn site into intravascular compartment causing the hematocrit to decrease (A decreased hematocrit may also reflect actual anemia due to red blood cell destruction at the burn site.)

POTASSIUM IMBALANCES

Tendency toward hyperkalemia (in early postburn period)

Massive cellular trauma (hemolysis and tissue necrosis) releases intracellular potassium into the bloodstream (This process is especially severe in rhabdomyolysis associated with electrical and incineration injuries.)

Contributing to tendency for hyperkalemia is reduced renal excretion of potassium in fluid accumulation phase

Hypokalemia

Possible causes
- Increased renal excretion of potassium associated with high aldosterone level (stress reaction)
- Inadequate dietary intake or pharmacological supplementation to replace losses incurred during diuresis
- Increased renal potassium wasting associated with use of certain antibiotics (such as sodium penicillin) to treat infection

SODIUM IMBALANCES

Hyponatremia

Possible causes
- Excessive free water intake (seen more commonly in children and can be severe enough to produce convulsions)
- Use of aqueous silver nitrate dressings (allows water absorption from burn site with dilutional hyponatremia)
- Loss of sodium during hydrotherapy (in addition to absorption of water from whirlpool treatment)
- Loss of sodium in urine during diuresis phase

Hypernatremia

Possible causes
- Inadequate free water intake to replace water vapor loss
- Overzealous administration of hypertonic sodium solutions

(continued)

TABLE 22–1.
(continued)

IMBALANCE	COMMENTS
ACID–BASE DISTURBANCES	
Metabolic acidosis	**Possible causes**
	▶ Develops within few hours due to accumulation of fixed acids released from injured tissues
	▶ Can also be associated with ineffective tissue perfusion
	▶ Can be a side effect of mafenide acetate (Sulfamylon) use as a topical burn agent
Respiratory acidosis	Inhalation burns can traumatize pulmonary tissue sufficiently to interfere with gas exchange
OTHER IMBALANCES	
Hypocalcemia	**Possible causes**
	▶ Hypoalbuminemia (total serum calcium level appears lower than it actually is due to reduced binding of calcium to albumin); if this is only cause for hypocalcemia, ionized calcium fraction will likely be normal
	▶ Actual decrease in serum calcium level may occur due to sequestration of calcium in the burned tissues
	▶ Inadequate dietary intake or inadequate pharmacological supplementation
Hypomagnesemia	**Possible causes**
	▶ Inadequate dietary intake or supplementation of this cellular electrolyte, particularly during anabolic phase
	▶ Possibly related to loss of magnesium during debridement and bathing of denuded tissue
	▶ Use of aminoglycoside antibiotics (such as gentamycin) can cause renal magnesium wasting
	▶ See Chapter 7
Hypophosphatemia	**Possible causes**
	▶ Inadequate dietary intake or pharmacological supplementation to replace losses incurred during catabolism
	▶ Excessive use of phosphate-binding antacids (to prevent gastric bleeding associated with hyperacidity)
	▶ See Chapter 8

ADH, antidiuretic hormone; ATN, acute tubular necrosis.

burns. These examples help demonstrate that nursing care during the acute phase of burn care must be adapted to often rapidly changing physiological states.

Depending on the part of the body burned and the severity of the injury, the following nursing diagnoses should also be considered when analyzing assessment data:

▶ Potential for infection (at the burn site or associated with any invasive procedures required)
▶ Pain (varies with type of burn)
▶ Disturbance in body image (may occur even with small burn areas)
▶ Impaired mobility (depending on site and severity of burns)
▶ Self-care deficit (depending on site and severity of burns)

▶ Ineffective individual coping
▶ Ineffective family coping

FLUID ACCUMULATION PHASE

Effective care of the burned patient depends on the health care team's knowledge of the physiological changes caused by the injury and on their collaborative ability to define accurately the priorities of care, make appropriate treatment choices, execute the plan, and maintain an ongoing evaluation of results.

Physiological Changes and Need for Early Interventions

Shift of fluid from the plasma to the interstitial space (third-space shift) is rapid and well under way by the

TABLE 22–2.
Examples of Nursing Diagnoses for Patients with Major Thermal Burns

NURSING DIAGNOSIS	ETIOLOGICAL FACTORS	DEFINING CHARACTERISTICS
Fluid volume deficit (intravascular) related to third-space fluid shift from vascular compartment to burn site (during first 36–48 hrs)	Plasma leakage through damaged capillaries at burn site, results in decreased circulating blood volume	Tachycardia Hypotension Decreased urinary output Decreased CVP and PCWP
Fluid volume excess (intravascular) related to fluid shift from interstitium to vascular space (about 48 hours postburn)	Edema fluid at burn site shifts back into vascular compartment as injured capillaries heal Aggravated by excessive fluid administration	Venous distention Hypertension If pulmonary edema is present: ▶ Shortness of breath ▶ Moist crackles ▶ Coughing of frothy sputum ▶ Cyanosis
Decreased tissue perfusion related to edema at burn site	Edema at burn site constricts peripheral circulation	Decreased distal pulse in burned extremity (as assessed by Doppler scan if necessary), since overlying soft tissue may prevent palpation of pulses Decreased sensation and motor function of affected extremity
Alteration in potassium balance (hyperkalemia) in early burn phase related to release of cellular potassium from traumatized tissue	Massive cellular trauma (hemolysis and tissue necrosis) releases intracellular potassium into bloodstream Intensified by poor renal excretion of potassium during oliguric phase	Ventricular arrhythmias Tall, peaked T waves Vague muscular weakness Paresthesias, flaccid muscles Nausea Serum $K^+ > 5.0$ mEq/L Often associated with acidosis
Impaired gas exchange related to inhalation injury from carbon monoxide poisoning	Altered oxygen-carrying capacity of blood related to affinity of carbon monoxide for hemoglobin	Signs of CO poisoning: cherry-red skin color, hypoxia, severe tachypnea, or respiratory arrest Hypoxemia, hypercapnia, confusion, restlessness

CVP, central venous pressure; PCWP, pulmonary capillary wedge pressure.

end of the first hour. The maximal speed of edema formation is reached during the first 6 to 8 hours; the shift continues until 36 to 48 hours post-burn. By this time, the injured capillaries have recovered sufficiently to control further fluid loss. The decreased plasma volume can lead to rapidly forming hypovolemic shock and renal depression caused by decreased renal blood flow unless quickly corrected by fluid replacement therapy. Oliguria or anuria can be particularly threatening during this phase because of the excessive amounts of potassium flooding the extracellular fluid (ECF). Because potassium is mainly excreted in the urine, decreased urinary output causes a dangerous buildup in the bloodstream. The sodium deficit requires prompt attention as does the acidosis so frequently found. Acute tubular necrosis may result from the hypovolemia of burn shock or the hemoglobinuria or myoglobinuria associated with unusually deep tissue damage. This is an entirely preventable complication with fluid replacement sufficient to keep the urine output at 0.5 to 1.0 mL/kg of body weight/hr. In the presence of severe hemoglobinuria or myoglobinuria, as is seen in major electrical injuries, careful administration of mannitol may be needed to flush out the tubules.

Initial Assessment and Interventions

When the burn victim first arrives in the emergency department, the main priorities of care must be to:

▶ Stop further damage to the skin
▶ Perform a systematic, thorough assessment while obtaining a detailed medical history and account of the burn accident
▶ Attend to the priorities of airway, breathing, and circulation
▶ Evaluate the burn wound while protecting it from further harm
▶ Provide emotional support

All of these factors deserve immediate attention and are often performed concurrently during the emergency treatment. They will be discussed together.

Stopping the damage to the skin includes removing all clothing and jewelry that could retain heat or cause constriction. Chemicals must be carefully irrigated from the skin. Melted products, such as tar, should be cooled and gently removed. Damaged tissue may be cooled using room-temperature normal saline solution; however, to avoid chilling the patient, provide warm, dry blankets and increase the room temperature as necessary. Remember that, when the body's natural barrier against heat and water loss is damaged, there will be increased heat and water vapor loss. Hypothermia can readily occur and must be guarded against because it will worsen the hypovolemia of the burn shock. Ideally, the room temperature should be between 82° and 87° F (28° to 31° C). Shivering increases the rate of metabolism, causing increased loss of water from the body. Maintaining an environment saturated with water vapor decreases the transcutaneous water loss; for example, wounds covered with dressings of aqueous topical agents and dry covers lose only half the amount of water vapor lost through exposed wounds.

The priorities of airway, breathing, and circulation are of vital importance, not only initially, but throughout the shock (fluid accumulation) phase. Be aware that edema can compromise the airway and breathing, as can inhalation injury caused by smoke or other inhaled toxins. Peripheral circulation in burned limbs must be evaluated. Fluid resuscitation to maintain the circulating blood volume is discussed later in this section.

Assessment of and Interventions for Inhalation Injury

A positive history (being trapped in or exposed to a smoke- or fume-filled closed space) may be the most important diagnostic clue to inhalation injury. Without the history, positive signs and symptoms include burns of the face and neck, any burn from the waist up, or any major thermal burn. Singed facial or nasal hair or carbon present in the nares or oropharynx is suggestive of inhalation injury. Carbon in the sputum is nearly always a positive sign. Oxygen must be started while further assessment is made. Carbon monoxide (CO) poisoning, thermal injury to the upper airway, and inhalation of poisonous toxins are three distinct components of the inhalation injury.

If the burn victim was exposed to smoke for a prolonged period, CO poisoning may result. Carbon monoxide is a colorless, odorless gas with an affinity for he-

moglobin molecules that is 200 times greater than that of oxygen. A cherry-red skin color is characteristic of carbon monoxide poisoning. Hypoxia may cause symptoms ranging from severe tachypnea to respiratory arrest. If suspected, the patient is started on 100% oxygen until the carboxyhemoglobin level in the blood is obtained. Ventilatory support may be needed.

True burns of the lower respiratory tract and lung tissue are rare. Most heat is lost in the nasopharynx and upper airway. Upper airway distress may occur with or without smoke poisoning. The response to heat injury involves swelling of the nasopharyngeal mucous membranes. Inspection of the mouth and pharynx is necessary in any patient with facial burns; if abnormal, the larynx must be examined. Intraoral and pharyngeal burns are indications for prophylactic placement of an endotracheal tube. Progressive edema may make later intubation dangerous or impossible. The tube remains until the edema subsides.

Circumferential third-degree burns of the neck and chest may contribute to respiratory distress as the inelastic burn tissue begins to tighten from the formation of underlying edema fluid. Pressure develops over the trachea, while chest and diaphragm movements are hindered. The patient begins to develop hoarseness, stridor, dyspnea, restlessness, and air hunger. Escharotomies (incisions made through the burn tissue) may be the only intervention needed to relieve this constriction.

Inhalation injury due to smoke poisoning usually appears within the first 24 to 48 hours after the burn. It is caused by inhaling the toxic products of combustion. Signs and symptoms may be present initially and can include increased mucous production, carbonaceous sputum, hoarseness, hacking cough, labored or rapid breathing, rales, rhonchi, wheezing, air hunger, or stridor. The patient may be restless, irrational, or unconscious, depending on the degree of hypoxia.

After the inhalation injury there is immediate loss of the bronchial epithelial cilia and decreased alveolar surfactant. Microatelectasis or macroatelectasis may result and is compounded by mucosal swelling in the small airways. In a few hours, tracheobronchitis develops. As the disease worsens, interstitial edema develops, resulting in the adult respiratory distress syndrome (ARDS). Later, bacterial pneumonia frequently develops. Patients with inhalation injury usually need endotracheal intubation and ventilatory support. A tracheostomy should not be done for emergency treatment.

Supplying highly humidified air, maintaining vigorous pulmonary toilet, elevating the head of the bed unless contraindicated, encouraging deep breathing, and turning the patient often are all important. Another part of the treatment is use of bronchodilators and monitoring of arterial blood gas analyses. Severe cases of inhalation injury may require the use of a Swan-Ganz catheter and cardiac output determinations to determine the adequacy of fluid resuscitation. Underresuscitation with fluids may be more detrimental than adequate or even overresuscitation.

Prophylactic antibiotics are not of value in treating chemical pneumonitis. Burn wound management and treatment of eventual bacterial pneumonias will be more difficult if resistant organisms develop from indiscriminate use of antibiotics.

Assessment of and Interventions for Burn Shock

Hypovolemia of burn shock must be detected and offset with replacement fluids as soon as possible. A delay in fluid resuscitation can severely complicate the patient's recovery or even result in an irreversible situation. Remember that a delay has already occurred at the scene of the accident. Hypovolemic shock may be well advanced when the patient arrives in the emergency department.

Symptoms of burn shock can include the following:

1. Extreme thirst caused by generalized cellular dehydration
2. Increasing restlessness; persistent slight to moderate restlessness may be due to apprehension and discomfort produced by the burn rather than to inadequate fluid resuscitation
3. Sudden high pulse rate; heart beats faster to compensate for decreased blood volume
4. Respiratory rate is often increased, but character of breathing should be normal unless there are complicating factors
5. Blood pressure either normal or low; the supine burned patient can often tolerate a large fluid volume deficit with little or no change in blood pressure, however, on sitting or standing, hypotension and even syncope may occur. Thus, the badly burned patient should be left supine until hemodynamically stable.)
6. Cool, pale skin in unburned areas is indicative of cutaneous vasoconstriction, a compensatory mechanism that helps preserve normal blood flow
7. Oliguria due to decreased renal blood flow and increased levels of aldosterone and antidiuretic hormone (ADH)
8. Delerium or coma, presumably due to inadequate cerebral blood flow and are serious signs
9. Seizures possibly due to cerebral ischemia

Intravenous (IV) fluids are lifesaving in the treatment of moderate and severe burns; they must be started promptly to prevent or correct the onset and advancement of shock. As a rule, any patient with more than 20% BSA burned will develop some degree of burn shock; children younger than 2 years and adults older than 60 years may need fluid replacement with only 10% to 15% of BSA burned.

An indwelling urinary catheter is inserted when the burn involves more than 20% of the BSA. The catheter is connected to a device for hourly measurement of urine flow. The discard specimen should be saved for an admission urine analysis. If there is bloody discoloration of the urine, a fresh sample should be sent for hemoglobin and myoglobin analysis. With deep full-thickness burns, red blood cell hemolysis at the site occurs, causing the release of hemoglobin. If muscle was destroyed, myoglobin is also released into the bloodstream. Both products are filtered out by the kidneys and may be potential threats to the already compromised renal function.

The aim of early fluid therapy is to give the least amount of fluid necessary to maintain the desired urinary output and keep the patient relatively free of burn shock symptoms. Consideration must be given to the insertion site of the IV lines. A high flow rate will be necessary; to provide for this, one large-bore cannula may be inserted for burns less than 40% BSA, and two large-bore cannulas for burns exceeding 40% BSA. Remember that infection rates are high with all central lines, and pneumothorax is associated with use of subclavian lines. Suppurative thrombophlebitis often accompanies IV cutdowns.

Intravenous Fluids

Physicians vary widely in their opinions about the IV fluids to be used in burn treatment. Many resuscitation formulas have been developed over the years to guide initial treatment. These formulas use a combination of crystalloids and colloids but differ greatly in the ratio prescribed. It is generally agreed, however, that the keystone of therapy is sodium. The optimal sodium concentration for resuscitation of burn shock is not known and is probably not an absolute value; both hyponatremia and hypernatremia must be avoided. Many physicians favor beginning treatment with a balanced salt solution, such as lactated Ringer's (LR) solution. It not only supplies sodium and water but helps correct the metabolic acidosis associated with burns: 1 L of LR contains 130 mEq of lactate (a bicarbonate precursor). Lactated Ringer's solution is similar in composition to the lost intravascular fluid. Less commonly used is isotonic saline (0.9% NaCl), which supplies 154 mEq/L of sodium and 154 mEq/L of chloride. It has the disadvantage of supplying an excessive amount of chloride ions, which contribute to metabolic acidosis. Both LR and 0.9% NaCl solutions are economical and readily available. A major disadvantage with each is increased edema formation.

Hypertonic crystalloid solutions were introduced to decrease the fluid volume needed to correct burn shock and thereby minimize edema formation. One L of hypertonic lactated saline (HLS) solution contains 250 mEq of sodium, 100 mEq of lactate, and 150 mEq of chloride; it supplies sodium in a minimal fluid volume, causing a sustained hypernatremia and increase in serum osmolality. Proponents of this therapy believe that it is associated with less tissue edema, and fewer pulmonary complications, making its use beneficial in inhalation injuries, circumferential burns or intracranial injuries. Many authors demonstrated that patients can be resuscitated adequately using 50% to 75% of the volume required with isotonic electrolyte fluids. However, patients resuscitated with HLS require careful observation for hypernatremia and hyperosmolality, as well as for alkalosis.

Use of colloids (plasma or plasma substitutes) remains controversial. Those physicians advocating colloids argue that plasma or related substances must be given to replace the plasma leaked through injured capillaries into the burn site. In addition, they believe that excessive administration of salt solutions (such as LR) further contributes to the hypoproteinemia by dilution effect, and that the decrease in colloidal pressure adds to the edema formation by favoring shifting of fluid from the vascular into the interstitial space. Fortunately, repair of the protein leak at the burn site occurs within 12 to 24 hours after the burn injury. Other considerations regarding crystalloid versus colloid use in resuscitation are discussed in Chapter 11.

Although many physicians incorporate colloids into the fluid regimen, the exact timing of their use cannot be rigidly set. In general, they are prescribed after the first 24 hours of fluid therapy. Plasma contains sodium and thus helps correct sodium deficit. However, use of plasma is associated with a high risk of serum hepatitis and other viral disease. Another frequently used colloid in burn treatment is albumin. Nonprotein colloids, such as dextran and hetastarch, have molecular size and increased oncotic pressure to maintain blood volume and cardiac output by borrowing water from the interstitial space of nonburned tissue.

Blood is usually not included in burn fluid therapy unless the patient has incurred blood loss from an associated injury; it should be given if the hematocrit is less than 30%.

A nonelectrolyte solution, usually 5% dextrose in water, may be used to replace the normal insensible water loss and the increased transcutaneous water vapor loss associated with damage to the skin barrier. Although free water is lost from the burn site, it is generally not replaced in the first 24 hours of treatment. During this early phase, water contributes little to the maintenance of normal cardiovascular function.

FORMULAS   Whenever IV fluids are given there is a danger of administering too much or not enough; both hazards are always present in burn therapy. Fluid requirements for the first 24 hours after injury vary from 2 to 4 mL/kg of body weight/percent of BSA burned. The exact amount depends on the type of fluid used, the age of the patient, the size and depth of the burn, and complicating factors such as inhalation injury, electrical burns, or multiple trauma. Fluids should be delivered at a constant rate avoiding fluid challenges. Prolonged tissue hypoperfusion and acidosis may require larger total fluid volumes be given. The ideal infusion rate maintains adequate perfusion, as reflected by a minimum urine output of 0.5 mL/kg of body weight per hour in the adult. Both crystalloid and colloid solutions have been shown to be effective; treatment choices should be individualized according to the needs of the patient and close monitoring of overall clinical response. To provide a guide for the amount of fluids needed by burn patients, numerous formulas have been devised (see Table 22-3).

MONITORING THERAPY   It is essential to remember that any formula serves only as a guide because there are many variations among individual patients; frequent clinical assessment is mandatory to allow adequate tailoring of fluid replacement to individual needs. There are many physiological parameters that can be observed. Recall that the burn patient also is immunocompromised after the skin destruction; any invasive procedure will bring an increased chance for sepsis.

Successful fluid resuscitation of the burned patient is signaled by the following:

▶ Adequate urine volume
▶ Normal sensorium
▶ Near-normal vital signs
▶ Normal central venous pressure (CVP)

Urine Volume: Hourly urine volume (collected by means of a Foley catheter) is generally considered the best clinical sign for the adequacy of fluid resuscitation. The ideal range is believed to be 30 to 50 mL per hour adults and 1.0 mL/kg of body weight per hour for children weighing less than 30 kg. Commercial devices are available for measuring small urine volumes; *any* error can be significant. Absent or decreased urinary output can be due to inadequate fluid replacement, gastric dilatation, or renal failure. Remember that a clogged catheter may falsely indicate oliguria. Patency of the catheter should be checked before assuming

TABLE 22–3.
Formulas for Fluid Replacement/Resuscitation

	FIRST 24 HOURS			SECOND 24 HOURS		
	ELECTROLYTE	COLLOID	GLUCOSE IN WATER	ELECTROLYTE	COLLOID	GLUCOSE IN WATER
Burn budget of F. D. Moore	1000–4000 mL lactated Ringer's solution and 1200 mL 0.5N saline	7.5% of body weight	1500–5000 mL	1000–4000 mL lactated Ringer's solution and 1200 mL 0.5N saline	2.5% of body weight	1500–5000 mL
Evans	Normal saline, 1mL/kg/% burn	1.0 mL/kg/% burn	2000 mL	One half of first 24-hr requirement	One half of first 24-hr requirement	2000 mL
Brooke	Lactated Ringer's solution, 1.5 mL/kg/% burn	0.5 mL/kg/% burn	2000 mL	One half to three quarters of first 24-hr requirement	One half to three quarters of first 24-hr requirement	2000 mL
Parkland	Lactated Ringer's solution, 4 mL/kg/% burn				20–60% of calculated plasma volume	
Hypertonic sodium solution	Volume to maintain urine output at 30 mL/hr (fluid contains 250 mEq Na/L)			One third of salt solution orally, up to 3500 mL limit		
Modified Brooke	Lactated Ringer's solution, 2 mL/kg/% burn				0.3–0.5 mL/kg/% burn	Goal: maintain adequate urinary output
Burnett Burn Center	Isotonic or hypertonic alkaline sodium solution/% burn/kg			D_5 1/4 NS maintenance	Colloid 0.5 mL/% burn/kg	D_5W (% burn) (TBSAm^2)

(Hudak C, Gallo B, Benz J. Critical Care Nursing, 5th ed, p 766. Philadelphia, JB Lippincott, 1990; with permission.)

oliguria is present. Extreme care should be taken to record accurately the amount of fluid instilled as an irrigant and the amount of fluid removed. If the oliguria is due to inadequate fluid replacement, the urine volume will increase when the fluid flow rate is increased. If it is due to renal failure, the output will remain small. In addition to oliguria, acute renal failure will manifest with a urine of low osmolality. Fortunately, unless access to therapy is delayed, initial resuscitation should virtually eliminate oliguric renal failure. However, it should be noted that patients who have suffered a hypovolemic insult from burns (not sufficient to produce acute tubular necrosis) may develop transient *polyuric* renal failure.

The physician should indicate the desired urinary volume plus the variations in either direction to be reported. The desired urinary volume should be realistic and approximate the minimum, not the maximum. Attempts to increase fluid input sufficiently to cause large urine volumes in the aged or the very young are dangerous.

Accurate recording of intake and output (I&O) is necessary for assessing the patient's fluid balance status during burn treatment. Daily weights are also an important tool for monitoring the amount of retained edema fluid. In patients with severe burns, a weight gain of 15% to 20% is likely during the initial resuscitation period. The body weight probably will return to the preburn level by the tenth postburn day if fluid management has been handled properly.

Sensorium: The patient's sensorium must be assessed frequently as the adequacy of tissue perfusion is measured. Is he or she alert and lucid? Does he or she respond in a normal fashion? With adequate fluid replacement, sensorium should remain normal unless precluded by other factors, such as head injury, drug intoxication, or CO poisoning.

Vital Signs: Vital signs should be taken at least hourly in the newly burned patient. Blood pressure should be near normal; as a general guideline, a systolic pressure less than 100 mmHg or greater than 200 mmHg should be reported to the physician. The patient's baseline "normal" blood pressure must be considered when evaluating his current status. The cuff must fit properly; if sound is muffled by peripheral edema, an ultrasonic Doppler scan may be helpful.

Temperature is usually slightly elevated in the burned patient; as a general guideline, a reading greater than 101.5° F (38.6 ° C) should be reported to the physician. Lower than normal temperatures may indicate excessive loss of body heat or sepsis and also must be reported.

Tachycardia is common in the first few hours after burn but should decrease to the upper limits of normal with fluid replacement. A sustained pulse greater than 160/min or less than 60/min should be brought to the physician's attention.

Cardiac monitoring may be necessary in the presence of large burns to detect arrhythmias resulting from hypoxia, hypovolemia, acidosis, or electrolyte imbalances. Electrical injury, associated trauma, or underlying medical conditions will also necessitate cardiac monitoring. If there is no unburned skin available for attaching the electrodes, they may be applied over the topical agent and secured in place by the burn dressings.

The rate and character of respirations must be carefully observed and auscultated. Serial arterial blood gas sampling and chest radiographs will be necessary in suspected cases of inhalation injury or associated problems. As edema forms, escharotomies may be necessary to release inelastic burn tissue surrounding the chest wall (limiting respirations).

Circulatory Checks: Peripheral pulses in the burned extremities should be checked every few hours, or hourly if circumferential burns are present. Overlying soft-tissue edema may prevent palpation of underlying arteries; if so, an ultrasonic Doppler scan is indicated. If arterial pulses become diminished, escharotomies may be needed to restore circulation in the limb. In addition to pulses, sensory-motor function should be noted. A pulse oximeter is also helpful in monitoring oxygenation of the extremity.

Capillary refill time of unburned skin should be carefully observed. Warm, pink skin that displays a normal capillary filling time after blanching is a sign of intact circulation and adequate oxygenation. Remember that vasoconstriction of unburned skin is a normal compensatory response to help preserve normal blood flow in the early hours after a severe burn, causing unburned skin to be cool and pale during this period. The nailbeds are good sites for observing capillary refill time.

Invasive Monitoring: Careful consideration is necessary before initiating invasive monitoring in previously healthy patients. As a result of burn injury, the patient's immunological responses are severely hampered and the presence of any indwelling lines are likely to result in sepsis.

Arterial and CVP monitoring are the simplest forms of invasive monitoring. Arterial pressure monitoring is often needed when the patient remains hypotensive or hypertensive and IV vasoactive drugs are required; they are also used when oxygenation problems exist.

Central venous pressure measurements can be obtained from any central line; the readings should remain within normal limits in the adequately resuscitated patient. Central venous pressure measurements are frequently used to monitor the effects of IV fluid replacement therapy, particularly in infants, the aged, and patients with cardiac and renal disease. A CVP line is generally indicated when the burned surface is greater than 50% or 60%. Frequent checks of venous pressure allow more aggressive fluid replacement without the risk of circulatory overload. Normal venous pressure is from 4 to 10 cm of water, and a level of 15 to 20 cm represents a significant elevation. When venous pressure becomes elevated above a point designated by the physician, the fluid infusion rate should be curtailed. If the patient is responding poorly to fluid replacement therapy, a Swan-Ganz catheter should be considered to measure pulmonary artery pressure, wedge pressure, and cardiac output.

In summary, the nurse must be alert for symptoms of inadequate or excessive fluid administration. Inadequate fluid therapy in burned patients is indicated by the following:

▶ Decreased urinary output
▶ Thirst
▶ Restlessness and disorientation
▶ Hypotension and increased pulse rate

The following are indicative of circulatory overload:

▶ Elevated CVP
▶ Shortness of breath
▶ Moist crackles

Assessment of and Interventions for Gastrointestinal Complications

Gastric dilatation resulting from stress is common in burned patients. When present, fluids taken orally become trapped in the distended stomach. Thus, although oral fluids are swallowed, they are not available for the body's use or for urine formation.

Reflex paralytic ileus will usually develop some time during the first 24 hours postburn in most patients with 20% BSA burned, even if there were active bowel sounds as long as 6 to 10 hours after the injury. Usual symptoms include nausea, effortless vomiting, hiccoughing, and abdominal distention. Vomiting carries a high risk of tracheal aspiration and must be prevented. Some physicians favor placing a nasogastric tube in all patients with major burns to decompress the stomach until normal bowel sounds have returned. Another purpose of inserting a nasogastric tube is to allow for observation of gastric secretions. Patients with major burns are at risk for hemorrhagic gastritis due to stress. Bleeding from the stomach may be visible in gastric secretions or, if a slow ooze is present, it may

be manifested by guaiac-positive stools and a gradual decrease in hematocrit. Gastric aspirates should be observed frequently for signs of bleeding; in addition, gastric pH can be monitored. Antacids may be added at hourly intervals to deter superficial erosions of the gastric mucosa. A common practice is to add an ounce of antacid through the tube every hour and clamp the tube for 30-minute intervals. The incidence of Curling's ulcer, a once common burn complication, has markedly diminished due to the use of antacids, enteral feedings, and H_2 receptor antagonists when needed.

The presence of abdominal distention after the first few days post burn may indicate the presence of invasive wound sepsis as ileus commonly occurs with this condition. Ileus due to wound sepsis may be associated with gastroduodenal perforation. Again, the prophylactic use of antacids and improved nutritional support (allowing for quicker healing of small eroded areas and overall improved general condition) have reduced the frequency of major wound sepsis and therefore the incidence of gastroduodenal ulcers.

Assessment of and Interventions for Pain

The amount of pain present varies with the depth of the burn, the extent of the surface area involved, and the patient's pain threshold. Third-degree (full-thickness) burns are technically painless because the nerve endings are destroyed; however, pain is experienced around the periphery where first- and second-degree burns are present. As a rule, the requirement for analgesics is inversely proportional to the depth of the initial injury.

After 48 hours, the requirements for analgesics are greatly diminished, except when wounds are being actively debrided or joint range-of-motion exercises are being carried out. Burned patients complaining of severe pain may be given small doses of meperidine or morphine sulfate through the IV cannula placed for fluid administration. Fluid resuscitation should be underway before analgesics are administered. The IV route assures rapid and dependable concentrations of the drug in the central nervous system. The subcutaneous or intramuscular route should not be used to administer narcotics to a burned patient with circulatory impairment. Peripheral tissue perfusion is erratic when shock is present; thus, absorption of the drug may not occur or may be delayed. Failure to achieve the desired effect may prompt repeated doses by the same route. When peripheral circulation is improved with fluid administration, there may be a rapid absorption and cumulative overdosage of the narcotic, resulting in respiratory narcosis and depression.

Do not confuse the restlessness of burn shock

with pain. A patient thrashing about in bed without complaining of pain may well be in burn shock, in which case a narcotic is contraindicated. Rather, an increased rate of parenteral fluid administration is usually indicated.

Assessment of and Intervention for Disrupted Skin Integrity

Assessment of initial skin changes caused by burns was addressed earlier in the chapter. However, assessment of skin changes must continue as secondary infection can increase injury to the skin.

A loss of antibacterial protection occurs due to disruption in skin integrity caused by burn injury. As a result, burn wound infection poses a great threat to the thermally injured patient. There is no perfect topical antibacterial agent available for use on the burn wound. A number of agents may be applied locally to burn wounds to prevent or control infection. Those frequently used include silver sulfadiazine (Silvadene), mafenide acetate (Sulfamylon), 0.5% silver nitrate solution, and 10% povidone-iodine, as well as a growing number of temporary biological and synthetic skin substitutes. These local agents are often effective in controlling infection while permitting healing. They may, in varying degrees, alter body fluid and electrolyte balance, or result in undesirable side effects and complications. For example, mafenide acetate (Sulfamylon) is a carbonic anhydrase inhibitor that leads to increased bicarbonate wasting and, thus, to metabolic acidosis. Silver nitrate must be applied as a 0.5% aqueous solution; accordingly, water may be absorbed from the dressing site, possibly causing electrolyte abnormalities (primarily hyponatremia). In addition, hypochloremia may result when silver binds with chloride and precipitates as silver chloride within the burn tissues. Thus, the burn patient treated with silver nitrate may manifest hyponatremia and hypochloremic metabolic alkalosis. When applying a prescribed topical agent, be aware of its characteristics and the risk for side effects or complications. The burn patient must be monitored carefully for problems or signs of treatment failure while meticulous wound care and proper nutrition are provided.

FLUID REMOBILIZATION PHASE

Remobilization of the edema fluid represents an interstitial-to-plasma fluid shift that generally begins by the second or third postburn day. This remobilization phase usually lasts another 24 to 72 hours. Renal failure must be considered if diuresis does not occur. Similarly, polyuric renal failure may be confused with the fluid remobilization phase.

As edema fluid reenters the circulation, the blood volume is greatly increased and large amounts of urine are excreted. At this point, the IV fluids should be sharply curtailed or discontinued. Infusion of large volumes of fluid could easily cause circulatory overload with pulmonary edema. Fatal pulmonary edema may occur if the reno-cardiovascular system is not capable of handling the volume of water and electrolytes shifting from the interstitial space into the plasma.

Signs of circulatory overload and pulmonary edema include the following:

▶ Venous distention
▶ Shortness of breath, moist rales, and wheezing
▶ Cyanosis and coughing of frothy fluid
▶ Restlessness
▶ Hypertension
▶ Tachycardia and tachypnea

Either oral intake or tube feedings should supply adequate fluid and nutrition once normal bowel sounds have returned. Moderate quantities of IV fluids may be necessary to meet daily needs until the gastrointestinal (GI) tract is able to tolerate fully the high protein diet needed to heal the wounds and maintain the normal preburn weight.

CONVALESCENT PHASE

Once the shock and diuresis phases of the burn injury have been resolved, the treatment and nursing interventions will focus on healing the wound, either by regeneration of surviving skin elements retained deep in the dermis of partial-thickness burns or by skin grafting of the full-thickness wounds.

Complications that may hinder the healing process or threaten the survival of the burn patient must be avoided or diagnosed promptly and treated aggressively without interruption of wound care and closure. To achieve these ends, meticulous daily wound care, proper nutrition, and diligent control of infections are vital. Changes in the patient's sensorium and wound will often reflect changes in the patient's systemic condition before other clinical symptoms appear or diagnostic studies confirm suspected complications.

Good nutrition is of primary importance to burned patients, all of whom have great nutritional needs as a result of the hypermetabolic response to the injury. Total daily energy consumption for major burns may be as high as 40 kcal/percent of BSA burned plus 25 kcal/kg of preburn body weight. There is also a marked catabolic response, resulting in weight loss, slowed wound healing, and negative nitrogen, potassium, sulfur, and phosphorus balances. A number of formulas are used to calculate the exact carbohydrate, fat, and protein calories needed by the burned patient. If the patient is unable to consume all of the designated calories orally, enteral feedings may be used. (Tube feedings are discussed in Chapter 13.) If the GI tract is unable to tolerate the oral or enteral feedings (usually due to sepsis), parenteral or central line hyperalimentation will be needed. (Hyperalimentation is discussed in Chapter 12.) Use of a central line should be undertaken cautiously as the burned patient has increased susceptibility to catheter sepsis.

The convalescent phase is often complicated by inadequate electrolyte intake from the diet; the metabolic response to injury also leads to changes in the metabolism of vitamins, minerals, and trace elements. If appropriate electrolyte supplements are not given, the patient may insidiously develop deficits of potassium, sodium, and calcium. Hypophosphatemia may occur when large amounts of antacids are used or the patient is in a poor nutritional state. Muscle cramps, arrhythmias, and hallucinations may result from low serum magnesium. Vitamin C, vitamin A, and zinc are important to wound healing; B complex vitamins may also be supplemented.

Frequent laboratory data must be obtained to monitor the ever-changing needs of the burn patient. Complete blood counts, electrolyte levels, blood urea nitrogen, and osmolality are among the more commonly ordered studies.

Patients with major burns need comprehensive and meticulous follow-up in all aspects of their care. This chapter has highlighted only certain portions of that care as it directly relates to water and electrolyte concerns. Nurses provide a vital service to the patient and family by identifying various needs, planning and executing appropriate nursing interventions, and coordinating the efforts of the burn team.

BIBLIOGRAPHY

Boswick J: *The Art and Science of Burn Care.* Rockville, MD, Aspen 1987

Demling R: Fluid replacement in burned patients. Surg Clin North Am 67:15–29, 1987

Demling, R, LaLonde C: *Burn Trauma.* New York, Thieme Medical Publishers, 1989

Demling R: Chapter 138. Management of the burn patient. In Shoemaker W et al (eds): Textbook of Critical Care, 2nd ed. Philadelphia, WB Saunders, 1989

Dyer C, Roberts D: Thermal trauma. Nurs Clin North Am 25:1:85–117, 1990

Fabri P: Monitoring of the burn patient. Clin Plas Surg 13:21–26, 1986

Herndon D et al: Pulmonary injury in burn patients. Surg Clin North Am 67:31–45, 1987

Kokko J, Tannen R: Fluids and Electrolytes, 2nd ed. Philadelphia, WB Saunders, 1990

Martyn J: Acute Management of the Burned Patient. Philadelphia, WB Saunders, 1990

McManus W, Hunt J, Pruitt B: Postburn convulsive disorder in children. J Trauma 14:396–401, 1974

Monafo W, Halverson J, Schechtman K: The role of concentration sodium solutions in the resuscitation of patients with severe burns. Surgery 95:129–135, 1984

Mosley S: Inhalation injury: A review of the literature. Heart Lung, 17:3–9, 1988

Rubin W, Mani M, Hiebert J: Fluid resuscitation of the thermally injured patient: Current concepts with definition of clinical subsets and their specialized treatment. Clin Plast Surg 13:9–20, 1986

Said R, Hussein M: Severe hyponatremia in burn patients secondary to hydrotherapy. *Burns* 3:327–329, 1987

Schwartz S, Shires G, Spencer F: Princ Surg, 5th ed. New York, McGraw-Hill, pp 285–305, 1989

Shires, G: Fluids, Electrolytes and Acid Bases. New York, Churchill Livingston, pp 103–120, 1988

23

Pregnancy

Although physiologically normal in pregnancy, changes in fluid retention and blood volume expansion and alterations in acid–base and electrolyte balance, would be considered abnormal in the nonpregnant woman or in the male. These changes are temporary and necessary adaptations to provide for the growing fetus and for maternal health needs during pregnancy. Despite alterations in water and electrolyte balance, pregnancy is considered a wellness state because the changes serve a useful function.

Changes in body water and electrolyte balance in normal pregnancy will be explored in this chapter, as will some abnormal disease or treatment states that directly affect fluid and electrolyte balances.

NORMAL PHYSIOLOGICAL WATER AND ELECTROLYTE CHANGES

INCREASED BLOOD VOLUME

In a woman pregnant with one fetus, a 48% plasma volume increase may be expected; an even greater increase occurs in a woman pregnant with twins.[1] Although both plasma and red cell volumes are increased, there is a relatively greater expansion of the plasma volume, resulting in the so-called "physiological anemia of pregnancy." A hematocrit of 33% to 38% and a hemoglobin of 11 to 12 g/100 mL may be observed.[2] However, when iron stores are adequate, the decline in blood values is minimal.

SODIUM AND WATER RETENTION

Although fluid retention has always been considered an alteration characteristic of pregnancy, the mechanisms of its production are poorly understood. Circulating aldosterone increases during pregnancy; this is believed to be related to physiological changes in the reproductive hormones and the renin–angiotensin system.

In normal pregnancy, retention of 900 to 1000 mEq of sodium and 6 to 8 L of water is expected.[3] It has been estimated that 300 to 400 mEq of the retained sodium is stored in the maternal extracellular fluid (ECF) space whereas the rest is stored in the fetus, placenta, and amniotic fluid. Sodium is retained gradually (20–30 mEq/wk) with a resultant mean weight gain of 12.5 kg (27.5 lbs).[4]

In the past, diuretics and salt restriction were used at the first sign of edema in pregnant women.[5] However, diuretic use currently is not routine because it is understood that diuretics can cause a number of problems during pregnancy (eg, electrolyte imbalance, hyperglycemia, and hyperuricemia). Also, it is now generally agreed that dietary sodium intake should not be restricted during normal pregnancy, although excessive use should be avoided because of the relationship of sodium to the development of hypertension in those at risk for this problem. Of note, the average dietary salt intake in the typical American diet is 8 to 10 g/day; this is far more than is needed. During pregnancy, it is wise to limit salt intake to a moderate level (such as 5 g/day).[6] Because sodium represents about 40% of the weight of salt (sodium chloride), 1 g of sodium chloride is equivalent to 0.4 g of sodium. Thus, 5 g of salt is equivalent to 2 g of sodium. See Chapter 4 for a discussion of low-salt diets.

Edema

By definition, *edema* refers to an expansion of the interstitial fluid volume. It has been demonstrated that interstitial fluid volume increases in pregnancy as a consequence of maternal sodium retention. In the absence of hypertension, or renal or cardiac impairment, edema in pregnancy can be considered a normal occurrence. In fact, from 35% to 85% of healthy normotensive women develop edema at some time during pregnancy.[7] Apparently, women with edema tend to have heavier infants and fewer infants of abnormally low birth weight.[8]

Edema can be dependent or generalized. Dependent edema of the ankles frequently occurs when the pregnant woman assumes an upright position and is of little physiological significance. Several factors predispose to dependent edema; most significant is venous pressure. Impingement of blood flow through the inferior vena cava by the pregnant uterus causes stagnation of blood in the lower extremities. Increased permeability of the capillary walls may also influence the rate of filtration. Generalized edema is manifested by rapid weight gain and edema of the hands and upper half of the body. This type of edema can also occur in normal pregnancy. However, when generalized edema is accompanied by a rise in blood pressure and proteinuria, it is considered a disease process.

In summary, sodium and water retention of normal pregnancy commonly causes mild peripheral edema, particularly in the third trimester when pressure on the inferior vena cava by the enlarged uterus has a contributory effect.[9] When the pregnant woman elevates her legs or lies on her side, the hydrostatic pressure is partially overcome and interstitial fluid is returned to the circulation.

Authors of one study suggested that immersion in water is preferable to bedrest in treating the edema associated with pregnancy.[10] In this study, 11 healthy pregnant volunteers in their third trimester either rested in bed (in a lateral supine position) or sat in a bathtub of waist-level water or a tank of shoulder-level water for treatment periods of 50 minutes. After the treatments, the urine outputs were compared. For bedrest patients, urine volumes ranged from 40 to 180 mL; in contrast, urine volumes of those patients in the bathtub group were 42 to 490 mL, and in patients in the immersion tank group were 55–510 mL. Apparently the outside water pressure, which rises proportionally to the depth of the water, forces the edema fluid back into the vascular space.

The dependent edema associated with normal pregnancy can be quite annoying. Table 23-1 gives an example of application of the nursing process to deal with this problem.

Plasma Sodium Concentration

The plasma sodium concentration falls approximately 5 mEq/L in almost all pregnant women within the first 2 months of pregnancy and then remains stable until delivery.[11] Studies have suggested that human chorionic gonadotropin may be important in this response.[12] Also, plasma osmolality falls approximately 10 mOsm/kg. These responses are partly due to increased release of antidiuretic hormone (ADH) (which in turn causes water retention) and the increased thirst common in

TABLE 23–1.
Example of Nursing Diagnosis and Nursing Process in Care of Patient with Pedal Edema
Problem: Discomfort Related to Pedal Edema

ASSESSMENT	INTERVENTIONS	EXPECTED OUTCOME
28-year-old sales clerk in last trimester of pregnancy complains of ankle swelling after standing for a few hours at work Pedal edema present; no edema in face or hands BP, 120/82 No proteinuria	1. Advise client to avoid constrictive garments around the legs 2. Recommend use of support hose 3. Advise against prolonged standing; suggest that she obtain a stool to sit on periodically during time at work 4. Instruct client regarding passive exercises to improve circulation 5. Advise frequent rest periods when feasible in which lateral position can be assumed (with legs slightly elevated to reduce venous pressure) 6. Advise ample fluid intake (8 to 10 glasses of water/day) 7. Encourage client to report increase in pedal edema or appearance of edema in face, hands, or other parts of body	Client will use self-care measures to increase comfort and decrease edema Client will verbalize decrease in discomfort Dependent edema will diminish or become no worse Client will be knowledgeable of possible abnormal developments

pregnant women.[13] The lowered plasma sodium level quickly returns to normal after delivery.[14]

CALCIUM BALANCE

Total serum calcium concentration begins to fall during the 2nd or 3rd month of pregnancy and reaches its lowest point between the 28th and 32nd weeks.[15] Total blood calcium reportedly falls by about 0.25 mEq/L in the last trimester.[16] This slight decrease is primarily due to a reduced serum albumin level, which in turn causes decreased calcium binding.[17]

Under normal circumstances, calcium balance in pregnancy is easily maintained by a normal diet. A pregnant woman requires 1.5 to 2 g of calcium daily (as opposed to approximately 0.5 g for nonpregnant women). Approximately 25 to 30 g of calcium are accumulated during pregnancy; most of this is required for fetal skeletal calcification.[18] Needed calcium is acquired during pregnancy through an increase in intestinal calcium absorption (secondary to an increase in plasma levels of $1,25(OH)D_3$) and increased rate of maternal bone turnover.

MAGNESIUM BALANCE

The serum magnesium levels fall by about 6% to 9% in pregnancy.[19] However, rather than reflecting actual hypomagnesemia, this small decrease probably represents the effects of plasma volume expansion and decreased protein binding associated with mild hypoalbuminemia.[20] Of course, actual magnesium deficiency may develop if dietary intake is inadequate. In pregnancy, formation of new tissues requires that dietary magnesium be higher than in nonpregnant women of the same age.[21]

POTASSIUM BALANCE

A cumulative retention of approximately 350 mEq of potassium occurs during pregnancy.[22] The retained potassium is stored in the fetus, uterus, breasts, and red blood cells.[23] This retention occurs in spite of increased circulating levels of mineralocorticoids and increased delivery of sodium to the distal nephron resulting from the increased glomerular filtration rate.[24] Concentration of potassium in the maternal plasma either remains at a prepregnancy level or is slightly decreased. Prolonged nausea and vomiting or the use of diuretics may lead to hypokalemia and metabolic alkalosis.

ACID–BASE CHANGES

Pregnancy is associated with a compensated respiratory alkalosis, which begins early and continues until delivery. The cause is hyperventilation, secondary to the potent stimulating effect of progesterone on the medullary respiratory center.[25] As a result of hyperventilation, the pCO_2 decreases from the normal 40 mmHg to approximately 30 mmHg during gestation, causing an arterial pH of 7.44 ± 0.003 compared with the normal measurement of 7.40.[26]

As with any form of chronic respiratory alkalosis, that occurring in pregnancy is compensated for by changes in the serum bicarbonate concentration. This metabolic compensation causes the bicarbonate level to drop to approximately 20 mEq/L by the third trimester (compared with the normal bicarbonate level of 24 mEq/L).[27] Because their total buffering capacity is reduced by this renal compensation, pregnant women are more likely to develop severe acidosis when conditions causing either ketoacidosis or lactic acidosis are present.[28] If the serum bicarbonate level is normal or elevated in late pregnancy, the possibility of a second imbalance (metabolic alkalosis) should be investigated.[29] Possible causes of the latter could be persistent vomiting or excessive use of potassium-losing diuretics.

ABNORMAL CONDITIONS AFFECTING OR AFFECTED BY FLUIDS AND ELECTROLYTES

PREGNANCY-INDUCED HYPERTENSION

In the past, the term "toxemia" was applied to a condition arising during pregnancy, or in the early puerperium, characterized by hypertension, proteinuria, edema, and convulsions (presumably caused by an unknown toxic agent). In 1972, the American College of Obstetricians and Gynecologists deleted the label *toxemia of pregnancy* and introduced the term *pregnancy-induced hypertension,* or PIH. The terms *preeclampsia* and *eclampsia* are included in the new classification. Preeclampsia is characterized by hypertension with proteinuria, edema, or both, and usually occurs after 20 weeks of gestation. If the pregnant woman develops convulsions, the term eclampsia is used.

Pregnancy-induced hypertension occurs in 5% to 7% of all pregnancies and is the third leading cause of maternal death in the United States. It is a disease of the nullipara usually involving women younger than 20 years or older than 35 years. It develops after the 20th week of gestation and has its highest incidence among women who have a strong predisposition to hypertension. There is a strong familial predisposition to the development of preeclampsia (one study reported that 25% of women whose mothers had had preeclampsia developed preeclampsia themselves). Preeclampsia occurs more frequently in black women and is associated with multiple pregnancy, polyhydramnios, vascular disease, trophoblastic disease, and abruptio placentae.

The pathogenesis of PIH is unknown; in fact, this condition has long been known as the "disease of theories." Evidently it is somehow related to the physiological changes of pregnancy as the condition improves and the disease apparently disappears after the termination of pregnancy. It has been conjectured that immunological changes, among other factors, have a pathogenetic role. The pathological changes associated with preeclampsia indicate that poor perfusion secondary to vasospasm is a major factor leading to the derangement of maternal physiological functions and increased perinatal morbidity.

Sodium Retention and Fluid Distribution Changes

As discussed earlier, sodium retention is expected with normal pregnancy; however, that which occurs with preeclampsia may be pathological. Although rapid weight gain and sodium retention are characteristic of preeclampsia, they are not universally present or, as indicated earlier, unique to preeclampsia. At most, these signs are a reason for closer observation of blood pressure and monitoring of urinary protein. The primary indicators of preeclampsia are hypertension and proteinuria.

Paradoxically, the plasma volume is often diminished in women with preeclampsia, despite the increase in total body sodium. The intense vasoconstriction that is characteristic of preeclampsia may result in a shift of the retained sodium and water from the vascular space to the interstitial space, causing a reduced plasma volume (reflected by a rising hematocrit) and increased interstitial fluid volume.

Clinical Indicators

Hypertension in the pregnant woman is defined as a blood pressure reading of greater than 140/90 or a reading that represents an increase over baseline readings of 30 mmHg systolic or 15 mmHg diastolic.[30] Two abnormal blood pressure readings taken at least 6 hours apart are required. Note that the typically accepted level of 140/90 may be inaccurate in a patient who normally has a low blood pressure. For example, in a woman with a normal baseline blood pressure of 90/50, a reading of 130/80 may well represent hypertension. Proteinuria is often the most valid clinical indicator of preeclampsia, although it tends to be a late change.[31] Significant proteinuria approximates a 2+ urinary protein. The definitive evaluation of the degree of proteinuria is a quantitative analysis of a 24-hour urine collection. (A level of 500 mg is accepted as the upper limit of normal in pregnancy.[32]) (See Table 23-2 for a summary of suggested nursing assessment parameters for abnormal fluid balance changes associated with preeclampsia and eclampsia.)

Therapeutic Measures

Although thiazide diuretics were given prophylactically in the past to prevent preeclampsia, their effectiveness for this purpose was not demonstrated.[34] Because plasma volume is already decreased in preeclamptic women, the naturesis associated with diuretic use may be counterproductive and adversely affect fetal outcome by decreasing placental perfusion.[35] Similarly, strict sodium restriction has no role in the prevention or therapy of preeclampsia and may actually be counterproductive (again because of the decreased plasma volume in preeclamptic women).[36] However, moderate sodium restriction may minimize the discomfort of women with significant edema.[37]

Antihypertensive therapy (usually hydralazine) is generally reserved for women with severe hypertension that could lead to intracranial bleeding.[38] When antihypertensive therapy of preeclampsia is directed at reduction of peripheral vascular resistance, a shift of excess sodium and water from the interstitial into the intravascular space may occur. As a result, excessive expansion of the intravascular space may cause an inadequate response to antihypertensive therapy. As fluid reenters the vascular space, the judicious use of diuretics may be appropriate to prevent the rebound sodium retention that occurs coincident with relief of vasoconstriction.[39] To monitor the volume status of seriously ill preeclamptic or eclamptic patients, it may be necessary to use a Swan-Ganz catheter to identify those patients with elevated wedge pressures who might benefit from the use of diuretics.

Preeclamptic women may develop oliguria, either because of a diminished intravascular volume or renal problems. Fluid administration in the presence of oliguria must be undertaken cautiously because if the oliguria is renal in origin, fluid overloading is likely to result. Although oliguria due to hypovolemia may be corrected by fluid infusion, excessive fluid administration can lead to congestive heart failure. Also, excessive fluid administration can lead to cerebral edema if the serum sodium level is very low. To avoid lowering the plasma osmolality, hypotonic fluids should not be used (particularly if oxytocin is being administered). Either isotonic electrolyte or colloid-containing fluids may be considered. For the woman with seriously decreased colloid oncotic pressure secondary to hypoalbuminemia, colloid-containing fluids may be indicated. The rate of fluid administration must be closely titrated to urine output and other clinical indicators such as central venous or, preferably, pulmonary wedge pressures.

Magnesium Sulfate as an Anticonvulsant

The therapeutic use of magnesium sulfate in preeclampsia-eclampsia is due to its pharmacological effects of central nervous system depression and vasodilatation. More specifically, magnesium ions block nerve transmission by presynaptic inhibition, causing a neuromuscular blockage.[40] Also, magnesium tends to block catecholamine release from the adrenal medulla and may cause peripheral vasodilatation.

Magnesium sulfate can be given intramuscularly (IM) or intravenously (IV); however, because the IM administration of large volumes of magnesium sulfate is painful, many clinicians advocate the IV route. Magnesium sulfate is commonly given IV with an initial bolus followed by a continuous slow infusion, titrating the rate of administration against maternal deep tendon reflexes.[41] The desired dosage of magnesium sulfate varies depending on renal status and the patient's response to the drug. Intravenous administration of magnesium at doses up to 2 g/hr appears to be safe for the patient with normal renal function.[42] However, doses exceeding this level require that serum magnesium concentrations be monitored at least every 2 hours until a steady state has been achieved.[43]

Most authorities agree that magnesium sulfate ($MgSO_4 \cdot 7H_2O$) is a safe and efficient agent to prevent convulsions. Eclamptic convulsions are usually prevented if plasma magnesium levels are maintained at 4 to 7 mEq/L.[44] (Recall that the normal plasma magnesium concentration is 1.3–2.1 mEq/L). Because deep tendon reflex depression occurs at a serum level lower than that associated with adverse respiratory and cardiac effects, the presence of deep tendon reflexes indicates that the serum magnesium concentration is not dangerously high[45] (see Table 7-3). However, in addition to monitoring patellar reflexes, rate and depth of respirations should be regularly observed. Because magnesium is primarily eliminated by the kidneys, the adequacy of renal function must be monitored during its administration. It is generally agreed that urine output should total at least 100 mL every 4 hours. If toxic symptoms occur from magnesium overdosage, calcium gluconate may be prescribed as an antidote. A commonly recommended dose is 1 g (10 mL of a 10% solution) given slowly over 3 minutes.[46] Mechanical respiratory support may also be needed if respirations are severely depressed.

Apparently neonatal serum magnesium levels are nearly identical to maternal levels. A study of 118 infants of mothers who received magnesium sulfate found that the average serum magnesium concentration was 3.7 mEq/L, and there was no correlation between magnesium concentrations and Apgar scores.[47]

Magnesium sulfate is not a perfect anticonvulsant; some women have convulsions even with high serum magnesium levels. Diazepam (Valium) is another possible choice because it has been used successfully to treat and prevent convulsions. In the United States, it is not often chosen as the primary anticonvulsant as it can have adverse effects on the fetus; however, diazepam is commonly used in Europe and other countries for the treatment of preeclampsia and eclampsia.[48] Some authors believe that the traditional use of magnesium deserves reexamination because it must be given in doses nearing those causing hypoventilation, and that diazepam may be a safer tranquilizer.[49]

Nursing Interventions

The following interventions are often indicated for patients with severe preeclampsia and eclampsia:

1. Maintain bedrest with patient in lateral recumbent position. (Bedrest in this position increases renal perfusion and, thus, urinary output. Placental perfusion is also increased.)
2. Monitor changes in blood pressure, degree of edema, and degree of proteinuria (Table 23-2). Frequency of these observations depends on the severity of

the patient's condition; for example, they may be needed hourly if the condition is advanced.
3. Provide a quiet, nonstimulating environment (preferably a private room.)
4. Monitor closely for development of labor; monitor fetal status (fetal monitor).
5. Keep airway at bedside and maintain seizure precautions. Have emergency tray immediately accessible.
6. Monitor for hyperreflexia.
7. Inquire about subjective symptoms such as headaches, epigastric pain, visual disturbances. Record results of daily funduscopic examinations; edema of the retina reflects retinal ischemia and is a serious development.
8. If prescribed, administer magnesium sulfate according to facility protocol as appropriate. The goal is to prevent convulsions without creating generalized central nervous system depression. To pre-

TABLE 23–2.
Summary of Nursing Assessment Parameters for Abnormal Fluid Balance Changes
Associated with Preeclampsia

ASSESSMENT PARAMETER	COMMENTS
Weight changes	Weigh on same scale each time, after voiding, and with same amount of clothing
	(Normal weight curve is a 10-lb weight gain at 20 weeks with a 0.5-lb/wk gain until 40 weeks. In patients with PIH, weight gain is usually greater than 30 lbs by the third trimester.[33])
BP changes	Establish baseline BP in early pregnancy
	Assess BP with client in same position and in same arm each visit; use cuff of appropriate size
	Although 140/90 serves as a rough baseline for hypertension, it is better to look for degree of elevation over baseline.)
	▶ As a rough rule of thumb, consider BP abnormal if systolic elevates > 30 mmHg or diastolic elevates > 15 mmHg.
	▶ Two abnormal readings taken at least 6 hours apart are required for a diagnosis of hypertension.
Edema*	+1 edema: minimal edema of lower extremities
	+2 edema: marked edema of lower extremities (as evidenced by inability to wear usual shoes)
	+3 edema: edema of lower extremities, face, and hands (as in inability to wear rings)
	+4 edema: generalized massive edema including the abdomen and face (puffy eyelids and blunted facial features)
Proteinuria	Obtain clean-catch voided specimen, avoid contamination with vaginal secretions (causes false positive)
	▶ Significant if 1+ or 2+ on two or more occasions or if greater than 500 mg in a 24-hour urine collection

* *Edema without other clinical indicators of preeclampsia can occur in normal pregnancy (see text).*
PIH, pregnancy-induced hypertension; BP, blood pressure.

vent overdose of magnesium, it is necessary to do the following:

A. Check patellar reflexes at regular intervals (if depressed, notify physician).

B. Check respirations (12 or less per minute is cause to notify physican).

C. Monitor urine output (if less than 30 mL/hr, notify physician).

D. Monitor serum magnesium levels, reporting elevations above the therapeutic range designated by physician. The reader is referred to Table 7-1 for nursing considerations in administering IV magnesium, and to Table 7-3 for clinical indicators of hypermagnesemia in approximate relationship to the degree of serum elevation.

9. Administer oxygen if needed after convulsion. Monitor breath sounds for signs of pulmonary edema.

HYPONATREMIA AS A COMPLICATION OF OXYTOCIN ADMINISTRATION

Labor induction with oxytocin delivered in an appreciable amount of an aqueous solutions (such as D_5W) can lead to water retention, severe hyponatremia, and seizures in both the mother and fetus.[50] Recall that the pharmacological action of oxytocin includes a potent antidiuretic effect causing increased water retention. Although the plasma sodium concentration may return to normal after the water diuresis that follows discontinuance of the infusion, permanent neurological sequelae or even death may occur.[51]

Symptoms of water intoxication (dilutional hyponatremia) include lethargy, headache, blurred vision, twitching, convulsions, and coma. See Chapter 4 for a more complete discussion of this topic.

This complication can be prevented by using an electrolyte solution instead of dextrose and water as a vehicle for oxytocin administration, and limiting the amount of water intake. Oxytocin should not be infused by gravity as the rate of flow by this method is too erratic to assure a steady delivery of the drug. Instead, it should be administered by a continuous infusion pump (such as a Harvard pump or a peristaltic-type pump). For induction of labor, the standard dilution is 1 mL (10 units) of oxytocin in 1 L of lactated Ringers (LR) solution or 0.9% sodium chloride.[52] Initial dose is usually 1 to 2 mU/min; the maximum dose rarely exceeds 20 mU/min.[53]

HYPEREMESIS GRAVIDARUM

Hyperemesis gravidarum is defined as severe vomiting occurring before the 20th week of gestation.[54] It is a relatively rare condition that reportedly occurs in three to four cases per 1000.[55] Excessive vomiting causes fluid volume deficit (FVD), starvational ketoacidosis, and, at times, metabolic alkalosis with hypokalemia. (These imbalances are commonly seen with excessive vomiting; see Chapter 16 for a discussion of fluid and electrolyte disturbances associated with gastric fluid loss.) Significant weight loss may occur and reflects fluid as well as lean tissue loss. Also indicative of FVD is decreased urinary output with a high specific gravity and a high blood urea nitrogen (BUN) level. Ketonuria can occur and is reflective of starvation; excessive ketones in the bloodstream cause metabolic acidosis. As stated above, metabolic alkalosis is also a possibility with the loss of gastric acid.

The cause of hyperemesis gravidarum is unknown; it has been postulated that it is related to several factors (eg, vitamin B_6 deficiency, impaired function of the adrenal cortex, hyperthyroidism and excess hCG secretion, change in gastrointestinal (GI) physiology, poor nutrition, and emotional state).[56]

Prognosis is good if proper management is instituted. Treatment usually includes hospitalization, often in a private room. In severe cases, parenteral nutrition is provided until vomiting ceases, oral intake can be initiated, and serum electrolytes return to normal. At times, total parenteral nutrition may be indicated to achieve adequate nutrient intake and allow the GI tract to rest. Careful use of antiemetics or mild sedatives may also be indicated for some patients. Attention should be given to handling any psychological component of the patient's illness. Monitoring needs of patients with hyperemesis gravidarum include daily weights, fluid intake and output, vital signs, and laboratory measures of electrolytes and general metabolic status (including potassium, sodium, BUN, glucose, and serum creatinine levels).

REFERENCES

1. Kokko J, Tannen R: Fluids and Electrolytes, 2nd ed, p 907. Philadelphia, WB Saunders, 1990
2. Maxwell M, Kleeman C, Narins R: Clinical Disorders of Fluid and Electrolyte Metabolism, 4th ed, p 851. New York, McGraw-Hill, 1987
3. Rose B: Clinical Physiology of Acid–Base and Electrolyte Disorders, 3rd ed. New York, McGraw-Hill, 1989
4. Kokko, Tannen, p 907
5. Creasy R, Resnik R: Maternal–Fetal Medicine: Principles and Practice, 2nd ed, p 175. Philadelphia, WB Saunders, 1989
6. Ibid
7. Ibid, p 911
8. Ibid
9. Rose, p 450

10. Katz et al: A comparison of bed rest and immersion for treating the edema of pregnancy. Obstet Gynecol 75(2):147, 1990
11. Rose, p 614
12. Davison et al: Serial evaluation of vasopressin release and thirst in human pregnancy: Role of human chorionic gonadotropin in the osmoregulatory changes of gestation. J Clin Invest 81:798, 1988
13. Maxwell et al, p 858
14. Rose, p 165
15. Maxwell et al, p 860
16. Kokko, Tannen, p 915
17. Ibid
18. Ibid, p 916
19. Ibid
20. Ibid
21. Maxwell et al, p 833
22. Ibid, p 857
23. Kokko, Tannen, p 914
24. Maxwell et al, p 857
25. Rose, p 583
26. Maxwell et al, p 860
27. Ibid, p 750
28. Ibid, p 860
29. Ibid, p 750
30. Rivlin M, Morrison J, Bates G: Manual of Clinical Problems in Obstetrics and Gynecology, 3rd ed, p 31. Boston, Little, Brown, 1990
31. Creasy, Resnik, p 804
32. May K, Mahlmeister L: Comprehensive Maternity Nursing, 2nd ed, p 512. Philadelphia, JB Lippincott, 1990
33. Ibid
34. Creasy, Resnik, p 805
35. Ibid
36. Ibid, p 803
37. Kokko, Tannen, p 912
38. Creasy, Resnik, p 809
39. Ibid
40. Brody S, Ueland K: Endocrine Disorders in Pregnancy, p 404. Appleton & Lange, 1989
41. Ibid
42. Creasy, Resnik, p 809
43. Ibid
44. Rivlin et al, p 32
45. Creasy, Resnik, p 807
46. Rivlin et al, p 32
47. Pritchard J, Stone S: Clinical and laboratory observations on eclampsia. Am J Obstet Gynecol 99:754, 1967
48. Brody, p 404
49. Thompson W: Hypertensive urgencies and emergencies. In: Shoemaker W et al (eds): Textbook of Critical Care, 2nd ed, p 401. Philadelphia: WB Saunders, 1989
50. Rose, p 613
51. Lillien A: Oxytocin induced water intoxication: A report of maternal death. Obstet Gynecol 32:171, 1968
52. Gahart B: A Handbook of Intravenous Medications, 6th ed, p 412. St. Louis, CV Mosby, 1990
53. Ibid, p 413
54. Rivlin et al, p 188
55. Ibid
56. Ibid

24

Oncologic Conditions

Maintaining fluid and electrolyte balance is often difficult in patients with cancer. In some situations, fluid and electrolyte problems may cause the initial symptoms exhibited by the undiagnosed patient. At other times they are related to the development of metastatic disease. Unfortunately, they may often be the consequence of aggressive therapy. Of the oncology patient population, 50% to 75% will experience a problem with fluid and electrolyte regulation during the course of their illness.[1] These fluid and electrolyte problems can be acute or chronic and vary significantly in degree of severity.

CAUSES OF FLUID AND ELECTROLYTE PROBLEMS IN ONCOLOGY PATIENTS

The underlying mechanisms for fluid and electrolyte imbalances may result directly from increased electrolyte loss or from decreased intake or they may be the indirect result of faulty hormonal regulation of body water and electrolytes. A summary of these fluid and electrolyte imbalances and their causes is given in Table 24-1.

TABLE 24–1.
Fluid and Electrolyte Imbalances in Cancer Patients

ELECTROLYTE IMBALANCE	PHYSIOLOGICAL PROCESS	UNDERLYING CAUSE/MALIGNANCY
Hypercalcemia	Increased osteolytic activity of tumor	Breast cancer Kidney cancer Non-small-cell lung cancer Multiple myeloma Thyroid cancer
	Ectopic PTH production	Epidermoid lung cancer Renal adenocarcinoma Oral cavity squamous cancer
	Increased osteoclastic activity	Immobility
		Ectopic OAF release: ▶ Lymphoma ▶ Multiple myeloma ▶ Leukemia
		E series prostaglandin: ▶ Lymphoma ▶ Leukemia
		Treatment with: ▶ Estrogens ▶ Progestins ▶ Androgens ▶ Antiestrogens Dehydration
Hypocalcemia	Increased calcium use	"Hungry bone syndrome" Metastases from prostate or breast cancer treated with hormonal therapy Rapid healing of bony lesions
	Decreased calcium intake	Starvation Hyperalimentation with inadequate calcium supplementation
	Decreased calcium absorption	Fistulae (with loss of fluid before absorption can occur) Lymphoma of small bowel
	Decreased serum albumin	Starvation Transudation of protein into third-space fluid accumulation
Hyperuricemia	Increase in uric acid precursors	Polycythemia vera Chronic granulocytic leukemia
	Rapid tumor dissolution with increased nucleic acid release	Induction therapy for leukemia Radiosensitive/chemotherapy-sensitive lymphomas
Hyponatremia	Loss of sodium	Fistulas Prolonged vomiting Prolonged nasogastric suction Small-cell lung cancer
	Ectopic ADH production (SIADH)	Thymoma Lymphoma

(continued)

TABLE 24–1.
(continued)

ELECTROLYTE IMBALANCE	PHYSIOLOGICAL PROCESS	UNDERLYING CAUSE/MALIGNANCY
		Chemotherapy-induced:
		▶ High-dose cyclophosphamide
		▶ Vincristine (Oncovin)
Hypernatremia	Increased water loss	Renal damage associated with multiple myeloma
Hyperkalemia	Increased release of potassium from cellular breakdown	Induction therapy for acute leukemia
Hypokalemia	Ectopic ACTH production	Small-cell lung cancer Thymoma Islet cell pancreatic cancer Bronchial carcinoid
	Increased GI loss of potassium	Prolonged vomiting, suction, diarrhea, fistulous drainage
	Increased renal tubular loss	Tubular damage from induction therapy in leukemia
Hypophosphatemia	Increased urinary loss	Multiple myeloma
	Respiratory alkalosis	Sepsis (Recall that fever causes hyperventilation, which in turn causes respiratory alkalosis.)
	Decreased intake	Starvation, hyperalimentation with inadequate PO_4
Hyperphosphatemia	Increased cellular release	Acute leukemia Sensitive lymphomas
Hypomagnesemia	Increased loss	Renal magnesium wasting from cisplatin therapy Chronic diarrhea
	Decreased intake	Hyperalimentation without adequate Mg supplementation Prolonged period of inadequate dietary intake

ACTH, adrenocorticotrophic hormone; OAF, osteoclast activating factor; PTH, parathyroid hormone; SIADH, syndrome of inappropriate antidiuretic hormone secretion.

FAULTY REGULATION OR AVAILABILITY OF ELECTROLYTES

Fluid and electrolyte problems associated with cancer are most commonly related to faulty regulation or availability of one of the following substances:

▶ Calcium
▶ Uric acid
▶ Sodium
▶ Potassium
▶ Phosphate
▶ Magnesium

ALTERED HORMONAL REGULATORY MECHANISMS

Electrolyte imbalance in oncology patients is frequently due to alterations in various hormonal regulatory mechanisms caused by a variety of tumors. These malignant tumors produce ectopic polypeptide hormones or pseudohormone substances that interfere with water and electrolyte balances. Involved hormones (or hormone-like substances) include the following:

▶ Antidiuretic hormone (ADH)
▶ Parathyroid hormone (PTH)

▶ Osteoclastic activating factor (OAF)
▶ Adrenocorticotrophic hormone (ACTH)

Production of these hormones is not regulated by normal suppression feedback loops; consequently, the ectopic hormone continues to be released by the tumor, often causing life-threatening electrolyte imbalances. The generally accepted theory that accounts for the production of ectopic hormones is faulty genetic regulation by the malignant tumor itself.[2]

THIRD-SPACE FLUID ACCUMULATION

Cancer patients frequently develop third-space fluid accumulations; these may be due to the following:

▶ Malignant effusions into the peritoneal, pericardial, or pleural compartments: Direct tumor involvement of the cavity's serous surface appears to be the most frequent cause of effusions in cancer patients.

▶ Edema: Trapping of excess fluid in the interstitial fluid space due to obstruction of lymphatic drainage or venous return secondary to tumor pressure. Protein seepage through the capillary bed in the edematous site pulls fluid with it, making the edema more severe. Reduced serum oncotic pressure due to reduced serum albumin along with extremity dependence contributes to ankle and leg swelling in oncology patients who sit for long periods.

Major shifts of water and electrolytes into potential fluid spaces results in an increase in total body fluid, although a clinically defined state of fluid volume deficit (FVD) is present. Recall that FVD is manifested by poor skin turgor, decreased urinary output, increased urinary specific gravity, and postural hypotension. Body weight does not decrease (as it does with actual fluid loss) because fluid is trapped inside the body; in fact, weight may increase with parenteral fluid replacement. Unfortunately, administration of intravenous (IV) fluids to correct the FVD also allows an increase in the fluid volume trapped in the third space, which only adds to the patient's discomfort.

TREATMENT-RELATED IMBALANCES

The treatment of malignancies can create fluid and electrolyte imbalances. Examples of treatment-induced imbalances include the following:

▶ Hypercalcemia associated with hormonal treatment (tamoxifen) for breast cancer
▶ Hyponatremia and hypokalemia associated with nausea and vomiting frequently caused by chemotherapy
▶ Hyponatremia (water intoxication) associated with the use of certain chemotherapeutic drugs (vincristine [Oncovin] and cyclophosphamide [Cytoxan])

▶ Hyperuricemia associated with destruction of cells, release of pools of nucleic acids that are metabolized to uric acid (seen in patients with acute leukemia, Burkitt's lymphona, diffuse histiocytic lymphoma, and preexisting renal disease)

▶ Hypomagnesemia associated with hypocalcemia that does not respond to calcium replacement therapy (magnesium deficits occur in patients receiving chronic diuretic therapy and cisplatin therapy, and in patients to whom parenteral hyperalimentation has been administered without adequate magnesium replacement)

▶ Tumor lysis syndrome associated with release of large amounts of intracellular electrolytes (phosphate and potassium) into the serum due to destruction of rapidly growing neoplasms (eg, acute leukemia, Burkitt's lymphoma, and diffuse histiocytic lymphoma). High levels of free phosphate radicals combine with ionized serum calcium creating hypocalcemia (Table 24-2).[3]

FLUID AND ELECTROLYTE DISTURBANCES

Fluid balance problems common to patients with cancer are described in this section. Mechanisms responsible for the imbalances, as well as the tumors (or associated problems) causing the imbalances are described. A summary of this information is presented in Table 24-1.

Treatment to correct common electrolyte imbalances is also described in this section. Note that treat-

---

TABLE 24−2.
Management of Tumor Lysis Syndrome

Prevention:

▶ Assessment of patients at risk: Those with leukemia, diffuse histiocytic lymphoma, and Burkitt's lymphoma
▶ Pretreatment IV hydration (3000 mL/m²)
▶ Urinary alkalinization with $NaHCO_3$ to maintain pH at 7.0 or greater
▶ Administration of allopurinol (220−500 mg/m²)
▶ Baseline serum electrolytes, BUN, calcium, phosphorus, creatinine with subsequent q. 6-hr monitoring

Treatment:

▶ Hemodialysis if renal failure occurs

BUN, blood urea nitrogen.

---

ment of tumor-related fluid and electrolyte problems is directed first at relieving immediate life-threatening problems and second at controlling the tumor underlying the basic physiological response.

HYPERCALCEMIA

One of the more common problems of malignant disease is hypercalcemia. About 10% to 20% of all persons with cancer will develop an elevated serum calcium during the course of their illness.[4] It is associated with virtually any type of malignancy, from solid tumors with or without bony metastases to hematological malignancies, and may include the following:

1. Solid tumors with bony metastases:
   - Breast
   - Lung
   - Renal
   - Colon
   - Ovary
   - Epidermoid cancers of the head and neck
2. Solid tumors without bony metastases:
   - Lung
   - Head and neck
   - Renal
   - Ovary
3. Select chemotherapeutic agents:
   - Androgens
   - Estrogens
   - Progestins
   - Antiestrogens

The hypercalcemia associated with solid tumors is most notable in patients with breast cancer. However, patients with hematological malignancies, ie, lymphoma, leukemia, and multiple myeloma, may also have profound elevations in serum calcium. The following brief review suggests a variety of pathways other than osseous metastases as a basis for hypercalcemia of malignant disease.

Mechanisms

The basic mechanism responsible for an elevated serum calcium level is an increase in calcium release from bone that exceeds calcium excretion from the renal tubules. The following physiological mechanisms may be responsible for the increase of calcium from bone in neoplastic states:

1. Tumor-related mechanisms
   - Direct
     - Tumor lysis of the bone
   - Indirect (humoral hypercalcemia of malignancy [HHM])
     - Prostaglandin activity

- Tumor release of PTH or pseudo-PTH substance
- Immune cell release of OAF
- Tumor release of vitamin D-like sterols
2. Treatment-related mechanisms
   - Treatment with androgens, estrogens, progestins, or antiestrogens
3. Non–tumor-related mechanisms
   - Coincidental primary hyperparathyroidism

Presence of malignant tumor cells in bony spaces has been demonstrated to cause an increased release of calcium from bone and a loss of skeletal integrity. This direct osteolytic action is commonly the mechanism for hypercalcemia in women with breast cancer. In addition to the direct resorption of bone by tumor cells, prostaglandin action has been proposed as a mechanism for increased calcium release from the bone.[5] Prostaglandins may be produced from one of the following:

- Tumor cells
- Immune cells
- Osteoclasts[6]

Animal models have shown that prostaglandins have osteolytic activities.[7] It is not known if this animal model principle can be transferred to humans.

Solid tumors without bony metastases have been associated with hypercalcemic states, as documented in patients with squamous cell carcinoma of the head and neck and carcinomas of the lung and kidney. Further investigation is needed to demonstrate the actual mechanisms responsible for hypercalcemic clinical syndromes in patients with radiographically negative skeletal series.

Immune cells (lymphocytes and monocytes) have also been implicated in the production of hypercalcemia. There are three possible mechanisms whereby monocytes may lead to the release of calcium from bone.[8]

- Release of prostaglandins
- Direct bone resorption through contact action
- Release of OAF

Monocytes, through direct contact with bony tissue, cause a dissolution of bone. Kahn and Stewart[9] demonstrated that monocytes, frequently present in metastatic bony lesions, release an enzyme that causes bone destruction. Bockman's model demonstrates the synergistic action between tumor cells and immune cells in producing hypercalcemia[10]:

1. Immediate
   - Tumor cells initiate osteolytic process at metastatic site.
   - Host cells (monocytes) and tumor cells cause active bone resorption.

2. Intermediate
  ▶ Bony resorption stimulates an increase in tumor cells and monocytic phagocyte migration to the lesion.
3. Late
  ▶ Tumor cell resorption is primarily a lytic process.

In addition to prostaglandin release and direct contact-mediated bone resorption, immunocytes may release an osteoclast-like activating factor that increases the release of calcium from bone.

The only treatment-related cause of hypercalcemia is that associated with use of androgens, estrogens, antiestrogens, and progestins. Metabolic alterations associated with use of these agents cause calcium release from bone. This results in an elevation of serum calcium. Obviously, patients should have their serum calcium levels closely monitored. Any marked elevation of the calcium level warrants discontinuation of therapy. Usually no additional treatment is required once hormonal therapy is stopped.

Clinical Presentation

The symptoms exhibited by the cancer patient experiencing hypercalcemia are the same as those in hypercalcemic patients with primary hyperparathyroidism (Table 24-3). (Table 24-3 also provides an example of nursing process application to the care of a hypercalcemic oncology patient.) Severity of symptoms is directly related to the development rate and level of serum calcium modified by age, other electrolyte disorders, and any other underlying problems. In review, symptoms of hypercalcemia may include anorexia, nausea and vomiting, constipation, muscular weakness and hyporeflexia, disturbance in behavior, confusion, psychosis, tremor, and lethargy. Differential diagnosis in a cancer patient with hypercalcemia should include primary hyperparathyroidism. In addition, the following factors should be considered in distinguishing a tumor-associated hypercalcemia from that seen in primary hyperparathyroidism[11]:

▶ Type of malignant tumor. Is it one commonly associated with hypercalcemia?
▶ Patient history. Was there a history of hypercalcemia before the diagnosis of a malignancy?
▶ Effect of anticancer therapy on the hypercalcemia. If hypercalcemia is a tumor-induced syndrome, anticancer therapy should alleviate it.

Treatment

Treatment for tumor-related hypercalcemia is similar to that for other clinical states of elevated serum calcium levels (Table 24-4). Isotonic saline (0.9% NaCl) administration facilitates calcium elimination by the kidneys by increasing the glomerular filtration rate. Furosemide (Lasix) may also be helpful because it selectively inhibits resorption of calcium. Salmon calcitonin may be of limited use in rapidly lowering serum calcium levels.[12] However, the decrease in serum calcium produced by calcitonin is generally small and is sometimes not sustained. Mithramycin, an antineoplastic antibiotic, lowers the serum calcium level by inhibiting osteoclast activity; however, its action does not begin until 18 to 24 hours after administration.[13] Unfortunately, it may cause a precipitous drop in platelet count. Glucocorticoids are helpful in the treatment of hypercalcemia secondary to osteolytic processes. A more thorough discussion of the treatment of hypercalcemia is given in Chapter 6. In patients in whom the calcium level is less than 13 mg/dL and symptoms are not clinically evident, treatment with traditional anticancer therapy may be all that is needed. If other therapy is required, the diphosphonates are considered to be strong antihypercalcemic agents.[14, 15] Drugs such as clodronate or didronel inhibit osteoclastic-induced resorption of bone. Use of diphosphonates for hypercalcemia may be considered before use of mithramycin, which may be associated with thrombocytopenia and bleeding diatheses. (Recall that the patient who has received previous chemotherapy may be thrombocytopenic before receiving the additional platelet insult of mithramycin.)

In addition to the immediate control of symptoms, long-term therapy for the cancer patient with tumor-induced hypercalcemia must be considered. Remember that, although cancer patients with hypercalcemia may respond rapidly to emergency treatment, the serum calcium level may return to an elevated state and remain a chronic management problem unless the malignancy is controlled with antineoplastic therapy.

Hypocalcemia

Malnutrition with resultant decrease in serum albumin is a major cause of hypocalcemia in cancer patients. For each decrease in serum albumin of 1 g/dL, serum calcium level will decrease approximately 0.8 mg/dL. Although it is uncommon in cancer patients, hypocalcemia may occur secondary to the following:

▶ Severe liver disease
▶ Malabsorption due to extensive bowel resection or tumor replacement (ie, tumor in small intestine of such magnitude that it interferes with bowel absorptive surface)
▶ "Hungry bone syndrome" due to rapid bone healing after successful treatment of bony lesions
▶ Magnesium depletion
▶ Tumor lysis syndrome: sudden release of free phos-

(text continues on page 330)

TABLE 24–3.
Clinical Care Guidelines: Alteration in Body Fluid Composition Related to Elevated Serum Calcium

GROUPS AT RISK

Persons with the following neoplasma (evidence of bony metastases need not be present):

Breast	Oral cavity
Kidney	Lymphoma
Lung	Multiple myeloma
Thyroid	Acute/chronic leukemia

Persons with cancer who are also immobile or volume depleted

Persons receiving treatment with estrogens, progestins, androgens, or antiestrogens

NURSING ASSESSMENT GUIDE

1. Evaluate laboratory data:
   ▶ Serum calcium
   ▶ BUN, creatinine
   ▶ Albumin
   ▶ Potassium
2. Assess for signs/symptoms of effects of elevated serum calcium:
   ▶ Renal: Polyuria, polydipsia, volume depletion
   ▶ CNS: Fatigue, weakness, decreased reflexes, confusion, agitation, obtundation leading to coma
   ▶ Cardiac: Elevated BP, arrhythmias, ECG changes (decreased Q–T interval, widened T wave)
   ▶ Gastrointestinal: Nausea, anorexia, distention, constipation, pain, paralytic ileus
   ▶ Altered comfort level: Pruritus and complaints of bony pain
3. Review medications and report:
   ▶ Coadministration of digitalis preparations
   ▶ Antiestrogens, estrogens, androgens, progestins
   ▶ Antacids
4. Evaluate fluid status:
   ▶ Intake and output
   ▶ Daily weight
   ▶ Vital signs
5. Evaluate mobility/activity status

NURSING DIAGNOSIS	ETIOLOGY	DEFINING CHARACTERISTICS	NURSING INTERVENTION	OUTCOMES
Alteration in bowel elimination: Constipation	Decreased GI motility related to calcium effect on smooth muscle Volume depletion related to polyuria	Abdominal pain Distention Anorexia Hard formed stool Altered pattern of bowel elimination Nausea	Obtain baseline elimination pattern and routine for elimination Establish pattern for elimination: q.2d., q.3d., etc. Provide privacy and regular time each day for elimination Increase fluid intake Encourage activity increase within limits Implement appropriate dietary changes: Bulk, natural stimulants, softeners, etc. Administer appropriate laxatives, softeners, enemas, etc. Record bowel elimination pattern observing for regularity, changes in stool, increasing constipation, impending ileus, etc.	Evacuates soft, formed stool with ease on days scheduled

(continued)

TABLE 24–3.
(continued)

NURSING DIAGNOSIS	ETIOLOGY	DEFINING CHARACTERISTICS	NURSING INTERVENTION	OUTCOMES
Actual/potential fluid volume deficit	Hypercalcemia interferes with tubular reabsorption of water leading to excretion of a dilute urine	Polydipsia Polyuria Nocturia	Monitor intake and output Monitor orthostatic BP, CVP, urine volume, SG Monitor q.d. weight Monitor skin turgor, mucous membranes for dryness Encourage p.o. fluids: Offer small amounts frequently at the preferred temperature Identify factors that interfere with fluid consumption or contribute to additional fluid loss, ie, environmental temperature, activity, etc. Monitor IV fluid administration to guard against overhydration Maintain oral hygiene	Demonstrates measures to maintain fluid balance Maintains adequate fluid volume
Alteration in cardiac output (decreased)	Impaired cardiac conduction with decreased rate and contractility due to calcium influence on myocardium	Arrhythmias Decreased Q–T interval Widened T wave Decreased S–T interval Increased BP	Monitor VS Ascultate lung sounds Promote bedrest in Fowler's position Monitor intake and output Monitor daily weights Encourage rest after meals; balance rest with all activities Monitor ECG pattern and observe for change	States has no SOB at rest Stable dry weight is maintained
Alteration in thought process, acute, reversible confusion	Increased calcium Metabolic dysfunction	Disorientation Failure to recognize others Incoherent communication Verbalizes confusion Agitation Aggression Anxiety Depressed state Delusion with withdrawal Climbing out of bed Incontinence Purposeless activity	Make call light available and reinforce use of call light Provide for safety Encourage use of eyeglasses, hearing aides, etc. Speak slowly, distinctly in a low-pitched voice Establish touch contact Orient to time and place Use calm, nonthreatening responses Encourage discussion of interest to patient Give simple, brief instructions just before occurrence of events Introduce new experiences slowly with participation in decision making Pace activities Monitor confusion for frequency and time of day Keep light on at night Provide consistent staffing Reduce distracting noises Provide clocks/calendars	Orientation Able to function in environment Interacts with others appropriately

BP, blood pressure; CVP, central venous pressure; ECG, electrocardiogram; SG, specific gravity; VS, vital signs.

TABLE 24–4.
Management of Hypercalcemia in the Patient with Cancer

Short-term/acute

Fluid replacement with NaCl solutions

Increase renal calcium excretion:
▶ NaCl repletion increases renal calcium clearance
▶ Administration of diuretics:
   Furosemide
   Ethacrynic acid

Reduce calcium intake by dietary manipulation

Withdraw medications that increase serum calcium levels:
▶ Thiazide diuretics
▶ Vitamins A and D
▶ Hormonal agents used to treat breast cancer (tamoxifen)

Inhibit bone resorption:
▶ Didronel
▶ Mithramycin
▶ Calcitonin

Directly reduce blood levels:
▶ Hemodialysis
▶ Peritoneal dialysis

Long-term/chronic

Decrease bone lysis/humoral stimulus
▶ Tumor ablation with radiation, chemotherapy, or surgical excision of the tumor

Decrease osteoclastic activity
▶ Increase mobility

Decrease intake

Decrease absorption from the gut:
▶ Phosphates
▶ Corticosteroids

---

phates associated with rapid cell lysis resulting in calcium phosphate salt precipitation and serum calcium reduction

Symptoms of hypocalcemia include weakness, fatigue, irritability, progressive paresthesia, carpopedal spasms, and tetany. Treatment of hypocalcemia consists of oral or IV calcium gluconate administration (using serial serum calcium levels until normal states are achieved).[16]

Hyperuricemia

Hyperuricemia and hyperuricosuria are significant problems for patients with myeloproliferative disorders, lymphomas, myeloma, or leukemia.[17] It is not usually a problem for patients with solid tumors. The serum uric acid elevation that occurs is usually related to the following:

▶ Rapid release of nucleic acids from the tumor cell lysis as a result of radiation therapy or chemother-

apy (This is most commonly noted in patients with lymphoma or leukemia.)
▶ Overproduction of uric acid precursors by tumor (this is most commonly noted in patients with polycythemia vera and chronic granulocytic leukemia.)
▶ Certain rapidly proliferating neoplasms with a high nucleic acid turnover that may present with hyperuricemia even in the absence of prior chemotherapy

Obviously, malignant tumors with high growth rates and a high cell mass release excessive amounts of nucleic acids when treated. Consequently, nucleic acid metabolism leads to elevation of the serum uric acid level. Diagnosis is established by measurement of serum and urine uric acid levels. The normal excretory rate for uric acid is 300 to 500 mg/day.

Untreated serum uric acid levels may reach 20 mg/dL. The patient may exhibit ureteral colic, oliguria, and azotemia. Hemodialysis should be considered in patients with urate nephropathy.[18]

Prevention of hyperuricemia is the cornerstone of management (Table 24-5). Prophylactic treatment of hyperuricemia consists of the following:

▶ Vigorous hydration
▶ Administration of allopurinol
▶ Alkalinization of the urine

Hyperuricemia must be viewed as a preventable complication rather than as an emergent condition.

HYPONATREMIA

Isaacs[19] reported that hyponatremia was the most common electrolyte imbalance seen in her patient popula-

---

TABLE 24–5.
Management of Hyperuricemia in the Patient with Cancer

Prevention:

▶ Allopurinol (Zyloprim) 300 mg q.d. Started 1 day before chemotherapy to inhibit uric acid formation

Emergency treatment:

▶ Decrease uric acid concentration in the urine by means of adequate hydration to achieve an output of 4 L/day
▶ Decrease uric acid production by administration of allopurinol 300 mg/day (more in severe cases)
▶ Increase uric acid solubility by increasing urine pH to 7.0 or above by means of sodium bicarbonate administration

If nephropathy is established, emergency hemodialysis or peritoneal dialysis may be indicated (fluid administration in the presence of renal failure is dangerous)

tion. Reasons cited for decreased serum sodium levels in cancer patients include the following:

▶ Ectopic release of an ADH-like substance from certain tumors, especially small-cell bronchogenic cancer
▶ Salt loss from the gastrointestinal (GI) tract as occurs in vomiting or fistulous drainage
▶ Hyperproteinemic states, including multiple myeloma and hyperglobulinemia

Secretion of inappropriate antidiuretic hormone (SIADH) syndrome may occur in persons with certain malignancies. These tumors produce an ectopic ADH-like substance in the presence of decreasing serum sodium and serum osmolality. Serum sodium level falls dangerously low and creates a myriad of clinical manifestations (see Table 4-4). Antitumor agents associated with SIADH include cyclophosphamide (Cytoxan) and vincristine (Oncovin). Cytoxan given in doses greater than 50 mg/kg will induce related hyponatremia, which will usually occur 4 to 8 hours after the drug is given and resolve within 24 hours of drug withdrawal. Patients receiving high-dose cyclophosphamide should be monitored for water intoxication. Hyponatremia associated with vincristine administration is usually accompanied by other signs of toxicity associated with the drug. The most common of these are ileus and peripheral neuropathy.[20]

Surgical removal of the tumor is the most direct treatment of SIADH. Chemotherapy and radiation therapy may be palliative and temporarily increase the sodium level by decreasing formation of the ectopic hormone. Other standard measures to control water excess and restore normal serum sodium concentrations are described in Chapter 4. On a short-term basis, fluid intake is restricted to the extent that negative water balance is induced; this may require restriction of as little as 400 to 700 mL/day. Administration of furosemide plus salt replacement has accomplished an increase in the serum sodium concentration. Use of demeclocycline (Declomycin) for long-term control of hyponatremia may be indicated, particularly in patients with uncontrolled malignancies; this agent inhibits the action of ADH on the kidneys, allowing increased urinary output and an increase in serum sodium. (Many patients find the long-term restriction of water extremely unpleasant.)

HYPERKALEMIA

Rapid cell destruction after successful treatment of large tumors may cause a precipitous release of cellular potassium and an increase in the serum potassium level. This is most frequently seen during induction therapy for acute leukemia. An increased serum potassium level can also result from acute renal failure due to untreated hyperuricemia.

A falsely high serum potassium level may be reported in the presence of high white blood cell counts. (Increased leukocyte fragility and lysis of cells after venous sampling may falsify the level in the clotted serum sample.) Validation of a supposed hyperkalemic state with the expected electrocardiographic changes and other clinical signs of hyperkalemia is needed to determine if the serum potassium level is truly elevated in a patient with a high white count due to a leukemic process.

HYPOKALEMIA

A decrease in serum potassium in patients with cancer may be associated with decreased intake or excessive loss of potassium ions. Excessive loss of potassium due to renal tubular damage occurs in 60% of patients during induction therapy for acute nonlymphocytic leukemia.[21] Renal tubular damage is attributed to two processes:

▶ Acute tubular necrosis due to antibiotic therapy during neutropenic states (Drugs that may produce this effect include gentamycin, carbenicillin, and cephalothin.)
▶ Elevated lysozymuria due to cellular breakdown

These mechanisms for increased potassium loss both revert to normal after the patient recovers from induction therapy.

Certain malignancies produce a decreased serum potassium level related to an ACTH-like substance released by cancer cells. These malignancies include the following:

▶ Small-cell carcinoma of the lung
▶ Thymoma
▶ Pancreatic islet cell carcinomas
▶ Medullary carcinoma of the thyroid
▶ Carcinoid tumors of the bronchus[22, 23]

Patients with ACTH-like tumor-related hypokalemia do not usually exhibit clinical signs associated with Cushing's disease. The main manifestations of ectopic ACTH tumor release include such things as elevated urinary 17-hydroxycorticosteroid content, decreased serum potassium, edema, and presence of ACTH in the tumor extract. High ACTH levels stimulate gluconeogenesis, which results in hyperglycemia. As with ectopic ADH production, normal feedback regulatory inhibition does not occur; thus, testing with normal-dose dexamethasone suppression is not successful. Only high-dose dexamethasone administration will depress ACTH levels due to ectopic tumor production. Surgical removal of the tumor is warranted to control the production of the ectopic ACTH. If this is not possible, surgical adrenalectomy or treatment with aminoglutethimide may be indicated. Potassium losses can be replaced with oral supplements, a difficult treatment that requires titration of potassium doses up to 120 mEq/day.

A decrease in serum potassium related to decreased intake may commonly be associated with anorexia or nausea related to cancer or prescribed therapy. Administration of potassium-free IV fluids exaggerates the potassium reduction further.

Excessive loss of potassium can be associated with excessive vomiting, fistulae drainage, diarrhea, prolonged GI mechanical suction, increased renal tubular loss due to damage, and ectopic ACTH production by malignant cells.

HYPERPHOSPHATEMIA

An elevated phosphate level alone does not cause symptoms. Hyperphosphatemia usually occurs along with hyperuricemia and hyperkalemia. It is an uncommon complication of therapy for certain malignancies (ie, leukemia and lymphoma). Massive tumor breakdown in those patients undergoing treatment releases large amounts of uric acid, potassium, and phosphate. Although the increase in phosphate levels may not be evident for several days after initiating therapy, this elevation may persist for several days after treatment and be as high as 20 mg/dL.

Renal damage or acute renal failure may be a serious problem resulting from the precipitation of calcium phosphate in the kidneys. If the patient's ionized calcium concentration is markedly reduced, tetany may develop. High phosphate levels must be reduced rapidly to prevent or to correct renal damage[24] (Table 24-6).

HYPOPHOSPHATEMIA

Hypophosphatemia may be associated with rapidly proliferating malignancies (eg, acute leukemia) pre-

TABLE 24–6.
Management of Hyperphosphatemia

Oral fluids, 2–4 L/day

Aluminum hydroxide gel (to bind phosphate in the intestine)

IV infusion of hypertonic dextrose and regular insulin (to force phosphate into cells)

IV infusion of half-normal saline at 100–200 mL/hr to expand the extracellular fluid volume

Dialysis (may be necessary for patients with renal failure)

sumably due to the consumption of phosphate by the tumor cells. Hypophosphatemia that is severe (less than 1 mg/dL) can result in hemolysis.[25] Hypophosphatemia associated with malignant disease occurs subsequent to nutritional deprivation and cancer cachexia. Prolonged hyperalimentation without appropriate phosphate additives, and respiratory alkalosis, which is associated with the septicemic episodes of neutropenic patients, may also result in hypophosphatemia. Therapy consists of phosphate replacement by either the oral or the IV route. Intravenous replacement is indicated in severe cases (see Chapter 8).

HYPOMAGNESEMIA

Cisplatin, a potentially nephrotoxic agent used against epithelial neoplasms, can cause hypomagnesemia.[26] Apparently, cisplatin causes renal-magnesium wasting in a dose-related manner.[27] The cause of the renal magnesium wasting is not clear, but among the possible causes are a direct effect of cisplatin on the renal absorption of magnesium, and interstitial nephritis due to the drug (causing damage to Henle's loop and reducing magnesium absorption).[28] Other causes of hypomagnesemia are those that can occur in any patient (eg, magnesium loss in chronic diarrhea or prolonged diuretic use, and inadequate magnesium supplementation during hyperalimentation). The reader is referred to Chapter 7 for a discussion of other causes of hypomagnesemia as well as its treatment.

SUMMARY OF TREATMENT

Traditionally, many fluid and electrolyte problems experienced by oncology patients are managed with replacement or restrictive treatment modalities. However, the underlying cause of the electrolyte problem must be considered or a chronic problem will develop. Tumor elimination or control is a primary consideration. Careful, continued observation of the patient is indicated to control the malignancy and its associated fluid/electrolyte problems effectively. See Chapter 2 for a review of assessment parameters associated with fluid and electrolyte balances and Chapters 3–9 dealing with specific imbalances.

REFERENCES

1. Dorr R, Fritz W: Cancer Chemotherapy Handbook, p 180. New York, Elsevier North-Holland, 1980
2. Lind J: Ectopic hormonal production: Nursing implications. Sem Onco Nurs 1(4):251, November 1985
3. Cunningham E: Fluid and electrolyte disturbances

associated with cancer and its treatment. Nurs Clin North Am 17(4):579, 1982

4. Fields A, Josse R, Bergsagel R: Metabolic emergencies. In DeVita et al (eds): Cancer Principles and Practices of Oncology, pp 1866–1877. Philadelphia, JB Lippincott, 1985

5. Singer F, Fernandez M: Therapy of hypercalcemia and malignancy. Am J Med 82:2A, 1987

6. Carlson H, Casciato D, Lowitz B: Manual of Clinical Oncology, 2nd ed, pp 411–426. Boston, Little, Brown, 1988

7. Bockman R: Hypercalcemia in malignancy. Clin Endocrinol Metab 9(2):317, 1980

8. Ibid, p 322

9. Kahn A, Stewart C, Teirtelbaum S: Contact medicated bone resorption by human monocytes in vitro. *Science* 199:988, 1978

10. Bockman, p 322

11. Dorr, Fritz, p 153

12. Carlon G, Turnbull A, Howland W: Intensive care of the cancer patient. In: Shoemaker W et al (eds): Textbook of Critical Care, 2nd ed, p 937. Philadelphia, WB Saunders, 1989

13. Ibid

14. Didronel IV Infusion for the Treatment of Hypercalcemia of Malignancy: A Monography, pp 4–9. Norwich, NY, Norwish-Eaton, May 1987

15. Bonjour J, Rizzoli R: Clodronate in hypercalcemia of malignancy. Calcif Tissue Int 46 (Suppl):520, 1990

16. Haskell C: Cancer Treatment, p 988. Philadelphia, WB Saunders, 1980

17. Haskell, p 998

18. See-Lasley K, Ignoffo R: Manual of Oncology Therapeutics, p 357. St. Louis, CV Mosby, 1981

19. Isaacs M: Life threatening fluid and electrolyte abnormalities in patients with cancer. Curr Probl Cancer 4 (3):8, 1979

20. Schilsky R: Renal and metabolic toxicities of cancer chemotherapy. Semin Oncol, 9 (1):75, 1982

21. See-Lasley, Ignoffo, p 314

22. Carlson, p 422

23. Lind, p 254

24. Carlson, p 416

25. Ibid, p 417

26. Kokko J, Tannen R: Fluids and Electrolytes, 2nd ed, p 641. Philadelphia, WB Saunders, 1990

27. Lam M, Adelstein D: Hypomagnesemia and renal magnesium wasting in patients treated with cisplatin. Am J Kidney Dis 8:164, 1986

28. Maxwell M, Kleeman C, Narins R: Clinical Disorders of Fluid and Electrolyte Metabolism, 4th ed, p 835. New York, McGraw-Hill, 1987

unit five

SPECIAL CONSIDERATIONS IN CHILDREN AND THE ELDERLY

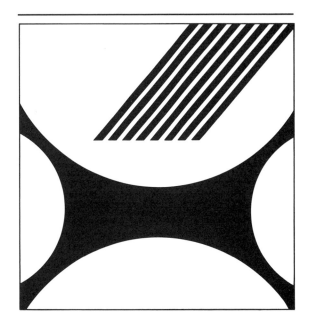

25

Fluid Balance in Infants and Children

An obvious difference between young children and adults is size. However, children are not merely miniature adults, for the child's body composition and homeostatic controls differ from those of the adult. The younger the child, the greater the differences. It is helpful to compare the child's body composition with that of the adult and review the salient characteristics of the child's homeostatic and metabolic functioning.

DIFFERENCES IN WATER AND ELECTROLYTE BALANCE IN INFANTS, CHILDREN, AND ADULTS

BODY WATER CONTENT

The premature infant's body is approximately 90% water; the newborn infant's body, 70% to 80%; the adult's body about 60%. Infants have proportionately more water in the extracellular compartment than do adults. For example, 40% of the newborn infant's body water is in the extracelluluar compartment, as compared with less than 20% in the case of the adult.

As the infant becomes older, the ratio of extracellular to intracellular fluid volume decreases. Loss of extracellular fluid (ECF) is attributed to the growth of cellular tissue and the decreasing rate of growth of collagen relative to muscle growth during the early months of life. The decrease is particularly rapid during the first few days of life, but continues throughout the first 6 months. After the first year, the total body water is about 64% (34% in the cellular compartment and 30% in the ECF compartment). By the end of the second year, the total body water approaches the adult percentage of approximately 60% (36% in the cellular compartment and 24% in the ECF compartment). At puberty, the adult body water composition is attained.

DAILY BODY WATER TURNOVER IN INFANTS AND ADULTS

The fact that infants have a relatively greater total body water content does not protect them from excessive fluid loss. On the contrary, infants are *more* vulnerable to fluid volume deficit (FVD) because they ingest and excrete a relatively greater daily water volume than adults do. An infant may exchange half of his or her ECF daily, whereas the adult may exchange only one sixth during the same period. Proportionately, therefore, the infant has a smaller reserve of body fluid than does the adult.

The daily fluid exchange is relatively greater in infants, in part because their metabolic rate is two times

higher per unit of weight than that of adults. Infants expend 100 kcal/kg of body weight, whereas adults expend only 40 kcal/kg. Owing to the high metabolic rate, the infant has a large amount of metabolic wastes to excrete. Because water is needed by the kidneys to excrete these wastes, a large urinary volume is formed each day. Contributing to this volume is the inability of the infant's immature kidneys to concentrate urine efficiently. In addition, relatively greater fluid loss occurs through the infant's skin because of the proportionately greater body surface area.

HOMEOSTATIC DIFFERENCES BETWEEN CHILDREN AND ADULTS

Young children have immature homeostatic regulating mechanisms that must be considered when planning water and electrolyte replacement.

Renal Function

The newborn's renal function is not yet completely developed. If infant and adult renal functions are compared on the basis of total body water, the infant's kidneys appear to become mature by the end of the first month of life. However, if body surface area is used as the criterion for comparison, the child's kidneys appear immature for the first 2 years of life. Because the infant's kidneys have a limited concentrating ability and require more water to excrete a given amount of solute, the infant has difficulty conserving body water when it is needed. Also, the infant has difficulty excreting an excess fluid volume.[1] Thus, infants are less able to adapt to too little, or too much, fluid. Although adults may be able to tolerate fluid imbalances for days, infants may tolerate similar disturbances for only hours before the situation becomes acute.

Acid–Base Homeostasis

Newborn and premature infants have less homeostatic buffering capacity than do older children. They have a tendency toward metabolic acidosis, with pH averages slightly lower (7.30–7.35) than normal.[2] The mild metabolic acidosis (base bicarbonate deficit) is believed to be related to high metabolic acid production and to renal immaturity. Because cow's milk has higher phosphate and sulfate concentrations than breast milk, newborns fed cow's milk have a lower pH than do breastfed babies.

Body Surface Area Differences

The skin represents an important route of fluid loss, especially in illness. This is an important concept when considering fluid balance in infants and young children because their body surface area is greater than that of older children and adults. For example, compared with the older child and adults, the premature infant has approximately five times as much body surface area in relation to weight, and the newborn, three times. Therefore, any condition causing a pronounced decrease in intake or increase in output of water and electrolytes threatens the body fluid economy of the infant. Because the gastrointestinal (GI) membranes are essentially an extension of the body surface area, their area is also relatively greater in the young infant than in the older child and adult. Hence, relatively greater losses occur from the GI tract in the sick infant than in the older child and adult. In comparing fluid losses in infants with those in adults, one might regard the baby's body as a smaller vessel with a larger spout.

Calcium–Phosphorus Regulation

Newborn infants are vulnerable to disrupted calcium homeostasis when stressed by illness or by an excess phosphate dietary load. Neonatal tetany with hypocalcemia was first described in the early 1900s. It is not clear if the disturbance is due to transient immaturity of parathyroid function or to other factors, such as vitamin D deficiency. It is known that the serum phosphate level is elevated in the early months of infancy (6.5–7.5 mg/dL) and remains somewhat above adult levels until puberty is reached. Phosphate retention is aggravated by the oliguria associated with FVD; of course, a high phosphate level contributes to hypocalcemia.

Electrolyte Concentrations

Plasma electrolyte concentrations do not vary strikingly among infants, small children, and adults. The plasma sodium concentration changes little from birth to adulthood. Potassium concentration is higher in the first few months of life than at any other time, as is the plasma chloride concentration. Magnesium and calcium are both low in the first 24 hours after birth. As stated above, the serum phosphate level is higher in infants and children than in adults, and inability of the premature infant to regulate calcium ion concentration can bring on hypocalcemic tetany.

NURSING ASSESSMENT

Initial assessment of the infant or child with a suspected or potential fluid and electrolyte imbalance includes a review of the history and laboratory data as well as systematic observation and physical inspection.

An infant or child who is ill appears flaccid, and the eyes lack their usual brightness and sparkle.

A history from the parents will usually reveal that the child has a decreased appetite, is less active, and is more irritable than usual. Additional information may reveal large losses of fluid through diarrhea or vomiting, and an inability to "get anything" into the child. The history should include the frequency and amount of voiding as well as the number and consistency of stools before admission. All this information should be carefully recorded in the child's record.

Additional objective assessments should be obtained and should include the child's weight and vital signs. A blood pressure reading in a young child is not always a reliable sign of fluid volume status because elasticity of the blood vessels may keep the blood pressure stable initially even when volume is diminished.[3] See Chapter 2 for a review of a systematic approach to assessment of fluid balance status. The following discussion is specific to children.

TISSUE TURGOR

Tissue turgor in the child is best palpated in the abdominal areas and on the medial aspects of the thighs. In a normal situation, pinched skin will fall back to its normal configuration when released. In a patient with FVD, the skin may remain slightly raised for a few seconds. Skin turgor begins to decrease after 3% to 5% of the body weight is lost as fluid. Severe malnutrition, particularly in infants, can cause depressed skin turgor even in the absence of fluid depletion.

Obese infants with FVD often have skin turgor that is deceptively normal in appearance. An infant with water loss in excess of sodium loss (hypernatremia, or sodium excess) has a firm, thick-feeling skin. This same phenomenon is observed in the child who has sodium excess owing to an excessive sodium intake such as occurs in salt poisoning. The thickened turgor is believed to be associated with pulling of water from the cells into the hypertonic interstitial fluid.

MUCOUS MEMBRANES

Dry mouth may be due to FVD or to mouth breathing. When in doubt, the nurse should run a finger along the oral cavity to feel the mucous membrane where the cheek and gums meet; dryness in this area indicates a true FVD. The tongue of the fluid-depleted child is smaller than normal. Mucous membranes in the child with sodium excess are dry and sticky. The absence of tearing and salivation is a sign of FVD that becomes obvious with a fluid loss of 5% of the total body weight.

BODY TEMPERATURE

Fluid volume deficit is often associated with a subnormal temperature because of reduced energy output. Depending on the underlying disease, however, fever can accompany FVD. If fever is present, its height should be recorded frequently. The rate of insensible water loss is greatly increased with fever; the amount of water loss depends on the height and duration of the fever. Fever may indicate excessive water loss from the body with resultant sodium excess, or it may indicate an infection. The extremities are cold to the touch in severe FVD, even when fever is present; this is due to decreased peripheral blood flow.

URINE VOLUME AND CONCENTRATION

When possible, all urine should be collected and measured in the child with a real or potential body fluid disturbance. Unfortunately, this is often difficult to do in infants and small children. In this situation, at least the frequency of voiding should be noted. In addition, the nurse should estimate the portion of the diaper saturated with urine. One would do well to weigh a dry diaper occasionally and compare its weight with that of the same diaper after the child has voided. The urine's concentration, as revealed by its color, should also be noted. When necessary, urinary specific gravity can be measured with a refractometer; fortunately, this device requires only a drop of urine for the test.

Hourly urinary output reflects the adequacy of hemodynamics and hydration. It will be zero if there is no perfusing pressure (< 70–80 mmHg systolic) and less than normal when there is an FVD of 20% or more of the blood volume.[4] As a general rule, normal urinary output is about 1 mL/kg of body weight per hour.[5] Because urine flow rates in sick newborns may vary considerably from hour to hour, the average output should be calculated every 6 hours. The urine output should average at least 5 mL/kg in each 6-hour period.[6]

When an accurate hourly recording of urine output is indicated, the nurse must devise a method to collect all the urine passed. A number of devices are available; regardless of the type used, check frequently for leakage and provide good skin care to prevent irritation of the genitalia.

A child with FVD has a decreased urinary output and an increased urinary specific gravity. If the FVD is severe, a child may go as long as 18 to 24 hours without voiding and still not have a distended bladder. If a child with a known FVD excretes large amounts of dilute urine, renal damage probably exists. If renal concentrating ability is impaired, or if the child is receiving a high-solute diet, the urine volume will be somewhat above normal to clear all the metabolic

wastes. The same is true if a hypercatabolic state (such as fever or infection or both) is present.

WEIGHT CHANGES

If possible, the child's weight before the onset of the illness should be obtained from the parents or from the family physician, who may have a record of the normal weight from a recent office visit.

Weight loss can be caused by loss of fluid or by catabolism of body tissues. The weight loss associated with FVD occurs more rapidly than that caused by starvation. A mild FVD in an infant or child entails a loss of from 3% to 5% of the normal body weight; a moderate FVD, from 5% to 9%; a severe FVD, 10% or more. (An acute loss of 15% of the body weight will likely cause hypovolemic shock.)

If weighing is not performed accurately, it is useless. Even a minor error is important when the patient is small. The child should be weighed at the same time each day, before eating, and after having voided. The same scales should be used each time. The child should be undressed and covered with a light blanket to protect against chilling while being weighed. (The same blanket should be used each time for consistency.)

OTHER CONSIDERATIONS

Additional assessment parameters pertaining to evaluation of fluid balance status are presented in other sections of the text. For example, evaluation of laboratory data is presented in Chapter 2; findings expected in specific imbalances are described in Chapters 3 through 9.

CONDITIONS IN CHILDREN PREDISPOSING TO FLUID AND ELECTROLYTE DISTURBANCES

See Chapters 10 through 24 for discussion of specific entities; although these chapters are primarily concerned with the care of adults, some information is also applicable to children. The discussion below concerns common fluid and electrolyte problems occurring in a pediatric population.

PYLORIC STENOSIS

Pyloric stenosis is a condition in which the circular muscle of the pylorus is elongated and hypertrophic. The condition produces progressive narrowing of the lumen of the outlet from the stomach to the duodenum and results in vomiting after feedings. The condition becomes evident in the first few weeks of life as vomiting becomes progressive and eventually projectile in nature. The condition affects approximately one in every 150 male infants and one in every 750 female infants.

Because of the repeated vomiting, the infants are poorly nourished. Although this condition can be corrected surgically, preoperative correction of the water and electrolyte disturbances caused by the prolonged vomiting is mandatory.[7]

Vomiting causes the same imbalances in children as it does in adults. These include metabolic alkalosis, potassium deficit, sodium deficit, and FVD. See Chapter 16 for a discussion of imbalances associated with vomiting.

The infant with hypertonic pyloric stenosis has the following symptoms:

► Difficulty in retaining feedings, which becomes progressively worse during the first few weeks of life; eventually, projectile vomiting follows each feeding
► Signs of malnutrition
► Signs of FVD (see Chapter 3)
► Constipation
► Decreased respiration (compensatory action of lungs to retain carbon dioxide and thus help counteract metabolic alkalosis)
► Tetany accompanying alkalosis (owing to decreased calcium ionization in an alkaline *p*H)
► Palpable pyloric mass
► Ketoacidosis (may appear if starvation is prolonged)

Once the infant's fluid and electrolyte balance is restored, surgical correction of the pyloric obstruction can be accomplished and oral feedings resumed.

DIARRHEA

Fluid and Electrolyte Disorders

Diarrhea is a common cause of water and electrolyte disturbances in infants and small children. A large loss of liquid stools can rapidly deplete the young child's ECF volume, especially when it is combined with vomiting. Usually water and electrolytes are lost in isotonic proportions (FVD or "isotonic dehydration"). However, water can be lost in excess of electrolytes (FVD with sodium excess or "hypertonic dehydration"), and electrolytes can be lost in excess of water (FVD with sodium deficit or "hypotonic dehydration"). Because sodium is the chief extracellular ion, its excess or deficit is of primary importance in producing symptoms.

Isotonic Dehydration (FVD)

Approximately 70% of patients with severe diarrhea undergo a proportionate loss of water and electrolytes. Symptoms of FVD due to infantile diarrhea include the following:

► History of large quantities of liquid stools
► Acute weight loss
► Dry skin with poor turgor (see Fig. 25-1)
► Diminished tearing
► Soft eyeballs with a sunken appearance (resulting from decreased intraocular pressure)
► Skin ashen or gray in color and extremities cold (owing to inadequate peripheral perfusion)
► Depressed body temperature, unless infection is present
► Lethargy

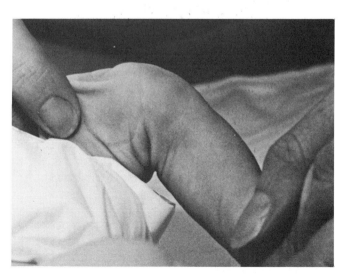

FIGURE 25–1.
Poor skin turgor in infant.

TABLE 25–1.
Nursing Care Plan for an 11-Month-Old Infant with Gastroenteritis (Vomiting and Diarrhea)

ASSESSMENT FINDINGS	GOAL	INTERVENTIONS	EVALUATION CRITERIA
NURSING DIAGNOSIS: FLUID VOLUME DEFICIT, ACTUAL, RELATED TO FLUID LOSS FROM DIARRHEA AND VOMITING			
History of diarrhea and vomiting: ▸ 20 stools in last 24 hr ▸ 4 vomits in 48 hr **Signs of fluid volume loss:** ▸ Last void 6 hr before admission ▸ Skin dry and gray ▸ Skin turgor poor ▸ Sunken fontanel ▸ Eyes sunken ▸ No tearing ▸ Drowsy and lethargic ▸ Weight was 10 kg one week before admission; current weight 9 kg ▸ Pulse 165/min ▸ Respirations 35/min ▸ BP 70/50 History of anorexia and poor intake (nothing by mouth for 12 hr before admission) **Laboratory values:** ▸ Na⁺ 137 mEq/L ▸ Cl⁻ 100 mEq/L ▸ K⁺ 4.1 mEq/L	Safely rehydrate infant (avoid accidental fluid overload during treatment) Maintain serum electrolyte levels within normal limits Decrease incidence of diarrhea and vomiting	Administer prescribed IV fluids and monitor response closely (record type, rate, and amount absorbed) Document hydration status at regular intervals (skin turgor, appearance of eyes and fontanels, vital signs) Maintain NPO status until diarrhea decreases Maintain accurate recording of I & O, weigh diapers if indicated; attach urine collection bag When oral fluids are given, note type and tolerance to the fluid Record weight daily, same time of day, same amount of clothing	Return to normal skin turgor, skin color, and facial appearance Vital signs within normal limits for 11-month-old (resp. 20–30/min, pulse 80–160/min, BP 89/60) Return to near-normal body weight with rehydration No signs of fluid overloading during IV fluid administration Return to normal stool pattern for infant Absence of vomiting, able to retain oral fluids (at this time parenteral route for fluid administration no longer needed) Return to normal, alert behavior Serum electrolyte levels remain within normal limits
NURSING DIAGNOSIS: ALTERATION IN COMFORT RELATED TO RESTRAINTS FOR IV INFUSION			
Prolonged crying; appears frustrated when attempts at movement are thwarted by restraints	Optimum emotional and physical comfort (in given situation)	Provide comfort for infant through holding and stroking, encourage parent participation Remove restraining devices from extremities as often as possible; assure they are not excessively tight; change position at regular intervals	Decreased fretful crying Return to happy, smiling infant Circulation to extremities remains good, as evidenced by normal skin color and temperature and peripheral pulses
NURSING DIAGNOSIS: IMPAIRED SKIN INTEGRITY RELATED TO FREQUENT LOOSE STOOLS			
Loss of superficial epidermis in perianal area	Promote healing	Change diaper frequently to keep the infant clean and dry; wash perianal area with mild soap after each stool, rinse well, pat dry, and apply protective ointment	Perianal area heals; skin integrity normal

(continued)

TABLE 25–1.
(continued)

ASSESSMENT FINDINGS	GOAL	INTERVENTIONS	EVALUATION CRITERIA
NURSING DIAGNOSIS: PARENTAL KNOWLEDGE DEFICIT RELATED TO INFANT DIARRHEA AND MANAGEMENT			
Parents asking questions regarding care of ill infant	Answer questions to parents' satisfaction	Provide information regarding physical care of infant (encourage parental involvement in care as much as possible)	Parents report understanding of infant's care
		Provide information regarding emotional care of infant (encourage holding, comforting, and stimulation)	Parents participate in both physical and emotional care of infant
Parents express concern about what to do the next time diarrhea occurs		Provide information regarding infection control techniques, handwashing, stool disposal, and dietary management	Parents report understanding of infection-control techniques, stool disposal, and dietary management
		Discuss need for follow-up care with pediatrician and need to report diarrhea early so that appropriate treatment can be initiated	Return visit to pediatrician established
			Parents express understanding of need to consult physician early if diarrhea recurs

▶ Signs of hypovolemia (weak, rapid pulse, decreased blood pressure)
▶ Oliguria, increased specific gravity
▶ Serum sodium concentration between 130 and 150 mEq/L

To assist the reader with application of the nursing process, a sample care plan for a child with FVD (isotonic dehydration) related to diarrhea is presented in Table 25-1.

Hypertonic Dehydration (FVD with Hypernatremia)

Approximately 20% of patients with severe diarrhea have suffered a relatively greater loss of water than of electrolytes. If the infant has ingested a high-solute-containing formula during illness or has been inadvertently given an overly concentrated electrolyte mixture, the resultant increased renal water loss will intensify the sodium excess already present. Recall that the infant cannot concentrate urine efficiently and thus needs a relatively large water intake to excrete solutes. The infant's need for water is further intensified by a large body surface area and resultant increased insensible water loss.

Symptoms of FVD and sodium excess (hypertonic dehydration) caused by diarrhea include the following:

▶ History of large quantities of liquid stools associated with a low water intake, high solute intake, poor renal function, or all three
▶ Weight loss
▶ Serum sodium > 150 mEq/L
▶ Thickened, firm-feeling skin (caused by fluid being pulled from cells into interstitial space)
▶ Avid thirst (hypertonic ECF draws water from cells, producing cellular dehydration)
▶ Irritability when disturbed: otherwise behavior is lethargic
▶ Tremors and convulsions
▶ Muscle rigidity
▶ Nuchal rigidity
▶ Pronounced signs of hypernatremia; signs of FVD are variable
▶ Brain injury (Hypernatremia causes the brain tissue to shrink; if the imbalance is severe and occurs rapidly, small blood vessels may rupture. See Chapter 4 for further discussions of hypernatremia.)

Hypotonic Dehydration (FVD with Hyponatremia)

Approximately 10% of patients with severe diarrhea experience a relatively greater loss of electrolytes than water in the stool. Bacillary dysentery and cholera are two diseases that may result in hypotonic dehydration because the concentration of sodium in the stool rises with the increasing volume of the stool.[8] Viral infections are not associated with such severe losses of sodium. However, hyponatremia can occur in children with viral enteritis if they are given electrolyte-free fluids to replace their losses. See the next sections for a discussion of oral rehydration therapy and the consequences of excessive water intake.

Because sodium is the chief extracellular ion, the primary symptoms in hypotonic dehydration are due to the sodium deficit. Symptoms include the following:

▶ Gray pallor
▶ Cold, clammy skin with poor turgor
▶ Slightly moist mucous membranes
▶ Sunken eyes
▶ Rapid pulse and low blood pressure
▶ Lethargy that may advance to coma
▶ Serum sodium < 130 mEq/L

Metabolic Acidosis

Metabolic acidosis usually accompanies frequent liquid stools. (Recall that the intestinal secretions are alkaline because of their high bicarbonate content; therefore, loss of alkaline secretions in diarrheal stools results in metabolic acidosis.) Decreased dietary intake contributes to metabolic acidosis; in the absence of adequate food intake, the body uses its own fats for energy purposes. The metabolism of these fats causes the accumulation of acidic ketone bodies in the blood, further contributing to the metabolic acidosis caused by bicarbonate loss.

A major symptom of metabolic acidosis is increased depth of respiration, a compensatory mechanism that blows off carbon dioxide, thus reducing the carbonic acid content of the blood and influencing the carbonic acid–base bicarbonate balance in the direction of an increased pH. If ketosis of starvation is present, an acetone odor may be noted on the breath.

Other Electrolyte Imbalances

Deficits of potassium and magnesium are also common disturbances with prolonged diarrhea. These imbalances are discussed in Chapters 5 and 7, respectively.

Treatment

Oral Rehydration

The dehydration that results from diarrhea in infants and children can be treated by the oral administration of a glucose-electrolyte solution. In many developing countries, oral rehydration therapy is the only form of treatment available, and it has been shown to reduce significantly the mortality rate from acute diarrhea.[9] The oral rehydration solution (ORS) recommended by the Diarrhea Disease Control Program of the World Health Organization contains sodium, potassium, chloride, base, glucose, and water. Table 25-2 presents the composition of ORS and several other commercial products. Glucose is the preferred sugar to use in oral rehydration solutions because it facilitates the transport of sodium across the bowel wall.[10]

The amount and rate of oral fluid administration are calculated according to the degree of volume depletion and the child's weight. Vomiting is not necessarily a

TABLE 25–2.
Oral Electrolyte Solutions: Concentration When Diluted

PRODUCT	Na (mEq/L)	K (mEq/L)	Cl (mEq/L)	BASE (mEq/L)	GLUCOSE g/L
Rehydration					
ORS (WHO)	90	20	80	30	20
Rehydralyte (Ross)	75	20	65	30	25
Maintenance					
Infalyte (Pennwalt)	50	20	40	30	20
Lytren (Mead Johnson)	50	25	45	30	20
Pedialyte (Ross)	45	20	35	30	25
Resol (Wyeth)	50	20	50	34	34

(Adapted from Feld LG, Kaskel FJ, Schoeneman MJ: The approach to fluid and electrolyte therapy in pediatrics. In Barness LA: Advances in Pediatrics, vol 35, p 520. Chicago, Year Book Medical Publishers, 1988.)

contraindication to oral rehydration therapy.[11] To minimize vomiting, the solution should be given slowly in small amounts and at frequent intervals. To evaluate the child's progress, skin turgor, body weight, and behavioral responses should be assessed frequently. Nursing strategies for administering oral fluids to infants and young children are discussed later in the chapter.

Parenteral Fluid Therapy

Infants and children with diarrhea who are in impending hypovolemic shock, or who are unable to drink because of lethargy or severe nausea, must have parenteral fluid therapy to replace their losses and restore their fluid and electrolyte homeostasis. See section on principles of parenteral fluid replacement in children later in this chapter.

CONSTIPATION

Undesirable effects of enemas for the treatment of constipation in infants and young children are discussed in Chapter 16. Serious electrolyte complications (primarily hyperphosphatemia, hypocalcemia, and hypernatremia) have been reported with the use of sodium phosphate (Fleet) enemas in young children. As indicated below, excessive absorption of water from tap-water enemas can lead to hyponatremia. Many clinicians favor the use of isotonic saline (0.9% NaCl) as an enema solution when enemas are needed in young children.[12]

EXCESSIVE WATER INTAKE

Healthy older children and adults can tolerate large increases in free water intake, but infants cannot. Because the urinary diluting capacity of infants is limited by a low rate of glomerular filtration,[13] excess water cannot be excreted efficiently. The accumulation of free water in the extracellular space produces acute dilutional hyponatremia (water intoxication), which is a very serious fluid and electrolyte problem.

Acute dilutional hyponatremia can develop in infants who are fed excessively diluted formula[14] or who swallow large amounts of water during swimming lessons.[15] The condition also can occur in infants who are given tap-water enemas because excessive water may be absorbed from the large intestine.[16] The inappropriate use of glucose solutions in water, either as oral or parenteral therapy, to treat infants with dehydration can result in acute dilutional hyponatremia.[17]

As the extracellular sodium dilutes, water shifts to the intracellular space, pulmonary and cerebral edema develop, and intracranial pressure increases. Signs of acute dilutional hyponatremia include the following:

▸ Lethargy and irritability
▸ Subnormal temperature
▸ Focal or generalized seizures
▸ Respiratory distress

Treatment is directed toward restricting free water intake and carefully elevating the serum sodium level.[18] With skilled medical and nursing care, the prognosis is good. In a report of 19 infants with acute dilutional hyponatremia, all of whom experienced seizures and six of whom required endotracheal intubation, all recovered without apparent sequelae.[19]

PRINCIPLES OF PARENTERAL FLUID REPLACEMENT IN CHILDREN

DAILY REQUIREMENTS

Daily requirements for water are related to both caloric consumption and expenditure. The normal water requirements per kilogram of body weight for healthy infants and children are listed in Table 25-3.

Infants and children who cannot tolerate oral feedings, particularly when abnormal losses are occurring, must receive parenteral fluid therapy to meet maintenance and replacement needs. Maintenance requirements can be computed in several ways. One common method is based on total body weight and uses the following formula:

100 mL/kg of body weight for the first 10 kg
50 mL/kg of body weight for the second 10 kg up to 20 kg
20 mL/kg of body weight for each kg above 20 kg

Another method for calculating maintenance fluid requirements is based on total body surface area in square meters (m^2) and the formula of 1500 mL/m^2/day. Body surface area (BSA) can be determined by plotting the child's height and weight on a nomogram (Fig. 25-2).

Maintenance requirements calculated by either of these formulas may have to be modified on the basis of assessment data. Factors such as an extremely humid environment or the ability to take and retain some oral fluids will reduce the amount of maintenance fluids to be delivered parenterally. Factors such as hyperventilation, an extremely dry environment, or a high body temperature will require an increase in the amount of maintenance fluids.

In addition to the rough guidelines described above, fluid volume replacement must be based on the history, on clinical assessment of circulatory impairment or changes in skin elasticity (discussed earlier), and on laboratory values such as serum electrolytes and osmo-

TABLE 25–3.
Range of Average Water Requirements of Children at Different Ages
Under Ordinary Conditions

AGE	AVERAGE BODY WEIGHT (KG)	TOTAL WATER IN 24 HOURS (ML)	WATER PER KG BODY WT IN 24 HOURS (ML)
3 days	3.0	250–300	80–100
10 days	3.2	400–500	125–150
3 mo	5.4	750–850	140–160
6 mo	7.3	950–1100	130–155
9 mo	8.6	1100–1250	125–145
1 yr	9.5	1150–1300	120–135
2 yr	11.8	1350–1500	115–125
4 yr	16.2	1600–1800	100–110
6 yr	20.0	1800–2000	90–100
10 yr	28.7	2000–2500	70–85
14 yr	45.0	2200–2700	50–60

(Adapted from Behrman RE, Vaughn VC: Nelson Textbook of Pediatrics, 13th ed, p 115. Philadelphia, WB Saunders, 1987.)

lality. See Chapter 2 for a discussion of laboratory tests and Chapter 11 for a discussion of water and electrolyte solutions and nursing considerations in their administration. In summary, the amount and type of parenteral fluid to be administered must be based on the degree and type of dehydration (isotonic, hypertonic, or hypotonic), serum electrolyte levels, and the nature of acid–base balance.

CORRECTION OF ISOTONIC DEHYDRATION (FVD)

Isotonic constriction of body fluids is observable by dry skin and mucous membranes as well as tachycardia when about 5% of the body weight has been lost over a 24-hour period. Marked circulatory impairment evidenced by mottled, cool, inelastic skin and sunken eyes occurs when the child has lost 10% of the body weight over a 1- to 2-day period. Losses of 15% of the body weight over this time can produce a moribund or near-moribund state.[20]

When the degree of fluid and electrolyte imbalance has been determined, therapy is administered in phases. The objective of the first phase (the emergency period) is to restore circulation by rapid expansion of the ECF volume, either to treat shock or prevent its occurrence. The repletion period lasts 6 to 8 hours and replaces ECF losses with half the estimated volume deficit. During the next 16 of the first 24 hours, the concern is with cellular fluid restoration, and the second half of the day's estimate plus any additional disease-related losses is administered.

CORRECTION OF HYPERTONIC DEHYDRATION (FVD WITH HYPERNATREMIA)

Recall that in this type of fluid loss, water loss has exceeded sodium loss. The child will likely have central nervous system involvement, evidenced by irritability, lethargy, nuchal rigidity, and convulsions. The principle of therapy is *very gradual* replacement of water over time so that the brain does not swell. A dilute sodium solution (eg, 20–30 mEq of sodium/L) to replace the estimated water deficit gradually over a 48-hour or longer period is sometimes recommended.

Some practitioners use a 0.3% NaCl solution to treat hypertonic dehydration. (See Chapter 4 for a discussion of safe correction of hypernatremia.)

Depression of the ECF calcium level may occur but is rarely of clinical significance. The mechanism is obscure; when necessary, calcium gluconate may be administered to abort symptomic hypocalcemia.[21]

Potassium losses may be extreme; their replacement is an important factor in restoring water to cells.

CORRECTION OF HYPOTONIC DEHYDRATION (FVD WITH HYPONATREMIA)

This condition tends to occur in patients with fluid loss replaced primarily with water; in such instances, the serum sodium level decreases below normal. Management of this condition depends on how low the serum sodium level becomes. If it is extremely low and neu-

WEST NOMOGRAM FOR ESTIMATING SURFACE AREA OF INFANTS AND YOUNG CHILDREN

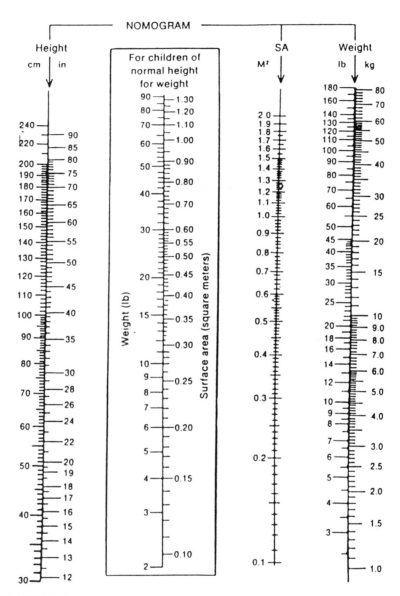

FIGURE 25-2.
The surface area is indicated where a straight line connecting the child's height and weight intersects the surface area (SA) column or, if the child appears to be of normal proportion, from the weight alone (enclosed area). (Nomogram modified from data of E Boyd by CD West. In Behrman RE, Vaughn VC: Nelson Textbook of Pediatrics, 13th ed, p 1521. Philadelphia, WB Saunders, 1987)

rological symptoms are present, it may be necessary to cautiously administer a small volume of hypertonic sodium solution. Half the calculated amount is usually given and then the clinical situation (including serum sodium measurement) is reevaluated. If results are as expected, the second half is given. See Chapter 4 for a discussion of treatment of hyponatremia, including principles for administering hypertonic sodium solutions.

Once the ECF volume has been restored, the child

is managed in the same manner as one with isotonic body fluid constriction. Potassium deficits should be considered and replaced as indicated. Nursing considerations in potassium administration are discussed in Chapter 5.

NURSING CONSIDERATIONS IN PARENTERAL FLUID REPLACEMENT

Emotional Preparation

Because children regard intravenous (IV) fluid replacement procedures as intrusive and threatening, they should be given adequate time to develop coping mechanisms. This will be facilitated if the procedure is explained at the child's cognitive level, if the child is given an opportunity to handle the equipment, and if opportunities are provided for play to reduce stress. The IV should be initiated in a quiet, private setting. The child should be encouraged to "hold still" during insertion; however, an adequate number of people must be available to help restrain the child if necessary. The parents should be offered the opportunity to remain with the child to provide emotional support if they so choose. Children feel more in control when they can sit up during the insertion procedure.

The most common sites for infusing fluids are the superficial veins located in the arm, wrist, and scalp (see Fig. 10-9). Ability to immobilize the area is an important consideration in children. The older child should be allowed site selection, when possible, to promote feelings of control and lessen interference with activities such as writing or coloring with the preferred hand. For the infant, scalp veins are convenient and accessible; because there are no valves in these veins, the IV can be infused in either direction. However, the head must be partially shaved for access to the site, and the parents must be prepared for this alteration in the infant's appearance. The nurse should also make certain that the parents understand that the fluid is to be administered into the infant's circulation and not into the brain. Some parents fear scalp vein infusions because of a mistaken association with "water on the brain" (hydrocephalus).

Equipment to Deliver Fluids Safely

Special equipment is used for infusing fluids into children as it is necessary to avoid overloading the smaller system with too large a volume at too rapid a rate. The danger of administering an excessive fluid volume must be a real consideration in all age groups. Infants and small children face special dangers simply because of their small size and the fact that fluids tend to be supplied in adult-sized containers. Children are more susceptible to pulmonary edema from excessive fluid overload than are adults because they have greater difficulty excreting excessive fluid volume. In fact, pneumonia from overhydration is believed to be one of the most common treatment-related diseases of hospitalized children.

One method to promote safety with gravity flow is to use a microdrip delivery set with a calibrated volume-control chamber that limits the amount of fluid that can be infused. The microdrip delivers a reduced-size drop (60 microdrops/mL) that is one fourth the size of a macrodrop (usually 15 macrodrops/mL). The calculation for infusion is simplified because the number of prescribed milliliters per hour equals the number of microdrips per minute; for example, 15 mL/hr equals a rate of 15 microdrops/min. Volume-controlled sets are favored to limit the amount of fluid available for administration in the event of an accident. It has been recommended that quantities exceeding 150 mL not be connected to children younger than 2 years, no more than 250 mL to children younger than 5, and no more than 500 mL to children younger than 10.

Infusion pumps that can be set at a prescribed rate per hour are an additional safety feature for infants and young children. Chapter 10 provides a description of infusion pumps and other IV equipment, as well as techniques for initiating fluids and assuring their safe delivery.

Monitoring Flow Rate

Although drop size adaptors, small containers, and infusion pumps are used to reduce the possibility of error, the nurse must still keep a close vigil on the flow rate as well as on the patient's response to the fluids. The flow rate should be counted at frequent intervals and adjusted as necessary. (Factors that can alter the flow rate are discussed in Chapter 10.) A pediatric parenteral fluid sheet should be kept at the bedside of infants and small children to record the observed flow rate, the amount of fluid absorbed each hour, and the amount of fluid left in the bottle. Such frequent observations and notations greatly reduce the risk of excessive fluid administration. Obviously, fluid monitoring is a major aspect of pediatric nursing.

APPROACHES FOR ORAL FLUID REPLACEMENT

When infants and children are able to take fluids by mouth and retain them, fluid replacement by the oral route is preferred over the parenteral route. Parenterally administered fluids pass directly into the cir-

TABLE 25-4.
Approximate Sodium, Potassium, and Caloric Content of Selected Beverages

BEVERAGE	SODIUM	POTASSIUM	CALORIES
Orange juice, canned, 8 fluid oz	6 mg (0.26 mEq)	436 mg (11.2 mEq)	104
Tomato juice, 6 fluid oz	658 mg (28.6 mEq)	400 mg (10.3 mEq)	32
Pineapple juice, canned, 6 fluid oz	2 mg (0.09 mEq)	280 mg (7.2 mEq)	103
Peach nectar, canned, 8 fluid oz	17 mg (0.74 mEq)	101 mg (2.6 mEq)	134
Pepsi Cola, 12 fluid oz	2 mg (0.09 mEq)	—	160
Coca Cola, 12 fluid oz	6 mg (0.26 mEq)	0	155
Sprite, 12 fluid oz	46 mg (2.0 mEq)	0	142
Thirst Quencher, bottled, 8 fluid oz	96 mg (4.2 mEq)	26 mg (0.67 mEq)	60
Tang, orange, from powder, 6 fluid oz	2 mg (0.09 mEq)	45 mg (1.2 mEq)	88
Kool-Aid from powder, all flavors, 8 fluid oz	8 mg (0.35 mEq)	1 mg (0.03 mEq)	98
Milk, 2% fat, 8 fluid oz	122 mg (5.3 mEq)	377 mg (16.4 mEq)	121

(Adapted from Pennington J: Bowes and Church's Food Values of Portions Commonly Used, 15th ed. Philadelphia, JB Lippincott, 1989.)

culation, while fluids taken into the GI tract are absorbed slowly. Thus, there is less risk of fluid overload with oral fluid replacement. Also, the child's freedom of movement is not impaired with oral replacement as it is with parenteral replacement.

Oral electrolyte solutions that are available as commercial products are listed in Table 25-2. These solutions may be prescribed by a physician for children who have mild fluid and electrolyte imbalances or for children who are recovering from acute imbalances that have been treated by parenteral therapy. Fruit juices and soda are usually acceptable to young children and generally provide at least some electrolytes as well as calories. Table 25-4 presents the sodium and potassium composition of various oral fluids.

Infants and children who are able to take and retain oral fluids may not be willing to do so. Illness often makes them irritable and anorexic, and they cannot understand why they are sick, why their distress cannot be alleviated promptly, and why they need to drink. Children who have gastroenteritis and those who have acute respiratory infections are usually restricted to clear liquids. They may react with frustration when an oral electrolyte solution or soda is offered when they expect and want milk. The phrase "force fluids" is often used in hospital settings, but fluids should *never* be forced on a child. Attempts to force a child to drink will only increase the child's distress and decrease the likelihood that the child will take and retain the fluid.

Efforts to encourage infants and children to take oral fluids should be gentle and persistent; the process requires patience, perseverance, and creativity. Some recommended approaches for meeting the oral fluid needs of infants and young children are listed below.

► Talk with the child's parents and learn about the child's usual experience in taking fluids at home. What type of fluids does the child usually drink? What amount? What temperature? How often? What method (bottle, cup, or special glass)? What are favorite fluids?

► Plan with the parents to meet the child's fluid needs and involve them in encouraging fluids, measuring amounts, and recording the intake accurately.

► Offer small amounts of favorite fluids in small containers at frequent intervals (at least every hour).

► Use measured containers for precise determination of intake and record the intake accurately.

► Promote the child's comfort before offering fluids. Make certain the child is clean and dry and the upper airway is clear of mucus. (A rubber syringe can be used to remove mucus from the nares.)

► Continue to offer fluids on a regular schedule, even though the infant or child may refuse to drink.

- Hold infants before and after offering fluids. Toddlers and preschool children may prefer to sit on the nurse's lap and hold the cup or glass.
- Toddlers may respond positively to a routine, such as offering a drink to a stuffed animal before offering the child a drink. Toddlers might also respond to the opportunity to feed themselves bite-sized pieces of frozen Popsicle, soda, or fruit juice.
- Young children like stories and may respond to the power of suggestion in stories about thirsty boys or girls who are looking for a drink.
- Some young children will drink if they have some solid food to hold or mouth, such as a saltine cracker or a vanilla wafer.
- Infants and children who are required to fast before surgery or diagnostic tests should have extra fluids just before the period of fasting to prevent dehydration. A pacifier helps relieve the distress that infants experience while oral feedings are withheld.

Nurses who are patient, perseverant, and creative will be successful in meeting the oral fluid needs of infants and children who are able to take and retain oral fluids.

REFERENCES

1. Yared A, Foose J, Ichikawa I: Disorders of Osmoregulation. In: Ichikawa I (ed): Pediatric Textbook of Fluids and Electrolytes, p 185. Baltimore, Williams & Wilkins, 1990
2. Ichikawa I, Narins R, Harris H Jr: Regulation of acid–base homeostasis. In: Ichikawa I (ed): Pediatric Textbook of Fluids and Electrolytes, p 84. Baltimore, Williams & Wilkins, 1990
3. Wong D, Whaley L: Clinical Manual of Pediatric Nursing, 3rd ed, p 273. St. Louis, C V Mosby, 1990
4. Pestana C: Fluids and Electrolytes in the Surgical Patient, 4th ed, p 47. Baltimore, Williams & Wilkins, 1989
5. Ibid
6. Avner et al: Fluid and electrolyte abnormalities in the stressed neonate. In: Ichikawa I (ed): Pediatric Textbook of Fluids and Electrolytes, p 403. Baltimore, Williams & Wilkins, 1990
7. Robson A: Parenteral fluid therapy. In: Behrman R, Vaughan V (eds): Nelson Textbook of Pediatrics, 13th ed, p 202. Philadelphia, WB Saunders, 1987
8. Ibid, p 200
9. Ibid
10. Ibid, p 201
11. American Academy of Pediatrics Committee on Nutrition: Use of oral fluid therapy and posttreatment feeding following enteritis in children in a developed country. Pediatrics 75:358, 1985
12. Foster R, Hunsberger M, Anderson J: Family-Centered Nursing Care of Children, p 1392. Philadelphia, WB Saunders, 1989
13. Kokko J, Tannen R: Fluids and Electrolytes, 2nd ed, p 166. Philadelphia, WB Saunders, 1990
14. Medani C: Seizures and hypothermia due to dietary water intoxication in infants. South Med J 80:421, 1987
15. Bennett J, Wagner T, Fields A: Acute hyponatremia and seizures in an infant after a swimming lesson. Pediatrics 73:125, 1983
16. Kokko, Tannen, p 166
17. Robson, p 205
18. Ibid, p 206
19. Medani, p 421
20. Feld L, Kaskel F, Schoeneman M: The approach to fluid and electrolyte therapy in pediatrics. In: Barness et al (eds): Advances in Pediatrics, vol 35, p 508. Chicago, Year Book Medical Publishers, 1988
21. Robson, p 199

26

Fluid Balance in the Elderly Patient

CHANGES IN WATER AND ELECTROLYTE HOMEOSTASIS ASSOCIATED WITH AGING

Because the percentage of elderly in the population is increasing, nurses in all settings must be aware of the risk in elderly people of developing fluid and electrolyte imbalances. Fluid balance in the elderly is marginal at best because of physiological changes associated with aging. Under normal conditions, elderly people can usually maintain homeostasis; however, they may require more time to return to normal when deficits or excesses are imposed by disease or environmental stress.[1] Elderly people do not possess the fluid reserves or ability to adapt readily to rapid changes. Alterations in fluid and electrolyte balance frequently accompany acute illness, particularly in aged persons. These alterations may delay recovery, prolong hospitalization, and result in loss of independence.[2, 3]

Normal aging changes that affect fluid and electrolyte balance are summarized in Table 26-1. Included also are nursing implications related to these changes.

Renal structural changes associated with aging result in a decreased glomerular filtration rate (GFR) and a decrease in the older person's ability to concentrate urine when fluid intake is restricted. The nurse must remain alert to this when aged patients are subjected to fluid restriction for any reason. It is also an important consideration when patients are disoriented and unaware of fluid needs, or are unable to provide for their own fluid needs.

Aged kidneys have a slower response to sodium and potassium imbalances. For example, half-time for reduction in urinary sodium after salt restriction is 17 hours in young people but increases to 31 hours in elderly people. Hyponatremia may occur in an older patient who is placed on a strict sodium-restricted diet. Hyperkalemia has been shown to develop quickly in the aged when IV potassium is administered.[4]

351

TABLE 26–1.
Normal Aging Changes Affecting Fluid Balance: Related Nursing Implications

PHYSIOLOGICAL COMPONENT	NORMAL AGING CHANGES	NURSING IMPLICATIONS
Total body water	Approximately 6% reduction in total body water	Increased risk for fluid volume deficit
	Decrease in ratio of intracellular to extracellular fluid	
Renal function	Reduction in weight by 50 g between ages 40 and 80	Greater difficulty in eliminating heavy solute loads (drugs, glucose, protein, electrolytes)
	Loss of 30% to 50% of glomeruli by age 70	
	Thickening of glomerular and tubular basement membranes	Slower conservation of fluids in response to fluid restriction
	46% decrease in glomerular filtration rate from age 20 to 90 (maximum serum creatinine increase is to 1.9 mg/100 mL)	
	Decrease in ability to concentrate urine (maximum ability to concentrate urine is 1.022–1.026)	
Regulatory functions	Decrease in secretion of aldosterone from adrenal cortex	Diminished ability to conserve sodium and excrete potassium
	Decreased response of zona glomerulosa	Reduced ability to correct an acid–base imbalance
	Decreased response of distal tubule to vasopressin	
	Decreased ability to form and excrete ammonia	Increased risk for hyperglycemia and osmotic diuresis
	Decreased glucose tolerance	
	Decreased sensation of thirst	Decreased ability to recognize a fluid deficit
Skin changes	Decreased skin elasticity	Skin turgor is poor indicator of state of hydration
	Atrophy of sweat glands	
	Diminished capillary bed	Skin is less effective in cooling body temperature
Cardiovascular function	Decreased baroreceptor sensitivity	Diminished ability to manage hypotension associated with shock
	Decreased cardiac output (1% per year from age 20–80)	Increased frequency of peripheral edema
	Decreased stroke volume (0.7% per year from age 20–80)	
	Decrease in renal plasma flow from 600 mL/min in 2nd decade to 300 mL/min by 8th decade	Increased risk for orthostatic hypotension, dizziness, falls
	Decreased elasticity of arteries	
	Increased vascular rigidity causing increased peripheral resistance	
Respiratory function	Decreased compliance of chest wall	Increased difficulty in regulation of pH if experiencing major illness, surgery, burns, or trauma
	Decreased elasticity of lung tissue	
	Decreased number of alveoli	
	Decreased strength of expiratory muscles	
	Decreased normal partial pressure of oxygen	
Gastrointestinal function	Decreased volume of saliva	Mouth may be dryer
	Decreased volume of gastric juice	Increased risk for hyponatremia and hypokalemia during vomiting and gastric suction
	Decreased calcium absorption	
		Increased need for dietary calcium and vitamin D

(Adapted from Burnside I: Nursing and the Aged, pp 83–94. New York, McGraw-Hill, 1988; Kenney R: Physiology of Aging, pp 113–121. Chicago, Year Book Medical Publishers, 1989; and Garner B: Guide to changing lab values in elders. Geriatr Nurs: 10:144, 1989.)

Cardiovascular and respiratory changes combine to contribute to a slower response to stress in the aged. As a result, the aged cannot respond as quickly to blood loss, fluid depletion, shock, and acid–base imbalances.

Current research indicates that thirst sensation diminishes with aging. In a comparison of 24-hour water deprivation in two age groups, the elderly group reported a lack of thirst sensation after the 24-hour period.[5] In another study comparing thirst sensation in normotensive young adults with that in healthy older adults, the older group failed to develop thirst after the administration of a hypertonic saline solution.[6] Decreased thirst has been demonstrated in elderly subjects with normal mental status, ability to communicate needs, and ability to physically obtain water.[7] Thus, the studies indicate that reduced sensitivity of the thirst mechanism to osmotic stimuli may be a problem in elderly persons. The elderly patient, therefore, may fail to drink sufficient amounts, even when fluids are readily available. It is important for the nurse to assess the adequacy of fluid intake in all elderly patients, but especially in those with an altered mental status because this may significantly interfere with the ability to recognize thirst.[8] Adding to the problem of decreased thirst is the conscious restriction of fluid by urinary-incontinent elderly patients in an effort to limit involuntary urination.

Elderly patients experience a decreased acuity for the taste of salt; thus, they may salt food heavily in an attempt to satisfy this taste sensation. For all of the above reasons, the aged are at risk for dehydration (hypernatremia) and hyperosmolarity.[9]

In summary, be aware that the elderly are often slow in adapting to change and may lack the physiological reserves to respond adequately to stress.

ASSESSMENT OF THE ELDERLY PATIENT

Fluid imbalances, particularly dehydration (hypernatremia), are seen quite frequently in aged clients in all settings. To make accurate nursing diagnoses, a thorough physical and functional assessment must be done.

Usual measures for assessing fluid balance may need to be altered for the elderly; for example, testing skin turgor on the forearm is not a valid measure for the elderly as skin loses elasticity with age. Skin turgor can best be observed in the older patient by tenting the tissue on the forehead or over the sternum because alterations in skin elasticity are less marked in these areas.

In younger individuals, a temperature elevation

above normal (98.6° F [37° C]) may be an indicator of dehydration (hypernatremia). However, when assessing aged patients, it is important to remember that their normal body temperature is often lower than 98.6° F (37° C), possibly closer to 97° F (36.1° C). Thus, a temperature of 98.6° F (37° C) may represent a significant elevation in an aged patient.

A more reliable physical measure of fluid balance in the aged is observation of the rate and degree of filling of small veins in the foot. A dorsal foot vein can be occluded by finger pressure at a distal point and emptied of its blood by stroking proximally with another finger. In a well-hydrated patient, the vein will fill instantly when the pressure is released. In a volume-depleted patient, the vein will fill slowly, over a period longer than 3 seconds. Researchers using this measure found that changes in the rapidity and degree of foot vein filling provided the best means for evaluating changes in hydration of elderly subjects.[10]

Although intake and output (I&O) records are often crucial in managing patients with fluid imbalances, research has indicated that frequent inaccuracies make these records less than reliable. According to Pflaum,[11] daily weights may be a more accurate measure of a patient's fluid status. However, one must be aware that inaccuracies also occur in measuring body weights. Therefore, *both* I&O and weight records should be maintained to monitor fluid status.[12] In general, a gain or loss of 1 kg body weight in a short period is equivalent to a gain or loss of 1 L of fluid.

Because of decreased salivation in elderly people, mucous membranes are less moist and shiny than in younger individuals. However, the center of the tongue should remain moist, and there should also be an observable pool of saliva beneath the tongue.[13] Research indicates that this method is useful in evaluating hydration in aged persons.[14]

Monitoring for positional changes in blood pressure is another measure that is helpful in assessing hydration. Research has indicated that a drop of at least 15 mmHg in the systolic pressure and 10 mmHg in the diastolic pressure occurs when volume-depleted patients are quickly shifted from a lying to a standing position.[15]

Functional assessment of an aged client's ability to obtain fluids is essential before determining nursing diagnoses and appropriate interventions. For example, one should assess the patient's ability to ambulate and use the arms and hands to obtain fluids. Also, is the patient able to swallow? Is he or she mentally clear? Is he or she able to participate independently in interventions to meet goals set up in the nursing care plan? Also, what are his or her fluid preferences?[16]

SPECIAL PROBLEMS IN THE ELDERLY PATIENT

Elderly patients with specific problems can be identified as having a potential for fluid imbalances. The care plans for these patients should include a nursing diagnosis reflecting this potential. Interventions should be employed to monitor for these imbalances and prevent them from occurring when possible.

HYPERNATREMIA RELATED TO POOR INTAKE OR INCREASED WATER LOSS

Hypernatremia associated with a decreased extracellular fluid (ECF) volume is a common problem in the elderly. It may be induced by free-water losses from diuresis, diarrhea, vomiting, and hyperglycemia. Usually it will not occur unless oral intake is restricted.[17, 18]

Synder et al[19] found a 1.1% incidence of serious hypernatremia (42% mortality rate) in elderly hospitalized patients. The causes were primarily treatment related.

Hypernatremia has been shown to be a common problem in long-term care facilities. Nursing home residents are often unable to ambulate, pour their own fluids, or express feelings of thirst. A study comparing fluid intake practices of institutionalized and non-institutionalized elderly found that the average daily intake for institutionalized persons was 1507 mL, as compared with 2115 mL for those not confined to institutions.[20] In addition, those not confined to institutions tended to consume water in greater amounts than the institutionalized subjects. Another interesting finding was that subjects outside institutions had greater access to very cold and very hot liquids; the extent to which this influenced fluid intake is not known.

Researchers have identified institutionalized residents at greatest risk for developing hypernatremia as those who are older than 85 years, have four or more chronic illnesses, take more than four medications, and are semidependent or require some skilled care.[21, 22]

A study by Himmelstein et al[23] examined the frequency of hypernatremia in patients admitted from nursing homes. When reviewing circumstances under which hypernatremia developed, no evidence of vomiting, diarrhea, or refusal of fluids was found. The researchers concluded that, with adequate observation and provision of fluids, this condition could have been prevented.

The role of the caregiver in preventing hypernatremia by early recognition of inadequate fluid intake and provision of needed fluids cannot be overemphasized.[24] See the case studies dealing with hypernatremia in Chapter 4 for further discussion of this topic.

Development of hypernatremia as a result of high-protein (hypertonic) tube feedings is not as common today because of the widespread use of isotonic tube feedings. However, fluid balance of tube-fed aged patients should be closely monitored as extra fluid may be needed even when isotonic feedings are used. Recall that elderly individuals are not as able to concentrate urine as their younger counterparts because of changes in renal structure. (See Chapter 13 for further discussion of this topic.)

Hypernatremia, superimposed on volume depletion, is one of the more common etiological factors related to the acute confusional states that are common in the aged. When an elderly client in any setting experiences a change in mental status, the nurse should immediately assess fluid status. The frequency of this problem is supported by current research. When fluid is limited for any reason, there is an increase in serum sodium concentration and mental functioning can be impaired. Using the case study method, Jana and Jana[25] studied four confused elderly dehydrated (hypernatremic) patients. With restoration of fluid volume, all subjects became oriented and cooperative. Seymour et al[26] examined 71 patients older than age 70 admitted to a hospital in acute confusional states. Assessment of mental status and fluid status was done on admission and 1 week later after measures to restore hydration. Results indicated a significant relationship between mental scores on admission and degree of dehydration. Because of the large number of subjects, the study provides strong evidence for the relationship between confusion and dehydration (hypernatremia). Another study found a significant change in mental status in elderly patients depleted of fluids in preparation for diagnostic procedures.[27] Table 26-2 is an example of a mental status questionnaire.

In a study of 71 hospitalized elderly medical patients, it was found that one third of them developed confusion.[28] The researchers found that hypernatremia, as well as hypokalemia, hypotension, elevated creatinine, and elevated blood urea nitrogen (BUN), were among the 10 factors significantly associated with confusion. Another study of 90 confused hospitalized patients found fluid and electrolyte imbalances to be confirmed, probable, or possible causes of confusional states in 20 patients.[29]

A care plan for an elderly client with a nursing diagnosis of altered mental status related to inadequate fluid intake is shown in Table 26-3.

Older adults should be cautioned not to use sodium bicarbonate antacids. These are readily absorbed and can result in hypernatremia.[30]

IMBALANCES ASSOCIATED WITH USE OF DIURETICS

Diuretics are the most frequently prescribed drugs for treatment of hypertension and congestive heart failure

TABLE 26–2.
Short Portable Mental Status Questionnaire (SPMSQ)

Instructions: Ask questions 1 through 10 in this list and record all answers. Ask question 4A only if patient does not have a telephone. Record total number of errors based on ten questions.

+	−

1. What is the date today? _____
   Month   Day   Year
2. What day of the week is it?_____
3. What is the name of this place? _____
4. What is your telephone number? _____
4A. What is your street address? _____
   (Ask only if patient does not have a telephone.)
5. How old are you? _____
6. When were you born? _____
7. Who is the President of the U.S. now? _____
8. Who was the President just before him? _____
9. What was your mother's maiden name? _____
10. Subtract 3 from 20 and keep subtracting 3 from each new number, all the way down.
   Total Number of Errors

Scoring: 0–2 errors = intact mental function
3–4 errors = mild intellectual impairment
5–7 = moderate intellectual impairment
8–10 errors = severe intellectual impairment
Allow one more error if subject had only grade school education.
Allow one fewer error is subject has had education beyond high school.

(Pfeiffer, E A short portable mental status questionnaire for the assessment of organic brain deficit in elderly patients. J Am Geriatr Soc 23:433, 1975; with permission.)

TABLE 26–3.
Nursing Care Plan for an 80-Year-Old Woman with a Nursing Diagnosis of Alteration in Thought Process Related to Inadequate Fluid Intake

ASSESSMENT	GOAL	INTERVENTIONS	EVALUATION CRITERIA
Disoriented	Restore normal mental status	Increase oral intake to 2000 mL/day	Score on Mental Status Questionnaire will improve
Score on Mental Status Questionnaire is 2 (normal is 10)		**Follow this schedule:**	Behavior will improve
Behavior changes			Oral intake will reach 2000 mL in 24 hours
Skin turgor poor on forehead		8:00 breakfast — 300 mL	
Tongue dry and furry		9:00 water — 120 mL	Physical assessment will reveal improved skin turgor, pool of saliva under tongue, normal vein filling, and absence of marked postural hypotension on position change
No pool of saliva under tongue		10:00 lemonade — 120 mL	
BP 160/80 (supine), 128/62 (standing)		11:00 water — 120 mL	
		12:00 lunch — 300 mL	
Foot vein fills in 6 seconds		1:00 water — 120 mL	
Oral intake 900 mL/day		2:00 water — 120 mL	
Able to swallow		3:00 orange juice — 120 mL	
Unable to pour fluids due to arthritis in hands		4:00 water — 120 mL	
		5:00 water — 120 mL	
Favorite fluids		6:00 supper — 300 mL	
▶ Water		7:00 water — 120 mL	
▶ Lemonade		8:00 water — 120 mL	
▶ Orange juice		Continue assessment of fluid and mental status every shift	

in the elderly. Both thiazides and furosemide (Lasix) are potassium-losing diuretics, having a greater tendency to induce hypokalemia in the aged than in the younger adult. Remember that hypokalemia potentiates the action of digitalis and can precipitate toxic symptoms. Use of a potassium-sparing diuretic such as spironolactone (Aldactone) or triamterene (Dyrenium) has been shown to produce a higher incidence of hyperkalemia in the aged.[31, 32]

Hyponatremia has also been attributed to thiazide diuretic use. Persons of small body mass, low fluid intake, or excessive intake of low-sodium nutritional supplements are at greater risk for effects of fluid and electrolyte imbalance caused by diuretics.[33, 34]

Because of the orthostatic hypotension associated with diuretic-induced *fluid volume deficit* (FVD), an older patient may become dizzy on position change and experience a fall. Indeed, use of diuretics has been identified as a characteristic of patients at risk for falls.[35]

Patients on diuretic therapy should be weighed daily. Serum electrolyte levels should be determined at regular intervals. In addition, older patients should be monitored closely for signs of weakness, lethargy, and postural hypotension. One should also monitor for confusion, thirst, and muscle cramps.[36]

IMBALANCES RELATED TO CONSTIPATION AND LAXATIVE ABUSE

Reduced motility of the intestinal tract and a lessened sense of the need to eliminate can lead to chronic constipation with laxative and enema dependency. Prolonged use of strong laxatives predisposes to hypokalemia and FVD. Metabolism of drugs by the aged person is generally slower than in a younger person. Abnormal prolongation of the effect of some "over-the-counter" laxatives containing phenolphthalein has been seen. There is an increase in the half-life of the drug and, thus, diarrhea may result as the drug's action continues.

It has been reported that persons over 70 years take laxatives twice as often as those in the 40- to 50-year age group. In addition to decreased gastrointestinal (GI) motility with aging, certain drugs, such as anticholinergics and antacids containing calcium carbonate or aluminum hydroxide, predispose to constipation. Unfortunately, use of laxatives in the aged often becomes habit forming, requiring larger and more frequent doses to achieve results.[37]

Increased fluid and bulk intake, plus regular exercise, should be encouraged to correct constipation. Stool softeners are useful physiological tools, and a glass of warm water or hot coffee first thing in the morning can stimulate the evacuation reflex. These nursing interventions are preferable to drugs in reducing the constipation problem and thereby preventing fluid and electrolyte problems associated with laxatives and enemas.

IMBALANCES ASSOCIATED WITH PREPARATION FOR DIAGNOSTIC TESTS

Standard colon-cleansing techniques for diagnostic studies usually include dietary restrictions (liquid diet several days before; NPO after midnight the day before the test), purgatives (such as castor oil, magnesium citrate, Dulcolax), and numerous cleansing enemas. These techniques constitute a threat to elderly persons who are only marginally hydrated. Studies have indicated that the rigorous catharsis associated with this kind of preparation leads to significant shifts of fluid among body compartments; if the shifts occur rapidly in an elderly person with cardiovascular disease, the results can be dangerous.[38]

In a study of elderly persons undergoing preparation for a barium enema, a significant number of indicators of fluid volume depletion were detected on nursing assessment.[39] In addition, there was a slowed response to restore fluid balance.

Elderly persons undergoing rigorous bowel preparation should be observed closely for adverse reactions. Based on current research, it is most appropriate to include a nursing diagnosis in the care plan that reflects the potential for fluid volume depletion related to bowel preparation. The need for close observation is reflected in the care plan in Table 26-4. Care should be taken to perform the procedure correctly the first time to avoid the need for repeated radiographs, requiring more cathartics, more enemas, and more fluid restrictions. The elderly can ill afford to undergo one test after another without a "rest period"; it is frequently up to the nurse to intervene in this area on the patient's behalf.

It should be noted that the radiocontrast agents used in diagnostic radiology (such as intravenous [IV] pyelography) are sodium rich. Because of the already reduced GFR, the older patient has difficulty excreting the increased solute load. This may cause osmotic diuresis and, thus, increased fluid loss.[40] The aged patient undergoing GI radiographs should probably receive IV fluids during the preparation period of reduced oral intake and increased fluid loss by catharsis and enemas.

OSTEOPOROSIS

Calcium deficiency has been associated with osteoporosis development in the elderly. In fact, 15 to 20 million aged individuals have been diagnosed as having this condition. Annually, 1.3 million fractures (mainly

TABLE 26–4.
Nursing Care Plan for an 84-Year-Old Man with a Nursing Diagnosis of at Risk for Hypernatremia with Fluid Volume Depletion Related to X-Ray Preparation

ASSESSMENT	GOAL	INTERVENTIONS	EVALUATION CRITERIA
To receive rigorous colon preparation on Tuesday Fluid restriction (NPO) after midnight Tuesday Decreased renal function, related to advanced age Alert and functionally able to obtain own fluids Baseline physical assessment of fluid balance within normal limits	To prevent hypernatremia with fluid volume depletion	Physical assessment of fluid balance every shift 2000 to 3000 mL of fluid orally the day before x-ray; give 150 mL/hr from 8:00 a.m. to 10:00 p.m. Obtain order for IV fluids if unable to drink above amount Force fluids (150 mL/hr) after x-ray until HS Explain need for fluids to patient; give schedule to him or her; assist as needed	Intake exceeds 2000 mL/day on day before x-ray Intake exceeds 2000 mL/day after x-ray No change in baseline physical assessment parameters

HS, hour of sleep (bedtime)

of the spine, wrist, and hip) are attributed to osteoporosis. The risk of developing osteoporosis increases with age. Postmenopausal osteoporosis is most common in smallframed white women older than 50.[41] Back pain is the most frequent symptom, and spinal deformity is the most common sign. "Dowager's hump" (a hunchback posture due to severe loss of anterior vertebral height) is a common finding. The patient's height may be 1 to 6 inches shorter than the arm span if multiple wedge-compression fractures have occurred. Loss of 2 inches in height has been found to be an accurate screening mechanism to detect osteoporosis.[42] Involutional bone alterations may reduce cortical bone mass of the femurs by a factor of 30% to 50%.

It should be noted that serum concentrations of calcium, phosphate, and alkaline phosphatase are normal even though deficits of total body calcium, phosphate, and nitrogen exist.

Reduced calcium intake seems to play a role in the development of postmenopausal osteoporosis. Also implicated are diminished physical activity, impaired intestinal calcium absorption, increased renal calcium loss, increased parathyroid hormone (PTH) effect, and reduced secretion of estrogen. Increased PTH secretion in postmenopausal osteoporosis may be related to a slightly decreased ionized calcium level owing to a number of hepatic, renal, and intestinal changes that accompany aging.[43]

Research has indicated that no single treatment is effective in preventing osteoporosis. Calcium supplements alone, even in amounts of 2000 mg daily, were not effective in protecting against accelerated trebecular bone loss of the spine and wrist. However, calcium in combination with estrogen or exercise did result in decreased bone loss.[44-46]

It seems that oral calcium, vitamin D, and estrogen can reverse negative calcium balance related to menopause and probably delay or prevent the onset of clinical osteoporosis. Women should consume at least 1000 mg/day of elemental calcium and 400 IU of vitamin D to increase calcium absorption and bone formation. If the elderly person is housebound, Vitamin D may be increased to 800 IU.

Oral estrogen administration has been shown to be the most effective treatment modality; it reduces negative calcium balance and stimulates positive calcium balance. It should be remembered, however, that large daily doses of estrogen have been shown to be associated with sodium retention, hypertension, myocardial infarction, and increased risk of endometrial carcinoma. Many physicians believe that the anticatabolic effect of estrogen, which reduces bone resorption, outweighs the risk of these untoward effects.[47] Research indicates that short-term use of calcitonin may be effective in slowing bone loss.[48]

Education in the areas of nutrition, proper exercise, and safety must be included in the care plans of patients with osteoporosis.

Nutrition

1. Encourage the intake of adequate calcium in the diet. One quart of skim milk daily is recommended; whole milk or cheese products may be used if the patient's physical condition allows. See Table 6-2 for a list of high-calcium foods. (Some sources recommend 1000–1500 mg of calcium for postmenopausal women and elderly men.)
2. Encourage adequate protein intake. For the older adult, the recommendation is 1 g of protein per kilogram of body weight.
3. Encourage intake of sufficient calories to maintain normal body weight.
4. For those unable to consume adequate calcium in the diet, consider use of calcium supplements. Caution elderly patients to take calcium 1 hour before or 2 hours after meals to ensure absorption.

Exercise

After assessing for abilities and disabilities, consider the following interventions:

1. Encourage patients who swim, golf, or bicycle to continue to do so. Jogging should be avoided because of the possibility of joint damage.
2. Teach individuals who have been habitually sedentary to avoid strenuous exercise. (Research indicates that simple exercises will help decrease bone mass loss.) The heart rate should not increase more than 60 beats/min over baseline.
3. Suggest the following exercises for sedentary individuals:
   A. Arm Circles
      i. Sit erect, arms extended
      ii. Form circles by moving arms backward and then forward
   B. Angle Stretch
      i. Lie on bed (not floor), legs straight, feet together, and arms at side
      ii. Slide arms and legs to a spread-eagle position and return
   C. Stationary Rocking
      i. Sit erect on chair, feet flat on floor, arms at side
      ii. Lean forward and press floor with toes
      iii. Lean back to upright position and press floor with heels
4. Recommend extension and isometric abdominal exercises for those diagnosed with spinal osteoporosis. Teach them to avoid any flexion exercises of the spine as this action may cause compression/fractures.[49]

Safety

1. Teach the patient to avoid sudden bending, twisting, lifting, or carrying of heavy objects.
2. Teach the patient to use assistive devices, such as canes or walkers, if needed, to prevent falls.
3. Teach the patient to wear well-fitted, low-heeled shoes (athletic shoes should be suggested).
4. Teach the patient to use long-handled utensils and cleaning tools if needed.
5. Assess the patient's environment. Make sure the home is well lighted, and obtain non-skid rugs. Look for objects that might cause falls.

HYPERTHERMIA

The greatest number of cases of heatstroke occur in the elderly. Sweating, the major mechanism for heat dissipation, is altered in the aged. Not only is the number of operative sweat glands decreased in aged persons, it takes longer for them to begin sweating, and they produce less sweat than in their younger years. Loss of subcutaneous adipose tissue reduces the effectiveness of the skin as an insulator and enhances water loss from the deeper tissues.

Elderly persons seem to have an impaired sense of warmth perception. Also, the elderly exhibit little change in cardiac output in response to heat stress. The circulatory system cannot efficiently dissipate the heat through peripheral vasodilatation and evaporation of perspiration.[50, 51] In addition, a number of medications frequently prescribed for aged patients can interfere in some way with thermoregulation (eg, diuretics, antiparkinsonian drugs, and propranolol).[52]

Mortality related to heat stress increases progressively in those older than 70 years. Because of their greater susceptibility to heat stress, it is important to teach these individuals to take the following precautions during a heat wave:

▸ Avoid excessive physical activity.
▸ Wear light-colored cotton fabrics to facilitate sweating.
▸ Increase dietary consumption of carbohydrates and fluids.
▸ Use air conditioners or fans when available.
▸ Contact health provider if cessation of sweating occurs.[53]

The nurse must be cautious when assessing the older person for heat stress. Normal body temperature decreases with age; as such, the older adult may be experiencing heat stress with a temperature of 99° F (37.2° C).[54]

SPECIAL CONSIDERATIONS RELATED TO PERIOPERATIVE PERIOD

Elderly persons tolerate major surgery and its complications less well than younger adults; therefore, preoperatively, every effort should be made to treat conditions likely to cause postoperative problems. Cardiac complications are a common cause of postoperative mortality; pneumonia and atelectasis also occur frequently.[55] Conscientious preoperative preparation often means the difference between success or failure of surgery in the aged as the decreased body homeostatic adaptability of these patients predisposes to difficulty when they are exposed to stress.

The following facts apply to the aged surgical patient:

▶ Moderate FVD and decreased circulating blood volume are not uncommon in the elderly *before* surgery. Fluid volume deficit predisposes to renal insufficiency, particularly in elderly individuals. Administration of adequate IV fluids before surgery improves renal blood flow and renal function; in contrast, administration of the same fluids after induction of anesthesia will have only minimal effect in increasing renal blood flow. It is important that parenteral fluids be started before surgery and an adequate urine volume established before induction of anesthesia. Urine flow should be at least 50 mL/hr (preferably 75–100 mL/hr).

In the operating room, the older patient is at risk for hypothermia. In addition to the cool environment, the patient is rapidly infused with cool IV fluids and possibly blood. Rinsing the skin with cool solutions also increases the risk of hypothermia. Use of a cap, warm gown, stockinette on unaffected limbs, and warmed flannelette blankets are recommended.[56-58]

▶ Because diminished respiratory function interferes with carbon dioxide elimination, many aged patients are in a state of impending respiratory acidosis. Because of this decline in pulmonary function, the nurse must help the aged patient achieve maximal ventilation. This can be accomplished by keeping the respiratory tract free of excessive secretions, providing maximal allowed activity, turning the bedfast patient from side to side at regular intervals, and avoiding restrictive clothing and chest restraints.

▶ Because renal response to pH disturbances is not as efficient in the aged, imbalances occur faster. There is a tendency toward metabolic acidosis as a result of decreased renal function. It behooves the health care team to detect imbalances early and to intervene early.

▶ Changes in pH are less well tolerated in the aged.

In addition to decreased renal and pulmonary reserves, presence of anemia, with its decreased hemoglobin, depletes one of the major buffer systems. Blood should be administered as needed to correct anemia, preferably several days before the operation. Emphysema is not uncommon in the aged and also disrupts pH control. Measures to improve pulmonary function should also be employed preoperatively.

▶ Hypotension is poorly tolerated by the aged, and, unless corrected quickly, is frequently complicated by renal damage, stroke, or myocardial infarct. Shock becomes irreversible earlier than in young patients.

▶ The aged patient will develop sodium deficit faster than younger adults; thus, the nurse should be particularly alert for this imbalance when the patient is losing body fluids containing sodium. Hyponatremia is particularly apt to occur when there is a free intake of water orally or when excessive volumes of 5% dextrose in water are administered IV.

▶ Hyponatremia may also result from excessive water retention associated with the stress of hospitalization and anticipation of surgery. Stress mediates the release of antidiuretic hormone (ADH). Research has shown that relocation and separation from loved ones, as occur with hospitalization, cause greater stress in the aged. This stress has been shown to contribute to the development of water intoxication (dilutional hyponatremia).[59]

▶ Malnutrition is more common in aged than in younger adults and contributes to the increased incidence of postoperative complications. Preoperative dietary management is particularly important. Optimal nutrition helps the aged patient withstand the electrolyte deficits and pH changes occurring with surgery. If the patient is unable to eat, tube feedings or parenteral nutrients are indicated to meet nutritional needs and build up operative reserves. (Tube feedings are discussed in Chapter 13 and parenteral nutrition is discussed in Chapter 12.)

▶ Ambulation and activity improve appetite and sleep and prevent the complications of bedrest. Bedrest in the preoperative period can be damaging to the aged patient because it predisposes to negative nitrogen balance, osteoporosis, muscle weakness, pneumonia, phlebitis, bedsores, bladder and bowel dysfunction, decrease in myocardial reserve, and diminished pulmonary ventilation and tidal volume.

In maintaining patency of the IV site in a restless elderly person, restraints should be avoided. Use of restraints creates anxiety and agitation, as well as respiratory and cardiovascular problems. A Posey mitt may prove useful in preventing pulling at the IV tubing while still allowing for movement. Because of the older person's increased skin fragility, excessive tape should be avoided in securing the IV site; also, extreme care should be taken when removing the tape.[60]

HYPEROSMOLAR HYPERGLYCEMIC NONKETOTIC COMA

Most patients who develop hyperosmolar hyperglycemic nonketotic coma (HHNC) are elderly with relatively mild (perhaps not-yet-detected) diabetes mellitus. Unconscious patients may present in the emergency room with a history of days or weeks of polyuria and increased thirst. Precipitating factors in the diabetic elderly may include medications such as osmotic diuretics, Dilantin, steroids, immunosuppressive agents, infections such as pneumonia, hyperosmolar tube feedings, and high carbohydrate infusion loads (as in total parenteral nutrition).[61, 62] Normal aging changes affecting kidney function create a greater potential for fluid imbalance in the older diabetic. Monitoring fluid intake adequacy in the elderly diabetic is an important nursing assessment that can lead to earlier detection of HHNC. A thorough discussion of HHNC is presented in Chapter 21.

REFERENCES

1. Leaf A: Dehydration in the elderly. N Engl J Med 311:791, 1984
2. Kositzke J: A question of balance: Dehydration in the elderly. Journal of Gerontological Nursing 16(5):4, 1990
3. Miller M: Fluid and electrolyte balance in the elderly. Geriatrics 42(11):65, 1987
4. Cape R, Coe R, Rossman I: Fundamentals of Geriatric Medicine, p 71–74. New York, Raven Press, 1983
5. Phillips et al: Reduced thirst after water deprivation in elderly healthy men. N Engl J Med 311:753, 1984
6. Menully G: Thirst threshold changes pose dehydration risk. Geriatrics 40(12):91, 1985
7. Miller et al: Hypodipsia in geriatric patients. Am J Med 72:354, 1982
8. Michaelsson E: Assessment of thirst among severely demented patients in the terminal phase of life: Exploratory interviews with ward sisters and enrolled nurses. Int J Nurs Stud 24(2):87, 1987
9. Matteson M, McConnel E: Gerontological Nursing: Concepts and Practice, p 323. Philadelphia, WB Saunders, 1988
10. Robinson S, Demuth P: Diagnostic studies for the aged: What are the dangers? Journal of Gerontological Nursing 11(6):6, 1985
11. Pflaum S: Investigation of intake-output as a means of assessing body fluid balance. Heart Lung 8:495, 1979
12. McCarthy D: Clinical utility of daily patient weights in the coronary care unit. Cardiovascular Nursing 20:31, 1984
13. Wolanin M, Phillips L: Confusion, p 117–118. St. Louis, CV Mosby, 1981
14. Robinson, DeMuth, p 8–9
15. Wolanin, Phillips, p 117
16. Adams F: How much do elders drink? Geriatr Nurs 9(4):218, 1988
17. Beck L, Lavizzo-Maurey R: Geriatric hypernatremia. Ann Intern Med 107:768, 1987
18. Sadat A, Paulman P, Mathews M: Hypernatrema in the elderly. Fam Pract 40:125, 1989
19. Snyder N, Feigal D, Arieff A: Hypernatremia in elderly patients: A heterogenous, morbid, and iatrogenic entity. Ann Intern Med 107:309, 1987
20. Adams, p 218
21. Lavizzo-Maurey R, Johnson J, Stotley P: Risk factors for dehydration among elderly nursing home residents. J Am Geriatr Soc 36(3):213, 1988
22. Gaspar P: What determine how much patients drink? Geriatr Nurs 9(4):221, 1988
23. Himmelstein D, Jones A, Wollhander S: Hypernatremic dehydration in nursing home patients: An indicator of neglect. J Am Geriatr Soc 31(8):466, 1983
24. Aaronson L, Seaman L: Managing hypernatremia in fluid deficient elderly. Journal of Gerontological Nursing, 15(7):29, 1989
25. Jana D, Jana L: Hypernatremic psychoses in the elderly: Case reports. J Am Geriatr Soc 31(10):473, 1983
26. Seymour et al: Acute confusional states and dementia in the elderly: The role of dehydration/volume depletion, physical illness, and age. Age-Ageing 9:137, 1980
27. Robinson, DeMuth, p 6–9
28. Foreman M: Confusion in the hospitalized elderly: Incidence, onset, and associated factors. Res Nurs Health 12(2):21, 1989
29. Francis J, Martin D, Kapoor W: A prospective study of delirium in hospitalized elderly. JAMA 263:1097, 1990
30. Todd B: Antacid alert. Geriatr Nurs 10(6):278, 1989
31. Todd B: Diuretics' danger. Geriatr Nurs 10(4):212, 1989
32. Lamy P: Hypertension, diuretics, and the elderly. Caring 6(2):58, 1987
33. Rudman et al: Hypernatremia in tube-fed elderly men. J Chron Dis, 39(2):73, 1986
34. Ashouri O: Severe diuretic induced hyponatremia in the elderly. Arch Intern Med 146:1355, 1986
35. Barbieri E: Patient falls are not patient accidents. Journal of Gerontological Nursing 9:165, 1983
36. Todd B: When the patient is on diuretics. Geriatr Nurs 2(2):149, 1981
37. Yakaborwich M: Prescribe with care: the role of laxa-

tives in the treatment of constipation. Journal of Gerontological Nursing, 16(7):7, 1990

38. Burbige E, Bourke E, Tarder G: Effect of preparation for colonoscopy on fluid and electrolyte balance. Gastrointest Endosc 24:286, 1978
39. Robinson, DeMuth, p 8–9
40. Cape et al, p 74
41. National Institute of Health: Osteoporosis. *Consensus Development Conference Statement* 5 3:2, 1984
42. Reed A, Burge S: Screening for osteoporosis. Journal of Gerontological Nursing, 14(7):18, 1988
43. Holm K, Walker J: Osteoporosis: Treatment and prevention update. Geriatr Nurs 11(3):140, 1990
44. Etinger B: Postmenopausal bone loss is prevented by treatment with low dosage estrogen with calcium. Ann Intern Med 106:40, 1987
45. Riis B, Thomsen K, Christianson C: Does calcium supplementation prevent postmenopausal bone loss? N Engl J Med 316:173, 1987
46. Dalsky G, Stocke K: Weight bearing exercise training and lumbar bone mineral content in postmenopausal women. Ann Intern Med 108:824, 1988
47. Holm, Walker, p 140
48. Madson S: How to reduce the risk of postmenopausal osteoporosis. Journal of Gerontological Nursing 15(9):20, 1989
49. Aisenbrey J: Exercise in the prevention and management of osteoporosis. Phys Ther 67:1100, 1987
50. Caruso P: Heat waves threaten the old. Geriatr Nurs 6(4):209, 1985
51. Robbins A: Hypothermia and heat stroke: Protecting the elderly. Geriatrics 44(1):73, 1989
52. Kolanowski A, Gunter L: Thermal stress and the aged. Journal of Gerontological Nursing 9:13, 1983
53. Ibid
54. Caruso, p 211
55. Latz P, Wyble R: Elderly patients perioperative nursing implications. AORN J 46(2):238, 1987
56. Jackson M: High risk surgical patient. Journal of Gerontological Nursing 14(1):8, 1988
57. White H, Thurston N, Blackmore K, Green S, Hannah K: Body temperature in elderly surgical patient. Res Nurs Health 10:317, 1987
58. Latz, Wyble, p 250
59. Booker J: Severe symptomatic hyponatremia in elderly outpatients. J Am Geriatr Soc 33(2):108, 1985
60. Mellema S, Ponialawski B: Geriatric I.V. therapy. Journal of Intravenous Therapy 11(1):56, 1988
61. Smokvina G, Givens R: Hyperglycemia in the aged. Journal of Gerontological Nursing 9:449, 1983
62. Cahill G: Hyperglycemia hyperosmolar coma: A syndrome almost unique to the elderly. J Am Geriatr Soc 31(2):103, 1983

Index

Page numbers followed by *f* indicate figures; those followed by *t* indicate tabular material; those followed by *b* indicate boxed material.